PRAISE FOR CLINICAL NEPHROLOGY IN CHINESE MEDICINE

A remarkably well written and scholastic book on clinical nephrology from a Chinese medicine perspective. It integrates the essence of traditional Chinese medicine with Western differential diagnosis, with comprehensive and well-organized content based on both Chinese medicine pattern identifications as well as Western clinical diagnosis. The first of its kind to be published in the English language, this book will be an indispensable resource not only for Chinese medicine practitioners and students, but also for any Western-trained physician interested in learning about the diagnosis and treatment of renal and urological diseases with Chinese medicine.

> —**Lawrence Lau**, M.D., L. Ac., Dipl. Ac.
> Academic Dean / Chief Administrator
> Yo San University, Los Angeles

Dr. Li is very knowledgable and has a lot of clinical experience regarding the differentiation and treatment of diseases in nephrology. More importantly, she is willing to share this experience throughout the many chapters of this book. I believe that this book will help its readers learn a lot.

> —**Wen-shuo Wu**, Dean of Acupuncture & Oriental Medicine
> Southern California University of Health Sciences

Clinical Nephrology in Chinese Medicine is a wonderful book. It clearly describes how to treat modern Westren medical kidney and bladder diseases with Chinese medicine. This book reflects Dr. Wei Li's extensive clinical experience from the perspectives of both Chinese and Western medicine. I highly recommend this book and I think it will definitely help practitioners' treatment of these diseases.

> —**Dr. Haihe Tian**, A.P., Ph.D., M.D.(China)
> Largo, FL

Dr. Wei Li's Clinical Nephrology in Chinese Medicine is comprehensive, well organized, and thoroughly indexed. Therefore, I found the material easy to access and, more importantly, easy to understand. The Clinical Tips sections are another excellent addition for a Western practitioner like myself. I can easily refer to this text when seeking concise herbal remedies and answers for my patients with nephrological diseases. This is a terrific addition to the reference resources for practitioiners such as myself who seek to assist our patients in attaining optimal health.

> —**Betty A. Ehrlich**, D.C., CCN, DACBN
> Essential Health, Los Angeles

This is an excellent, much needed book on Chinese medicine and nephrology in which the authors discuss various common kidney disorders in depth. Those who read this book will benefit many patients suffering from common but often difficult-to-treat illnesses of the kidneys and other organs. Without hesitation, I strongly recommend this book to all students and practitioners of Eastern medicine.

> —**Young K. Park**, D.O.
> Westview Center for Integrated Medicine, Indianapolis

CLINICAL NEPHROLOGY IN CHINESE MEDICINE

Clinical Nephrology in Chinese Medicine

By

Wei Li, L. Ac. & David Frierman, L. Ac.
with Ben Luna, N.D., L. Ac. & Bob Flaws, L. Ac

Published by:
BLUE POPPY PRESS
A Division of Blue Poppy Enterprises, Inc.
5441 Western Ave., Suite 2
Boulder, CO 80301
www.bluepoppy.com

First Edition, October 2003

ISBN 1-891845-23-3
LCCN # 2003106541

Cover & page design: Eric J. Brearton

COMP Designation: Original work

10 9 8 7 6 5 4 3 2 1

Printed at Thomson-Shore Inc., Dexter, Michigan

TABLE OF CONTENTS

Acknowledgements..ix
Preface...xi

Part 1. General Theory...1

  1. The Kidney in Western and Chinese Medicine...................................3
  2. Disease Causes & Mechanisms 17
  3. Important Treatment Principles in Chinese Nephrology 25
  4. Safety Issues When Using Chinese Medicinals and Chinese
      Medicinal-Western Drug Interactions 33

Part 2. Chinese Medical Diseases in Nephrology & Urology 37

  1. Kidney Wind 39
  2. Block & Repulsion 49
  3. Dribbling Urinary Block 59
  4. Bloody Urine 67
  5. Water Swelling 75
  6. Kidney Taxation & Taxation Wind 87
  7. Phlegm Rheum 97
  8. Lumbar Pain 105
  9. Strangury...115
 10. Turbidity Condition 125
 11. Abdominal Distention 129
 12. Dizziness 133
 13. Blood Stasis 141

Part 3. The Chinese Medical Treatment of Kidney & Bladder Diseases 149

1. Urinary Tract Infections (UTI) 151
2. Interstitial Cystitis (IC) 173
3. Nephrotic Syndrome (NS) 183
4. Acute Nephritis 197
5. Chronic Nephritis 209
6. Acute Renal Failure (ARF) 227
7. Chronic Renal Failure (CRF) 239
8. Tubulointerstitial Nephritis 265
9. Polycystic Kidney Disease (PKD) 273

Part 4. Integrating Western & Chinese Medicine 279

General Index 303

Formula Index 319

Acknowledgments

I wish to express my appreciation and gratitude to my parents for their encouragement and vision. My mother encouraged my father to teach me Chinese medicine while supporting me in these studies. My father taught me a deep respect for Chinese medicine. When Chinese universities reopened after the Cultural Revolution, my parents insisted I study Western medicine as well as Chinese medicine. They felt that the future of medicine would involve a combination of the two. They also encouraged me to write books intended to integrate the Chinese and Western perspectives on disease and treatment. I am pleased that I have been able to fulfill their desire.

Wei Li, L.Ac.

I would like to thank my students and friends for their suggestions on content and language and Subhuti Dharmananda for suggesting the inclusion of certain caveats. Benjamin Luna, N.D., L.Ac., deserves special mention. I could not have coauthored this book without his assistance.

David Frierman, L.Ac.

PREFACE

This book is a Chinese medical textbook and clinical manual of nephrology and urology. It has been written by Dr. Wei Li with the assistance of David Frierman, Ben Luna, and Bob Flaws. It is divided into four main parts or sections. Part 1 reviews the general Chinese medical theory and strategies when dealing with diseases of the kidneys and urinary bladder. Part 2 presents 13 Chinese medical disease categories which traditionally cover kidney and bladder diseases. These are presented as building blocks for understanding how to treat modern Western medical kidney and bladder diseases with Chinese medicine. If one knows how to reframe any modern Western nephrological disease into its component traditional Chinese medical disease categories, one should be able to understand how to diagnose and treat any modern Western kidney or bladder disease with Chinese medicine. However, to make that process even clearer, Part 3 consists of a discussion of nine modern Western medical nephrological diseases and Part 4 covers six modern Western medical conditions that are associated with kidney disease. These conditions are all commonly seen in clinical practice, yet their Chinese medical treatment is inadequately covered in currently existing English texts. Under each disease, we discuss its pattern identification, treatment principles, and treatment with acupuncture and Chinese medicinals as well as present a number of clinical tips based on Dr. Li's extensive clinical experience.

Because this book addresses the treatment of disease from the point of view of both modern Western medical disease diagnosis and Chinese medical pattern identification, it is an example of the on-going contemporary attempt to integrate these two great and paramount medical systems. Part 4 discusses certain specific clinical issues in the treatment of kidney-bladder diseases with integrated Chinese-Western medicine. For instance, in Part 4, you will find specific advice on how to deal with hypertension and kidney disease, edema and kidney disease, proteinuria and kidney disease, etc., including which Chinese medicinals are especially indicated and contraindicated.

Dr. Li has been integrating Chinese and Western medicine for close to 30 years. In her view, each medicine has its own unique strengths. On the one hand, Chinese medicine provides a deep perspective on a multiplicity of treatment strategies, while Western medicine primarily focuses its attention on attacking evils and pays scant attention to supporting the righteous. In Dr. Li's experience, this overemphasis on a single treatment strategy limits Western medicine's effectiveness. A typical example is the ubiquitous use of antibiotics for infections. From a Chinese medical perspective, the use of antibiotics is limited to the treatment principles of clearing heat, eliminating dampness, and resolving toxins and rarely is an infection merely an issue of damp heat and toxins. Therefore, professional practitioners of Chinese medicine typically add other treatment principles when attacking such evils, such as clearing heat, draining fire, and cooling the blood. They also commonly support the righteous with strategies such as nourishing yin, engendering fluids, and supplementing the qi. In Chinese doctors' experience, use of such multifaceted treatment principles speeds recovery and prevents recurrences. On the other hand, Western medicine provides a scientific analysis of medicinals. This analysis leads to a deeper understanding of Chinese medicinals and opens the door to new research and treatment possibilities. Dr. Li believes the continuing integration of the two medicines will provide new treatments for difficult diseases.

This book provides information that can be used by inexperienced practitioners. The chapter on urinary tract infections is a good example. When the diagnosis is evident, the beginning practitioner may read this chapter and find the correct pattern identification, treatment principles, and formula. However, some of the material demands more analysis from the practitioner. Many kidney diseases are complicated and serious, even life-threatening. It is not enough to know the Western medical diagnosis and look for a pattern identification that seemingly matches the patient's signs and symptoms. Clinical presentations rarely match abstract categories. In order to understand kidney disease patterns, it is essential that one have a broader understanding of Chinese kidney diseases and their Western counterparts. This includes Chinese and Western etiology, disease mechanisms, risks, and complications as well as the Chinese historical perspective on kidney disease. Furthermore,

one must develop an advanced understanding of the use of medicinals and formulas. This includes some knowledge of drug-medicinal interactions.

If one is planning to treat serious kidney diseases, one should read this entire book. This text provides Chinese historical accounts of kidney diseases and their treatments. It provides a thorough discussion of the historical and modern Chinese theories of kidney physiology. It discusses etiology and disease mechanisms. It recommends the most appropriate medicinals for particular kidney diseases and patterns. It reviews modern Chinese kidney research. However, based on the saying:

> If one reads 1000 books, one will find no patients in them. If one sees 1000 patients, one will find none in a book

this text also provides classical and modern case histories in order to give the reader a sense of how Chinese physicians actually treat kidney disease in clinic. These case histories illustrate how Chinese doctors have analyzed diseases through pattern identification and modified standard formulas to fit the treatment principles and peculiarities of each case.

Once practitioners have a greater understanding of theory, historical and modern treatment strategies, formulas, and single medicinals, they can approach pattern identification and the treatment of difficult kidney diseases with confidence. They will then be able to prescribe formulas with ingenuity and flexibility.

We hope this book adds a small bit to the growing English language literature on Chinese medicine. Like every book, we know it is not perfect. Consequently, we take full responsibility for all the shortcomings of this book, and we invite our readers to point out any mistakes or errors so that we can make future editions even better.

PART 1
GENERAL THEORY

CHAPTER 1
THE KIDNEY IN WESTERN
AND CHINESE MEDICINE

WESTERN ANATOMY & PHYSIOLOGY
OF THE KIDNEYS

The urinary tract includes the kidneys, ureters, bladder, and urethra. Together, these organs serve to produce and excrete urine and regulate fluid and electrolyte content in the body. Urine is a by-product of blood, water, salts, and toxins. The genitourinary system is one of the principal organ systems responsible for waste management and reduction in the body. The other systems include the lungs, skin, and gastrointestinal tract. The kidneys are a highly vascularized, paired organ system. They are bean-shaped and approximately the size of a child's fist. They lie just above the waist behind the abdominal cavity. This area is defined as retroperitoneal.

The inner structure of the kidney reveals an outer layer or cortex and an inner layer or medulla. Within the cortex and medulla are approximately a dozen medullary pyramids which contain upwards of a million nephrons. These nephrons are the functional units of the kidneys. They are responsible for filtering, secreting, and reabsorbing waste products of the body. Although it was once thought that the kidneys do not have the ability to regenerate damaged or lost nephrons, recent research indicates that nephrons

can regenerate. In addition, individual nephrons may enlarge or hypertrophy in order to assume a greater burden in filtration and secretion.

Two main arteries, the right and left renal arteries, carry approximately 25% of the resting cardiac blood supply to the kidneys. This amounts to greater than 1000ml/min of blood that pass through them. Within the kidneys, as previously mentioned, there is a vast network of progressively narrowing blood vessels. The capillary end-point of blood entering the kidney is called the glomerulus, and it is in this region that the most significant filtration and re-absorption occur. Blood eventually exits the kidney via a single vein, the renal vein.

The amount of filtrate that forms every minute within the renal structures is called the glomerular filtration rate (GFR). In adults, the GFR is approximately 120ml/min. Three unique processes regulate GFR: 1) kidney self-regulation, 2) hormones, and 3) neural regulation. The glomerulus is acutely sensitive to input from the entire body. It uses this information to continuously monitor and optimize the filtration rate.

The kidneys have the ability to set their own blood

pressure if the body's systemic blood pressure experiences stress and/or dysfunction. This self-regulation is vital for the health of the entire body.

Two active hormones play key roles for the kidneys. These are angiotensin II and atrial diuretic peptide (ADP). Angiotensin II is produced at the conclusion of a cascade of events beginning with the release of an enzyme, rennin. Rennin is released from within the cells of the kidney. With the eventual production of angiotensin II, four essential processes occur. First, the efferent arterioles, (those that exit the kidney) are constricted, thus raising the internal kidney blood pressure. Second, the adrenal cortex is stimulated to release aldosterone. Aldosterone serves to increase the amount of reabsorbed sodium, also raising the blood pressure. Third, the thirst center in the hypothalamus in the brain is stimulated. The body is encouraged to drink more water. This also increases blood volume and pressure. Finally, the posterior pituitary gland in the brain is stimulated to release antidiuretic hormone. This process encourages water retention within the kidneys.

Atrial diuretic peptide serves the kidneys in the opposite manner. As the heart stretches, for instance, in the case of increased blood volume, cells within the atria of the heart release ADP. Atrial diuretic peptide promotes both diuresis (the excretion of water from the kidneys) and natriuresis (the excretion of sodium). Together, this serves to lower internal blood pressure in the kidneys.

The third form of GFR regulation is neural. The sympathetic, fight or flight division of the autonomic nervous system supplies vasoconstricting input to the blood vessels of the kidneys. When the body enters into a sympathetic dominant state, as with exercise, stress, trauma, etc., the fibers are activated, thus constricting the renal blood vessels. This process serves to decrease the GFR and allows for increased blood flow to other areas of the body.

Apart from the nephrons, the rest of the urinary tract is fairly mechanical in nature. The medullary pyramids empty into the initial collecting spaces for the urine, the minor and major calyces. From the calyces, urine flows to the bladder via the right or left ureter. Peristalsis within the ureters allows urine to flow into the bladder. Each ureter is an extension of the kidney and is approximately one foot in length.

The bladder is a hollow organ, described as pear- or triangular-shaped. As with the kidneys, it is retroperitoneal. In males, it lies just in front of the rectum, and, in females, it lies in front of the vagina and below the uterus. Males tend to have larger bladders than females.

Micturition refers to the expulsion of urine from the bladder. Though the average adult bladder may hold up to 800ml of fluid, when the bladder exceeds 200-400ml, stretch receptors are activated, sending signals to the lower spinal cord. These nerve impulses are both voluntary and involuntary. As humans grow in age, from toddler to child, they are able to actualize their voluntary impulse and control the urge for involuntary release. Ultimately, however, if prolonged long enough, the involuntary aspect of the micturition reflex will dominate regardless of the willful, voluntary control.

The urethra is the single, final vessel of the urinary tract. It exits at the exterior of the body. In males, it is approximately eight inches in length and is comprised of three distinct sections: 1) prostatic urethra, 2) membranous urethra, and 3) spongy urethra. Initially, the urethra passes through the prostate. It then transverses the urogenital diaphragm, and, finally, it enters the penis. For the male, the urethra serves the dual purpose as conduit for urine from the bladder and for semen from the prostate. In females, the urethra is approximately one inch and a half in length. It lies just behind the pubic symphysis and in front of the vagina. The external opening is between the clitoris and the vaginal opening.

THE KIDNEY IN CHINESE MEDICINE

The *Huang Di Nei Jing Su Wen (Yellow Emperor's Inner Classic, Simple Questions)*, Chapter 17, "*Mai Yao Jing Wei Lun* (On the Finest Essence of the Essentials of Pulse [Examination])," states, "The lumbus is the mansion of the kidneys." *Su Wen*, Chapter 9, "*Liu Jie Zang Xiang Lun* (Treatise on the

Relationship Between the Six Nodes & the Viscera)," states, "[The kidney is] of the water phase in the lower burner . . ." The kidney resides in the lower burner and connects physically with the urinary bladder, its paired bowel, by channels (and the ureters), and thus to the urethra. The kidney system is composed of the kidney, the life-gate, the bladder, the marrow, the ears (via the sea of marrow or the brain), the two lower orifices (and, by implication, the testes, ovaries, and prostate), and the channels that connect them. The kidney is intimately connected to the heart. They are part of the same *shao yin* organ network. It is also connected to the root of the tongue (via channels) and the head hair (via the brain).

The leg *shao yin* kidney channel starts beneath the little toe where the *tai yang* bladder channel ends. It crosses the sole of the foot, emerges at the medial side of the foot at the navicular tuberosity, circles the medial malleolus, enters the heel and continues upward along the medial aspect of the lower leg. It intersects the spleen and liver channel three *cun* above the medial malleolus. It continues upwards, traversing the medial aspect of the popliteal fossa and the medial posterior aspect of the thigh, to the base of the spine. Here, it intersects the governing vessel. It proceeds inward and upward to home to its organ, the kidney, and to communicate with the bladder. It intersects the conception vessel on the lower abdomen and then ascends parallel to the linea alba to the root of the tongue. A branch ascends directly from the kidney, crosses the liver, proceeds up through the diaphragm to enter the lung, and continues up the throat to the root of the tongue. Another branch separates in the lung, connects to the heart and disperses in the chest.

"The kidney is the water viscus." Much of Chinese medical kidney theory flows from this statement. In Daoism, water is the first offspring of the *tai ji* or supreme ultimate, the heavenly oneness that is the source of all that unfolds. In the body, the kidney is the source of water, essence,[1] source qi (also called original qi), and ministerial fire.[2] It stores the fundamental yin and yang[3] and is the root of yin and yang for all the organs and the entire body. When kidney yin and yang are balanced, the kidney's source qi can

maintain the harmony of yin and yang in the other organs and the entire body. Conversely, disharmony of yin and yang in any organ will eventually affect the kidney.

Lao Zi ascribes great power to the softness and malleability of water and uses it as a metaphor for following the Dao. In Chapter 8 of the *Dao De Jing* (*The Classic of the Way [& Its] Power*), he states:

> The best attitude is like water.
> Water benefits the myriad things without
>   competing.
> It seeks out the lowest position.

The kidney, as the water viscus, takes the lowest position of the viscera in the body. In Chapter 66, Lao Zi states, "The river and sea rule the myriad valleys by making the lower position an asset;" and in Chapter 78, he continues:

> Nothing in the world is softer and more
>   supple than water.
> Yet when attacking the hard and the strong,
>   nothing can surpass it.
> The supple overcomes the hard.
> The soft overcomes the strong.

Since water drains downward, the kidney's low position allows it to "govern water." It does this through its function of storage and qi transformation. It is the kidney's source qi that powers the qi transformation necessary to produce and regulate the body's water.

Kidney yin consists of former heaven yin (or congenital essence) and latter heaven yin (or acquired essence) and is called true yin or true water. Kidney yang, or life-gate fire, an immaterial fire, is called true yang or true fire. True fire steams true water to produce source qi. Source qi is stored in the kidney and the cinnabar field. It travels through the triple burner, reaching all the organs and enabling all qi transformation. All other forms of qi in the body are derivatives of source qi. While all viscera contain source qi, the kidney stores the surplus.

Governing water refers to the kidney's close physical and functional relation to the urinary bladder. This bowel is also associated with water and resides, along with the kidney, in the lowest part of the body. The saying that "the kidney governs opening and closing" is usually interpreted to mean that the kidney controls the urinary bladder's storage and release of urine. (The relationship between the kidney and bladder will be discussed more fully in a following section.)

Because the kidney is in the lowest position, kidney qi can easily control the two lower orifices. This includes control of urinary continence, sexual functions, and fecal continence. Food or "water and grain" enters the stomach and must finally pass out of the two lower orifices. Thus the kidney is described as the bar or gate of the stomach. Fear affects the kidney and may cause it to lose control of the lower orifices, hence resulting in urinary and fecal incontinence.

The water phase corresponds to winter, a cold, dark season. Winter's coldness and darkness necessitate but also facilitate the preservation and storage of seeds which are full of essence. Hibernating within these stored seeds is the immaterial fire that will generate new life in the spring. In winter, things go underground to hibernate, and the kidney pulse is sinking. As water and winter are associated with coldness and darkness, the kidney is particularly sensitive to excess cold, and kidney pathology may show up in a darkened or black complexion. As the water viscus, "the kidney is averse to dryness" that desiccates the body's fluids, marrow, and bones, "wearing" or consuming yin and essence.

Kidney yang is especially important in pathologies of water, dampness, and cold. Water dampness tends to accumulate, to seek its own level, and to stagnate. Cold is congealing and can cause stagnation. *Su Wen*, Chapter 14, "*Tang Ye Lao Li Lun* (On Rice Soup, Aged & Sweet Wine)*" states:

> Some evils do not invade at the skin level. They may come from yang vacuity of the five viscera. When the yang is vacuous, the qi cannot propel the flow of the water and the water is retained in the skin, causing water swelling.

Ye Tian-shi has said, "When dampness prevails, yang

is debilitated." Conversely, it is kidney yang, the kidney's warming, activating aspect, that provides the yang qi transformation necessary to dispel cold and water dampness.

The *Nan Jing* (*The Classic of Difficulties*) associated kidney yang with the life-gate and the life-gate fire. Difficulty 36 states:

> The two kidneys are not both kidneys. The left one is the [true] kidney, while the right one is the life-gate. The life-gate is the abode of the spirit essence. Original qi is tied to it. It stores the essence [sperm] in males. It supports the uterus in females.

Difficulty 39 states that, "The life-gate's qi and the kidney's qi communicate."

All Chinese scholars accepted and employed this theory from the time of the *Nan Jing* until the Song dynasty. However, in the Ming dynasty, Zhang Jing-yue challenged this idea. In the *Lei Jing* (*Systematic [Compilation of the Inner] Classic*), he stated that the life-gate is between the kidneys and connects them. He theorized that the life-gate is the *tai ji* or supreme ultimate in the human body. The supreme ultimate generates both fire and water. When it moves, it generates yang; when it is quiet, it generates yin. It is the mansion of water and fire, the abode of yin and yang, and the sea of essence. It holds the key to life and death.[4]

Zhao Xian-ke further developed the theory of the life-gate in the *Yi Guan* (*[Key] Link of Medicine*) published in1687. In this work, he stated that the life-gate has a small orifice on each side of it. The triple burner springs from the right orifice and spreads ministerial fire to the five viscera and six bowels. The left sends true water, which has no form, up the spine to the sea of marrow, the brain.[5] True water secretes the fluids that enter the channels, nourish the four extremities, and enter the five viscera and six bowels. It moves with ministerial fire to fill the entire body. He believed the life-gate fire initiates processes. For instance, it is the spark that ignites or initiates the spleen's function of transforming food. In the *Yi Guan*, Zhao Xian-ke states:

The spleen's ability to transform depends completely on the insubstantial ministerial fire of *shao yin*, steaming from the lower [burner]. Only with this can it begin to transform and transport.

THE KIDNEY'S FUNCTIONS & RELATIONSHIPS

1. THE KIDNEY STORES ESSENCE AND GOVERNS THE FORMER HEAVEN CONSTITUTION, GROWTH, AND MATURATION.

Su Wen, Chapter 4, "*Jin Gui Zhen Yan Lun* (Treatise on the Truth from the *Golden Cabinet*)" states, "The sage knows that essence is the most precious [thing] in the human body." *Su Wen*, Chapter 9, states:

The kidney is the place of storage of the true yang and the root of all storage in the body. The kidney stores the essence qi of the five viscera and six bowels. It manifests its abundance and health in the head hair. It fills the bones and the marrow. Being of the water phase in the lower burner, the kidney is considered yin. It is the *shao yin* of the three yin and corresponds to winter.

Storage of essence includes storage of former heaven essence and later heaven essence. Former heaven essence is congenital, while later heaven essence is derived from food and air transformed by the spleen and lung. Former heaven essence is the foundation of later heaven essence but is dependent on the later heaven for continual nourishment. Later heaven essence supplies all the organs, and its excess is stored in the kidney. *Su Wen*, Chapter 1, "*Shang Gu Tian Zhen Lun*" (Preceding Ancients' Heavenly Truth)" states,

Kidney qi is the former heaven qi of the human body, but it can only bring its functions into play when it is nourished by latter heaven qi. The essence of the five viscera and six bowels is supplied from the finest essence of water and grains. It is only after receiving and storing the essence of food that the five viscera and six bowels can provide essence for the kidney. The kidney is water. It receives and stores the essence and qi from the five viscera and six bowels. Therefore, the kidney can only spread its essence and qi to the whole body when the five viscera and six bowels are substantially filled with essence.

The *Ling Shu* (*Spiritual Axis*), Chapter 10, "*Jing Mai* (The Channels & Vessels)" states:

In the beginning of human life, essence is formed first. It then develops into the brain and spinal cord, and finally the human body is formed.

The kidney governs the former heaven constitution, growth, and maturation through its storage of essence. *Su Wen*, Chapter 1, describes the waxing and waning of the human life-cycle:

In general, [the reproductive physiology of] a woman is [such that] at seven years of age, her kidney qi becomes full, her permanent teeth come in, and her hair grows long. At two [times] seven years, the heavenly water [6] is exuberant, the controlling [vessel] is freely flowing, and the great penetrating [vessel] is effulgent, menstruation begins, and conception is possible. At three [times] seven years, the kidney energy is strong and healthy, the wisdom teeth appear, and the body is vital and flourishing. At four [times] seven years, the sinews and bones are well developed and the hair and secondary sex characteristics are complete. This is the height of female development. At five [times] seven years, the *yang ming* stomach and large intestine channels that govern the major facial muscles begin to deplete, the muscles begin to atrophy, facial wrinkles appear, and the hair begins to thin. At six [times] seven years, all three yang channels [*tai yang, shao yang,* and *yang ming*,] are exhausted, the entire face is wrinkled, and the hair begins to turn gray. At seven [times] seven years the conception and penetrating [vessels] are completely empty, the heavenly water is exhausted, the passages of the earth are cut, the body deteriorates, and she can no longer bear children.

In the male, at eight years of age, the kidney energy becomes full, the permanent teeth appear, and the hair becomes long. At two [times] eight, the kidney qi is exuberant, the heavenly water is effulgent, and the essence is ripe, so procreation is possible. At three [times] eight, the kidney qi is abundant, the sinews and bones grow strong, and the wisdom teeth come in. At four [times] eight, the body is at the peak of strength, and functions of the male are at their height. At five [times] eight, the kidney qi begins to become depleted, the teeth become loose, and the hair starts to fall. At six [times] eight, the yang energy of the head begins to deplete, the face becomes sallow, the hair grays, and the teeth deteriorate. By seven [times] eight years, the liver qi weakens, causing the sinews to stiffen. At eight [times] eight, the heavenly water dries up and the essence is drained, resulting in kidney exhaustion, fatigue, and weakness. When the qi of all organs is full, the excess energy stored in the kidney is excreted for the purpose of conception. But now, the organs have aged and their qi has become depleted, the sinews and bones have become frail and stiff, and movement is hampered. The kidney reservoir becomes empty, marking the end of the power of conception.

Menstrual blood and sperm are called heavenly water because they represent the descending of the true qi of heaven in liquid form into maturing women and men. Many scholars have theorized about the source and origin of heavenly water. In the Qing dynasty work *Yi Zong Jin Jian* (*The Golden Mirror of Ancestral Medicine*), Wu Qian *et. al.* state that heavenly water is passed by parents to the embryo and is the same as former heaven source qi. Heavenly water combines each parent's essence and

blood and sperm, it also controls and stores them.

In Western medicine, heavenly water corresponds with the hormonal functions of the hypothalamus-pituitary-thyroid-adrenal-sex glands axis. (See Figure 1.1.)

2. THE KIDNEY GOVERNS THE BONES AND ENGENDERS MARROW.

Su Wen, Chapter 10, "*Wu Zang Sheng Cheng Lun* (Treatise on the Engenderment & Production of the Five Viscera)" states, "The bones and marrow correspond with the kidney."[7] *Su Wen,* Chapter 44, "*Wei Lun* (On Wilting)" states, "The kidney governs the bone and engenders bone marrow." Chapter 5, "*Yin Yang Ying Xiang Da Lun* (Great Treatise on the Corresponding Manifestations of Yin & Yang)" states:

> The north corresponds to cold and water. Cold is invisible and water is visible, and, as visible things are produced from invisible things, water is produced from cold. The flavor corresponding with the kidney is salty, water produces saltiness,

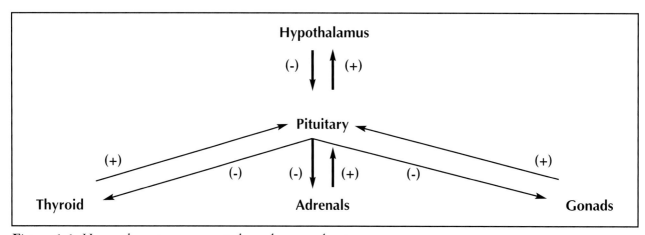

Figure 1.1. Heavenly water represented as a hormonal axis

blood, which is derived from food. When kidney qi is developed and strong, at 16 years of age in men and 14 years of age in women, heavenly water matures. The mature heavenly water combines with menstrual blood and sperm starting the menstrual cycle and the ability to conceive. Although one can say that heavenly water is a precursor to menstrual

and saltiness produces the kidney. When the kidney obtains water essence, it produces fat, fat produces marrow, and thus the kidney produces marrow.

. . . Of the six environmental (qi) in heaven, the north is cold. In the five phases on earth, it is water. In the human body, it is bone. In the five viscera, it is the kidney.

Su Wen, Chapter 17, states, "The bones are the palace of the marrow." Marrow is differentiated into bone marrow (which promotes the bones and the surplus of the bones, the teeth), spinal marrow, and the brain, the sea of marrow. Kidney essence, the brain, marrow, and the bones (as well as the source qi) give the body and mind agility.

Ling Shu, Chapter 36, "*Wu Long Jin Ye Bie Lun* (A Divergent Treatise on the Five Infirmities and Fluids & Humors)" states:

> [If essence is lost, this] lessens not only the essence but also the marrow. Once this passes a certain degree, vacuity results, vacuity that causes pain in the lower and upper back as well as aching in the shins.

3. THE KIDNEY GOVERNS AGILITY.

Su Wen, Chapter 8, "*Ling Lan Mi Dian* (Magic Orchid Secret Teachings)" states, "The kidney holds the office of labor from whence agility emanates." Agility includes agile thinking as well as agile movement. Agile movement is related to the bones and bone marrow, and agile thinking is related to the brain. *Su Wen*, Chapter 17, states:

> The head is where the spirit is located. If the head hangs down or tilts with the eyes caving in, it shows the spirit will decline soon.

Kidney essence generates the bones and marrow, while life-gate fire warms the marrow and keeps it functioning properly. The quality of the individual's essence determines how the bones and brain develop and flourish. *Ling Shu*, Chapter 33, "*Si Hai Lun* (On the Four Seas)," states:

> When the sea of marrow is replete, one will feel light and vigorous and will be able to undertake unusually hard work. When the sea of marrow is vacuous, one's brain will spin and one will have tinnitus, sore legs, and dizziness. One will be unable to see clearly and be enervated and sleepy.

This theory, that diseases associated with the head and brain are related to weakness of kidney essence or life-gate fire is borne out in clinic. One must often treat the kidney for chronic memory problems, insomnia, and dizziness. In renal failure, the kidney is too weak to excrete toxins, and patients may have insomnia, headache, impaired memory, and dizziness, and may even have hallucinations or become comatose. Although toxins cause some of these symptoms, kidney vacuity is also responsible. Once one supplements and improves the functioning of the kidney, toxins will be excreted and all these symptoms will improve.

4. THE KIDNEY GOVERNS THE EARS, [AND] ITS EFFLORESCENCE IS IN THE HAIR [OF THE HEAD].

Su Wen, Chapter 4, states, "The kidney governs the ears." *Su Wen*, Chapter 17, states:

> . . . the kidney communicates with the ear orifices. When the qi of the ear is harmonious, the ears can hear the five tones.

The ears are connected to the brain and thus are dependent on the kidney essence. *Ling Shu*, Chapter 30, "*Jue Qi* (Concerning Qi)" states, "When one's essence is vacuous, one's ears will be deaf." As people age, they inevitably deplete their kidney essence. The depleted kidney essence is less able to nourish the brain, thus causing hearing loss.[8]

Su Wen, Chapter 9, states, "The kidney manifests its abundance and health in the head hair." An ancient theory posited that hair is a direct outgrowth of the sea of marrow or the brain. Hair growth depends on essence and blood. The kidney stores the essence, essence generates blood, and hair is the surplus of the blood.

5. THE KIDNEY GOVERNS THE TWO YIN [I.E., THE TWO LOWER ORIFICES].

Su Wen, Chapter 4, states, "The kidney opens at the two yin [the two lower orifices]." Therefore, the proper functioning of the anus, urethra, and, by extension, the reproductive organs depends on kidney qi.

Kidney qi transformation controls water metabolism. Qi transformation distributes fluids throughout the body. The turbid descends to the bladder to become urine. If there is kidney vacuity, the qi transformation may not completely separate the clear from the turbid, causing urinary turbidity. If there is kidney yin vacuity, vacuity heat may burn the network vessels in the lower burner causing bloody urine. If there is kidney qi vacuity, the kidney may not maintain control of lower orifices, causing incontinence or dribbling urinary block. In addition, many patterns of strangury involve the kidney. For example, taxation strangury is exacerbated by sexual taxation. In this case, the loss of essence compromises the kidney's control of the lower orifices.

The kidney is also in control of the posterior yin, the anus. The kidney is described as the bar or gate of the stomach. Food entering the stomach must finally pass out of one of the two lower orifices. If there is kidney yang vacuity, the life-gate fire may become too weak to generate earth, causing yang vacuity constipation or diarrhea. (This constipation is a result of fluid loss through copious urination.) Again, kidney yin vacuity may cause dryness in the intestines with resultant constipation.

6. THE KIDNEY INFLUENCES THE UTERUS AND THE PENETRATING AND CONCEPTION VESSELS.

Kidney essence governs heavenly water and influences the penetrating and conception vessels. Only when heavenly water matures can the conception and penetrating channels flow freely allowing menarche and conception. With age, kidney essence declines and there is a corresponding decline in heavenly water. The penetrating and conception vessels become empty, menopause begins, and menstruation ends.

The penetrating vessel originates in the uterus, emerges at the perineum, and then ascends through the spinal column. A superficial branch passes through the region of *Qi Chong* (St 30) and joins the kidney channel. Through *Qi Chong,* it connects with the *yang ming* channel. It harmonizes the qi and blood of the 12 channels and is, therefore, called the sea of

blood. The conception vessel originates in the uterus and emerges from the perineum. In the lower abdomen, it communicates with all three foot yin channels. It controls and harmonizes all the yin channels and is called the sea of yin channels. The conception vessel can be full and strong only when the 12 channels have an abundance of qi and blood, and the uterus can support menstruation only after the penetrating and conception vessels harmonize the qi and blood. The exuberance of the penetrating and conception vessels is controlled by heavenly water. If the kidney becomes vacuous, heavenly water becomes vacuous, causing insufficiency and disharmony in the penetrating and conception vessels. Women may experience infertility as well as irregular menstruation, amenorrhea, and other menstrual disorders.

7. THE KIDNEY STORES THE WILL (OR MIND), AND FEAR IS THE AFFECT CORRESPONDING TO THE KIDNEY.

Su Wen, Chapter 5, states:

> . . . the kidney stores the mind. Excessive fear damages the kidney . . .

The quality of the essence is reflected in the strength of the will and determination seen as a soul or mind "housed" in kidney essence. Essence is the stuff of life, and while fear is an emotion necessary to preserve life, an excess of fear (often described as "dark and cold") can blunt will power, damaging the will and essence. It is common clinical experience to see testicular changes in patients who have experienced car accidents, gun shot wounds, or acute epidemic diseases.[9]

8. THE KIDNEY & URINARY BLADDER

The kidney stands in an interior-exterior relationship with the urinary bladder. They both belong to water in terms of the five phases, the bladder being the yang aspect. Channels of each organ connect to the other organ.

In normal fluid metabolism, the urinary bladder receives the body's turbid fluids. (The small intestine, triple burner, and lung are the principal organs involved in passing these fluids to the bladder.) Kidney qi transformation then separates the clear fluids from the turbid. The kidney sends the clear fluids up to the lung; the bladder excretes the turbid fluids. Because normal fluid metabolism requires this process, kidney yang and its source qi must first pass through the urinary bladder before circulating in the triple burner. *Su Wen*, Chapter 8, states:

> The bladder holds the office of gathering, it stores the water and fluid, after the body fluid is transformed into water by (kidney) qi, it can be excreted.

Some scholars interpret this to mean that the bladder as well as the kidney "governs opening and closing," *i.e.*, the storage and discharge of urine. However, because the bowels transport but do not store, most scholars believe it is the kidney that is responsible for the bladder's ability to store urine. The kidney, along with the bladder, is also responsible for the qi transformation necessary for the discharge of urine.

Kidney source qi empowers qi transformation throughout the body. Bladder qi transformation is limited and refers only to the bladder controlling the normal discharge of urine. When this function is compromised or damaged, it is called "inhibited bladder qi transformation" or "bladder qi transformation failure." Symptoms include urinary frequency, urgency, inhibition, dribbling, pain, and/or stones.

Pathology of the kidney and bladder are usually interrelated. Problems with urination are often ascribed to impairment of kidney qi transformation and/or failure of bladder qi transformation without a clear distinction between the two. Since the kidney stores essential substances and there can be no excess of these, kidney patterns are usually ones of vacuity. Bladder patterns often involve damp heat and other substantial evils and are usually replete.

9. THE KIDNEY & HEART

In the course of kidney disease, dual patterns such as heart-kidney qi, yang, or yin vacuity often arise. The heart, the sovereign of all of the organs residing in the upper burner, corresponds to fire.[10] The kidney, the water viscus, resides in the lower burner. Heart yang descends to warm kidney yang, while kidney yin ascends to nourish heart yin.

Heart fire and kidney water balancing each other is called "heart and kidney interacting" or "heart and kidney communicating." This communication is especially important for sleep. Insomnia usually involves disharmony between heart yang and kidney yin to some degree. This is called "noninteraction of the heart and kidney" or "heart and kidney not communicating."

A common disease mechanism begins with loss or damage to essence. This depletes kidney water and vacuous kidney water cannot balance heart fire. Therefore, it flares upward with symptoms of vexation and insomnia. Heart and kidney not communicating may also start with a heart pattern. Replete heart fire, from any cause, burns up kidney water and results in vexation and insomnia. Loss of kidney essence may also lead to both yin and yang vacuity. This may affect the heart and cause hypersomnia.

10. THE KIDNEY & LIVER

"The liver and kidney are of the same source." Although kidney yin is the basis of the yin of all the organs, the kidney water is the mother of the liver wood in the five phase cycle. Thus liver yin is especially dependent on kidney yin, with vacuity of kidney yin easily leading to vacuity of liver yin. If there is liver yin vacuity, liver yin cannot control liver yang and it may rise out of control. On the other hand, excesses of the son can easily draw qi from the mother. Since liver wood is the son of kidney water, hyperactivity of liver yang can easily damage the kidney.

The liver stores blood and the kidney stores essence, and blood and essence are mutually convertible and interdependent. Therefore, vacuity of either will eventually wear on the other. Normal menstruation relies on the liver properly governing the sea of blood, *i.e.*, the liver viscus, the penetrating vessel, and the conception vessel. Proper storage of blood is also necessary for a normal pregnancy. Liver and kidney yin vacuity leads to emptiness of blood in the channels. In men, this may result in lack of sperm; in women, it may result in problems with menstruation and pregnancy.

The ministerial fire inhabiting both the liver and kidney has its source in the life-gate. Decline of life-gate fire may lead to weakening of the liver's coursing and discharge of the qi. The liver governs coursing and discharge, and the kidney governs storage. These "contrary" functions are dependent on, and must balance each other.

11. THE KIDNEY & SPLEEN

In five phase theory, the spleen and stomach correspond to the earth phase. The spleen is "wet" (yin) earth and abhors dampness, while the stomach is "dry" (yang) earth and abhors dryness. These balance one another. Although earth restrains water in the five phase control cycle, this can only be done by dry earth. Therefore, stomach yang qi must be strong for earth to restrain water. On the other hand, the kidney is water and too much dryness can desiccate kidney water. This is repletion of dry earth overwhelming water.

"The kidney governs the former heaven [and] the spleen governs the latter heaven." The kidney stores former heaven (or congenital) essence and is the basis of the congenital constitution, while the spleen produces latter heaven (or acquired) essence from the transformation of food and water and is the basis for the acquired constitution. In five phase theory, fire engenders earth. Life-gate fire is necessary to initiate and maintain the spleen's transformation of food and water into latter heaven essence. Latter heaven essence nourishes former heaven essence and is also stored in the kidney. Because spleen and stomach vacuity or middle burner disharmony may cause kidney essence vacuity, one often supplements both the spleen and kidney at the same time.

Both the spleen and kidney are responsible for the production of blood. The spleen produces blood through the normal metabolism of food, and the kidney produces blood through its governance of

bone marrow.

12. THE KIDNEY & LUNG

In five phase theory, metal (lung) generates water (kidney). "The lung is the governor of qi [and] the kidney is the root of qi," i.e., the kidney is the source of water and the lung distributes it. The lung receives and absorbs the qi, controls breathing, and produces true qi but can only do so if the kidney helps absorb the qi and provides source qi to transform the gathering qi.

"The kidney governs water, [while] the lung is the upper source of water [and] governs regulation of the water passageways." The lung controls the movement of water by its function of diffusing and depurative downbearing, and the kidney receives water and sends water back up to the lung through its action on bladder fluids. Because of their relationship to qi and water, "the lung and kidney are mutually engendering."

Kidney yin and essence nourish and maintain lung yin. A vacuity of kidney yin and essence often causes lung yin vacuity.

Five phase theory and viscera-bowel theory give different accounts of the kidney's relation to the other viscera. These are summarized in Table 1.1.

13. THE KIDNEY & TRIPLE BURNER

Ancient and modern scholars have disagreed as to the exact nature of the triple burner. Different sources state that it refers to discreet body spaces similar to, but not exactly the same as, the modern thoracic, abdominal, and pelvic cavities; that it refers to the organs contained within these spaces; that it is a purely functional idea ("The triple burner has a name but not a form"); or that it refers to some other Chinese (or Western) anatomical entity such as the greater omentum.

Ling Shu, Chapter 18, "Ying Wei Sheng Hui (The Engenderment & Meeting [or Distribution] of the Constructive & Defensive)" describes the triple burner's location as follows:

FIVE PHASE THEORY	VISCERA-BOWEL THEORY
The kidney (water) restrains the heart (fire).	"The heart and kidney communicate." The kidney as water is the body's root yin and stands in the fundamental yin/yang relation to the body's root yang, the heart as fire.
The kidney (water) engenders the liver (wood).	"The liver and kidney are of the same source." Liver yin is rooted in kidney yin, and kidney essence and liver blood are mutually engendering.
Kidney water is engendered by lung metal.	"The lung and kidney are mutually engendering." Fluids reach the kidney after the lung diffuses and depuratively downbears them. The lung as well must flow freely in order for the kidney to function properly, especially to excrete water from the body. The kidney governs the absorption of qi that enters the lung and must function properly for the lung to function properly.
Kidney water is restrained by spleen earth.	"The kidney is the root of former heaven, the spleen is the root of latter heaven." The spleen supplies latter heaven qi to the kidney. The kidney houses the life-gate fire that is necessary to promote the spleen's function of digestion.

Table 1.1. The kidney's relation to the other viscera

> The upper burner emerges from the upper mouth of the stomach and ascends with the esophagus, passing through the diaphragm and spreading through the chest . . . The middle burner also comes out of the stomach and emerges behind the upper burner . . . The lower burner separates from the large intestine and pours over the bladder and seeps into it.

Thus according to the authors of the *Nei Jing*, the upper burner refers to the area above the diaphragm containing the heart and lung. The middle burner refers to the area below the diaphragm and above the umbilicus, containing the spleen, stomach, and part of the large and small intestines. The lower burner refers to the area below the umbilicus and above the external genital organs containing the kidney, liver, bladder, and part of the large and small intestines.

Although it may refer to the body cavities, the triple burner's location is sometimes metaphorical. For example, in cold damage theory, the triple burner's

location has to do with the *shao yang* stage. It is "half exterior and half interior," "midstage," or the "pivot" between exterior and interior disease. This location can be seen as between the interior (*i.e.*, the viscera and bowels) and the exterior (or the skin, flesh, sinews, and channels). From this location, the triple burner connects the interior organs to the exterior of the body. It springs from the kidney and bladder, connects to the organs, and is contiguous with the interstices.[11] The triple burner's connection of the kidney to the interstices helps explain the kidney's relation to defensive qi discussed in the next section.

Su Wen, Chapter 8, describes the triple burner's function as follows:

> The triple warmer holds the office of dredging water in the watercourse of the body. It takes charge of the qi transformation of the body fluid and the regulation and the dredging of fluids.

Ling Shu, Chapter 18, states, "The upper burner is like mist, the center burner is like foam, and the lower burner is like a sluice." "The upper burner is like mist" refers to the lung's function of diffusion of qi and fluids. "The center burner is like foam" refers to the reception, ripening, and extraction of the finest essence of food and water by the spleen and stomach. "The lower burner is like a sluice" refers to the elimination of waste by the intestines, kidney, and bladder. *Nan Jing,* Difficulty 31, states:

> The triple burner is the pathway for water circulation and food transportation and transformation. It is the beginning and end of qi circulation.

Later scholars expanded the triple burner's function to include the smooth operation of the body's passageways for qi, blood, water, and fire. The triple burner mirrors the role of the channels as the passageway for source qi, water, and ministerial fire. For example, the spleen's transformation of food is dependent on the life-gate fire that must pass through the triple burner. Similarly the grain essence extracted by the spleen is transported to the lung via the triple burner. Likewise, it is the passageway for turbid fluids to drain into the bladder and for clear fluids to travel from the urinary bladder back up to the body. Both these types of fluids are a result of the qi transformation of source qi directed through the triple burner. Even though the kidney and heart are part of the same *shao yin* channel, it is often stated that heart yang descends to the kidney and kidney yin ascends to the heart through the triple burner. The triple burner as a passageway explains certain disease mechanisms. It also suggests the use of certain medicinals and formulas in triple burner pathology.

The triple burner is associated with the kidney as it springs from the life-gate and is one of the organs that controls ministerial fire. It also separates or directs kidney source qi into different channels and organs as stated in *Nan Jing,* Difficulty 66:

> The triple burner is the director of separation for the source qi. It rules the free movement of the three qi through the five viscera and six bowels.

In cold damage theory, the triple burner has a role not only in *shao yang* disease but also in *shao yin* disease. In warm disease theory, the triple burner helps explain four aspect theory and is itself used as a means of pattern identification.

The kidney and triple burner are often closely involved in pathology, especially water pathology. The kidney governs water, but water must pass through the triple burner. The triple burner must be freely flowing for water to flow normally. The distribution of source qi and kidney yang also depends on the triple burner.

14. THE KIDNEY & DEFENSIVE QI

The kidney is involved in the production of defensive qi both directly and indirectly. The kidney's source qi enables the qi transformation in every phase of the production of true qi, a portion of which becomes the defensive qi. The kidney directly produces the defensive qi when kidney yang steams fluids in the bladder. A portion of bladder fluids becomes defensive qi through this qi transformation. The defense qi enters the triple burner, which springs from the kidney and bladder, and follows its pathway, spreading on the surface of the organs and in the interstices. The defensive qi also enters the *tai yang* bladder channel. The *tai yang* channel, along with the lung, is responsible for spreading the defensive qi on the surface (through the interstices) where it regulates the opening and closing of the pores. Because the kidney produces defensive qi and defensive qi regulates the pores, the phrase "the kidney governs opening and closing" has been taken to mean the kidney has some responsibility for regulating the opening and closing of the pores.

Because of the kidney's close connection to defensive qi, kidney vacuity makes the individual more susceptible to an external evil attack. Moreover, defensive qi is only one aspect of right qi. Once in the body, evil qi struggles with various aspects of this right qi. Since the kidney is necessary for the production and maintenance of all aspects of right qi, a prolonged struggle between evil qi and right qi will eventually damage the kidney.

15. KIDNEY HEALTH

The Chinese in general, and the sages of Chinese medicine in particular, have valued disease prevention for millennia. *Su Wen*, Chapter 2, "*Si Qi Tiao Shen Da Lun*" ("The Great Treatise on Regulating the Spirit [Through] the Four Seasons)," states:

> In ancient times, the sages treated disease by preventing illness before it began, just as a good government or emperor was able to take the necessary steps to avert war. Treating an illness after it has begun is like suppressing revolt after it has broken out. If someone digs a well when thirsty, or forges weapons after becoming engaged in battle, one cannot help but ask, "Are not these actions too late?"

In the course of discussing kidney disease, we have included information about maintaining and preserving kidney health. The following are a few introductory remarks.

Kidney health depends on diet, exercise, lifestyle choices, and spiritual practices. The life of the sage is the model: simple, moderate, contemplative, and generous.

A good diet is essential to kidney health, as well as general health. There are several books on Chinese dietetics available in English, and we refer the reader to them. There are also certain Daoist long-life medicinals that target the kidney. These supplementing medicinals can be taken safely for long periods of time. One can make a tea of *Sang Ji Sheng* (Sangjisheng, Ramulus) or *Sang Shen* (Mori Albi, Fructus) or make cordials of *He Shou Wu* (Polygoni Multiflori, Radix) or *Sang Shen*. One can also cook *Sang Shen* with congee.

A sedentary life harms the bones, while over-taxation harms the kidneys. Regular exercise that is not too strenuous is ideal. One should avoid exposing oneself to cold during exercise, including swimming in icy water, and one should avoid becoming dehydrated. *Tai ji quan* is an excellent exercise for maintaining kidney health that can be practiced at any stage of life.

In general, one's lifestyle should be moderate and in harmony with the seasons. The kidney governs storage, and it abides in contemplation. A tumultuous life, full of excitement and diversions, drains the kidneys. Certain recreational drugs are especially damaging to the kidney.

The number of spiritual disciplines is legion. *Su Wen*, Chapter 1, contains the following dialogue between Huang Di and Qi Bo:

> Huang Di inquired: I've heard of people in ancient times, spoken of as the immortals, who knew secrets of the universe and held yin and yang, and the world, in the palms of their hands. They extracted essence from nature and practiced various disciplines, such as *dao in* and *qi gong*, breathing and visualization exercises, to integrate the body, mind, and spirit. They remained undisturbed and thus attained extraordinary levels of accomplishment. Can you tell me about them?

> Qi Bo responded: The immortals kept their mental energies focused and refined, and harmonized their bodies with the environment. Thus, they did not show conventional signs of aging and were able to live beyond biological limitations. . . . Achieved beings were also able to preserve their life spans and live in full health. . . . Sages . . . adapted to society without being swayed by cultural trends. They were free from emotional extremes and lived a balanced and contented existence. . . . They abided in calmness, recognizing the empty nature of phenomenological existence. . . . [Naturalists] lived in accordance with the rhythmic patterns of the seasons . . . They . . . lived plainly and [thus] enjoyed long life.

Many spiritual practices, including *dao in* and *qi gong*, profoundly increase one's ability to conserve and restore former heaven kidney essence. These are beyond the scope of this book, and we must refer readers to books specifically on this subject. To fully devote oneself to a spiritual discipline, however, one must have an accomplished teacher.

Endnotes

[1] *Jing* means both essence and semen. Seminal fluid, vaginal fluids, blood, breast milk, and "spittle," *i.e.,* dense fluid essences, are all regarded as transformations of *jing*.

[2] Life-gate fire, original yang, and ministerial fire are, in a certain sense, synonymous with kidney yang, but these different terms stress different aspects or relationships of kidney yang. Original yang or original fire is kidney yang seen as the metabolic foundation of life, complimenting original yin or original water. The term "ministerial fire" is used to distinguish the kidney yang fire from the heart's yang fire, called "sovereign fire." It is also the life-gate fire as employed by or "inhabiting" the liver, gallbladder, and triple burner.

[3] The definitions of and relationships between kidney qi, yin, yang, and essence are not consistent in the literature. Various sources give primacy to essence or source qi, some saying that essence is derived from source qi, while others say the opposite is true. Essence is usually thought of as part of kidney yin but may act as both kidney yin and yang. Kidney yin may refer to water in general, to essence, or to substance and form. Some sources equate kidney qi with source qi, while others make a distinction between them. In the following discussion we have tried to present a view consistent with most Chinese medical theory.

[4] In the *Zhong Yi Za Zhi* (*Journal of Chinese Medicine*), issue #1, 1997, p. 49, Zi Yi-shen describes the results of autopsies performed in Military Hospital No. 157. It was found that those patients who had had kidney yang vacuity symptoms had pathological changes in their adrenal, thyroid, and sexual glands. There were no pathological changes in those patients who had not had kidney yang vacuity. Research was also conducted on living people, comparing middle-aged patients with kidney yang vacuity with randomly selected patients over 65. It was found that the younger patients with kidney yang vacuity had thyroid and sexual hormone functions similar to the older group. In other words, these kidney yang vacuity patients' hormone secretions declined 18-30 years earlier than normal individuals.

[5] This suggests a correlation with Western endocrinology.

[6] Wiseman translates (*tian gui*) "heavenly tenth." Although *gui* refers to the tenth heavenly stem, this stem pertains to water. Therefore we have decided to translate *tian gui* as "heavenly water".

[7] *Zhong Yi Za Zhi* (*Journal of Chinese Medicine*), issue #10, 1997, p. 621, reports that Dr. Yin Yu-shi conducted animal experiments on the connection between kidney conditions and bone metabolism using farm animals. He started with the Western idea that there are two kinds of blood cells involved in bone metabolism, cells that produce new bone, and cells that dissolve old bone. The formulas he used most were *You Gui Wan* (Restore the Right [Kidney] Pills), *Jin Gui Shen Qi Wan* (*Golden Cabinet* Kidney Qi Pills), *Liu Wei Di Huang Wan* (Six Flavors Rehmannia Pills), and *Zhi Bai Di Huang Wan* (Anemarrhena & Phellodendron Rehmannia Pills). He concluded that formulas that supplement kidney yang stimulate the production of blood cells that produce new bones, while formulas that nourish kidney yin depress the production of cells that dissolve bone. Formulas that supplement kidney yin and yang have both actions, and animals given these formulas had greater bone density and bone strength. He also found that medicinals that clear heat such as *Zhi Mu* (Rhizoma Anemarrhenae Asphodeloidis) and *Huang Bai* (Cortex Phellodendri) depress both types of cells. He concluded that, for diseases with bone loss such as osteoporosis, one should use formulas that supplement kidney yin and kidney yang.

[8] Xi Ming-wang, *Zhong Yi Ling Chuan Shen Zang Bing Xue* (*Clinical Nephrology in Chinese & Western Medicine*), Chinese Medicine Publishing Co., Beijing, 1997, p. 28, reports that animal experiments conducted by Xi Ming-wang had positive results using kidney-supplementing kidney formulas such as *Liu Wei Di Huang Wan* (Six Flavors Rehmannia Pills) to protect the inner ear against gentamicin's toxic side effects.

[9] *Ibid.*, p. 27. Xi Ming-wang conducted animal experiments that show that fear causes pituitary and testicular changes. In these experiments cats were used to frighten mice, humans were asked to frighten cats, and fireworks were used to frighten dogs. These animals were then examined and all three groups had testicular and pituitary pathologies.

[10] Some scholars assert that the kidney's ministerial fire is a "borrowed" fire of the heart. Others believe that because the kidney stores essence (the yin that is the basis of all yang), governs former heaven, and because its yang is the root of other organ yang, kidney fire is more primordial.

[11] The *Jin Gui Yao Lue* (*Essentials from the Golden Cabinet*), Chapter 1, states, "The crevices (*cou*) in the surface tissues on the exterior of the body and in the viscera and bowels are the place where the triple burner moves and gathers the true qi." Zhou Xue-hai, in the *Du Yi Sui Bi* (*Random Notes While Reading Medicine*), states, ". . . Openly traveling the interior and exterior, corresponding to the crevices (*cou*) of the exterior and interior (*li*) and influencing the half-interior half-exterior portion of the whole body, is the *shao yang* triple burner qi . . ."

CHAPTER 2
DISEASE CAUSES & MECHANISMS

INTRODUCTION

Su Wen, Chapter 5, "*Yin Yang Ying Xiang Da Lun* (Great Treatise on the Corresponding Manifestations of Yin & Yang)" states:

> Yin and yang in the body must always be kept in balance. Repletion of yang causes yin diseases, and repletion of yin causes yang diseases.

Various pathogenic factors are mentioned throughout this work, but there is no consistent classification of them. For example, in the same chapter it states:

> Exterior evils invade the body from the exterior to the interior, moving from the superficial to the deep, finally [damaging] the viscera. Improper diet mainly affects the six bowels. . . . Overindulgence in the five affects, joy, anger, sadness, worry or fear, and fright, may damage the viscera. Emotions injure the qi, while seasonal elements attack the physical body.

In *Su Wen*, Chapter 14, "*Tang Ye Lao Li Lun* (On Rice Soup, Aged & Sweet Wine)," it states:

> Some evils do not invade at the skin level. They may come from yang vacuity of the five viscera.

In *Su Wen*, Chapter 21, "*Jing Mai Bie Lun* (A Divergent Treatise on the Channels & Vessels)," it states, "Within the context of the yin and yang changes of the four seasons, the etiology of disease is often determined by one's constitution, taxation fatigue, diet, exercise, and emotions." In *Ling Shu*, Chapter 4, "*Xie Qi Zang Fu Bing Xing* (On Viscera & Bowel Diseases Caused by Evil Qi)," it states, "High falls may cause blood stasis." *Su Wen*, Chapter 71, "*Liu Yuan Zheng Ji Da Lun* (Great Treatise on the Six Origins & Correct Periods)" states, "When pestilential qi (*li qi*) comes strongly, populations will tend to die suddenly." Finally, *Su Wen*, Chapter 72, "*Ci Fa Lun* (On Needling Methods)" discusses toxins as a cause of epidemic disease.

Zhang Zhong-jing in the *Jin Gui Yao Lue* (*Essentials from the Golden Cabinet*) divides causes into three broad categories. In Chapter 1, "On the Pulse, Patterns & Transmission of Diseases of the Viscera, Bowels, Channels & Network Vessels," he states:

> When humans are strongly influenced by external evils, they perish. All human catastrophes fall within the following three causes. The first, internal causes, consist of evils attacking the channels and network vessels and being trans-

mitted into the viscera and bowels. The second, external causes, consist of external evils invading the four extremities and nine orifices and then circulating through the blood vessels obstructing the normal flow of qi. The third cause consists of sexual intemperance, various traumas, and animal and insect bites. These cover the causes of all diseases.

In the Southern Song dynasty, Wu Ze-chen (a.k.a. Chen Yan) developed the theory of three categories: external, internal, and neither external nor internal causes in the *San Yin Ji Yi Bing Zheng Fang Lun* (*A Unified Treatise on Diseases, Patterns & Remedies According to the Three Causes*). In his view, the external category includes the six excesses. The internal category consists of the affects. The neutral (literally "neither external nor internal") category includes sexual intemperance, trauma, and animal and insect bites. (The development of warm disease theory in the Qing dynasty added two other external evils to the external category: pestilential qi and warm toxins. Scholars have had different opinions on the scope of the neither external nor internal category.)

In modern Chinese medical theory, causes of disease are categorized as primary or secondary. The three primary causes are external, internal, and neither external nor internal causes. The external causes include the six external evils, toxins, and pestilential qi. The internal causes are the seven affects. Neither external nor internal causes include various types of congenital factors, trauma (knocks and falls, drowning, incised wounds, burns and scalds, animal bites,

poisonous reptile bites, and insect bites and stings), dietary irregularities, sexual intemperance, taxation fatigue, and parasites. The three primary causes produce the secondary causes of disease: phlegm and static blood.

Some causes may attack or damage the kidney directly, while others damage the kidney only indirectly or as a consequence of damage to other organs. For example, cold may directly attack and damage the kidney. On the other hand, dietary irregularities may only indirectly damage the kidney by first damaging the spleen. A weakened spleen may then produce dampness that hampers the yang qi of the kidney.

External evils often combine. *Su Wen*, Chapter 3, "*Sheng Qi Tong Tian Lun* (The Union of Heaven & Living Beings)" states, "Wind is the spearhead of a thousand diseases." Wind combines with and facilitates the entrance of other evils into the body. In clinic, one commonly sees wind combined with cold, heat, dryness, and damp. Summerheat may be viewed as a combined pathogen. It is a type of heat that is always mixed with a certain amount of dampness. The following figure shows some common combinations of external evils.

THE PRINCIPLE CAUSES OF KIDNEY DISEASE

A. EXTERNAL CAUSES

Although any external evil may cause kidney disease

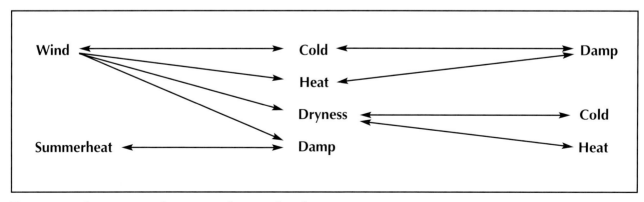

Figure 2.1. Common combinations of external evils

directly or indirectly, the most common are wind (in combination with cold, heat, or damp), cold damp, damp heat, and dry heat.

1. WIND

Su Wen, Chapter 42, "*Feng Lun* (Treatise on Wind)" states, "when a person is injured by wind on the *ren* and *gui* days in winter, it is kidney wind." Later in this chapter, the following description is found:

> The symptoms of the kidney wind are profuse sweating, aversion to wind, water swelling of the face, pain in the loin and spine, inability to stand very long, a black facial complexion like the smoke from burning coal, and inhibited urination. During inspection, take note of the cheeks. They should be of a black hue.

Wind cold is a combination of the two evils. Wind is a yang evil that tends to attack the upper burner and outer layers of the body first. Cold is a yin evil that tends to attack the lower burner. In kidney wind, wind cold first attacks the exterior and constrains the lung and then the cold moves down to the kidney. This is called "lung cold moves to the kidney."

Cold belongs to yin and readily damages kidney yang, compromising the kidney's qi transformation and leading to water accumulation. Kidney yang vacuity eventually damages kidney yin, leading to complicated patterns of yin and yang vacuity. Cold may damage the kidney's control of the lower orifices, inhibiting urination and compromising the kidney's storage of essence. With essence diminished, the marrow and bones are damaged.

Wind cold causes several diseases associated with the kidney. Kidney wind involves water swelling. A wind cold attack on the chest and abdomen may cause block and repulsion. A wind cold attack on the back may cause lumbar pain. Long-term damage to kidney yin and yang by wind cold can eventually result in kidney taxation.[1] Wind cold may also exacerbate already existing kidney diseases.

Wind heat is a combination of two yang pathogens. Wind heat tends to move quickly, penetrating deeply.

When wind heat causes kidney wind, the disease mechanism is somewhat different than wind cold. In wind heat, wind constrains the lung qi, inhibiting the dispersing and depurative downbearing function of the lung, while heat constrains the spleen and middle burner, inhibiting the upbearing of the clear qi of the spleen and the downbearing of the stomach qi. This middle burner dysfunction leads to dampness that stagnates and damages the true qi. Because the true qi is debilitated, it cannot contain the evils in the upper burner and, thus, the heat moves down to the kidney. Although the classical literature does not mention this latter mechanism, we feel this should be called "lung heat moving to the kidney," being similar to lung cold moving to the kidney.

Jin Gui Yao Lue, Chapter 2, "On the Pulses, Patterns & Treatment of Tetany & Heatstroke" states:

> When wind and dampness invade, the patient will suffer acute body pain, and moving around will be difficult. . . . Wind and dampness cause acute pain in the joints that impairs the movement of joints due to egregious referred pain. The pain is aggravated with pressure. The patient is short of breath, sweats, fears wind, is reluctant to remove clothing, suffers from painful urination, and has slight water swelling.

Wind damp is similar to wind cold in its effect on the kidney. Both cold and damp are yin evils. Damp as well as cold can hamper kidney yang and the kidney's qi transformation. Kidney qi transformation failure leads to more damp and water accumulation. Dampness is sticky and tenacious by nature. It tends to linger, causing heaviness in the body and intractable water swelling.

Jin Gui Yao Lue, Chapter 2, warns against inducing profuse sweating to treat wind damp.

> [Inducing] profuse sweating will dispel wind evils but not dampness, and the pattern remains. To disperse wind and dampness simultaneously, only a light perspiration should be induced.

In this book, we use the term "proper sweating" to indicate correctly releasing the exterior. A proper sweat is a light sweat over the entire body with, perhaps, a little heavier sweating on the nose.

2. COLD DAMP

In kidney diseases with patterns of cold damp, the body feels heavy, the waist is cold, and there is profuse urination. *Jin Gui Yao Lue*, Chapter 14, "*Shui Zhong* (Water Swelling)" states, "When yang qi fails to circulate normally, cold prevails in the body." *Jin Gui Yao Lue*, Chapter 2 states:

> Patents with a chronic disease caused by dampness will sweat only from the head, have a stiff back, prefer heavy clothing and prefer to remain near a fire. …There are also signs and symptoms of fullness in the chest or painful urination.

Dampness affecting the kidney is described in the *Jin Gui Yao Lue*, Chapter 11, "Accumulation of Wind & Cold" as follows:

> A pattern affecting the kidney…has the following signs and symptoms…heaviness in movement and cold in the lumbar region as if the patient were sitting in water. …The etiology of this pattern is as follows: The patient has performed work and sweated causing the patient's clothes to become wet and cold. If this continues for a long period of time, the patient will be affected by cold with a painful sensation below the waist and by a feeling of heaviness in the abdomen as if the patient were carrying a thousand coins around the waist.

Both cold and dampness are yin evils. When yin is exuberant, water prevails and transforms into cold damp. Cold is contracting by nature, while damp is clammy, viscous, lingering, and tends to stagnate. Cold damp is especially damaging to kidney yang qi and is intractable.

3. DAMP HEAT

The most important of the evils in kidney disease is damp heat. Damp heat is a combination of a yin evil and a yang evil. Dampness easily compromises the kidney qi transformation, while heat burns yin fluids. The combination of dampness and heat damages both kidney yang and yin, with symptoms of qi vacu-

ity and heat. Diseases caused by damp heat tend to become chronic and intractable.

Damp heat may be externally contracted[2] or internally engendered. External damp heat is an invasion of the combination of the two external evils, fire (a type of heat) and dampness, or a manifestation of summerheat.[3] Internally generated damp heat is usually due to viscera and bowel disharmony. These two are often linked.

Internally engendered damp heat is usually generated by disharmonies of the kidney, spleen, and lung and involves the triple burner. The most common pathology is that of the spleen and triple burner as in the following example. Irregular diet or contaminated food damages the spleen causing spleen qi vacuity. Spleen qi vacuity compromises the spleen's function of movement and transformation of water in the triple burner resulting in damp accumulation. Dampness is a "hothouse," *i.e.*, dampness easily causes stagnation that results in heat and can "wrap" the heat preventing it from dispersing. The dampness and heat combine to form damp heat. For any evil to invade, the right qi must be vacuous. Internally engendered damp heat damages the right qi and facilitates an invasion of external damp heat.

4. DRY HEAT

Dry heat is a combination of two yang evils. The kidney is the water viscus and is adverse to dryness. Dry heat tends to burn up kidney yin and desiccate fluids, therefore leading to kidney yin vacuity. When resolving dry heat, one must be careful to supplement kidney yin, moisten dryness, and safeguard fluids.

B. INTERNAL CAUSES

The normal emotions do not cause disease. Only when emotions are especially strong and/or long lasting will they cause organ disharmonies that lead to disease. *Su Wen*, Chapter 5, states, "Excessive fear damages the kidney." Although fear directly damages the kidney, other emotions may indirectly damage the kidney.

Excessive anger may damage the liver leading to liver

depression qi stagnation. Liver depression qi stagnation, in turn, may lead to fire that damages kidney yin. Liver depression can damage the blood. The liver stores blood and the kidney stores essence. Because essence and blood are mutually convertible, liver blood vacuity may cause kidney essence vacuity.

Excessive thinking may damage the spleen leading to spleen qi vacuity. If the spleen is vacuous, it cannot govern movement and transformation. Therefore, it also cannot send latter heaven essence and qi to the kidney for storage. Without this replenishment, the kidney becomes vacuous.

Excessive joy may damage the heart leading to heart fire. Heart fire may then desiccate kidney water. Shock may cause heart qi or yang vacuity. Heart yang descends to warm kidney yang as part of its interaction with the kidney. If heart yang is vacuous, this may affect kidney yang.

Excessive sorrow may damage the lung leading to lung qi vacuity. The lung is the upper source of water which depurates and downbears water to the kidney. If the lung is vacuous, it cannot downbear the necessary water to the kidney leading to vacuity. The lung governs the regulation of the water passageways. Thus lung vacuity may also lead to water accumulation. Water accumulation is yin and readily damages the yang qi of the kidney. In terms of the five phases, metal engenders water. Metal must be strong to engender water.

C. NEITHER EXTERNAL NOR INTERNAL CAUSES

Some of the neither external nor internal causes are especially important in kidney disease, and the former heaven (or inherited) constitution is paramount. *Ling Shu*, Chapter 6, "*Shou Yao Gang Rou* ([On the Relation Between] Firmness & Softness, Longevity & Premature Death)" refers to former heaven in the statement:

> Human bodies are different in character. Some are firm and some are soft. In constitution, some are strong and some are weak . . .

The constitution, age, and health of the parents plus

any problems during pregnancy are factors that can affect the fetus and thus the offspring's constitution. The kidney houses the former heaven essence made up of the parents' essence. If the parents' essence is vacuous or damaged, this may cause kidney essence and qi vacuity in their children. Parents with kidney yang or yin vacuity may pass this particular vacuity to their children.

The depletion of kidney essence after birth is ascribed to several neither external nor internal causes. First there is the wear of the normal life cycle, itself controlled by kidney essence. The control of the cycles of life by the kidney is described in *Su Wen*, Chapter 1, "*Shang Gu Tian Zhen Lun* (Preceding Ancients' Heavenly Truth)" and has been presented above in full. This famous section describes the impact on the waxing and waning kidney's essence on growth, maturation, aging, and decline. However, the rate of the decline of essence is also dependent on one's lifestyle. If one leads a moderate and conscious life, being careful of one's diet, sleep, and exercise, living in harmony with the seasons, and using relaxation and meditation to conserve one's essence, one can slow down the consumption of kidney essence and the debility and decline it entails. If one lives a profligate life, indulging in rich food, alcohol, excessive sex, or if one worries excessively, overworks, and does not live in harmony with nature, one speeds up the consumption of essence.

One of the neither external nor internal causes especially deleterious to the kidney is over-indulgence in sex. This is especially true in men since kidney essence is the basis for sperm. In fact, in Chinese the term *jing* denotes both sperm and essence. Therefore, the loss of sperm directly causes loss of kidney essence. This, in turn, can cause kidney qi vacuity, since kidney qi is dependent on kidney essence. Women, on the other hand, lose essence through abnormal, excessive menstruation. Menstrual blood, heavenly water, is directly produced from kidney essence, but all blood and essence are mutually convertible. Loss of blood in excessive childbearing is especially damaging to the kidney.

Taxation fatigue is caused by overexertion or lack of

exercise. Overexertion may damage the bones, while a sedentary lifestyle may cause a lack of circulation of qi and blood to the marrow, both related to the kidney. Both taxation fatigue and lack of exercise also damage the spleen, leading to a reduction of latter heaven essence.

Dietary irregularities may indirectly damage the kidney. *Su Wen*, Chapter 43, "*Bi Lun* (On Impediment)" states, "If food and drink are taken excessively, the intestines and stomach will be injured." If the middle burner is injured, the spleen will be unable to produce qi and blood. In that case, latter heaven essence is diminished and cannot supplement former heaven essence. Indulgence in alcohol causes heat and fire that burns the fluids and damages kidney water. Rotten food may be toxic and directly damage the kidney.

Toxins,[4] such as poisonous mushrooms, fish's gallbladder, pufferfish poison, snakebites, insect stings, and certain chemicals, may directly damage the kidney. These may damage kidney qi, yin, yang, and essence. Other chemicals and heavy metals may first damage the liver or lung and then indirectly damage the kidney.

D. PHLEGM & BLOOD STASIS

As stated above, phlegm and blood stasis are so-called secondary causes of disease. They do not arise independent of primary causes, but, once formed, they may cause further disease. They are mutually engendering, each causing stagnation that facilitates the formation of the other.

The source of phlegm is water. If water is not transformed and moved, it congeals into dampness and phlegm. Dysfunction of the major viscera involved in water metabolism, the lung, spleen, and kidney, leads to phlegm formation. Heat "boiling" and thus concentrating water, or cold "congealing" water also form phlegm. Once formed, phlegm impairs qi and blood circulation and may exacerbate kidney disease. In clinical fact, phlegm is typically found in difficult kidney diseases. The signs and symptoms of phlegm are legion since phlegm may accumulate anywhere in the body, causing stagnation and

impediment. Phlegm is associated with asthma, nausea, vomiting, water swelling, nodules, accumulations, etc.

Jin Gui Yao Lue, Chapter 12, "*Tan Ke* (Phlegm & Coughing)" states, "Phlegm patterns can be cured by warm medicinals." Warm medicinals refers to interior-warming and yang-invigorating medicinals. Yang qi, especially kidney yang qi, transforms water and disperses dampness. Boosting yang qi to transform phlegm has remained a basic treatment strategy for transforming phlegm.

Ling Shu, Chapter 81, "*Yong Ju* (On Welling & Flat Abscesses)" states, "If cold invades the channels, the channels will become obstructed and the blood becomes stagnant..." Again, in Chapter 62 of the *Su Wen*, "*Tiao Jing Lun* (Treatise on Regulating the Channels)," it states, "...repletion evils in the minute network vessels may overflow and cause the retention of blood in the network vessels." These and other statements in the *Nei Jing* suggest that any of the three causes may cause blood stasis. In damp heat invasions, the heat burns the network vessels causing extravasation of blood leading to blood stasis. Cold and dampness block qi and blood circulation leading to blood stasis. The affects cause visceral disharmony that leads to stagnation and heat and ultimately to blood stasis. Likewise, knocks and falls cause damage, impediment, and extravasation of blood leading to blood stasis.

Blood stasis can obstruct the flow of water causing or exacerbating water swelling, while water swelling can cause obstruction that leads to blood stasis. As the *Jin Gui Yao Lue* succinctly states, "Water diseases affect the blood." In water swelling, symptoms such as dry mouth, dry lips, rough skin ("crocodile skin"), purple tongue, and a choppy pulse indicate blood stasis. Symptoms of blood stasis affecting fluids are described in *Jin Gui Yao Lue*, Chapter 16, "On the Pulse, Patterns & Treatment of Convulsions & Palpitation, Hematemesis, Epistaxis, Hematochezia, Chest Fullness & Blood Stasis":

> The patient experiences a sense of fullness in the chest, withered lips, a bluish tongue, and parched mouth. He is thirsty but merely holds the water in

his mouth with no intention of swallowing it.[5] He has no fever and chills. He has no abdominal distention but claims to be suffering from this. His pulse is feeble, huge, and slow. This is a case of blood stasis.

Blood stasis often causes bleeding. If this is the case, prescribing only astringent or blood-stanching medicinals may cause more stasis which may, in turn, cause more bleeding. A better strategy is to employ medicinals whose secondary function is to stanch bleeding. Examples of such medicinals include *Han Lian Cao* (Ecliptae Prostratae, Herba), *Sheng Di Huang* (Rehmanniae Glutinosae, uncooked Radix), *Bai Shao* (Paeoniae Lactiflorae, Radix Albus), *Mu Dan Pi* (Moutan, Cortex Radicis), *Long Gu* (Draconis, Os), *Mu Li* (Ostreae, Concha), and *E Jiao* (Asini, Gelatinum Corii).

Blood stasis may also be caused by underlying vacuity of qi, blood, yang, or yin. "Qi is the commander of the blood," *i.e.*, qi engenders and moves (as well as contains) the blood. Thus qi vacuity can lead to blood stasis. "Blood is the mother of qi," *i.e.*, blood vacuity may lead to qi vacuity, qi stagnation, and to blood stasis. Yin vacuity may desiccate the fluids, including the blood, or cause heat that damages the blood leading to blood stasis. Yang vacuity may result in cold or damp blockage or water swelling that leads to blood stasis.

Blood stasis can exacerbate kidney diseases by blocking the kidney's network vessels and/or compromising the kidney qi transformation. In fact, blood stasis has become a major focus of modern Chinese research on kidney disease.

ENDNOTES

[1] Kidney taxation may present as the Western diseases renal failure and nephritis.

[2] Many Western infectious diseases present patterns of damp heat. A partial list includes malaria, encephalitis B, staphylococcus infections of the skin, urinary tract infections, streptococcal sore throat, and infectious hepatitis.

[3] Summerheat, which occurs in the summer or autumn in humid climates, presents with symptoms of red face, swollen body, yellow-green nasal discharge or sore throat, sloppy stool or constipation, and painful scanty urine. The tongue is red with yellow, slimy fur, and the pulse is soggy. Some scholars distinguish two types of summerheat—summerheat heat and summerheat dampness— as well as several summerheat disease patterns. However, in all of these, there is an admixture of heat and dampness.

[4] The term "toxins" has several meanings in Chinese medicine. It can refer to the toxic nature of medicinals, toxic animal and plant products, particular patterns in dermatology, or external evils. In this book, we include environmental exposure or ingestion of toxic chemicals or heavy metals in the neither external nor internal category of causes along with toxic reactions to prescription drugs, alcohol, street drugs, poisonous mushrooms, etc. However, in certain instances we have categorized these toxins as external causes to better explain a particular etiology.

[5] The phrase, "He is thirsty but merely holds the water in his mouth with no intention of swallowing it," indicates that the thirst is due to blood stasis blocking the distribution of fluids, not to fluid exhaustion. The patient only needs to hold the water in his mouth to moisten dryness due to local blockage of fluids, not to swallow it to replenish vacuous internal fluids.

CHAPTER 3

IMPORTANT TREATMENT PRINCIPLES IN CHINESE NEPHROLOGY

In general, the treatment principles should adhere to the cardinal principle in Chinese medicine: "Determine treatment by patterns identified." Many treatment principles are used in treating patterns in kidney diseases. The most important ones follow.

A. TIP TREATMENT STRATEGIES

1. CLEAR HEAT, ELIMINATE DAMPNESS & RESOLVE TOXINS

Since damp heat is one of the two most important evils in kidney disease, clearing and eliminating damp heat and any associated toxins is a priority. This treatment strategy employs several treatment methods and varied medicinals from many medicinal categories. For instance, a distinction is made between externally contracted and internally engendered damp heat when choosing the appropriate treatment method. If the damp heat and/or toxins are in the exterior, one can employ the sweating method. However, in clinic, one usually sees these factors after they have penetrated more deeply. Thus, the most common methods are the clearing method and the dispersing method. The clearing method may be used for heat or damp heat in any aspect or burner. Using the dispersing method, it is common

to employ the principles of clearing heat and percolating dampness, freeing the flow of strangury, and dispersing qi stagnation and blood stasis. In some cases, the precipitating method is necessary to precipitate heat toxins and expel water.

Although formulas used for clearing and eliminating dampness and heat and resolving toxins vary widely according to the location of the damp heat within the body and the specific treatment method chosen, a general representative formula is *Huang Lian Jie Du Tang* (Coptis Toxin-resolving Decoction):

Huang Lian (Coptidis Chinensis, Rhizoma), 10g
Huang Qin (Scutellariae Baicalensis, Radix), 10g
Huang Bai (Phellodendri, Cortex), 10g
Zhi Zi (Gardeniae Jasminoidis, Fructus), 10g

All the medicinals in this formula clear heat, eliminate dampness, and resolve toxins. *Zhi Zi* also cools the blood, stanches bleeding, and disperses blood stasis.

A more specific formula, one for strangury with damp heat, is *Ba Zheng San* (Eight [Ingredients] Rectification Powder):

Mu Tong (Akebiae Mutong, Caulis), 9g

Qu Mai (Dianthi, Herba), 9g
Bian Xu (Polygoni Avicularis, Herba), 9g
Hua Shi (Talcum), 6g
Deng Xin Cao (Junci Effusi, Medulla), 9g
Che Qian Zi (Plantaginis, Semen), 9g
Zhi Zi (Gardeniae Jasminoidis, Fructus), 9g
processed *Da Huang* (Rhei, Radix Et Rhizoma), 9g
Gan Cao (Glycyrrhizae Uralensis, Radix), 9g

In this formula, the emphasis is on clearing damp heat via urination using the first six cool, water-disinhibiting, dampness-percolating medicinals. The last three medicinals resolve the toxins directly.

One of the hallmarks of Chinese medicine is that it attempts to treat the root of disease, not just alleviate the tip or symptoms. Clearing and eliminating dampness and heat and resolving toxins treats the tip. Even when there is egregious external evils and the initial strategy is to attack these evils, one must support the righteous to treat the root. One should be careful not to damage the true qi by using medicinals inappropriate for the patient's constitution, and one should be especially careful to protect the yin when employing drying, heat-clearing, or water-disinhibiting medicinals.

2. DIFFUSE THE LUNG

We have used the metaphor "making a hole in the teapot's lid"[1] throughout this text to explain what is meant by diffusing the lung in terms of nephrology. This phrase refers to the potter's practice of making a teapot's lid with a hole in it in order to facilitate the pouring of tea. The hole releases pressure that allows the tea to flow out of the spout unobstructed. The lung governs the qi and the regulation of the water passageways. Inhibition of the lung's diffusion and depurative downbearing can cause qi transformation failure in other organs and inhibit urination. When dealing with inhibited urination, it is often not enough to simply disinhibit urination. One must also diffuse the lung to regulate the water passageways. One may use medicinals from the warm or cool, acrid, exterior-resolving categories and/or the cough-suppressing, panting-leveling category for this strategy. Many exterior-resolving formulas may be

used. A representative formula for wind water from the *Jin Gui Yao Lue* is *Yue Bi Tang* (Maidservant from Yue Decoction):

Ma Huang (Ephedrae, Herba), 18g
Shi Gao (Gypsum Fibrosum), 48g
Sheng Jiang (Zingiberis Officinalis, uncooked Rhizoma), 9g
Gan Cao (Glycyrrhizae Uralensis, Radix), 6g
Da Zao (Zizyphi Jujubae, Fructus), 15 pieces

One may also see this strategy at work in *Shen Ling Bai Zhu San* (Ginseng, Poria & Atractylodes Powder):

Ren Shen (Panacis Ginseng, Radix), 9g
Bai Zhu (Atractylodis Macrocephalae, Rhizoma), 9g
Fu Ling (Poriae Cocos, Sclerotium), 9g
mix-fried *Gan Cao* (Glycyrrhizae Uralensis, Radix), 3g
Shan Yao (Discoreae Oppositae, Radix), 9g
Bai Bian Dou (Dolichoris Lablab, Semen), 9g
Lian Zi (Nelumbinis Nuciferae, Semen), 9g
Yi Yi Ren (Coicis Lachryma-jobi, Semen), 9g
Sha Ren (Amomi, Fructus), 3g
Jie Geng (Platycodi Grandiflori, Radix,) 6g

Most of the medicinals in this formula supplement the qi and percolate dampness. *Jie Geng* is an arrow to the lung. Its acrid flavor disperses and its bitter flavor downbears. *Jie Geng* is included in *Shen Ling Bai Zhu San* to reinforce the lung's functions of diffusion and depurative downbearing and, therefore, its regulation of the water passageways. This action increases the effectiveness of the formula to eliminate dampness.

Diffusing the lung treats the tip, and one must also address the root to achieve real success. When employing the sweating method, one must always gauge the patient's constitution and strength. Too much sweating weakens the true. The sweating method is contraindicated in great blood loss. One must also take into account the geography and weather when employing exterior-resolving medicinals. For instance, one must lower the dosage or eliminate *Ma Huang* (Ephedrae, Herba) if a patient is weak or lives in the south where the weather is hot.

3. DISINHIBIT WATER & PERCOLATE DAMPNESS

The kidney is the water viscus, and most kidney diseases inhibit kidney qi transformation of water resulting in water accumulation. Water is a yin evil and often damages yang qi, especially kidney yang qi. However, inhibited yang qi is less able to transform water, thus leading to a vicious cycle. Water and dampness resulting from spleen, lung, and triple burner dysfunction and contraction of external evils may also overwhelm and inhibit the kidney's qi transformation, leading to even greater water accumulation.

In order to disinhibit water and percolate dampness you need to employ the dispersing method to eliminate water accumulation via urination. It is said, "Without disinhibiting urination, dampness cannot be cured." The most common medicinals used for this strategy come from the water-disinhibiting, dampness-percolating category. However, medicinals from other categories are also used for this strategy. Important medicinals in the stasis-dispelling, blood-quickening category include *Ze Lan* (Lycopi Lucidi, Herba), *Xiao Ji* (Cephalanoplos Segeti, Herba), and *Yi Mu Cao* (Leonuri Heterophylli, Herba). In the heat-clearing, toxin-resolving category, *Yu Xing Cao* (Houttuyniae Cordatae, Herba Cum Radice), *Hai Jin Sha* (Lygodii Japonici, Spora), and *Lu Dou* (Phaseoli Radiati, Semen) also disinhibit water and percolate dampness. In the spirit-quieting category, there is *Hu Po* (Succinum), while in the phlegm-transforming category, there are both *Hai Zao* (Sargassii, Herba) and *Kun Bu* (Algae, Thallus). And finally, in the qi-supplementing category, we should never forget *Huang Qi* (Astragali Membranacei, Radix).

A representative formula based on this treatment method is *Wu Ling San* (Five [Ingredients] Poria Powder):

Ze Xie (Alismatis Orientalis, Rhizoma), 4g
Fu Ling (Poriae Cocos, Sclerotium), 2.3g
Zhu Ling (Polypori Umbellati, Sclerotium), 2.3g

Bai Zhu (Atractylodis Macrocephalae, Rhizoma), 2.3g
Gui Zhi (Cinnamomi Cassiae, Ramulus), 1.5g

The first three medicinals in this formula disinhibit water and percolate dampness. *Bai Zhu* fortifies the spleen and transforms dampness, while *Gui Zhi* warms the life-gate and dispels evils from the exterior.

When employing the water-disinhibiting, dampness-percolating strategy, one must be careful not to damage yin. In order to prevent this, one can add medicinals that safeguard yin, as in *Zhen Wu Tang* (True Warrior Decoction) from the *Shang Han Lun (Treatise on Damage [Due to] Cold)*:

Fu Zi (Aconiti Carmichaeli, Radix Lateralis Praeparatus), 9g
Bai Zhu (Atractylodis Macrocephalae, Rhizoma), 6g
Fu Ling (Poriae Cocos, Sclerotium), 9g
Bai Shao (Paeoniae Lactiflorae, Radix Albus), 9g
Sheng Jiang (Zingiberis Officinalis, uncooked Rhizoma), 9g

This formula treats the tip and the root simultaneously. It warms kidney and spleen yang and eliminates cold, boosts the spleen qi and disinhibits urination. Zhang Zhong-jing included *Bai Shao* in this formula in order to safeguard yin. Some scholars contend that *Bai Shao* also "separates the yin complex." Cold damp is a combination of two yin evils. If they are separated, one can deal with each more easily.

Three other formulas important in kidney diseases, *Wu Pi San* (Five Peels Powder), *Wu Pi Yin* (Five Peels Beverage), and *Fang Ji Huang Qi Tang* (Stephania & Astragalus Decoction), disinhibit water and percolate dampness while also fortifying the spleen. They are discussed later in this book.

4. MOVE THE QI, QUICKEN THE BLOOD & DISPEL STASIS

As mentioned above, water and blood stasis are mutually engendering. Water may also block the qi, resulting in qi stagnation, and qi stagnation can lead to blood stasis. In kidney disease, it is common for external evils, especially damp heat, to invade and impede the free flow of the qi and blood. When the qi is stagnant and the blood is static, one should employ the principles of moving the qi, quickening the blood, and dispelling stasis. However, moving the qi, quickening the blood, and dispelling stasis are all species of the attacking, draining method. Therefore, when choosing medicinals from the qi-moving, stasis-dispelling, and blood-quickening categories, one must pay attention to the strength of the patient. One must choose medicinals with the appropriate strength and qi and be aware of the area affected by the medicinal. One can also employ the secondary functions of the medicinal. For instance, *Yi Mu Cao* (Leonuri Heterophylli, Herba) and *Ze Lan* (Lycopi Lucidi, Herba) quicken blood but also disinhibit water.

Qi-moving, blood-quickening, and stasis-dispelling medicinals can also be found in other categories. For instance, in the acrid, exterior-resolving category, one finds *Chai Hu* (Bupleuri, Radix) and *Bo He* (Menthae Haplocalycis, Herba). In the aromatic, dampness-transforming category, one finds *Hou Po* (Magnoliae Officinalis, Cortex). In the interior-warming category, there is *Wu Zhu Yu* (Evodiae Rutacarpae, Fructus). Blood-quickening medicinals listed in the heat-clearing category include *Mu Dan Pi* (Moutan, Cortex Radicis) and *Chi Shao* (Paeoniae Lactiflorae, Radix Rubrus). In the draining precipitation category, there is *Da Huang* (Rhei, Radix Et Rhizoma), and, in the spirit-quieting category, one has *He Huan Pi* (Albizziae Julibrissinis, Cortex), *Ye Jiao Teng* (Polygoni Multiflori, Caulis), and *Hu Po* (Succinum).

The most famous formula representing this treatment method is Wang Qing-ren's *Xue Fu Zhu Yu Tang* (Blood Mansion Dispel Stasis Decoction):

Tao Ren (Pruni Persicae, Semen), 10g
Hong Hua (Carthami Tinctorii, Flos), 7g
Chuan Xiong (Ligustici Wallichii, Radix), 15g
Dang Gui (Angelicae Sinensis, Radix), 10g
Chi Shao (Paeoniae Lactiflorae, Radix Rubrus), 10g
Niu Xi (Achyranthis Bidentatae, Radix), 9g
Chai Hu (Bupleuri, Radix), 3g
Sheng Di (Rehmanniae Glutinosae, uncooked Radix), 10g

Jie Geng (Platycodi Grandiflori, Radix), 9g
Zhi Ke (Citri Aurantii, Fructus), 6g
Gan Cao (Glycyrrhizae Uralensis, Radix), 3g

The first six medicinals in the above formula quicken and harmonize the blood. *Chai Hu* and *Zhi Ke* rectify the qi. *Gan Cao* harmonizes the formula. *Jie Geng* and *Zhi Ke* upbear and downbear the qi in the chest, thus facilitating the movement of blood in the "blood mansion." This is a strong formula and must be used cautiously for weak patients and those with bleeding problems. Although it nourishes the blood and yin to some degree, one must also determine and address the root.

5. TRANSFORM PHLEGM RHEUM & DISPEL STASIS

This is a combination strategy of transforming phlegm on the one hand and dispelling stasis on the other. Both of these are species of the draining method. This strategy is used for accumulations and gatherings as seen in polycystic kidney disease. The cysts are thought to be a combination of phlegm-rheum and static blood. Phlegm necessarily implies qi stagnation; hence the saying, "if there is free flow of the qi, there can be no phlegm formation." In addition, qi stagnation easily leads to blood stasis.

Dispelling stasis has been discussed above. Three prominent theories about transforming phlegm are: 1) To transform or disperse phlegm, one must rectify qi. 2) One must use the warming method to treat the root, and 3) to completely eliminate phlegm, one must disinhibit the urination.

Important medicinals for transforming phlegm can be found in other than the phlegm-transforming, cough-suppressing, panting-leveling category of medicinals. In the qi-rectifying category, these include *Chen Pi* (Citri Reticulatae, Pericarpium) and *Zhi Shi* (Citri Aurantii, Fructus Immaturus). In the blood-rectifying category, there are *Hu Zhang* (Polygoni Cuspidati, Radix Et Rhizoma) and *Yu Jin* (Curcumae, Tuber). In the food-dispersing category, there are *Lai Fu Zi* (Raphani Sativi, Semen) and *Mai Ya* (Hordei Vulgaris, Fructus Germinatus). In the dampness-dispelling category, one has *Fu Ling* (Poriae Cocos, Sclerotium) and *Wei Ling Xian*

(Clematidis Chinensis, Radix). In the heat-clearing, toxin-resolving category, consider *Niu Huang* (Bovis, Calculus) and *She Gan* (Belamcandae Chinensis, Rhizoma). In the exterior-resolving category, there is *Sheng Jiang* (Zingiberis Officinalis, uncooked Rhizoma), and, in the heat-clearing category, there are *Xia Ku Cao* (Prunellae Vulgaris, Spica) and *Xuan Shen* (Scrophulariae Ningpoensis, Radix).

A representative formula for transforming phlegm is *Er Chen Tang* (Two Aged [Ingredients] Decoction):

Ban Xia (Pinelliae Ternatae, Rhizoma), 5g
Chen Pi (Citri Reticulatae, Pericarpium), 4g
Fu Ling (Poriae Cocos, Sclerotium), 5g
mix-fried *Gan Cao* (Glycyrrhizae Uralensis, Radix), 1g
Sheng Jiang (Zingiberis Officinalis, uncooked Rhizoma), 3g
Wu Mei (Pruni Mume, Fructus), 1 piece

In this formula, both *Ban Xia* and *Chen Pi* are bitter and acrid. The bitter flavor dries, and the acrid flavor disperses, drying the phlegm and rectifying qi. This is based on the saying, "If the qi moves, phlegm moves." Acrid *Sheng Jiang* warms and transforms phlegm. *Fu Ling* disinhibits urination to help transform phlegm-rheum. Mix-fried *Gan Cao* boosts the spleen, the root source of the engenderment of phlegm, and *Wu Mei* is an opposing assistant, countering the draining tendency of the formula.

An important formula for rheum, especially in kidney disease, is *Shi Pi Yin* (Bolster the Spleen Beverage):

Fu Zi (Aconiti Carmichaeli, Radix Lateralis Praeparatus), 30g
Gan Jiang (Zingiberis Officinalis, dry Rhizoma), 30g
Fu Ling (Poriae Cocos, Sclerotium), 30g
Bai Zhu (Atractylodis Macrocephalae, Rhizoma), 30g
Mu Gua (Chaenomelis Lagenariae, Fructus), 30g
Hou Po (Magnoliae Officinalis, Cortex), 30g
Mu Xiang (Aucklandiae Lappae, Radix), 30g
Da Fu Pi (Arecae Catechu, Pericarpium), 30g
Cao Guo (Amomi Tsao-ko, Fructus), 30g
mix-fried *Gan Cao* (Glycyrrhizae Uralensis, Radix), 15g

These medicinals are ground into powder and 12 gram doses are administered as a draft with five slices of *Sheng Jiang* (Zingiberis Officinalis, uncooked Rhizoma) and one piece of *Da Zao* (Zizyphi Jujubae, Fructus). This formula treats the tip and root simultaneously. *Fu Zi* and *Gan Jiang* warm and invigorate spleen and kidney yang. *Fu Ling, Bai Zhu,* and mix-fried *Gan Cao* boost spleen qi and disinhibit water. *Mu Gua, Hou Po, Mu Xiang, Da Fu Pi,* and *Cao Guo* warmly transform dampness and rheum and rectify the qi.

Internal cysts often present a pattern of blood stasis and phlegm or blood stasis and phlegm-rheum. An important formula for fluid-filled cysts is *Gui Zhi Fu Ling Wan* (Cinnamon Twig & Poria Pills):

Gui Zhi (Cinnamomi Cassiae, Ramulus), 9-12g
Fu Ling (Poriae Cocos, Sclerotium), 9-12g
Chi Shao (Paeoniae Lactiflorae, Radix Rubrus), 9-15g
Mu Dan Pi (Moutan, Cortex Radicis), 9-12g
Tao Ren (Pruni Persicae, Semen), 9-12g

Warm, sweet, and acrid *Gui Zhi* invigorates the yang qi to disperse phlegm and rheum and quickens the blood in the vessels. Bland *Fu Ling* transforms phlegm-rheum, percolates dampness, and supplements the spleen. *Chi Shao* and *Mu Dan Pi* quicken and harmonize the blood and clear any blood aspect heat. *Tao Ren* dispels blood stasis.

This formula focuses on the tip, and one should be careful to also treat the root. Blood-quickening medicinals and water-disinhibiting, dampness-percolating medicinals can damage the qi and blood. One must take the patient's constitutional strength into consideration when prescribing medicinals such as these.

B. ROOT TREATMENT STRATEGIES

1. NOURISH KIDNEY YIN, INVIGORATE KIDNEY YANG & BOOST THE KIDNEY QI

This treatment strategy employs the supplementing

method as well as the warming method. When supplementing the kidney, it is important to recognize the interdependence of kidney yin, yang, and qi. *Su Wen*, Chapter 5, "*Yin Yang Ying Xiang Da Lun* (Great Treatise on the Corresponding Manifestations of Yin & Yang)" states, "The interdependence of yin and yang is reflected in all things and cannot be separated." Yin and yang are rooted in each other, *i.e.*, they are mutually dependent.

The kidney is the viscus of fire and water, of original yin and original yang, as well as of original qi. It is said that, "The doctor who knows how to supplement yang must know how to gain yang from supplementing yin," and, "The doctor who knows how to supplement yin must know how to gain yin from supplementing yang." Kidney original qi is a product of kidney yang steaming kidney yin.

While there are several medicinals in the yin- and yang-supplementing category that supplement the kidney, there are a few medicinals that are said to boost the kidney qi directly. *Shan Yao* (Dioscoreae Oppositae, Radix) and *Xi Yang Shen* (Panacis Quinquefolii, Radix) are two, and *Ren Shen* (Panacis Ginseng, Radix), although it does not enter the kidney channel, is said to boost the original qi. However, since the time of the *Jin Gui Yao Lue*, practitioners attempting to supplement kidney yin, yang, and especially kidney qi, have relied on *Jin Gui Shen Qi Wan* (*Golden Cabinet* Kidney Qi Pills):

Fu Zi (Aconiti Carmichaeli, Radix Lateralis Praeparatus), 3g
Gui Zhi (Cinnamomi Cassiae, Ramulus; now usually replaced with *Rou Gui*, Cinnamomi Cassiae, Cortex), 3g
Sheng Di (Rehmanniae Glutinosae, uncooked Radix; now usually replaced with *Shu Di*, Rehmanniae Glutinosae, cooked Radix), 24g
Shan Yao (Dioscoreae Oppositae, Radix), 12g
Shan Zhu Yu (Corni Officinalis, Fructus), 12g
Ze Xie (Alismatis Orientalis, Rhizoma), 9g
Fu Ling (Poriae Cocos, Sclerotium), 9g
Mu Dan Pi (Moutan, Cortex Radicis), 9g

This formula and its derivatives, especially *Liu Wei Di Huang Wan* (Six Flavors Rehmannia Pills), are among the most discussed in the Chinese medical literature. For our purposes, it is enough to point out that *Jin Gui Shen Qi Wan* fulfills the above treatment principles. *Shu Di* and *Shan Zhu Yu* nourish and secure kidney yin and essence. *Fu Zi* and *Rou Gui* invigorate kidney yang.[2] Now the reinvigorated kidney yang can resume steaming kidney essence to produce kidney qi. *Shan Yao* boosts the kidney qi. Although the remaining medicinals are not in the supplementing category and largely attack and drain, they work synergistically with the first three medicinals to facilitate supplementation. They balance the formula by percolating dampness, clearing any pathological heat, and dispelling any blood stasis. This formula treats the root but also contains medicinals that treat water accumulation, the tip. It is a very balanced formula that can be used for extended periods of time as long as the pattern identification is correct. However, one should make appropriate modifications to address the peculiarities of the patient.

C. COMBINED TREATMENT STRATEGIES

Combining treatment strategies, especially combining supplementing and draining strategies, is the key to the successful treatment of most kidney diseases. However, this is complicated, and several factors must be considered. One must carefully ascertain the degree of vacuity and repletion and weigh the treatment strategy accordingly. One must ascertain the proper time to supplement and drain. One must choose the correct type of supplementation and drainage. Finally, one must decide whether to treat the root or tip first or both simultaneously.

One must pay special attention to the tongue and pulse as well as understanding the patient's signs and symptoms. When supplementing, for example, if a patient's pulse is vacuous and the tongue small, this usually indicates liver-kidney vacuity and one must nourish the liver and kidney. A thin pulse usually indicates blood and yin vacuity, while a large and empty pulse usually indicates qi vacuity. If a patient's pulse is vacuous but his or her tongue is swollen, puffy, and big, this usually indicates qi vacuity with dampness and one must supplement the spleen and kidney qi to transform dampness. When draining or dispersing, one must employ a similar process. Since draining always weakens the patient, one must always decide how much to drain and carefully observe the patient's tongue and pulse to ascertain if the right qi has been weakened.

In real life, there are no pure cases of repletion or vacuity; these are always combined. When trying to combine strategies, if one supplements inappropriately, it will cause more stagnation. If one drains inappropriately, it will weaken the patient. One should weigh the treatment strategy according to the degree or percentage of vacuity and repletion. If there is 30% vacuity and 70% repletion, one should supplement 30% and drain 70%. If one is unsure of the percentages, one can start with 50% supplementation and 50% draining and carefully monitor the patient. If the patient gets weaker, one must supplement more. If the patient shows more repletion, one must drain more.

Although the phrase, "disease should be treated from the root," has been a major guiding principle in Chinese medicine for millennia, one must always consider whether it is first necessary to dispel evils. One may first dispel evils, first support the right, or combine these strategies in an appropriate way. The following case illustrates how Dr. Li chose the appropriate course by relying on the pulse and tongue diagnoses.

CASE HISTORY FROM DR. WEI LI'S PRIVATE PRACTICE: JIM, A 45 YEAR-OLD MALE

Two years previous to visiting Dr. Li, X had been diagnosed with IgA nephritis. His protein was 1-2+ even after Western medical treatment. He could not make any further improvement. Both X's pulse and tongue indicated egregious heat and toxins. Though he complained of tiredness, Dr. Li felt that the thrust of the treatment strategy and formula must be to clear heat and resolve toxins. Her prescription consisted of: *Huang Lian* (Coptidis Chinensis, Rhizoma), 6g, *Xuan Shen* (Scrophulariae Ningpoensis, Radix), 6g, *Jin Yin Hua* (Lonicerae

Japonicae, Flos), 15g, *Lian Qiao* (Fructus Forsythiae Suspensae), 10g, *Ban Lan Gen* (Isatidis Seu Baphicacanthi, Radix), 10g, *Sheng Di* (Rehmanniae Glutinosae, uncooked Radix), 10g, *Shan Yao* (Dioscoreae Oppositae, Radix), 10g, *Fu Ling* (Poriae Cocos, Sclerotium), 10g, *Bai Zhu* (Atractylodis Macrocephalae, Rhizoma), 10g, *Dang Shen* (Codonopsitis Pilosulae, Radix), 10g, and *Chuan Xiong* (Ligustici Wallichii, Radix), 6g.

This formula strongly clears heat and resolves toxins while mildly supplementing the right qi. X took this formula for three weeks. Each week he felt better. After three weeks, he felt very good and his urine protein was negative. Even after strenuous labor, X's urine protein would vary only slightly up and down, not even a full point. Even though X was better, Dr. Li found that his pulse was still a bit slippery, indicating lingering damp heat. She decided she must continue clearing damp heat toxins until X's tongue and pulse were completely without heat signs. Only then could she supplement as well as address any stasis.

The number of combined treatment strategies is legion. The following are a few of the most important ones; more are to be found later in the text. These examples combine supplementing and draining as well as treatment of the root and tip.

1. BOOST THE QI & DISINHIBIT WATER

Medicinals for this strategy are chosen mainly from the qi-supplementing and water-disinhibiting, dampness-percolating category. A representative formula is *Shen Ling Bai Zhu San* (Ginseng, Poria & Atractylodes Powder) described above. The first five medicinals boost the qi, but some also disinhibit water. These include *Fu Ling* and *Yi Yi Ren*. *Lian Zi* supplements and astringes the qi. *Sha Ren* aromatically transforms damp by penetrating it but also by arousing the spleen. *Jie Geng*'s role in diffusing the lung to regulate the water passageways has been described above.

Two other important formulas for disinhibiting water and boosting the qi when it is spleen qi that is vacuous are *Fang Ji Huang Qi Tang* (Stephania & Astragalus Decoction) and *Ling Gui Zhu Gan Tang* (Poria, Cinnamon, Atractylodes & Licorice Decoction). These are discussed later in the book. As implied above, *Jin Gui Shen Qi Wan* (*Golden Cabinet* Kidney Qi Pills) also fulfills this combined treatment strategy and is more appropriate than *Shen Ling Bai Zhu San* when kidney qi is vacuous.

In the modern Chinese medical clinic, uncooked powdered *Huang Qi* (Radix Astragali Membranacei) has been used alone to fulfill the treatment strategy, especially for chronic nephritis. *Huang Qi* is in the qi-supplementing category but also disinhibits urination and disperses water swelling. Please see Chapter 7 for an account of recent research using this medicinal.

2. WARM THE SPLEEN & DISINHIBIT WATER

To fulfill this treatment strategy, medicinals from the interior-warming category are added to the qi-supplementing and water-disinhibiting, dampness-percolating category. A representative formula is *Zhen Wu Tang* (True Warrior Decoction) described and analyzed above.

3. WARM THE KIDNEY & DISINHIBIT WATER

When warming the kidney, one often combines interior-warming and yin-supplementing medicinals. Representative formulas include *Zhen Wu Tang* (True Warrior Decoction) and *Jin Gui Shen Qi Wan*

(*Golden Cabinet* Kidney Qi Pills) described and analyzed above.

One can see from reviewing these representative formulas that fulfilling combined treatment strategies involves flexibility and a large view. To disinhibit water, for instance, one must not only rely on the medicinals in the water-disinhibiting, dampness-percolating category, even if some of these also boost the qi. The doctors that created the most revered formulas took such a large view and included medicinals from other categories that furthered those processes that help the principle medicinals disinhibit water. For instance, they included medicinals that warm yang or rectify the qi. They also addressed the root and tip with the same formula. One must strive to see the large view and use these precious formulas with flexibility.

ENDNOTES

[1] Dr. Li prefers this metaphor: "raising the pot and removing the lid."

[2] Many scholars and prominent textbooks contend that *Jin Gui Shen Qi Wan* (*Golden Cabinet* Kidney Qi Pills) supplements kidney yang. However, *Fu Zi* (Aconiti Carmichaeli, Radix Lateralis Praeparatus) and *Rou Gui* (Cinnamomi Cassiae, Cortex) are in the interior-warming category, not the yang-supplementing category. [Note that the treatment strategy employs the word "invigorate" (*zhuang*), which means to supplement but also means to "stimulate" or "awaken."] *Fu Zi* and *Rou Gui* warm and stimulate kidney yang, but many scholars contend they do not supplement kidney yang. *Jin Gui Shen Qi Wan* takes advantage of the fact that kidney yang is dependent on kidney yin. In this case, yang is gained from supplementing yin and re-establishing the kidney's normal physiology.

CHAPTER 4
SAFETY ISSUES WHEN USING CHINESE MEDICINALS AND CHINESE MEDICINAL-WESTERN DRUG INTERACTIONS

In the last few years, the public at large, and physicians in particular, have expressed concern about herb-drug interactions. While a great deal of research is being conducted and published in the West, this is still a nascent field. Although the Chinese have long combined Western and Chinese medicines, their research is not easily obtained. Unfortunately, a thorough discussion of Chinese medicinal-Western drug interactions is beyond the scope of this book. Nevertheless, we have included some important caveats about specific drug-medicinal interactions, toxic medicinals, and high dosages. In addition, we would like to provide the following general recommendations.

1. To use Chinese medicinals safely, one should follow standard dosages. We refer readers to texts by Bensky and Gamble[1] and Yeung.[2] Standard dosages are the safest dosages. When one uses them, one can be sure that toxic side effects are not due to Chinese medicinals.

2. Standard dosages change with the patient's age. For example, infants should receive only 1/8 of the standard adult dose. A three year-old should receive 1/4, a six year-old 1/2, a ten year-old 3/5, and so on. Again, if a patient is above 65 years old,

one should use 1/2-1/3 of the standard adult dose.

3. In many ancient and some modern case histories, large doses of medicinals are employed. We question these high dosages because standard pharmaceutical curves indicate that, at a certain high dosage, therapeutic effects diminish, while toxic effects increase. (See Figure 4.1.)[3]

4. *Su Wen*, Chapter 70, *"Wu Chang Zheng Da Lun* (Great Treatise on the Five Righteous Administrators)"* has this to say about using toxic medicinals:

> In diseases, some are protracted and some are newly contracted. In prescriptions, some are large and some are small. In decoction, some medicinals are toxic and some are not, and there are certain rules in taking them. The medicinals with the greatest toxicity should be discontinued when the disease is six parts cured. The medicinals with low toxicity should be discontinued when the disease is eight parts cured, and medicinals without any toxicity should be discontinued when the disease is nine parts cured.

In other words, one should try to discontinue prescribing toxic medicinals as soon as possible.

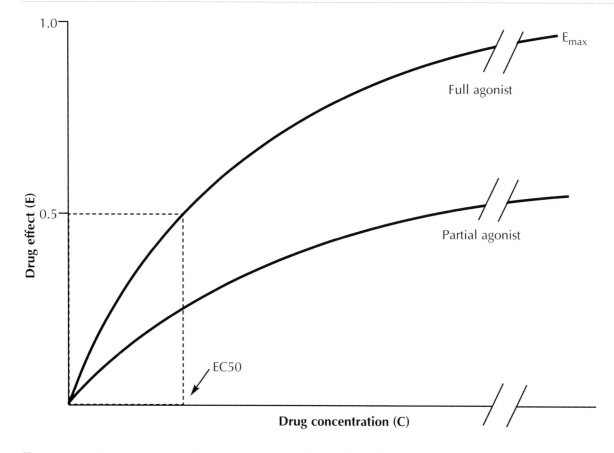

Figure 4.1. Relation between drug concentration and drug effect. The concentration at which the effect is half-maximal is denoted EC50. If the receptor-bound drug is plotted against drug concentration, a similar curve is obtained, and the concentration at which 50% of the receptors are associated with drug is denoted K_D. (Modified and reproduced, with permission, from Katzung B.G. [editor]: *Basic & Clinical Pharmacology*, 5th ed. Appleton & Lange, 1992.)

5. The practitioner should be conscious of and apply the 19 antagonisms, the 18 incompatibilities, and the seven interactions of medicinals in combinations.

The 19 antagonisms are as follows:
Liu Huang (Sulphur) antagonizes *Po Xiao* (Glabueris, Sal). *Shui Yin* (Hydrargyum) antagonizes *Pi Shuang* (Arsenicum). *Lang Du* (Euphorbiae Fischerianae, Radix) antagonizes *Mi Tuo Seng* (Lithargyum). *Ba Dou* (Crotonis Tiglii, Semen) antagonizes *Qian Niu Zi* (Pharbiditis, Semen). *Ya Xiao* (Nitrum) antagonizes *San Leng* (Sparganii Stoloniferi, Rhizoma). *Ding Xiang* (Caryophylli, Flos) antagonizes *Yu Jin* (Curcumae, Tuber). *Wu Tou* (Aconiti, Radix) antagonizes *Xi Jiao* (Rhinocerotis,

Cornu). *Ren Shen* (Panacis Ginseng, Radix) antagonizes *Wu Ling Zhi* (Trogopterori Seu Pteromi, Excrementum). *Rou Gui* (Cinnamomi Cassiae, Cortex) antagonizes *Chi Shi Zhi* (Hallyositum Rubrum).

The 18 incompatibilities are as follows:
Gan Cao (Glycyrrhizae Uralensis, Radix) is incompatible with *Gan Shui* (Euphorbiae Kansui, Radix, *Da Ji* (Cirsii Japonici, Herba Seu Radix), *Yuan Hua* (Daphnis Genkwae, Flos), and *Hai Zao* (Sargassii, Herba). *Wu Tou* (Aconiti, Radix) is incompatible with *Bei Mu* (Fritillariae Thunbergii, Bulbus or Fritillariae Cirrhosae, Bulbus), *Gua Lou* (Trichosanthis Kirlowii, Fructus), *Ban Xia* (Pinelliae Ternatae, Rhizoma), *Bai Lian* (Ampelopsis, Radix),

and *Bai Ji* (Bletilla Striatae, Rhizoma). *Li Lu* (Veratri, Radix Et Rhizoma) is incompatible with *Ren Shen* (Panacis Ginseng, Radix), *Sha Shen* (Adenophorae Seu Glehniae Littoralis, Radix), *Dan Shen* (Salviae Miltiorrhizae, Radix), *Ku Shen* (Sophorae Flavescentis, Radix), *Xi Xin* (Asari, Herba Cum Radice), and *Bai Shao* (Paeoniae Lactiflorae, Radix Albus).

The seven interactions are:
Mutual accentuation involves combinations of medicinals with similar functions that accentuate their therapeutic action. Examples include *Shi Gao* (Gypsum Fibrosum) and *Zhi Mu* (Anemarrhenae Aspheloidis, Rhizoma) to clear heat and drain fire and *Da Huang* (Rhei, Radix Et Rhizoma) and *Mang Xiao* (Mirabilitum) to precipitate.

Mutual enhancement involves combinations of medicinals with different functions in which one or more enhance the effects of the other(s) in specific situations. Examples include *Fu Ling* (Poriae Cocos, Sclerotium) and *Huang Qi* (Astragali Membranacei, Radix) for edema and *Da Huang* (Rhei, Radix Et Rhizoma) and *Huang Qin* (Scutellariae Baicalensis, Radix) for red, painful eyes.

Mutual counteraction involves combinations in which one medicinal reduces the toxicity or side effects of another. An example is that the toxicity of *Ban Xia* (Pinelliae Ternatae, Rhizoma) is reduced by *Sheng Jiang* (Zingiberis Officinalis, uncooked Rhizoma).

Mutual suppression is the opposite of mutual counteraction. Here *Sheng Jiang* (Zingiberis Officinalis, uncooked Rhizoma) reduces the toxicity of *Ban Xia* (Pinelliae Ternatae, Rhizoma).

Mutual antagonism involves combinations of medicinals that weaken the functions of each other. An example is *Lai Fu Zi* (Raphani Sativi, Semen) which weakens the function of *Ren Shen* (Panacis Ginseng, Radix) to supplement the qi.

Mutual incompatibility involves combinations of medicinals that increase side effects or toxicity.

Examples are the 19 antagonisms and 18 incompatibilities.

Single effect involves the use of a single medicinal. An example is the use of *Ren Shen* (Panacis Ginseng, Radix) to supplement qi vacuity and rescue yang desertion.

6. Aristolochic acid is a constituent of several Chinese medicinals.[4] Overdoses of aristolochic acid have been implicated in renal failure. Therefore, one should avoid medicinals containing this constituent. The most commonly used medicinals containing aristolochic acid are *Qing Mu Xiang* (Aristolochiae, Radix), *Guang Fang Ji* (Aristolochiae Seu Cocculi, Radix), *Mu Fang Ji* (Aristolochiae Fangchi, Radix), *Ma Dou Ling* (Aristolochiae, Fructus), and *Guang Mu Tong* (Aristolochiae Manshuriensis, Caulis). Note that *Han Fang Ji* (Stephanies Tetrandrae, Radix) and *Mu Tong* (Akebiae Mutong, Caulis) do not contain aristolochic acid when correctly identified.

7. Practitioners should advise patients to consume Chinese medicinals and Western prescription drugs at different times.

8. Certain Western medications are especially interactive. They are particularly susceptible to either potentiation or diminishment when taken with other substances, including Chinese medicinals. Practitioners should acquaint themselves with these medications and be aware of patients who are taking them.

9. Practitioners should acquaint themselves with Chinese medicinals that are primarily metabolized by the kidneys.

10. In certain situations, practitioners may opt to use medicinals that are metabolized by the liver instead of the kidneys.

11. If the patient expresses concern about the use of Chinese medicinals and adverse reactions, practitioners must explain honestly that adverse reactions to any medicinal are a possibility. Practitioners should recommend, never demand, that a patient use Chinese medicinals and must not insist that the use of Chinese medicinals is absolutely risk free.

12. Although certain medicinals elicit some uncomfortable therapeutic effects, if practitioners or patients notice an adverse reaction to a formula, they should stop the formula immediately. The practitioner should re-examine the formula and its specific medicinals.

ENDNOTES

[1] Bensky, Dan and Gamble, Andrew, *Chinese Herbal Medicine: Materia Medica*, Eastland Press, Seattle, 1986
[2] Yeung, Him-che, *Handbook of Chinese Herbs and Formulas*, Vol. 1, Institute of Chinese Medicine, LA, 1983
[3] Katzung B. G. & Trevor, Anthony J., *Pharmacology, Examination & Board Review*, 3rd edition, Appleton & Lange, Norwalk, CT, 1993, p. 9
[4] Subhuti Dharmananda lists 19 plants currently used in China which contain aristolochic acid in his paper titled, "Are Artistolochia Plants Dangerous?" Institute of Traditional Medicine, Portland, OR.

PART 2
CHINESE MEDICAL DISEASES IN NEPHROLOGY & UROLOGY

Nephrology and urology have been included as specialties in Chinese medicine only relatively recently, largely due to the influence of modern Western medicine. Historically, kidney and bladder diseases were often in the list of so-called miscellaneous diseases of internal medicine. The Chinese have always treated kidney and bladder diseases under different rubrics and nosology. Therefore, instead of simply proceeding to the Chinese medical treatment of modern Western medical nephrological and urological disease categories, we believe that a review of these traditional Chinese disease categories is in order. In modern Western medicine, most of these disease categories are simply considered symptoms and are not diseases in their own right. Typically, the clinical symptoms of any Western designated kidney or bladder disease will consist of one or more of these traditional Chinese disease categories. Thus the traditional Chinese disease categories can be seen as the building blocks of modern Chinese nephrological and urological diseases. As such, if one understands the traditional Chinese disease's causes and mechanisms, pattern identification, treatment principles, and treatment, it is much easier to understand the modern Chinese medical treatment of Western designated kidney-bladder diseases. This becomes especially important when dealing with the complex, multipattern presentations so common with difficult kidney diseases. Here the practitioner must be flexible and have the insight and information necessary to modify treatment plans to fit varied, individual presentations.

CHAPTER 1
KIDNEY WIND

In *Su Wen*, Chapter 42, "*Feng Lun* (Treatise on Wind)," kidney wind is described as follows:

> The symptoms of kidney wind are profuse sweating, aversion to wind, water swelling of the face, pain in the loin and spine, inability to stand very long, a black facial complexion like the smoke from burning coal, and obstructed urination. During inspection, take note of the cheeks. They should be of a black hue.

In *Su Wen*, Chapter 47, "*Qi Bing Lun* (Treatise on Extraordinary Diseases)" is the following exchange between the Yellow Emperor and Qi Bo:

> What is the disease if someone has swelling of the face and eyes, a pulse that is surging and tight, no pain in the body, is not emaciated but cannot eat, or can eat only a little? The root of this disease is in the kidney and is called kidney wind.

In the *Jin Gui Yao Lue*, Chapter 14, "On the Pulse, Patterns & Treatment of Water Swelling," kidney wind is called wind water and is classified as one of the five types of water swelling. The symptoms are described as follows: "In wind water, there is floating pulse, joint pain, and aversion to cold..." The *Zhu Bing Yuan Hou Zong Lun (Treatise on the Source &*

Symptoms of All Diseases) also discusses wind water. It declares, "Wind water is caused by spleen and kidney qi vacuity." These different sources give different accounts of kidney wind with emphasis on either the underlying visceral vacuity or on the contraction of external evils. It follows that one must employ pattern identification with a clear understanding of the relative importance of the various causes and pathogenic factors to treat this disease effectively.

DISEASE CAUSES & MECHANISMS

Kidney wind is divided into two main types: acute and chronic. Acute kidney wind is more replete, and chronic kidney wind is more vacuous. The primary organs involved are the kidney, spleen, lung, and triple burner. Acute kidney wind usually presents patterns of wind cold, wind heat, and damp heat. Chronic kidney wind usually presents a pattern of cold dampness.

As stated above in Part 1, wind cold is a combination of two evils. Wind is a yang evil that tends to attack the upper burner and exterior of the body first. Cold is a yin pathogen that tends to attack the lower burner. In kidney wind, wind first attacks the exterior and constrains the lung and then cold moves down to the kidney. This is called "lung cold moves to the kidney." In wind heat kidney wind, the wind constrains the lung qi, inhibiting the dispersing and depurative downbearing function of the lung. Heat constrains the spleen and middle burner, inhibiting the upbearing of the clear qi of the spleen

damp. In this pattern, the life gate fire is vacuous. If this vacuity of life gate fire is not addressed, kidney wind becomes chronic and can lead to kidney exhaustion and failure. On the other hand, if damp heat burns up yin, chronic kidney wind will present a pattern of damp heat with yin vacuity. Please see Figure 1.1.

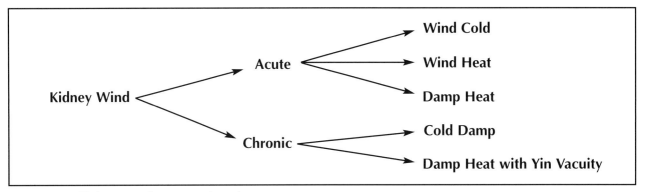

Figure 1.1. Kidney wind pattern identification

and the downbearing of the stomach qi. This middle burner dysfunction leads to dampness that stagnates and damages the true qi. Because the true qi is debilitated, it cannot contain the evils in the upper burner, and the heat moves downward to the kidney. Although the premodern literature does not mention this latter mechanism, we feel this should be called "lung heat moving to the kidney."

Chronic kidney wind usually involves spleen and kidney vacuity. Dietary irregularity, taxation fatigue, obsessive thinking, or excessive worrying—any of these can cause spleen qi vacuity and spleen qi stagnation. The spleen is unable to move and transform water, resulting in spleen qi vacuity with dampness. To use a common simile, the spleen is like the governor of a canal used for transporting grain. If the governor is weak and loses control and/or cannot maintain the canal, it may get holes in it and water can then leak out. This uncontrolled water may then cause damage, while the empty canal can no longer be used to transport grain. From the five phase perspective, the spleen is earth. If earth cannot control water in the restraining cycle, water overflows.

If vacuity causes debilitation of spleen and kidney yang, cold combines with dampness to form a pattern of cold

TREATMENT BASED ON PATTERN IDENTIFICATION

ACUTE KIDNEY WIND

1. WIND COLD

SIGNS & SYMPTOMS: Severe chills, nasal congestion, lung congestion, water swelling, loose stools, and difficult urination. The tongue is pale and swollen, and the pulse is floating and tight.

TREATMENT PRINCIPLES: Expel wind, scatter cold and percolate water

REPRESENTATIVE FORMULA: Modified *Ma Huang Jia Zhu Tang* (Ephedra Plus Atractylodes Decoction) plus *Wu Pi Yin* (Five Peels Beverage)

Ma Huang (Ephedrae, Herba), 9g
Gui Zhi (Cinnamomi Cassiae, Ramulus), 9g
Xing Ren (Pruni Armeniacae, Semen), 9g
mix-fried *Gan Cao* (Glycyrrhizae Uralensis, Radix), 3g
Cang Zhu (Atractylodis, Rhizoma), 9g
Chen Pi (Citri Reticulatae, Pericarpium), 9g
Fu Ling Pi (Poriae Cocos, Cortex Sclerotii), 15g

Da Fu Pi (Arecae Catechu, Pericarpium), 15g
Sang Bai Pi (Mori Albi, Cortex Radicis), 15g
Sheng Jiang Pi (Zingiberis Officinalis, Cortex Rhizomatis), 6g

MODIFICATIONS: If there is hematuria, add *Bai Mao Gen* (Imperatae Cylindricae, Rhizoma), *Che Qian Cao* (Plantaginis, Herba), *Ou Jie* (Nelumbinis Nuciferae, Nodus Rhizomatis), and *Xue Yu Tan* (Crinis Carbonisatus). For severe edema, add *Chi Xiao Dou* (Phaseoli Calcarati, Semen) and *Li Yu* (Cyprinus Carpio). These last two ingredients, along with *Sang Bai Pi* (Mori Albi, Cortex Radicis), form part of *Li Yu Tang* (Carp Decoction) from Wei Yi-lin's *Shi Yi De Xiao Fang* (*Effective Formulas from Generations of Physicians*). In this book, Wei discourages the addition of salt to flavor this "soup."

ACUMOXIBUSTION: Choose from *Da Zhui* (GV 14), *Feng Men* (Bl 12), *Fei Shu* (Bl 13), *He Gu* (LI 4), *Lie Que* (Lu 7), and *Fu Liu* (Ki 7).

2. WIND HEAT

SIGNS & SYMPTOMS: Fever, slight chills, nasal congestion, sore throat, coughing up of yellow phlegm, dark, scanty urination or bloody urination (the color of soy sauce or microscopic), constipation, and water swelling. The tongue is red with yellow fur, and the pulse is slippery, fast, and replete.

TREATMENT PRINCIPLES: Expel wind, clear heat and percolate water

REPRESENTATIVE FORMULAS: *Yin Qiao San* (Lonicera & Forsythia Powder), *Ma Huang Lian Qiao Chi Xiao Dou Tang* (Ephedra, Forsythia & Red Bean Decoction), or *Yue Bi Tang* (Maidservant from Yue Decoction) modified according to the peculiarities of the case

Modified *Yin Qiao San* (Lonicera & Forsythia Powder)

Jin Yin Hua (Lonicerae Japonicae, Flos), 9-15g
Lian Qiao (Forsythiae Suspensae, Fructus), 9-15g
Jing Jie (Schizonepetae Tenuifoliae, Herba Seu Flos), 6g

Fu Ping (Lemnae Seu Spirodelae, Herba), 9g
Ban Lan Gen (Isatidis Seu Baphicacanthi, Radix), 9-15g
Da Qing Ye (Daqingye, Folium), 9-15g
Shi Gao (Gypsum Fibrosum), 6g
Huang Qin (Scutellariae Baicalensis, Radix), 9g
Che Qian Zi (Plantaginis, Semen), 9g
Bai Mao Gen (Imperatae Cylindricae, Rhizoma), 9-15g

Modified *Ma Huang Lian Qiao Chi Xiao Dou Tang* (Ephedra, Forsythia & Red Bean Decoction)

Ma Huang (Ephedrae, Herba), 6-9g
Lian Qiao (Forsythiae Suspensae, Fructus), 9-15g
Chi Xiao Dou (Phaseoli Calcarati, Semen), 9-15g
Da Fu Pi (Arecae Catechu, Pericarpium), 9g
Che Qian Cao (Plantaginis, Herba), 9-12g
Han Fang Ji (Stephaniae Tetrandrae, Radix), 6g
Fu Ling (Poriae Cocos, Sclerotium), 9g
Huang Lian (Coptidis Chinensis, Rhizoma), 6-9g
Jin Yin Hua (Lonicerae Japonicae, Flos), 9-15g
Ban Lan Gen (Isatidis Seu Baphicacanthi, Radix), 9-15g
Da Qing Ye (Daqingye, Folium), 9-15g
Bai Mao Gen (Imperatae Cylindricae, Rhizoma), 9-15g

Modified *Yue Bi Tang* (Maidservant from Yue Decoction)

Ma Huang (Ephedrae, Herba), 9g
Shi Gao (Gypsum Fibrosum), 48g
Sheng Jiang (Zingiberis Officinalis, uncooked Rhizoma), 9g
Gan Cao (Glycyrrhizae Uralensis, Radix), 6g
Da Zao (Zizyphi Jujubae, Fructus), 10 pieces

MODIFICATIONS: For hematuria, add *Zhi Zi* (Gardeniae Jasminoidis, Fructus) or *Xiao Ji* (Cephalanoplos Segeti, Herba) and *Hu Po* (Succinum). However, because medicinals which stop bleeding can cause blood stasis, it is also a good idea to add *Chi Shao* (Paeoniae Lactiflorae, Radix Rubrus), *Yi Mu Cao* (Leonrui Heterophylli, Herba), and *Mu Dan Pi* (Moutan, Cortex Radicis) to quicken the blood and dispel stasis.

ACUMOXIBUSTION: Choose from *Da Zhui* (GV 14), *Feng Men* (Bl 12), *Fei Shu* (Bl 13), *Wai Guan* (TB 5), *Qu Chi* (LI 11), *Chi Ze* (Lu 5), *Lie Que* (Lu 7), and *Fu Liu* (Ki 7).

3. DAMP HEAT

SIGNS & SYMPTOMS: Fever, thirst, sore throat, fatigue, no appetite, dark urine, constipation, local red swollen skin, water swelling. The tongue is reddish purple with thick, yellow fur, and the pulse is fast, slippery, and replete.

TREATMENT PRINCIPLES: Clear heat and eliminate dampness

REPRESENTATIVE FORMULA: *Qing Shen Xiao Du Yin* (Kidney-clearing & Toxin-dispersing Beverage)

Lian Qiao (Forsythiae Suspensae, Fructus), 7g
Jin Yin Hua (Lonicerae Japonicae, Flos), 9g
Da Qing Ye (Daqingye, Folium), 9g
Pu Gong Ying (Taraxaci Mongolici, Herba Cum Radice), 9g
Hua Shi (Talcum), 9g
Dong Kui Zi (Abutili Seu Malvae, Semen), 9g
Di Fu Zi (Kochiae Scopariae, Fructus), 9g
Mu Dan Pi (Moutan, Cortex Radicis), 5g
Zhi Zi (Gardeniae Jasminoidis, Fructus), 9g
Dan Zhu Ye (Lophatheri Gracilis, Herba), 9g

MODIFICATIONS: If there is constipation add *Da Huang* (Rhei, Radix Et Rhizoma). If there is bloody urine, add *Sheng Di* (Rehmanniae Glutinosae, uncooked Radix), *Xiao Ji* (Cephalanoplos Segeti, Herba), and *Bai Mao Gen* (Imperatae Cylindricae, Rhizoma).

ACUMOXIBUSTION: Choose from *Da Zhui* (GV 14), *Qu Chi* (LI 11), *He Gu* (LI 4), *Zhi Gou* (TB 6), *Wei Yang* (Bl 53), *Zhong Wan* (CV 12), and *Yin Ling Quan* (Sp 9).

CHRONIC KIDNEY WIND

1. COLD DAMP

SIGNS & SYMPTOMS: Cough with phlegm, water swelling, abdominal distention, nausea, vomiting, low back pain, scanty urination. The tongue is puffy and pale with thin, white fur, and the pulse is slippery.

TREATMENT PRINCIPLES: Warm cold and eliminate dampness

REPRESENTATIVE FORMULA: *Shi Pi Yin* (Bolster the Spleen Beverage)

Fu Zi (Aconiti Carmichaeli, Radix Lateralis Praeparatus), 6g
Gan Jiang (Zingiberis Officinalis, dry Rhizoma), 6g
Fu Ling (Poriae Cocos, Sclerotium), 6g
Bai Zhu (Atractylodis Macrocephalae, Rhizoma), 6g
Mu Gua (Chaenomelis Lagenariae, Fructus), 6g
Hou Po (Magnoliae Officinalis, Cortex), 6g
Mu Xiang (Aucklandiae Lappae, Radix), 6g
Da Fu Pi (Arecae Catechu, Pericarpium), 3g
Cao Guo (Amomi Tsao-ko, Fructus), 3g
mix-fried *Gan Cao* (Glycyrrhizae Uralensis, Radix), 3g
Da Zao (Zizyphi Jujubae, Fructus), 5 pieces

MODIFICATIONS: For poor appetite, add *Shan Zha* (Crataegi, Fructus), *Mai Ya* (Hordei Vulgaris, Fructus Germinatus), *Ji Nei Jin* (Gigeriae Galli, Endothelium Corneum), and *Shen Qu* (Massa Medica Fermentata). For insomnia, add *He Huan Pi* (Albizziae Julibrissinis, Cortex) and *Tian Mu* (Gastrodiae Elatae, Rhizoma). For hypertension, add *Huai Niu Xi* (Achyranthis Bidentatae, Radix) and *Shi Jue Ming* (Haliotidis, Concha).

ACUMOXIBUSTION: Choose from *Yin Ling Quan* (Sp 9), *San Yin Jiao* (Sp 6), *Zu San Li* (St 36), *Pi Shu* (Bl 20), *Zhong Wan* (CV 12), and *He Gu* (LI 4).

2. DAMP HEAT WITH YIN VACUITY

SIGNS & SYMPTOMS: A warm or hot feeling, thirst, chronic sore throat, fatigue, no appetite, dark urine, constipation, dry skin and local red swollen skin, water swelling. The tongue is red with little or no fur, and the pulse is fine, bowstring, and often slippery.

TREATMENT PRINCIPLES: Clear heat, eliminate dampness, and supplement yin

REPRESENTATIVE FORMULA: Modified *Zhi Bai Di Huang Wan* (Anemarrhena & Phellodendron Rehmannia Pills)

Zhi Mu (Anemarrhenae Asphodeloidis, Rhizoma), 9g
Huang Bai (Phellodendri, Cortex), 9g
Sheng Di (Rehmanniae Glutinosae, uncooked Radix), 9g
Shan Yao (Dioscoreae Oppositae, Radix), 9g
Shan Zhu Yu (Corni Officinalis, Fructus), 9g
Fu Ling (Poriae Cocos, Sclerotium), 9g
Ze Xie (Alismatis Orientalis, Rhizoma), 9g
Mu Dan Pi (Moutan, Cortex Radicis), 5g

MODIFICATIONS: To help supplement the essence, take each dose with one tablespoon of honey (*Feng Mi*, Mel). For dry stools, add *Yu Zhu* (Polygonati Odorati, Rhizoma), *Hu Ma Ren* (Sesami Indici, Semen), and/or *Dang Gui* (Angelicae Sinensis, Radix). For night sweats, add *Di Gu Pi* (Lycii Chinensis, Cortex Radicis) and *Qing Hao* (Artemisiae Annuae, Herba). For hematuria, add *Han Lian Cao* (Ecliptae Prostratae, Herba), *Nu Zhen Zi* (Ligustri Lucidi, Fructus), and *Sheng Di Huang* (Rehmanniae Glutinosae, uncooked Radix).

ACUMOXIBUSTION: Choose from *Qu Chi* (LI 11), *He Gu* (LI 4), *Zhi Gou* (TB 6), *Wei Yang* (Bl 53), *Yang Ling Quan* (GB 34), *Yin Ling Quan* (Sp 9), *Tai Xi* (Ki 3), and *Zhao Hai* (Ki 6).

REPRESENTATIVE CASE HISTORIES

Case history 1: Xu, a 54 year-old man[1]

Xu's first visit was in November 1978. Xu had been traveling when he caught cold with symptoms of fever and chills, a heavy feeling in his joints, and discomfort throughout his entire body. Three days later, his eyelids became swollen. The edema spread to his entire face and then to his entire body. His tongue had thin, white fur, and his pulse was floating and tight. The Western medical diagnosis was acute nephritis, and his Chinese medical diagnosis was wind cold kidney wind. The treatment principles were to diffuse the lung and resolve the exterior, eliminate dampness and percolate water. He was prescribed *Ma Huang Jia Zhu*

Tang (Ephedra Plus Atractylodes Decoction) plus *Wu Pi Yin* (Five Peels Powder) with modifications:

Ma Huang (Ephedrae, Herba), 15g
Gui Zhi (Cinnamomi Cassiae, Ramulus), 15g
Xing Ren (Pruni Armeniacae, Semen), 10g
Cang Zhu (Atractylodis, Rhizoma), 15g
Chen Pi (Citri Reticulatae, Pericarpium), 20g
Fu Ling Pi (Poriae Cocos, Cortex Sclerotii), 25g
Da Fu Pi (Arecae Catechu, Pericarpium), 20g
Sang Bai Pi (Mori Albi, Cortex Radicis), 20g
Sheng Jiang Pi (Zingiberis Officinalis, Cortex Rhizomatis), 15g
Di Fu Zi (Kochiae Scopariae, Fructus), 20g
Fu Ping (Lemnae Seu Spirodelae, Herba), 20g

Xu took this prescription for three days and had a mild sweat over his entire body. His urine began to flow easily, his edema disappeared, but he was still fatigued. His tongue fur was slimy, and his pulse was now slow. Dr. Li changed the prescription to transform dampness:

Fu Ling Pi (Poriae Cocos, Cortex Sclerotii), 15g
Sang Bai Pi (Mori Albi, Cortex Radicis), 20g
Che Qian Zi (Plantaginis, Semen), 20g
Shi Wei (Pyrrosiae, Folium), 10g
Bai Mao Gen (Imperatae Cylindricae, Rhizoma), 25g
Chen Pi (Citri Reticulatae, Pericarpium), 15g
Dan Zhu Ye (Lophatheri Gracilis, Herba), 10g

Xu took this prescription for three days and the slimy tongue fur disappeared, but he was still fatigued. Dr. Li prescribed a formula that harmonized the middle burner and transformed dampness and directed Xu to take it for one week. By the time Xu finished this last formula, he had completely recovered. A follow-up on May 15, 1981 found no recurrence.

Case history 2: Huang, a 12 year-old boy[2]

Huang's first visit was in April 1980. He caught cold and had symptoms of chills, fever, and sore throat for one week. Then his whole body became edematous. Urinalysis showed protein 2+ and RBCs 2+. Granular casts were 0-1. The Western medical diagnosis was acute nephritis. Huang was referred to a Chinese medical clinic for treatment during which he presented with symptoms of fever without sweating, sore throat, generalized edema, yellow, scanty urination, and constipation. His tongue had thin, yellow, slimy fur, and his pulse was floating and fast. The Chinese medical diagnosis was wind heat kidney wind. The treatment strategy was to clear and diffuse the lung, transform water and percolate dampness. The prescription was *Ma Huang Lian Qiao Chi Xiao Dou Tang* (Ephedra, Forsythia & Red Bean Decoction) plus *Huang Lian Jie Du Tang* (Coptis Toxin-resolving Decoction) with modifications:

Ma Huang (Ephedrae, Herba), 10g
Lian Qiao (Forsythiae Suspensae, Fructus), 20g
Sang Bai Pi (Mori Albi, Cortex Radicis), 20g
Xing Ren (Pruni Armeniacae, Semen), 8g
Huang Qin (Scutellariae Baicalensis, Radix), 10g
Zhi Zi (Gardeniae Jasminoidis, Fructus), 10g
Da Huang (Rhei, Radix Et Rhizoma), 5g
Jie Geng (Platycodi Grandiflori, Radix), 15g
Bo He (Menthae Haplocalycis, Herba), 10g
Gan Cao (Glycyrrhizae Uralensis, Radix), 8g
Chi Xiao Dou (Phaseoli Calcarati, Semen), 20g

After two days, Huang experienced a slight sweat over his entire body and his fever disappeared. He was able to pass more urine, the edema greatly decreased, and his constipation abated. His doctor removed *Da Huang* from Huang's prescription, and, after taking this new prescription for two more days, the edema completely dissipated. His doctor gave him a different prescription to harmonize the middle burner and clear heat. He took this for another three weeks and staged a complete recovery.

Case history 3: Sun, a 10 year-old boy [3]

Sun's first visit was in May 1977. He had mumps with a sore throat for eight days. Then, when the facial swelling had almost disappeared, his face suddenly became edematous and pitting edema spread throughout his entire body. He had a fever, thirst, headache, and low back pain. His urination was scanty and the color of red tea. His tongue was red with yellow, slimy fur, and his pulse was slippery and fast. Urinalysis showed protein 3+ and RBCs 4+. The Chinese medical diagnosis was damp heat kidney wind. The treatment principles were to clear heat

and resolve toxins, cool the blood and percolate dampness. The prescription was modified *Qing Shen Xiao Du Yin* (Kidney-clearing & Toxin-dispersing Beverage). A one-day dose consisted of:

Lian Qiao (Forsythiae Suspensae, Fructus), 20g
Zhi Zi (Gardeniae Jasminoidis, Fructus), 10g
Huang Bai (Phellodendri, Cortex), 10g
Da Qing Ye (Daqingye, Folium), 15g
Jin Yin Hua (Lonicerae Japonicae, Flos), 20g
Sheng Di (Rehmanniae Glutinosae, uncooked Radix), 15g
Mu Dan Pi (Moutan, Cortex Radicis), 10g
Xiao Ji (Cephalanoplos Segeti, Herba), 15g

Sun took this prescription for three days and had a proper sweat.[4] His urine and stool returned to normal, and the water swelling also greatly reduced. After six days of taking this formula, the edema was completely gone. He was then given a prescription to clear heat and percolate dampness. Sun took this prescription for three weeks and completely recovered. Subsequent urinalysis was normal.

Case history 4: Lee, a 56 year-old man [5]

Lee's first visit was in February 1973. Lee had recently caught a cold, and then, when he got up one morning, he found that his eyelids were swollen. Gradually his whole body became edematous. His lower extremities were especially swollen. He experienced fever, chills, difficult urination, fatigue, and his trunk and extremities felt heavy. His tongue was pale with teeth-marks on its edges and thin, white fur, and his pulse was forceless and fine. His doctor felt that Lee had constitutional yang vacuity because he always felt cold and had to wear a lot of clothes. The Chinese diagnosis was cold damp kidney wind. The treatment strategy was to diffuse the lung and percolate water, warm the interior and expel cold. The prescription was *Ma Huang Fu Zi Xi Xin Tang* (Ephedra, Aconite & Asarum Decoction) plus *Wu Ling San* (Five [Ingredients] Poria Powder) with modifications:

Ma Huang (Ephedrae, Herba), 10g
Fu Zi (Aconiti Carmichaeli, Radix Lateralis Praeparatus), 10g

Xi Xin (Asari, Herba Cum Radice), 3g
Zhu Ling (Polypori Umbellati, Sclerotium), 15g
Ze Xie (Alismatis Orientalis, Rhizoma), 15g
Cang Zhu (Atractylodis, Rhizoma), 15g
Fu Ling (Poriae Cocos, Sclerotium), 20g
Gui Zhi (Cinnamomi Cassiae, Ramulus), 15g
Ren Shen (Panacis Ginseng, Radix), 10g
Sheng Jiang (Zingiberis Officinalis uncooked Rhizoma), 5g

Lee took this formula for four days and the edema began to dissipate. After two weeks, it had completely disappeared. This formula was modified, and, after a month of taking it, Lee staged a complete recovery.

Case history 5: Gua, a 32 year-old woman[6]

Gua's first visit was in September 1978. A couple of weeks prior to this visit, after sweating with overexertion, she caught cold. She had fever, dry mouth, and irritability. One week later, she became edematous. Urinalysis showed protein 2+, RBCs 2+, and granular casts 0-1. On her first visit, she still had fever, aversion to wind, generalized edema, low back pain, and scanty, red urination. Her tongue was red and without fur, while her pulse was fine and fast.

Gua also had premenstrual syndrome, the principle symptom being heat in the five hearts. This convinced the doctor that Gua had constitutional yin vacuity. The Chinese medical diagnosis was yin vacuity kidney wind. The treatment principles were to diffuse the lung and percolate water, nourish yin and clear heat. The prescription was *Qing Hao Bie Jia Tang* (Artemisia Annua & Carapax Amydae Decoction) with modifications:

Qing Hao (Artemisiae Annuae, Herba), 20g
Bie Jia (Amydae Sinensis, Carapax), 20g
Sheng Di (Rehmanniae Glutinosae, uncooked Radix), 25g
Mu Dan Pi (Moutan, Cortex Radicis), 10g
Bai Wei (Cynanchi Baiwei, Radix), 20g
Sang Bai Pi (Mori Albi, Cortex Radicis), 20g
Di Gu Pi (Lycii Chinensis, Cortex Radicis), 15g
Fu Ling Pi (Poriae Cocos, Cortex Sclerotii), 15g
Fu Ping (Lemnae Seu Spirodelae, Herba), 15g

Bai Mao Gen (Imperatae Cylindricae, Rhizoma), 15g
Che Qian Zi (Plantaginis, Semen), 22g

After six days, Gua's fever was gone and her water swelling abated. The doctor removed *Bie Jia, Mu Dan Pi,* and *Fu Ping* from her prescription and directed Gua take this modified formula for one more week. After finishing this formula, her water swelling completely disappeared. The doctor prescribed a formula to nourish yin and blood and clear heat to consolidate the treatment. Gua took this prescription for a month and completely recovered.

Case history 6: Zou, a 45 year-old man[7]

Ten years before his first visit, Zou was sent to a rural area to receive re-education. He gradually became edematous due to overtaxation and living in a damp environment. Urinalysis showed protein and blood in his urine. The Western medical diagnosis was acute nephritis. He received some treatment, but the condition did not resolve.

In April 1982, after Zou overexerted himself, his whole body became edematous. He was tired and had low back soreness. Urinalysis showed protein 4+. The Western medical diagnosis was chronic nephritis. Zou was given immunosuppressant drugs, cortisone, and a diuretic with no results. He then came to see a Chinese physician.

At that point, Zou's symptoms included a pale facial complexion, generalized pitting edema, feeling cold, lack of appetite, and loose stools. His tongue was big and puffy with white, glossy fur, and his pulse was deep and fine. Urinalysis showed protein at 3+, granular casts at 2+, 24 hour urine protein at 8.65 gm/dl, blood protein at 4.08 gm/dl, and blood cholesterol at 346 mg/dl. The Chinese medical pattern identification was spleen-kidney yang vacuity with damp accumulation. The treatment strategy was to fortify the spleen, warm the kidney, and percolate dampness. There were two prescriptions. The patient was to cook *Hong Shen* (Panacis Ginseng, Radix Rubrus), 6g, and drink this instead of tea. He was also to take the following formula:

Huang Qi (Astragali Membranacei, Radix), 30g

Fu Zi (Aconiti Carmichaeli, Radix Lateralis Praeparatus), 12g
Gui Zhi (Cinnamomi Cassiae, Ramulus), 6g
E Zhu (Curcumae Zediariae, Rhizoma), 9g
Fu Ling (Poriae Cocos, Sclerotium), 15g
Xian Mao (Curculinginis Orchioidis, Rhizoma), 9g
Yin Yang Huo (Epimedii, Herba), 9g
Ba Ji Tian (Morindae Officinalis, Radix), 12g
Bai Shao (Paeoniae Lactiflorae, Radix Albus), 9g
Hu Lu Ba (Trigonellae Foeni-graeci, Semen), 6g,
Che Qian Zi (Plantaginis, Semen), 15g
Sheng Jiang (Zingiberis Officinalis, uncooked Rhizoma), 3g

Zou took this prescription for 14 days. Upon returning, his edema was completely gone, his appetite was better, his urine had increased, his cold feeling had dissipated, and his stool was firmer. His urinalysis showed protein at 1+, the granular casts had disappeared, the 24 hour urine protein was 0.63 gm/dl, and his blood protein was up. Therefore, the doctor removed *Che Qian Zi* and added *Shan Yao* (Radix Dioscoreae Oppositae), 9g and *Chen Pi* (Pericarpium Citri Reticulatae), 6g to his prescription. Zou continued on this new prescription for 21 days.

On his next visit Zou's water edema was completely gone, and all his other symptoms were almost gone. His tongue was pale red and his pulse was soggy. Urinalysis showed protein negative, his 24 hour urine protein at 0.15 gm/dl, and his blood protein and cholesterol were normal. Zou was given *Jin Gui Shen Qi Wan* (*Golden Cabinet* Kidney Qi Pills) along with *Zi He Che Wan* (Placenta Pills)[8] to consolidate the results.

CLINICAL TIPS

1. Kidney wind is a commonly seen condition in clinic. To treat this disease effectively, one must always apply basic yin-yang theory, *i.e.*, if the patient has heat, one must clear heat, if the patient is cold, one must warm the interior. In addition, one must always combine these strategies with percolating dampness. If one applies these basic but essential diagnostics and treatment strategies, one will have good results.

2. To successfully clear heat in this condition, one must employ four treatment principles—three to clear the heat and one to supplement yin. These four treatment principles are 1) drain fire, 2) clear heat from the four aspects, 3) discharge heat, and 4) nourish yin. If one simply clears four apsect heat, the flame may be extinguished but the ashes are still smoldering and can easily flare up again. If one drains fire at the same time, it lessens the time needed to clear heat and fire is less likely to recur. Discharging heat gives yet another way to clear heat and is specific to organs. For instance, in the lungs, depressive heat should be dispersed. In the spleen and stomach, one needs to clear and disperse depressive heat. In the large intestine, one must precipitate replete heat. However, since in this instance, we are concerned with the kidneys, one should drain heat through urination. No matter what aspect the heat is in, we must still employ all three heat-clearing methods. For example, *Yin Qiao San* (Lonicera & Forsythia Powder) is for defensive aspect heat, but it contains *Dan Zhu Ye* (Lophatheri Gracilis, Herba) to drain fire and discharge heat via urination. Furthermore, vacuity of yin and body fluids causes dryness and vacuity heat may facilitate the invasion of engenderment of replete heat. Therefore, one must also be sure to nourish yin and safeguard fluids. See Figure 1.2.

3. In cold damp chronic kidney wind, the root is yang vacuity. One must treat the root by warming the interior. However, one must also percolate dampness and rectify the qi. In Dr. Li's experience, if one just drains dampness, one can expect less than a 5% improvement. If one adds interior-warming medicinals, one will achieve up to a 60% improvement. If one adds qi-rectifying medicinals, one can achieve 80-90% improvement. Qi is the leader (of the other humors). Therefore, if the qi moves, everything else moves. One must move the qi to eliminate dampness. However, dampness is yin and is, thus, associated with coldness and heaviness. Therefore, one must always invigorate yang qi to completely transform dampness. When yang qi is strong and invigorated, one can eliminate dampness and prevent recurrences. See Figure 1.3.

METHOD	STRATEGY	REPRESENTATIVE MEDICINALS
Clearing Heat	**Clear heat from the four aspects**	**Defensive:** *Lian Qiao* (Forsythiae Suspensae, Fructus), *Jin Yin Hua* (Lonicerae Japonicae, Flos), etc. **Qi:** *Huang Lian* (Coptidis, Rhizoma), *Huang Qin* (Scutellariae Baicalensis, Radix), etc. **Construction:** *Sheng Di Huang* (Rehmanniae Glutinosae, Radix), *Xuan Shen* (Scrophulariae Ningpoensis, Radix), etc. **Blood:** *Xi Jiao* (Rhinoceri, Cornu), *Sheng Di Huang* (Rehmanniae Glutinosae, Radix), etc.
	Drain fire	*Shi Gao* (Gypsum), *Zhi Mu* (Anemarrhenae Asphodeloidis, Rhizoma), *Dan Zhu Ye* (Lophatheri Gracilis, Herba), etc.
	Discharge heat	*Dan Zhu Ye* ((Lophatheri Gracilis, Herba), *Che Qian Zi* (Plantaginis, Seman), *Mu Tong* (Mutong, Caulis), etc.
	Nourish yin, Safeguard fluids	*Mai Men Dong* (Ophiopogonis Japonici, Tuber), *Zhi Mu* (Anemarrhenae Asphodeloidis, Rhizoma), etc.

Figure 1.2. Clearing heat

OBJECTIVE	METHOD	MEDICINALS
To Eliminate Dampness	**1. Warm the Interior**	*Shi Gao* (Gypsum), *Fu Zi* , (Aconiti Carmichaeli, Radix Lateralis), *Rou Gui* (Cinnamomi Cassiae, Cortex), *Gan Jiang* (Zingiberis Officinalis, Rhizoma), etc.
	2. Percolate Dampness	*Fu Ling* (Poriae Cocos, Sclerotium), *Zhu Ling* (Polypori Umbellati, Sclerotium), *Yu Mi Xu* (Zeae Maydis, Stylus), etc.
	3. Rectify Qi	*Chen Pi* (Citri Reticulatae, Pericarpium), *Xiang Fu* (Cyperi Rotundi, Rhizoma), *Wu Yao* (Radix Linderae Strychnifoliae), etc.

Figure 1.3. Eliminating dampness

4. Damp heat with yin vacuity is a complicated combination of yin and yang evils, repletion and vacuity. In this case, the practitioner must skillfully employ three major treatment principles: 1) clearing heat, 2) draining and drying dampness, and 3) supplementing yin. In order to clear heat, one must apply the three strategies mentioned above. One must also drain and dry dampness, but one must also supplement yin essence to address the yin vacuity. Yin vacuity may coexist with damp heat. In fact, damp heat often burns yin causing yin vacuity in the first place. When attempting to dry dampness, one may inadvertently desiccate the body fluids and yin. Yin vacuity is like dry wood. Any spark may make it flare up, and lingering and smoldering damp heat often supplies that spark. Since essence is yin, one must also supplement essence to fully supplement yin.

One can see this thinking at work in Zhu Dan-xi's famous formula *Da Bu Yin Wan* (Greatly Supplementing Yin Pills). In it, pulverized *Shu Di Huang* (Rehmanniae Glutinosae, cooked Radix), deep-fried *Gui Ban* (Testudinis, Plastrum), stir-fried *Huang Bai* (Phellodendri, Cortex), and wine stir-fried *Zhi Mu* (Anemarrhenae Aspheloidis, Rhizoma) are cooked with pork marrow and formed into pills with honey. *Shu Di Huang* and *Gui Ban* supplement yin and fill essence, *Huang Bai* dries dampness, and *Zhi Mu* drains fire and engenders fluids. But one must not overlook the pork marrow and honey. These are also important ingredients to supplement yin and foster essence. Marrow is directly related to kidney essence, and honey can be thought of as the essence of flowers. As to the representative formula *Zhi Bai Di Huang Wan* (Anemarrhena & Phellodendron Rehmannia Pills), this formula is skillfully crafted to employ the three major principles in a balanced formula appropriate for extended use. But one must modify it appropriate to the relative strengths of the evils and righteous qi.

5. Although one can choose medicinals by category, the first choice should be those medicinals from any category that accomplish more than one relevant function. For instance, *Gui Zhi* (Cinnamomi Cassiae, Ramulus) and *Sheng Jiang* (Zingiberis Officinalis, uncooked Rhizoma) warm the interior and free the flow of the bladder. *Da Fu Pi* (Arecae Catechu, Pericarpium) and *Hou Po* (Magnoliae Officinalis, Cortex) move the qi and eliminate dampness. *Bai Zhu* (Atractylodis Macrocephalae, Rhizoma) and *Fu Ling* (Poriae Cocos, Sclerotium) supplement the spleen and eliminate dampness, and *Wu Yao* (Linderae Strychnifoliae, Radix) both rectifies the qi and warms the kidneys.

ENDNOTES

[1] Yu Wong-shi, *Dong Dai Ming Yi Ling Zhen Jing Hua* (*A Collection of the Clinical Experience of Famous Modern Doctors*), Chinese Ancient Book Publishing Company, Beijing, 1991, p. 6
[2] *Ibid.*, p. 8
[3] *Ibid.*, p. 9
[4] In this book, we use the term "proper sweat" to indicate correctly releasing the exterior. A proper sweat is a light sweat over the entire body with, perhaps, a little heavier sweating on the nose.
[5] Yu Wong-shi, *op. cit.*, p. 10
[6] *Ibid.*, p. 12
[7] Qing He-chen, *Dong Dai Ming Lao Zhong Yi Ling Zheng Hui Cui* (*Modern Famous Doctors Clinical Collection*), Guandong Science & Technology Publishing Company, Guanzou, 1991 p. 361
[8] This formula was not given.

CHAPTER 2
BLOCK & REPULSION

Block and repulsion can refer to any of four symptom complexes: 1) urinary stoppage (block) and continuous vomiting (repulsion) caused by insufficiency of the spleen and kidney with depressed lodged damp turbidity transforming into heat and thrusting upward; 2) vomiting with gradual appearance of fecal and urinary stoppage accompanied by a sense of blockage in the throat; 3) exuberance of both yin and yang. (When yin qi is overexuberant [sic] and yang qi is not nourished, this is called block. When yang qi is overexuberant and yin qi is not nourished, this is called repulsion. When yin and yang are both overexuberant and fail to nourish each other, this is called block and repulsion.); and 4) extremely exuberant wrist and *Ren Ying* pulses which are a sign of impending separation of yin and yang.[1] *Su Wen*, Chapter 17 "*Mai Du* (The Length of the Vessels)" states:

> . . . the kidney communicates with the ear orifices, and, when the energy of the ear is harmonious, the ears can hear the five tones. When the five viscera are inharmonious, the seven orifices will be obstructed. When the six bowels are inharmonious, carbuncles will occur due to the stagnation of the blood . . . When the evil is in the six bowels, the yang channels become disorderly, causing stagnation of yang. Therefore there is repletion in the yang channels. When the evil is in the five viscera, the yin channels become disorderly, causing stagnation of the yin. Therefore there is repletion in the yin channels. When yin is replete, it inhibits yang and is called block. When yang is replete, it inhibits yin and it is called repulsion. When both yin and yang are replete and inhibit one another, this is called block and repulsion, in which the exterior and interior fail to maintain their independence. When the patient appears to have block and repulsion, he will not be able to live his natural life and dies early.

In *Su Wen*, Chapter 9, "*Liu Jie Zang Xiang Lun* (Treatise on the Relationship Between the Six Nodes & the Viscera)," it states:

> If the *Ren Ying* pulse and wrist pulse are four fold greater than normal, it indicates both yin and yang are so replete as to cause the severing of them. This is called block and repulsion. The block and repulsion pulse indicates such a lack of mutual support that yin and yang will fail to communicate with the essence of heaven and earth. The patient with such a pulse will die.

For our purposes, block is very scanty or complete blockage of urine; repulsion is constant vomiting.

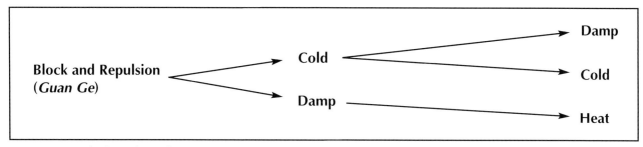

Figure 2.1. Block and repulsion

Together they are called block and repulsion. (See Chart 2.1.) Block and repulsion is a serious disease process. It is seen in late stages of water swelling, dribbling urinary block, and strangury. Patients usually have pattern identifications of spleen-kidney yang vacuity with damp accumulation. This dampness eventually obstructs the triple burner.

DISEASE CAUSES & MECHANISMS

Spleen and kidney vacuity are the root of this condition, while dampness and turbidity congestion and obstruction of the triple burner are the tip.

TREATMENT BASED ON PATTERN IDENTIFICATION

EARLY STAGE BLOCK & REPULSION

1. SPLEEN-KIDNEY YANG VACUITY

SIGNS & SYMPTOMS: Feeling cold, a somber white facial complexion, pale lips, somber white fingernails, lassitude of the spirit, lack of strength, lack of warmth in the four limbs, low back and knee soreness and limpness, devitalized eating and drinking, constipation and/or scanty or blocked urination, nausea and vomiting. The pulse is deep and fine, and the tongue is pale with thin fur.

TREATMENT PRINCIPLES: Fortify the spleen and warm the kidneys while also transforming turbidity

REPRESENTATIVE FORMULA: Modified *Wen Pi Tang* (Warm the Spleen Decoction) plus *Gui Lu Er Xian Jiao* (Turtle & Deer Two Immortals Gelatin)

Tai Zi Shen (Pseudostellariae Heterophyllae, Radix), 15-30g
Fu Zi (Aconiti Carmichaeli, Radix Lateralis Praeparatus), 5-10g
processed *Da Huang* (Rhei, Radix Et Rhizoma), 5-15g
stir-fried *Bai Zhu* (Atractylodis Macrocephalae, Rhizoma), 10g
Fu Ling (Poriae Cocos, Sclerotium), 9-18g
Shan Yao (Dioscoreae Oppositae, Radix), 1-15g
Gui Ban Jiao (Testudinis, Gelatinum Plastri), 15-30g
Lu Jiao Jiao (Cervi, Gelatinum Cornu), 5-10g
uncooked *Long Gu* (Draconis, Os), 15-30g
uncooked *Mu Li* (Ostreae, Concha), 15-30g
Dan Shen (Salviae Miltiorrhizae, Radix), 30g
mix-fried *Gan Cao* (Glycyrrhizae Uralensis, Radix), 5g

MODIFICATIONS: For difficult urination, add *Da Fu Pi* (Arecae Catechu, Pericarpium), *Ze Xie* (Alismatis Orientalis, Rhizoma), *Che Qian Zi* (Plantaginis, Semen), and *Shi Wei* (Pyrrosiae, Folium). For constipation, add *Da Huang* (Rhei, Radix Et Rhizoma) and *Rou Cong Rong* (Cistanchis Deserticolae, Herba). For nausea, add *Huo Po* (Magnoliae Officinalis, Cortex), *Ban Xia* (Pinelliae Ternatae, Rhizoma), and *Huo Xiang* (Agastachis Seu Pogostemi, Herba) or *Zhu Ru* (Bambusae, Caulis In Taeniis). However, if there is constipation, one must precipitate first to avoid causing more dryness.

ACUMOXIBUSTION: Moxibustion *Pi Shu* (Bl 20), *Wei Shu* (Bl 21), *Shen Shu* (Bl 23), *Ming Men* (GV 4), *Zhong Wan* (CV 12), *Shen Que* (CV 8), and *Guan Yuan* (CV 4), and needle *Nei Guan* (Per 6) and *Yin Ling Quan* (Sp 9).

2. YIN & YANG DUAL VACUITY

SIGNS & SYMPTOMS: A lusterless facial complexion, reversal chilling of the four extremities, occasional facial flushing, a dry mouth with a bitter taste, and nausea. The pulse is fine and rapid, while the tongue is pale and swollen with teeth-marks on its edges and thin, yellow fur.

TREATMENT PRINCIPLES: Warm the kidney and enrich yin, clear fire, and downbear turbidity

REPRESENTATIVE FORMULA: Modified *Da Huang Ling Pi Tang* (Rhubarb Magical Spleen Decoction)

processed *Da Huang* (Rhei, Radix Et Rhizoma), 9-15g
Yin Yang Huo (Epimedii, Herba), 30-60g
Tai Zi Shen (Pseudostellariae Heterophyllae, Radix), 15-30g
uncooked *Long Gu* (Draconis, Os), 30g
uncooked *Mu Li* (Ostreae, Concha), 30g
Dan Shen (Salviae Miltiorrhizae, Radix), 30g
Huang Bai (Phellodendri, Cortex), 9g
Zhi Mu (Anemarrhenae Aspheloidis, Rhizoma), 9g
Shan Yao (Disocoreae Oppositae, Radix), 9g
Sheng Di Huang (Rehmanniae Glutinosae, uncooked Radix), 15g
Xuan Shen (Scrophulariae Ningpoensis, Radix), 15g
Gou Qi Zi (Lycii Chinensis, Fructus), 9g

MODIFICATIONS: For nausea and vomiting, one can add *Zi Su Geng* (Perillae Frutescentis, Caulis), processed *Ban Xia* (Pinelliae Ternatae, Rhizoma), and *Chen Pi* (Citri Reticulatae, Pericarpium). For high blood pressure, add *Xian Mao* (Cuculiginis Orchioidis, Rhizoma) and *Dang Gui* (Angelicae Sinensis, Radix). If the kidney is swollen and enlarged or there are lumps in the lower abdominal region, add *San Leng* (Sparganii Stoloniferi, Rhizoma), *E Zhu* (Curcumae Zedoariae, Rhizoma), and *Che Qian Zi* (Plantaginis, Semen) to quicken the blood and dispel stasis, disinhibit water and disperse swelling.

ACUMOXIBUSTION: Needle *Tai Xi* (Ki 3), *San Yin Jiao* (Sp 6), *Yin Ling Quan* (Sp 9), *Nei Guan* (Per 6), and *Zhao Hai* (Ki 6), while moxaing *Pi Shu* (Bl 20), *Wei Shu* (Bl 21), *Shen Shu* (Bl 23), *Guan Yuan* (CV 4), and *Zhong Wan* (CV 12)

LATE STAGE BLOCK & REPULSION

1. TURBID EVILS ENCUMBERING THE SPLEEN

SIGNS & SYMPTOMS: Lassitude of the spirit, lack of strength, heaviness and encumbrance of the four limbs, a lusterless facial complexion, nausea and vomiting, indigestion, abdominal distention, possible glomus lumps in the abdomen, and a slimy-feeling mouth with a sweet taste. There is thick, slimy tongue fur, the tongue itself is pale and may be swollen with teeth-marks on its edges, and the pulse is deep and fine or soggy and fine.

TREATMENT PRINCIPLES: Warm yang and fortify the spleen, move the qi, and transform turbidity

REPRESENTATIVE FORMULA: Modified *Shi Pi Yin* (Bolster the Spleen Beverage)

Tai Zi Shen (Pseudostellariae Heterophyllae, Radix), 9-30g
Bai Zhu (Atractylodis Macrocephalae, Rhizoma), 9-30g
Fu Ling (Poriae Cocos, Sclerotium), 9-30g
Fu Zi (Aconiti Carmichaeli, Radix Lateralis Praeparatus), 3-6g
Hou Po (Magnoliae Officinalis, Cortex), 3-6g
Gan Jiang (Zingiberis Officinalis, dry Rhizoma), 3-6g
Mu Xiang (Auklandiae Lappae, Radix), 4.5-9g
Cao Dou Kou (Alpiniae Katsumadai, Semen), 6-9g
Da Fu Pi (Arecae Catechu, Pericarpium), 9-15g
Ze Xie (Alismatis Orientalis, Rhizoma), 9g
Shan Yao (Dioscoreae Oppositae, Radix), 9g
Mu Dan Pi (Moutan, Cortex Radicis), 4.5-6g

MODIFICATIONS: If there is simultaneous edema, add uncooked *Huang Qi* (Astragali Membranacei, Radix) and *Han Fang Ji* (Stephaniae Tetrandrae, Radix). After dampness has been disinhibited, remove *Fu Zi* and *Gan Jiang* so as to protect against damaging fluids. If turbid evils spill over above, add *Zi Su Geng* (Perillae Frutescentis, Caulis), ginger-processed *Ban Xia* (Pinelliae Ternatae, Rhizoma), and *Chen Pi* (Citri Reticulatae, Pericarpium).

ACUMOXIBUSTION: Needle *Tai Xi* (Ki 3), *San Yin Jiao* (Sp 6), *Yin Ling Quan* (Sp 9), *Nei Guan* (Per 6), and *Zhao Hai* (Ki 6), while moxaing *Pi Shu* (Bl 20), *Wei Shu* (Bl 21), *Shen Shu* (Bl 23), *Guan Yuan* (CV 4), and *Zhong Wan* (CV 12).

2. TURBID EVILS ASSAILING THE STOMACH

SIGNS & SYMPTOMS: Nausea, dry heaves or repeated vomiting, torpid intake, and abdominal distention. If there is transformation of heat, there is constipation, slimy, yellow or dry, sticky tongue fur and a fine, rapid or bowstring, rapid pulse. If there is transformation of cold, there will be loose stools or diarrhea up to 10 times per day with a swollen, pale tongue and a soggy, fine pulse.

TREATMENT PRINCIPLES: Harmonize the stomach, downbear counterflow, and transform turbidity

REPRESENTATIVE FORMULA: Modified *Xiao Ban Xia Tang* (Minor Pinellia Decoction) plus *Xuan Fu Dai Zhe Tang* (Inula & Hematite Decoction)

Ban Xia (Pinelliae Ternatae, Rhizoma), 6-9g
Sheng Jiang Zhi (Zingiberis Officinalis, Succus Rhizomatis), 5-10 drops
Tai Zi Shen (Pseudostellariae Heterophyllae, Radix), 9-30g
Xuan Fu Hua (Inulae Racemosae, Flos), 9g
Dai Zhe Shi (Haemititum), 9-15g
Da Zao (Zizyphi Jujubae, Fructus), 10 pieces
mix-fried *Gan Cao* (Glycyrrhizae Uralensis, Radix), 6g
uncooked *Long Gu* (Draconis, Os), 15-30g
uncooked *Mu Li* (Ostreae, Concha), 15-30g
Dan Shen (Salviae Miltiorrhizae, Radix), 30g
Bai Feng Mi (Mel, honey), 30g

MODIFICATIONS: If there is heat transformation, add *Huang Lian* (Coptidis Chinensis, Rhizoma), *Chen Pi* (Citri Reticulatae, Pericarpium), *Fu Ling* (Poriae Cocos, Sclerotium), *Zhu Ru* (Bambusae In Taeniis, Caulis), and *Zhi Shi* (Citri Aurantii, Fructus Immaturus). If there is cold transformation, add *Wu*

Zhu Yu (Evodiae Rutecarpae, Fructus), *Gan Jiang* (Zingiberis Officinalis, dry Rhizoma), and scorched *Bai Zhu* (Atractylodis Macrocephalae, Rhizoma). If there is diarrhea with numerous bowel movements per day, add *Chi Shi Zhi* (Hallyositum Rubrum).

ACUMOXIBUSTION: Needle *Zhong Wan* (CV 12), *Nei Guan* (Per 6), *Zu San Li* (St 36), *Yin Ling Quan* (Sp 9), *Tian Shu* (St 25), and *Da Chang Shu* (Bl 25).

MODIFICATIONS: If there is heat transformation, add *Nei Ting* (St 44), *He Gu* (LI 4), and *Qu Chi* (LI 11). If there is cold transformation, moxibustion *Zhong Wan, Zu San Li, Tian Shu,* and *Da Chang Shu* and add moxibustion on *Qi Hai* (CV 6) and *Guan Yuan* (CV 4).

REPRESENTATIVE CASE HISTORIES

Case history 1: Wang, a 27 year-old male[2]

Prior to Wang's first visit on July 21, 1982, he was diagnosed with chronic nephritis and chronic renal failure. His symptoms included headache, dizziness, chills, heat in the five hearts, thirst without desire to drink, fatigue, lethargy, loose stools 1-2 times per day, and turbid urine. His pulse was deep and fine, and his tongue had a red tip with a purple body. Urinalysis showed urine protein at 3+, RBCs at 3-5, and a few white blood cells. A blood test showed RBCs at 22450000, HB at 7, BP at 160/70mmHg, BUN at 71, and creatinine at 6.47. Based on these signs and symptoms, the pattern identification was spleen-kidney yang vacuity, liver-kidney yin vacuity, ascendant liver yang hyperactivity, and enduring blood stasis. The treatment principles were to supplement the kidney and nourish yin, fortify the spleen and supplement the qi. The basic formula was *Fu Gui Ba Wei Wan* (a.k.a. *Shen Qi Wan*, Kidney Qi Pills). However, because of middle burner dampness (the patient had nausea, vomiting, and could not eat), medicinals were added to the prescription to harmonize the stomach and descend the qi and dampness. These last ingredients were from *Xuan Fu Dai Zhe Tang* (Inula & Hematite Decoction). The complete formula was as follows: *Fu Zi* (Aconiti Carmichaeli, Radix Lateralis Praeparatus), *Rou Gui*

(Cinnamomi Cassiae, Cortex), *Shan Zhu Yu* (Corni Officinalis, Fructus), *Shan Yao* (Dioscoreae Oppositae, Radix), *Shu Di* (Rehmanniae Glutinosae, cooked Radix), *Mu Dan Pi* (Moutan, Cortex Radicis), *Fu Ling* (Poriae Cocos, Sclerotium), *Ze Xie* (Alismatis Orientalis, Rhizoma), *Ban Xia* (Pinelliae Ternatae, Rhizoma), *Xuan Fu Hua* (Inulae Racemosae, Flos), *Dai Zhe Shi* (Haematitum), *Sheng Jiang* (Zingiberis Officinalis, uncooked Rhizoma), *Ren Shen* (Panacis Ginseng, Radix), mix-fried *Gan Cao* (Glycyrrhizae Uralensis, Radix), *Da Zao* (Zizyphi Jujubae, Fructus), and *Fu Long Gan* (Terra Flava Usta). (No dosages given.)

Along with this, the patient had an enema of *Da Huang* (Rhei, Radix Et Rhizoma), 15g, every night. He also had intravenous injections of *Dan Shen* (Salviae Miltiorrhizae, Radix) in order to quicken the blood and dispel stasis, 10 injections constituting one course of treatment. After one course of these medicinals, the patient's nausea was better and all his other symptoms improved. *Bai Zhu* (Atractylodis Macrocephalae, Rhizoma) was added to the prescription in order to fortify the spleen. The patient's diet was restricted to low salt and protein and no fat or beans. He was also instructed to eat more fruit. After one month, Wang's kidney function was much improved. Blood urea nitrogen was reduced to 49.8 and creatinine to 5.12. All his symptoms had abated.

Case history 2: Qiao, a 19 year-old female[3]

Qiao had been vomiting for over one and a half years and could only drink one cup per day of human milk. She had not had a bowel movement for a month before her first visit. She looked normal, but her left pulse was bowstring, while her right pulse was weak. She had tried over 300 packets of Chinese medicinals, including *Huang Lian Tang* (Coptis Decoction), *Xuan Fu Dai Zhe Tang* (Inula & Hematite Decoction), *Si Mo Yin* (Four Milled [Ingredients] Beverage), and *Wu Zhi Yin* (Five Juices Beverage). She had taken a total of three pounds of *Yu Jin* (Curcumae, Tuber) and a half pound each of *Chen Xiang* (Aquilariae Agallochae, Lignum) and *E Zhu* (Curcumae Zedoariae, Rhizoma). None of these had helped. On the contrary, she had severe vacuity,

especially fluid vacuity, because some of the medicinals had damaged her fluids leading to the block and repulsion.

The family finally consulted Dr. Yu. He theorized that wood was too strong, while earth was weak leading to liver overwhelming the stomach and spleen. Thus when Qiao ate, she would get nauseous and vomit. He gave her an herbal prescription to course the liver and resolve depression, supplement the middle burner, descend the qi and dampness, and stop nausea and vomiting. The next day when she returned, her father reported that she had vomited all the medicinals. Dr. Yu then tried *Da Ban Xia Tang* (Major Pinellia Decoction) with additions: *Ban Xia* (Pinelliae Ternatae, Rhizoma), *Ren Shen* (Panacis Ginseng, Radicis), *Bai Mi* (Mel, honey), *Rou Cong Rong* (Cistanchis Deserticolae, Herba), *Niu Xi* (Achyranthis Bidentatae, Radix), and *Gan Cao* (Glycyrrhizae Uralensis, Radix). (No dosages given.) This was to be taken concurrently with *Jin Gui Shen Qi Wan*.

Ban Xia descends qi and dampness. *Gan Cao* and *Ren Shen* generate fluids and nourish the stomach. *Feng Mi* moistens. *Gan Lan Shui* (Aqua Preparata used in making the above-mentioned pills) serves as a channel-guiding medicinal, directing the other medicinals downward. *Rou Cong Rong* moistens the intestines. *Niu Xi* descends and settles yang. *Jin Gui Shen Qi Wan* supplements kidney yang. The combination of these two formulas supplements both lower burner yang and upper burner yin.

Qiao tried to take these medicinals but also vomited them all. Dr. Yu asked Qiao's father how she was able to drink the human milk. The father replied that a cup had to be divided into 3-5 parts for her to drink it. She could also take 3-5 small pills of *Jin Gui Shen Qi Wan* if they were dry and without water. In view of this, Dr. Yu then instructed the father to cook the herbal prescription using very little water to condense it and to keep it warm in a teapot. He instructed Qiao to drink it in little sips all day long and to take 3-5 little pills of *Jin Gui Shen Qi Wan* at a time throughout the day, up to 12 grams per day. He also advised Qiao to sit in a doorway and look outside to keep up her spirits. Using this method, Qiao could take the medication without vomiting.

After 3-4 days, Qiao suddenly felt tired, her face turned yellow, and she had a bowel movement consisting of a very dry stool two meters long. She went to bed and was unable to get up. Her family was alarmed. Dr. Yu, on the other hand, felt that this extraordinary bowel movement was a good sign indicating that Qiao's lower burner had opened up. His concern now centered on the upper burner. He surmised that it was still closed and food could not be absorbed. Because Qiao could eat a few dry pills, he thought that the prognosis was hopeful.

To continue the therapy, he instructed the family to mix 12 grams of *Shen Qi Wan* with 200 grams of steamed rice and smash them together to form pills. He instructed Qiao to take them little by little. After a few days, because her stomach began to absorb the qi of the steamed rice and her esophagus was slowly moistened, she could add three more grams of *Shen Qi Wan*. Every day, she added another three grams, and, gradually, she could also consume more rice. Day by day she got stronger and could eat more until one day she was able to eat 200 grams of rice in one meal. This signified that the upper burner had opened up. Dr. Yu then gave her moistening, supplementing-yin medicinals for three months and she was cured.

Case history 3: Gu, a 30 year-old male[4]

Gu liked to eat greasy food and drink alcohol. He went to a doctor because he had vomited blood, a whole basin full, causing severe damage to his body fluids. That doctor thought the pattern identification was kidney vacuity causing liver vacuity fire and ascendant liver yang hyperactivity. Therefore, he used cooling medicinals to stop the vomiting, but, after one year of treatment, Gu became constipated and did not have a bowel movement for an entire month. He also continued to vomit immediately after eating or he would eat in the morning and vomit in the evening. Gu decided to try other doctors, but they tended to give him warm, dry medicinals that just exacerbated his symptoms.

Gu finally came to see Dr. Yu. Dr. Yu reasoned that if vomiting the large amount of blood had caused severe damage to Gu's body fluids, the use of warm and dry medicinals had only damaged the fluids more. This had then led to liver blood vacuity. The insufficiency of yin-blood deprived the liver of nourishment and led to liver depression qi stagnation. The liver depression damaged the stomach, spleen, and intestines, resulting in block and repulsion. Moreover, the liver blood vacuity caused dryness that closed the bowels. Dr. Yu decided that *Huang Lian Tang* (Coptis Decoction) with additions would address this pattern: *Huang Lian* (Coptidis Chinensis, Rhizoma), mix-fried *Gan Cao* (Glycyrrhizae Uralensis, Radix), *Gan Jiang* (Zingiberis Officinalis, dry Rhizoma), *Gui Zhi* (Cinnamomi Cassiae, Ramulus), *Ren Shen* (Panacis Ginseng, Radix), *Ban Xia* (Pinelliae Ternatae, Rhizoma), *Da Zao* (Zizyphi Jujubae, Fructus), *Rou Cong Rong* (Cistanchis Deserticolae, Herba), *Gou Qi Zi* (Lycii Chinensis, Fructus), *Dang Gui* (Angelicae Sinensis, Radix), *Bai Shao* (Paeoniae Lactiflorae, Radix Albus), *Sha Yuan Zi* (Astragali Complanati, Semen), *Tu Si Zi* (Cuscutae Chinensis, Semen), *Ba Zi Ren* (Biotae Orientalis, Semen), *Hu Ma Ren* (Sesami Indici, Semen), *Niu Xi* (Achyranthis Bidentatae, Radix), *Rou Gui* (Cinnamonmi Cassiae, Cortex), and *Sheng Jiang* (Zingiberis Officinalis, uncooked Rhizoma). (No dosages given.)

These additions are warming and moistening. Gu took this formula for five days and was able to have a bowel movement and the vomiting also decreased. Therefore, Dr. Yu added *Lu Jiao Shuang* (Cervi, Cornu Degelatinum) and *Yu Jiao* (Piscis, Gelatinum). Gu took this new formula for 20 days and completely recovered. Eight years later, his symptoms started to recur, but Dr. Yu gave him a warm, sweet, moistening formula and the symptoms quickly abated.

Case history 4: Chen, male[5] (age not given)

A few years before his first visit to Dr. Yao, Chen almost drowned. Subsequently, he developed symptoms of block and repulsion. He tried some 30-40 herbal prescriptions, all with bitter, cold medicinals, without success. Chen might vomit immediately after eating, but usually, if he ate in the afternoon, he would vomit in the evening, or, if he ate in the evening, he would vomit in the morning. The vomit would contain lots of phlegm and had a very strong, bad odor. He would have a bowel movement only once in 10-17 days and this would resemble horses' stool. Chen's face was yellow and his urine was red and rough. Both his bar pulses were slippery, big, slow, and forceless, and the other positions could not be felt.

Based on the above, Dr. Yao thought that Chen did not really have block and repulsion but stomach qi vacuity. Because of the stomach qi vacuity, qi and dampness could not descend and would stagnate in the stomach. Food in the stomach would get wrapped or surrounded by the phlegm and would not be available to be digested. Dr. Yao explained the fact that Chen seldom vomited immediately after eating as follows: "The stomach likes fresh food and tries to hold it for digestion. Only when the food starts to turn and smell bad will the stomach throw it up." The scanty, rough urination was the result of the body not receiving enough fluids because grain and water could not descend to the large intestine. Therefore, Dr. Yao decided to use modified *Li Zhong Wan* (Regulate the Center Pills) as a decoction in order to boost stomach yang so it would descend the stomach qi. His prescription consisted of: *Dang Shen* (Codonopsitis Pilosulae, Radix), 15g, *E Zhu* (Curcumae Zedoariae, Rhizoma), 15g, *Fu Zi* (Aconiti Carmichaeli, Radix Lateralis Praeparatus), 9g, *Gan Jiang* (Zingiberis Officinalis, dry Rhizoma), 6g, *Gan Cao* (Glycyrrhizae Uralensis, Radix), 4.5g, and *Chi Shi Zhi* (Halloysitum Rubrum), 15g.

The news of Dr. Yao's novel approach spread throughout the hospital where he worked and was generally questioned and criticized as follows: "If the patient is constipated, why give him a qi-supplementing and securing and astringing prescription? This will make him worse." But Dr. Yao told Chen, "Do not listen to this criticism. Just take your herbs." Chen took the prescription for three days and his urination improved. In six days, he had bowel movements 10 times per day with lots of phlegm and water

mixed in with the stool. He was able to eat some porridge but nothing solid. His bar pulse was better and the others were palpable, although still soggy and weak.

Now both Dr. Yao and Chen felt hopeful, but a question still remained. Why was Chen unable to eat solid food? Dr. Yao theorized that, when the yin evils in the stomach had been discharged through the stool, they made the stomach "brand new," *i.e.*, it was weak and fragile like new skin under a scab or a scar. Chen's stomach needed time to heal and become strong enough to digest solid food. Therefore, Dr. Yao decided that Chen should continue on the same prescription to heal his stomach. Chen took this prescription for 10 more days and his middle burner qi completely recovered.

Case history 5: Zou, a 64 year-old man[6]

Zou had nausea and vomiting for two weeks. By April 12, he had a high fever. He went to a hospital and was treated with gentamicin, an antibiotic. After a week, his fever was gone, but he still had nausea and vomiting. His face became edematous and his urination decreased. The doctors continued to give him gentamicin, but then his low back became sore and blood was found in his urine. His blood analysis showed creatinine at 12mg/dL and BUN at 86mg/dL. Urinalysis showed protein at 1+ and granular casts at 0-1/HP. Ultrasound showed that both kidneys were swollen. The Western medical diagnosis was renal failure with uremia.

Zou was apathetic and had a dark facial complexion, very bad breath, nausea, no appetite, a low-grade fever, sore throat, and insomnia. His pulse was fine and fast, and his tongue was dark with thin, yellow fur. Based on these signs and symptoms, Dr. Jin's diagnosis was wind heat attacking the shao yin, causing kidney dysfunction with damp accumulation, virulent heat toxins damaging the middle burner, obstructing the clear from being upborne and the turbid from being downborne. Zou's was a severe case of block and repulsion. Dr. Jin's formula consisted of: *Bai Zhu* (Atractylodis Macrocephalae, Rhizoma), 9g, *Chi Shao* (Paeoniae Lactiflorae, Radix Rubrus), 9g,

Bai Shao (Paeoniae Lactiflorae, Radix Albus), 9g, *Tu Fu Ling* (Smilacis Glabrae, Rhizoma), 15g, *Liu Yue Xue Ye* (Eupatorii Chinensis, Folium), 30g, *Huang Lian* (Coptidis Chinensis, Rhizoma), 3g, *Gan Cao* (Glycyrrhizae Uralensis, Radix), 3g, *Chen Pi* (Citri Reticulatae, Pericarpium), 6g, *Yin Chai Hu* (Stellariae Dichotomae, Radix), 6g, *Lian Qiao* (Forsythiae Suspensae, Fructus), 9g, *Can Sha* (Bombycis Mori, Excrementum), 9g, *Hei Da Dou* (Phaseoli Vulgaris, Semen), 30g, *Ban Xia* (Pinelliae Ternatae, Rhizoma), 6g, *Yi Yi Ren* (Coicis Lachryma-jobi, Semen), 30g, *Shi Wei* (Pyrrosiae, Folium), 15g, *Da Ji* (Cirsii Japonici, Herba Seu Radix), 30g, *Shan Zha* (Crataegi, Fructus), 9g, and *Bai Hua She She Cao* (Oldenlandiae Diffusae, Herba Cum Radice), 30g.

Zou took this formula for one month and felt much better. His nausea and vomiting abated, but his appetite did not improve. His tongue had yellow, slimy fur. Dr. Jin removed *Hei Da Dou*, *Lian Qiao*, *Shan Zha*, and *Yin Chai Hu* from Zou's formula and added *Yin Chen Hao* (Artemisiae Capillaris, Herba), 30g, *Xuan Fu Hua* (Inulae Racemosae, Flos), 9g, *Huang Qin* (Scutellariae Baicalensis, Radix), 9g, and *Dai Zhe Shi* (Haematitum), 15g. Zou took this new formula for two months and his appetite improved, his nausea disappeared, and his urine and stool returned to normal, but he was still fatigued. His pulse was fine, and he had slimy tongue fur. Dr. Jin changed the prescription to: *Tai Zi Shen* (Pseudostellariae Heterophyllae, Radix), 12g, *Bai Zhu* (Atractylodis Macrocephalae, Rhizoma), 9g, *Shan Yao* (Dioscoreae Oppositae, Radix), 9g, *Bai Bian Dou* (Dolichoris Lablab, Semen), 9g, *Nu Zhen Zi* (Ligustri Lucidi, Fructus), 9g, *Han Lian Cao* (Ecliptae Prostratae, Herba), 15g, *Hei Da Dou* (Phaseoli Vulgaris, Semen), 30g, *Chi Shao* (Paeoniae Lactiflorae, Radix Rubrus), 9g, *Bai Shao* (Paeoniae Lactiflorae, Radix Albus), 9g, *Yi Yi Ren* (Coicis Lachryma-jobi, Semen), 30g, *Shi Wei* (Pyrrosiae, Folium), 15g, *Da Ji* (Cirsii Japonici, Herba Seu Radix), 30g, *Ban Xia* (Pinelliae Ternatae, Rhizoma), 6g, *Shan Zha* (Crataegi, Fructus), 9g, *Bai Hua She She Cao* (Oldenlandiae Diffusae, Herba Cum Radice), 30g, and *Gu Ya* (Oryzae Sativae, Fructus Germinatus), 12g. By June, Zou's kidney function was back to normal.

CLINICAL TIPS

1. As stated above, spleen and kidney vacuity are the roots of this condition, while damp stagnation and obstruction of the triple burner are the tips. Therefore, the treatment strategy should include warming and supplementing the spleen and kidney. Here "warming" means to invigorate yang and "supplementing" means to boost the qi. When invigorating yang, yang must be derived from yin as in formulas such as *Jin Gui Shen Qi Wan* (*Golden Cabinet Kidney Qi Pills*). However, because qi and yang have the same root, if there is egregious yang vacuity, one cannot use medicinals that invigorate yang alone. One must also employ medicinals that boost the qi such as *Ren Shen* (Panacis Ginseng, Radix). Similarly, if there is egregious yin vacuity, one must use medicinals that nourish yin as well as boosting the qi, such as *Xi Yang Shen* (Panacis Quinquefolii, Radix).

To reiterate, block and repulsion has vacuity at the root and repletion at the tip. The cause of the repletion is dampness accumulation. Dampness is a yin evil that can easily damage yang, and, if dampness is not transformed, yang cannot recover ("dampness winning, yang weakening"). Even if yang is vacuous and needs supplementation, one must still attack and eliminate dampness. In other words, one must treat both yang vacuity and dampness at the same time. To accomplish this, one usually uses combinations of *Jin Gui Shen Qi Wan* plus medicinals such as *Da Huang* (Rhei, Radix Et Rhizoma) and *Hei Da Dou* (Glycinis, Semen Atrum). *Da Huang* drains turbid dampness and frees the flow of the channels. One should use a low dosage so that there are only two or three bowel movements a day. *Hei Da Dou* is sweet, goes to the spleen and kidney channels, moves the blood and percolates dampness, expels wind and resolves toxins.

2. A traditional treatment strategy for block and repulsion is to "free the flow of yang [bowels] and drain the turbid." For this purpose, one may use *Da Huang* (Rhei, Radix Et Rhizoma), 30g, and *Mang Xiao* (Mirabilitum), 15g, cooked in 150ml of water and given as an enema once a day. The enema should be retained in the colon for one hour or more. For nausea accompanying the vomiting, one can use *Er Chen Tang* (Two Aged [Ingredients] Decoction): *Ban Xia* (Pinelliae Ternatae, Rhizoma), 5g, *Chen Pi* (Citri Reticulatae, Pericarpium), 4g, *Fu Ling* (Poriae Cocos, Sclerotium), 5g, mix-fried *Gan Cao* (Glycyrrhizae Uralensis, Radix), 1g, *Sheng Jiang* (Zingiberis Officinalis, uncooked Rhizoma), 3g, and *Wu Mei* (Pruni Mume, Fructus), 1 piece. To this, one should add *Fu Long Gan* (Terra Flava Usta) or modified *Xuan Fu Dai Zhe Tang* (Inula & Haematitum Decoction): *Xuan Fu Hua* (Inulae Racemosae, Flos), 9g, *Dai Zhe Shi* (Haematitum), 9-15g, *Ren Shen* (Panacis Ginseng, Radix), 6g, and *Da Zao* (Zizyphi Jujubae, Fructus), 4 pieces.

3. The *Jin Gui Yao Lue* states, "Water diseases affect the blood." Water and dampness stagnating for a long time underlie block and repulsion. One can see the effect they have on blood through symptoms such as dry mouth, dry lips, purple tongue, and a choppy pulse. The skin is often very rough, "crocodile skin," a common sign of blood stasis. These symptoms become more frequent in the late stages of this disease. Blood stasis may also cause bleeding. If there is bleeding, one cannot just use astringent or blood-stanching medicinals. These may cause more stasis which, in turn, may cause more bleeding. In this case, one must use medicinals whose secondary function is to stanch bleeding. Examples for use with concurrent yin vacuity include *Han Lian Cao* (Ecliptae Prostratae, Herba), *Sheng Di* (Rehmanniae Glutinosae, uncooked Radix), *Bai Shao* (Paeoniae Lactiflorae, Radix Albus), *Mu Dan Pi* (Moutan, Cortex Radicis), *Long Gu* (Draconis, Os), *Mu Li* (Ostreae, Concha), and *E Jiao* (Asini, Gelatinum Corii).

4. A useful formula for blood stasis in block and repulsion is modified *Gui Zhi Fu Ling Wan* (Cinnamon Twig & Poria Pills): *Gui Zhi* (Cinnamomi Cassiae, Ramulus), 9g, *Fu Ling* (Poriae Cocos, Sclerotium), 9g, *Chi Shao* (Paeoniae Lactiflorae, Radix Rubrus), 9g, *Mu Dan Pi* (Moutan, Cortex Radicis), 9g, *Tao Ren* (Pruni Persicae, Semen), 9g, *Yi Mu Cao* (Leonuri Heterophylli, Herba), 9g, *Bai Mao Gen* (Imperatae Cylindricae, Rhizoma), 15g, and *Liu Ji Nu* (Artemisiae Anomalae, Herba), 15g. To this, one can add *Shui Zhi* (Hirudo Seu Whitmania), using one piece per day. If *Shui Zhi* is ground into a powder, one can use nine grams per day divided into two servings. Some scholars also add *Da Huang* (Rhei, Radix Et Rhizoma) and *San Qi* (Notoginseng, Radix).

5. In any kidney disease, if the tongue is big or swollen, it is easier to treat. Conversely, if the tongue is small or shrunken, the case is more difficult because the disease is deeper.

ENDNOTES

[1] Wiseman and Ye, *A Practical Dictionary of Chinese Medicine*, Paradigm Publications, 1998, Brookline, MA, p. 24
[2] Yu Guan-shi, *Shen Yan Liao Du Zhen Zhuan Ji (Treatise on Nephritis and Chronic Renal Failure)*, Ancient Chinese Medical Book Publishing Co., Beijing, 1991, p. 303
[3] This case comes from a Qing dynasty book without a title or publishing information.
[4] This case comes from a Qing dynasty book without a title or publishing information.
[5] This case comes from a Qing dynasty book without a title or publishing information.
[6] *Shui Zhong Guan Ge Jun (Water Swelling and Block & Repulsion)*, Volume 2, Chinese Medicine Publishing Company, Beijing, 1998, p. 263

CHAPTER 3
DRIBBLING URINARY BLOCK

Long means dribbling urine or blockage of urine. *Bi* means urinary difficulty or complete blockage of urine. *Long* is chronic, while *bi* is acute. Together *long bi* or dribbling urinary block indicates both chronic and acute diseases with symptoms of blockage of the urine. Dribbling urinary block and block and repulsion are two different diseases. Block and repulsion can have blockage of urination and/or defecation and is accompanied by nausea and vomiting. Dribbling urinary block only indicates blockage of urination. (See Chart 3.1.)

DISEASE CAUSES & MECHANISMS

Dribbling urinary block can be caused by any of the six evils and seven affects and is located in the urinary bladder. *Su Wen*, Chapter 8, "*Ling Lan Mi Dian Lun* (Magic Orchid Secret Teaching)" states:

> The bladder takes the office of gathering, it stores water and fluids. After the body fluid goes through qi transformation, it can be excreted.

The triple burner is also involved in urination. The triple burner springs from the kidney and connects to the urinary bladder. It connects above with the lung and, in the middle, with the spleen and stomach. *Ling Shu*, Chapter 2, "*Ben Shu* (Root Transport [Points])" implicates the triple burner as well as the bladder in dribbling urinary block:

> When the triple burner is replete, painful urination will occur . . . When treating painful urination that is replete, precipitating therapy should be applied.

The urinary bladder's connection to the triple burner implicates several other viscera in this disease, the liver, kidney, spleen, and lung. For example, *Su Wen*, Chapter 48, "*Da Qi Lun* (Treatise on Greatly Strange [Diseases])" states that, "When one contracts a liver abscess, distention of the two rib-sides, fright during sleep, and painful urination will occur. . ." Dribbling urinary block is also associated with the five phase cycles. *Su Wen*, Chapter 70, "*Wu Chang Zheng Da Lun* (Treatise on the Five Invariable Administrators)" correlates it with:

> . . . injury of water by earth . . . When earth overwhelms water, wood [the son of water] will retaliate for its mother . . .

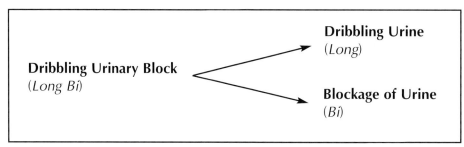

Chart 3.1. Dribbling urinary block

TREATMENT BASED ON PATTERN IDENTIFICATION

1. BLADDER DAMP HEAT

SIGNS & SYMPTOMS: Urinary dribbling and dripping and non-free flow or extremely scanty urination which is short and red and accompanied by burning pain, lower abdominal distention and fullness, a bitter taste and sticky feeling in the mouth, possible oral thirst but no desire to drink, and possible unsmooth or uneasy defecation. The root of the tongue is covered in slimy, yellow fur, while the tongue itself is red and the pulse is rapid.

TREATMENT PRINCIPLES: Clear and transform dampness and heat, free the flow and disinhibit urination

REPRESENTATIVE FORMULA: Modified *Ba Zheng San* (Eight [Ingredients] Rectification Powder)

Qu Mai (Dianthi, Herba), 9g
Bian Xu (Polygoni Avicularis, Herba), 9g
Zhi Zi (Gardeniae Jasminoidis, Fructus), 9g
Mu Tong (Akebiae Mutong, Caulis), 3-6g
Hua Shi (Talcum), 9-12g
Che Qian Zi (Plantaginis, Semen), 15-30g
Gan Cao Xiao (Glycyrrhizae Uralensis, Radix Tenuis), 3-6g
processed *Da Huang* (Rhei, Radix Et Rhizoma), 6-9g

NOTE: Commonly, the use of water-disinhibiting, dampness-percolating medicinals is discouraged in the treatment of dribbling urinary block due to bladder dysfunction. However, in the case of damp heat, the root is heat and, therefore, we must still use the three major principles for clearing heat. This includes discharging heat via urination. However, this method is only used for burning urination indicating heat, where we have a definite reason to clear heat via urination. If the cause of dribbling urinary block is qi stagnation, cold, or yang vacuity, one must be careful with water-disinhibiting, dampness-percolating medicinals.

MODIFICATIONS: If there is replete heat causing the body to be hot and constipation, use uncooked *Da Huang* instead of processed and add *Pu Gong Ying* (Taraxaci Mongolici, Herba Cum Radice) and *Jin Yin Hua* (Lonicerae Japonicae, Flos) to clear heat and resolve toxins. If the tongue is covered in thick, yellow fur, add *Cang Zhu* (Atractylodis, Rhizoma) and *Huang Bai* (Phellodendri, Cortex) to increase the clearing of heat and transformation of dampness. If there is simultaneous heart vexation and the tongue has sores and ulcers on it, add *Sheng Di Huang* (Rehmanniae Glutinosae, uncooked Radix) and *Dan Zhu Ye* (Lophatheri Gracilis, Herba) to clear heart fire. If damp heat has endured for a long time in the lower burner, and has damaged kidney yin, one can add *Sheng Di Huang* (Rehmanniae Glutinosae, uncooked Radix) and *Niu Xi* (Achyranthis Bidentatae, Radix) to enrich kidney yin.

ACUMOXIBUSTION: Needle *Yin Ling Quan* (Sp 9), *San Yin Jiao* (Sp 6), *Zhong Ji* (CV 3), *Pang Guang Shu* (Bl 28), and *Ci Liao* (Bl 32).

MODIFICATIONS: If there is simultaneous constipation, add *Tian Shu* (St 25), *Da Chang Shu* (Bl 25), *Zhao Hai* (Ki 6), *Yang Ling Quan* (GB 34), and *Zhi Gou* (TB

6). If enduring damp heat has damaged yin, add *Tai Xi* (Ki 3), *Zhao Hai* (Ki 6), and *Shen Shu* (Bl 23).

2. LUNG HEAT CONGESTION & EXUBERANCE

SIGNS & SYMPTOMS: Dribbling and dripping urination, a dry throat, vexatious thirst and a desire to drink, short, hasty breathing, and possible cough. The tongue fur is thin and yellow and the pulse is rapid.

TREATMENT PRINCIPLES: Clear and discharge lung heat in order to disinhibit the water passageways

REPRESENTATIVE FORMULA: Modified *Qing Fei Yin* (Clear the Lung Beverage)

Fu Ling (Poriae Cocos, Sclerotium), 12g
Huang Qin (Scutellariae Baicalensis, Radix), 9g
Sang Bai Pi (Mori Albi, Cortex Radicis), 9g
Mai Men Dong (Ophiopogonis Japonici, Tuber), 9g
Che Qian Zi (Plantaginis, Semen), 15-30g
Zhi Zi (Gardeniae Jasminoidis, Fructus), 9g
Mu Tong (Akebiae Mutong, Caulis), 3-6g

MODIFICATIONS: If there is heart fire effulgence with a red tongue tip, add *Huang Lian* (Coptidis Chinensis, Rhizoma) and *Dan Zhu Ye* (Lophatheri Gracilis, Herba) to clear heart fire. If lung yin is insufficient, one can add *Sha Shen* (Glehniae Littoralis, Radix) and *Bai Mao Gen* (Imperatae Cylindricae, Rhizoma) to enrich and nourish lung yin. If the stools are not freely flowing, one can add *Da Huang* (Rhei, Radix Et Rhizoma) and *Xing Ren* (Pruni Armeniacae, Semen) to diffuse the lung and free the flow of the stools. If the nose is congested and there is headache with a floating pulse, add *Bo He* (Menthae Haplocalycis, Herba) and *Jie Geng* (Platycodi Grandiflori, Radix) to resolve the exterior and diffuse the lung.

ACUMOXIBUSTION: Needle *Chi Ze* (Lu 5), *Feng Men* (Bl 12), *Fei Shu* (Bl 13), *Ying Ling Quan* (Sp 9), *Zhong Ji* (CV 3), and *Pang Guang Shu* (Bl 28).

MODIFICATIONS: If there is an exterior pattern, add *He Gu* (LI 4) and *Feng Chi* (GB 20). If there is nasal congestion, add *Ying Xiang* (LI 20). If there is consti-

pation, add *Yang Ling Quan* (GB 34), *Zhi Gou* (TB 6), *Tian Shu* (St 25), and *Da Chang Shu* (Bl 25).

3. LIVER DEPRESSION QI STAGNATION

SIGNS & SYMPTOMS: Emotional depression, pronounced vexation, irascibility, non-freely flowing urination or uneasily flowing urination, and rib-side and abdominal distention and fullness. The tongue is red with thin or thin, yellow fur, and the pulse is bowstring.

TREATMENT PRINCIPLES: Course and disinhibit the qi mechanism, free the flow and disinhibit urination

REPRESENTATIVE FORMULA: Modified *Chen Xiang San* (Aquilaria Powder)

Chen Xiang (Aquilariae Agallochae, Lignum), 1-3g
Chen Pi (Citri Reticulatae, Pericarpium), 6-9g
Dang Gui (Angelicae Sinensis, Radix), 9g
Wang Bu Liu Xing (Vaccariae Segetalis, Semen), 9g
Dong Gua Zi (Benincasae Hispidae, Semen), 9g
Hua Shi (Talcum), 9-15g

MODIFICATIONS: To rectify the qi even more strongly, add *Xiang Fu* (Cyperi Rotundi, Rhizoma), *Yu Jin* (Curcumae, Tuber), and *Wu Yao* (Linderae Strychnifoliae, Radix).

ACUMOXIBUSTION: Needle *Tai Chong* (Liv 3), *He Gu* (LI 4), *Zhong Ji* (CV 3), *Yin Ling Quan* (Sp 9), and *Pang Guang Shu* (Bl 28).

MODIFICATIONS: If there is rib-side and abdominal distention, add *Zhang Men* (Liv 13) and *Zhong Wan* (CV 12). If depression has transformed heat, add *Xing Jian* (Liv 2) and *Yang Ling Quan* (GB 34).

4. URINARY NETWORK VESSEL OBSTRUCTION & BLOCKAGE

SIGNS & SYMPTOMS: Dribbling and dripping urination, a possibly fine urine stream or complete blockage, and lower abdominal distention and pain. The tongue is purple and dark and the pulse is choppy.

TREATMENT PRINCIPLES: Move stasis and scatter nodulation, free the flow and move the water passageways

REPRESENTATIVE FORMULA: *Dai Di Dang Wan* (Substitute Resistance Pills)

Dang Gui Wei (Angelicae Sinensis, Extremitas Radicis), 6-9g
Chuan Shan Jia (Manitis Pentadactylis, Squama), 6-9g
Tao Ren (Pruni Persicae, Semen), 6-9g
Mang Xiao (Mirabilitum), 3-9g

MODIFICATIONS: To increase the quickening of the blood and dispelling of stasis, add *Hong Hua* (Carthami Tinctorii, Flos) and *Niu Xi* (Achyranthis Bidentatae, Radix). If enduring disease has resulted in damage to the qi and blood with a lusterless facial complexion, add *Huang Qi* (Astragali Membranacei, Radix) and *Dan Shen* (Salviae Miltiorrhizae, Radix) and replace *Dang Gui Wei* with *Dang Gui* (Angelicae Sinensis, Radix). If there are stones within the urinary passageways, one can add *Jin Qian Cao* (Lysimachiae, Herba), *Hai Jin Sha* (Lygodii Japonici, Spora), *Dong Gua Zi* (Benincasae Hispidae, Semen), *Qu Mai* (Dianthi, Herba), and *Bian Xu* (Polygoni Avicularis, Herba) to free the flow of strangury and disinhibit urination. If there is hematuria, add powdered *San Qi* (Notoginseng, Radix) and *Hu Po* (Succinum).

ACUMOXIBUSTION: *Xue Hai* (Sp 10), *He Gu* (LI 4), *San Yin Jiao* (Sp 6), *Yin Ling Quan* (Sp 9), *Zhong Ji* (CV 3), and *Guan Yuan* (CV 4).

MODIFICATIONS: If there is accompanying liver depression, add *Tai Chong* (Liv 3) and *Yang Ling Quan* (GB 34).

5. CENTRAL QI INSUFFICIENCY

SIGNS & SYMPTOMS: Lower abdominal sagging and distention, a desire to urinate but inability to discharge the urine, possible scanty amount which exits uneasily, lassitude of the spirit, devitalized eating and drinking, shortness of breath, disinclination to speak and/or a weak voice. The tongue is pale with thin fur and the pulse is fine and weak.

TREATMENT PRINCIPLES: Upbear the clear and downbear the turbid, move the qi and disinhibit water

REPRESENTATIVE FORMULA: Modified *Bu Zhong Yi Qi Tang* (Supplement the Center & Boost the Qi Decoction) plus *Chun Ze Tang* (Spring Pond Decoction)

Dang Shen (Codonopsitis Pilosulae, Radix), 9g
Huang Qi (Astragali Membranacei, Radix), 9g
Bai Zhu (Atractylodis Macrocephalae, Rhizoma), 9g
mix-fried *Gan Cao* (Glycyrrhizae Uralensis, Radix), 3-4.5g
Dang Gui (Angelicae Sinensis, Radix), 9g
Chen Pi (Citri Reticulatae, Pericarpium), 9g
Sheng Ma (Cimicifugae, Rhizoma), 3-4.5g
Chai Hu (Bupleuri, Radix), 3-4.5g
Rou Gui (Cinnamomi Cassiae, Cortex), 1.5-3g
Fu Ling (Poriae Cocos, Sclerotium), 3g

MODIFICATIONS: If there is qi and yin vacuity, add *E Jiao* (Asini, Gelatinum Corii) and *Hua Shi* (Talcum).

ACUMOXIBUSTION: Moxibustion *Bai Hui* (GV 20), *Qi Hai* (CV 6), *Guan Yuan* (CV 4), and *Zu San Li* (St 36). Needle *Zhong Ji* (CV 3) and *Yin Ling Quan* (Sp 9).

6. KIDNEY YANG VACUITY

SIGNS & SYMPTOMS: Non-freely flowing urination which dribbles and drips but does not exit with force, a somber white facial complexion, lassitude of the spirit, fatigue, fear of cold, low back and knee chill, pain, and lack of strength. The tongue is pale with white fur, and the pulse is deep, fine, and forceless.

TREATMENT PRINCIPLES: Warm yang and boost the qi, supplement the kidney and disinhibit urination

REPRESENTATIVE FORMULA: Modified *Shen Qi Wan* (Kidney Qi Pills)

Rou Gui (Cinnamomi Cassiae, Cortex), 1.5-3g
Fu Zi (Aconiti Carmichaeli, Radix Lateralis Praeparatus), 9g
Shu Di Huang (Rehmanniae Glutinosae, cooked Radix), 12g
Shan Zhu Yu (Corni Officinalis, Fructus), 4.5g
Mu Dan Pi (Moutan, Cortex Radicis), 6-9g
Shan Yao (Dioscoreae Oppositae, Radix), 12g

Ze Xie (Alismatis Orientalis, Rhizoma), 12g
Niu Xi (Achyranthis Bidentatae, Radix), 9g
Du Zhong (Eucommiae Ulmoidis, Cortex), 9g
Yin Yang Huo (Epimedii, Herba), 9g
Tu Si Zi (Cuscutae Chinensis, Semen), 9g

MODIFICATIONS: If the patient develops asthma, add *Dong Chong Xia Cao* (Cordyceps Sinensis) and *Ren Shen* (Panacis Ginseng, Radix). For nausea, add *Huo Xiang* (Agastachis Seu Pogostemi, Herba) and *Hou Po* (Magnoliae Officinalis, Cortex). If there is edema after the bladder's qi transformation has been restored, one can then add water-disinhibiting, dampness-percolating medicinals, such as *Che Qian Zi* (Plantaginis, Semen), *Fu Ling* (Poriae Cocos, Sclerotium), and *Zhu Ling* (Polypori Umbellati, Sclerotium).

ACUMOXIBUSTION: Moxibustion *Guan Yuan* (CV 4), *Qi Hai* (CV 6), *Shen Men* (Bl 23), *Ming Men* (GV 4), and *Pang Guang Shu* (Bl 28) and needle *San Yin Jiao* (Sp 6) and *Yin Ling Quan* (Sp 9).

7. KIDNEY YIN VACUITY

SIGNS & SYMPTOMS: Occasional desire to urinate but inability to urinate, dry throat, heart vexation, heat in the hearts of the hands and feet (or hands, feet, and heart). The tongue is bright red and the pulse is fine and fast.

TREATMENT PRINCIPLES: Enrich and supplement kidney yin in order to disinhibit urination

REPRESENTATIVE FORMULA: Modified *Liu Wei Di Huang Wan* (Six Flavors Rehmannia Pills) plus *Zhu Ling Tang* (Polyporus Decoction)

Sheng Di Huang (Rehmanniae Glutinosae, uncooked Radix), 12-15g
Shan Yao (Dioscoreae Oppositae, Radix), 12g
E Jiao (Asini, Gelatinum Corii), 9g
Shan Zhu Yu (Corni Officinalis, Fructus), 4.5g
Fu Ling (Poriae Cocos, Sclerotium), 3g
Ze Xie (Alismatis Orientalis, Rhizoma), 3g
Hua Shi (Talcum), 5g
Mu Dan Pi (Moutan, Cortex Radicis), 6g

MODIFICATIONS: If there is heat in the lower burner,

add *Zhi Mu* (Anemarrhenae Asphodeloidis, Rhizoma) and *Huang Bai* (Phellodendri, Cortex) to clear heat and strengthen yin. If there is qi and yin vacuity, add *Huang Qi* (Astragali Membranacei, Radix) and *Dang Shen* (Codonopsitis Pilosulae, Radix).

ACUMOXIBUSTION: Needle *Tai Xi* (Ki 3), *San Yin Jiao* (Sp 6), *Yin Ling Quan* (Sp 9), *Guan Yuan* (CV 4), *Shen Shu* (Bl 23), and *Pang Guang Shu* (Bl 28).

MODIFICATIONS: If there is qi and yin vacuity, add *Zu San Li* (St 36) and *Pi Shu* (Bl 20).

REPRESENTATIVE CASE HISTORIES

Case history 1: Jian, a 71 year-old female farmer[1]

Jian's first visit was on February 9, 1939 [sic]. Four years before this visit, she was caught in the rain and soaked while working in a field. Soon after this, she developed urinary impediment. She could not urinate at all and had to be catheterized every day. She was treated for six months in two different hospitals. All tests were negative. Western pharmaceuticals did not help; instead, they exacerbated the problem. She saw many famous Chinese medical doctors and took prescriptions for the interior and the exterior. In fact, she had tried over 300 different formulas. Then she stopped all treatment for one year except for catheterization three times a day. After being catheterized, she could work as normal. Her appetite, stool, and sleep were normal and her tongue and pulse seemed normal.

Su Wen, Chapter 17, "*Mai Yao Jing Wei Lun* (Treatise on the Essentials of the Finest Essence of the Pulse)" gives directions on taking the pulse when it appears normal in a patient who obviously has a disease:

> The palpation of the pulse should be taken in the calm dawn[2] when the yang qi has not yet been stirred, the yin qi has not yet been completely dispersed, and food and drink have not yet been consumed. At this time, the channel qi is not overactive, the qi of the network vessels is in harmony, and the qi and blood have not been disturbed. In this situation, the pulse condition can be diagnosed effectively.

Following this advice, Jian was asked to come in the next day, February 10, at 5:00 A.M. to have her pulse examined. Both the inch and bar were normal, but the cubit pulse was bowstring and big. At 6:10 A.M., she was not catheterized and her lower abdomen became very distended. Then her pulse was examined again. This time all three pulses on the left were bowstring and replete and all three pulses on the right were soggy and slow. She was then catheterized, her abdominal distention disappeared, and her abdomen appeared flat. After an hour, her pulse was examined again and it was normal.

Ling Shu, Chapter 35, "*Zhang Lun* (Treatise on Distention)" states, "In the distention of the urinary bladder, the patient will have distention and fullness in the lower abdomen and urine blockage with qi stagnation." When Jian was not catheterized, she experienced urine blockage with qi stagnation with severe distention in the lower abdomen. Jian's doctor analyzed her disease as follows: The disease started with Jian getting wet in the rain and contracting dampness. These damp evils had moved to the liver and kidney. The liver channel runs in the genital area and can cause bladder dysfunction, leading to blockage of urine. With this in mind, the treatment principle must be to disperse liver qi. However, Jian's doctor decided it was important to treat her kidney at the same time. Jian was given modified *Da Chai Hu Tang* (Major Bupleurum Decoction): *Chai Hu* (Bupleuri, Radix), 24g, *Ban Xia* (Pinelliae Ternatae, Rhizoma), 15g, stir-fried *Zhi Shi* (Citri Aurantii, Fructus Immaturus), 12g, *Huang Qin* (Scutellariae Baicalensis, Radix), 9g, *Bai Shao* (Paeoniae Lactiflorae, Radix Albus), 9g, *Da Huang* (Rhei, Radix Et Rhizoma), 6g, *Sheng Jiang* (Zingiberis Officinalis, uncooked Rhizoma), 15g, and *Da Zao* (Zizyphi Jujubae, Fructus), 6 pieces.

The amounts above were for one day and were given in two doses. The first dose was given at 10:00 A.M. and her 2:00 P.M. catheterization was interrupted. The second dose was given at 6:00 P.M. The next day, February 11, the patient reported that, after taking the prescription, she had felt the desire to urinate at 2:00 P.M., but that she could not pass any urine. However, at 2:30 P.M., she had only slight distention in her abdomen. She was then catheterized. After the

second dose (given at 6:00 P.M.), she had dribbling urine at 11:00 P.M., but, because she wanted to go to sleep, she was catheterized again. On February 12, she was given the same prescription and reported that, by 2:00 P.M., she could urinate a little but the flow was not strong. At 4:00 P.M., she urinated again. By evening, she had urinated a small amount 4-5 times.

On February 13, the doctor decided to modify the formula. Because the condition had begun with a cold damp contraction, the formula needed medicinals that strongly fortify the spleen and eliminate dampness. He removed some medicinals and added *Fu Ling* (Poriae Cocos, Sclerotium), *Bai Zhu* (Atractylodis Macrocephalae, Rhizoma), and mix-fried *Gan Cao* (Glycyrrhizae Uralensis, Radix). The new prescription read: *Fu Ling* (Poriae Cocos, Sclerotium), 12g, *Bai Zhu* (Atractylodis Macrocephalae, Rhizoma), 12g, *Bai Shao* (Paeoniae Lactiflorae, Radix Albus), 9g, mix-fried *Gan Cao* (Glycyrrhizae Uralensis, Radix), 6g, *Sheng Jiang* (Zingiberis Officinalis, uncooked Rhizoma), 9g, and *Da Zao* (Zizyphi Jujubae, Fructus), 6 pieces.

On February 15, after taking this formula one time, Jian's urination became freely flowing. She urinated four or five times a day, her stool returned to normal, her appetite and sleep were good, and her tongue and pulse returned to normal. She took this prescription five more days and staged a complete recovery. A checkup a few months later found her in good health. She lived until she was 80 years old.

Case history 2 from Dr. Wei Li's private practice: Annie, an 18 year-old female

Annie had two operations for a recurring mucoid tumor on her spine. After the second operation, she developed urinary retention. She retained 200-250ml of urine in her bladder after urinating and had to be catheterized four times a day. Her condition did not improve over the next two months. Annie was very pale and fatigued. She had nausea and lack of appetite. Her tongue was big, puffy, and pale with thick, white fur, and her pulse was forceless, bowstring, deep, and fine. Dr. Li's principle pattern identification was yang vacuity. Therefore, she prescribed modified *Suo Quan Wan* (Shut the Sluice Pills): *Yi Zhi Ren* (Alpiniae Oxyphyllae, Fructus), 9g, *Wu Yao*

(Linderae Strychnifoliae, Radix), 9g, *Shan Yao* (Dioscoreae Oppositae, Radix), 9g, *Dang Shen* (Codonopsitis Pilosulae, Radix), 15g, *Bai Shao* (Paeoniae Lactiflorae, Radix Albus), 9g, *Bai Zhu* (Atractylodis Macrocephalae, Rhizoma), 9g, *Gan Jiang* (Zingiberis Officinalis, dry Rhizoma), 9g, and *Dang Gui* (Angelicae Sinensis, Radix), 7g. Annie took this formula for one week, and her urine retention decreased to 50ml. She took it for one more week and her Western doctor found that catheterization was no longer necessary, her urination was normal.

Case history 3: Li, a 78 year-old male[3]

Li's first visit was in 1980. He had suffered with hypertension and urinary incontinence for a few years. Suddenly, about one year prior to this visit, Li was unable to urinate and had to go to an emergency room. The Western medical diagnosis was benign prostate hypertrophy. Surgery was contraindicated because of Li's hypertension and he had to be catheterized. The doctors tried many types of treatment short of surgery without success. Li was catheterized for a year. During this time, he had several urinary tract infections, and he had to be admitted to the hospital a few times because of them. Li appeared skinny and depressed. His tongue had thick, yellow fur, and his pulse was bowstring and replete. Dr. Hui's pattern identification for Li was damp heat in the lower burner with qi stagnation and blood stasis. His treatment principles were to course the liver and rectify the qi, soften the hard and scatter nodulation. His prescription consisted of: *Chai Hu* (Bupleuri, Radix), 10g, *Niu Xi* (Achyranthis Bidentatae, Radix), 10g, uncooked *Mu Li* (Ostreae, Concha), 30g, *Dan Shen* (Salviae Miltiorrhizae, Radix), 15g, *Dang Gui* (Angelicae Sinensis, Radix), 15g, *Chi Shao* (Paeoniae Lactiflorae, Radix Rubrus), 15g, *Hai Fu Shi* (Pumice), 15g, *Hai Zao* (Sargassii, Herba), 15g, *Kun Bu* (Algae, Thallus), 15g, *Xia Ku Cao* (Prunellae Vulgaris, Spica), 15g, *Xuan Shen* (Scrophulariae Ningpoensis, Radix), 15g, powdered *Chuan Bei Mu* (Fritillariae Cirrhosae, Bulbus), 3g, *Shen Jing Zi*,[4] 5 pieces wrapped in *Long Yan Rou* (Euphoriae Longanae, Arillus).[5] After two days on this formula, Li felt better and had the urge to urinate. After three

days, he did not need the catheter. After five days, his urine flowed easily. This made Li feel confident. He took another five day dose on his own and completely recovered. Follow-ups showed no recurrence.

Case history 4: Ren, an 84 year-old male[6]

Ren's first visit was in 1980. He experienced urinary difficulty for 2-3 years. The symptoms had worsened in the few months before his visit. Ren experienced painful distention in his bladder, it was difficult for him to urinate, and he would dribble. He needed 2-3 hours to empty his bladder. The Western medical diagnosis was benign prostate hypertrophy. The Western doctor told Ren that his only option was surgery, but Ren wanted to avoid an operation and decided to try Chinese medicine. Therefore, Dr. Hui's treatment strategy was to course the liver and rectify the qi, soften the hard and scatter nodulation. His formula consisted of: *Chai Hu* (Bupleuri, Radix), 15g, *Dang Gui* (Angelicae Sinensis, Radix), 15g, *Dan Shen* (Salviae Miltiorrhizae, Radix), 15g, *Chi Shao* (Paeoniae Lactiflorae, Radix Rubrus), 15g, *Hai Fu Shi* (Pumice), 15g, *Hai Zao* (Sargassii, Herba), 15g, *Kun Bu* (Algae, Thallus), 15g, *Xia Ku Cao* (Prunellae Vulgaris, Spica), 15g, *Xuan Shen* (Scrophulariae Ningpoensis, Radix), 15g, uncooked *Mu Li* (Ostreae, Concha), 30g, powdered *Chuan Bei Mu* (Fritillariae Cirrhosae, Bulbus), 3g, *Niu Xi* (Achyranthis Bidentatae, Radix), 10g, and *Shen Jing Zi*, 5 pieces wrapped in *Long Yan Rou* (Euphoriae Longanae, Arillus). After Ren took this formula, he reported that he actually felt the medicinals go directly to his prostate and stimulate it. In other words, he felt movement in his prostate. The same day, his urine flowed easily. He took this prescription for five days and completely recovered. A two month follow-up showed no recurrence. He returned home and later visited Japan without a problem.

CLINICAL TIPS

1. Although dribbling urinary block can be quite complicated because of its many causes and the involvement of several viscera, this disease is located in the urinary bladder, one of the bowels. Since the bowels transport and do not store, the treatment strategy is to free the flow of the bladder. There are

OBJECTIVE	STRATEGY	MEDICINALS
Warm the Interior	**1. Eliminate cold (replete)**	*Gan Jiang* (Zingiberis Officinalis, dry Rhizoma), *Gao Liang Jiang* (Alpiniae Officinari, Rhizoma), etc.
	2. Invigorate kidney yang	*Shu Fu Zi* ((Aconiti Carmichaeli, Radix Lateralis Praeparatus), *Rou Gui* (Cinnamomi Cassiae, Cortex), etc.
	3. Supplement kidney yang	*Du Zhong* (Eucommiae Ulimoidis, Cortex), *Yin Yang Huo* (Epimedii, Herba), etc.
	4. Supplement kidney yin to generate kidney yang and qi	*Shu Di Huang* (Rehmanniae Glutinosae, cooked Radix), *Shan Yao* (Discoreae Opposiate, Radix), etc.

Chart 3.2. Warming the interior

many theories on how to accomplish this, but they all promote one of two strategies: 1) directly freeing the flow of the bladder or 2) indirectly freeing the flow of the bladder.

To directly free the flow of the bladder, one can make the patient sneeze, vomit, or both. This opens the upper orifices and lung. A freely flowing lung promotes the opening of the lower orifices to disinhibit urination. This is "making a hole in a teapot's lid." Another method to directly free the flow of the bladder is to catheterize. Catheterization lets the urine directly flow out. The ancient Chinese would use hollow goose quills or green onions for this purpose.

The indirect method treats the root cause and then frees the flow of the bladder. For example, if the root is blood stasis, one quickens the blood and then promotes sneezing or vomiting. For qi stagnation, one disperses the qi and promotes sneezing or vomiting. For qi vacuity, one supplements the qi and promotes sneezing or vomiting.

2. Although dribbling urinary block is located in the bladder, it can be due to either a kidney or bladder dysfunction. With bladder dysfunction, the kidney is sending water to the bladder, but the bladder cannot discharge it. The use of water-disinhibiting, dampness-percolating medicinals in that case just increases the amount of urine. It does not help the bladder excrete the urine. In this case, one must rectify the

failure in bladder qi transformation. When the disease is due to kidney insufficiency, one may use water-disinhibiting, dampness-percolating medicinals along with supplementing medicinals to increase the flow of water to the bladder.

3. In the case of kidney yang vacuity, one must use four principles to warm the interior: 1) dispel cold, 2) invigorate (kidney) yang, 3) supplement the kidneys, and 4) supplement yin in order to engender yin and qi. This last principle is based on the sayings, "The doctor who knows how to supplement yang must know how to gain yang from supplementing yin," and, "The doctor who knows how to supplement yin must know how to gain yin from supplementing yang." The original qi of the kidneys is a product of kidney yang steaming kidney yin, and both must be supplemented. See Chart 3.2 above.

ENDNOTES

[1] Qing He-chen, *Dong Dai Ming Lao Shong Yi Ling Zheng Hui Cui (A Collection of the Clinical Experience of Famous Modern Doctors)*, Guagdong Science Technology Publishing Company, Guanzhou, 1991, p. 76
[2] The "calm dawn" is the period between 3-5 A.M.
[3] Qing He-chen, *op. cit.*, p. 418
[4] The authors have not been able to find the Latin name of this medicinal.
[5] *Shen Jing Zi* is very small and can stick on the teeth. To avoid this, one can take the pit out of *Long Yan Rou* (Arillus Euphoriae Longanae), insert *Shen Jing Zi* in it and wrap the *Long Yan Rou* around it. One can also put *Shen Jing Zi* in a capsule.
[6] Qing He-chen,. *op. cit.*, p. 419

CHAPTER 4
BLOODY URINE

In bloody urine, there is blood in the urine unaccompanied by pain. In current practice in China, this includes blood that is visible only under a microscope as well as blood that is visible to the naked eye. Bloody urine and blood strangury are different diseases. The principal distinguishing symptom is pain. In blood strangury, there is pain. In bloody urine, there is no pain. Bloody strangury is usually caused by external evils, while bloody urine is caused by internal causes or internal damage. (See Chart 4.1.) In Western medical terms, blood strangury is usually diagnosed as a type of urinary tract infection. Bloody urine is a result of what might be designated autoimmune diseases, benign tumors, or aplastic anemia among other diseases in Western medicine.

DISEASE CAUSES & MECHANISMS

Heat is often the cause of bloody urine. *Su Wen*, Chapter 37, "*Qi Jue Lun* (Treatise on Qi Reversal)" states, "When heat…is transferred into the urinary bladder, the patient will have bloody urine." The *Jin Gui Yao Lue*, Chapter 11, "On the Pulse, Patterns & Treatment of Wind & Cold in the Five Viscera" states, "When heat invades the lower burner, bloody urine, urinary disturbance, and constipation result." However, although heat is the principal cause of bloody urine, there are other causes as well. *Su Wen*, Chapter 44, "*Wei Lun* (Treatise on Wilting)" states, "When one has excessive sorrow, the pericardium will be damaged and the yang energy will stir inside to cause bloody urine."

	SYMPTOMS	CAUSE
Bloody urine (*Niao Xue*)	Blood in the urine without pain	Internal damage
Bloody strangury (*Xue Lin*)	Blood in the urine with pain	External evils

Chart 4.1. Differences between bloody urine & blood strangury

The *Zheng Zhi Zhun Shen* (*Standard Differentiation of Patterns & Treatments*) provides a fuller account of the causes of bloody urine:

> Heat in the five viscera can move into the blood and cause bloody urine. Lung (metal) is the mother of the kidney (water) and one of its functions is to harmonize water. If the lung has stagnant heat, this can transmit down to the urinary bladder and cause bloody urine. Spleen damp can transform heat and this heat can affect the kidney and urinary bladder and damage the yin channels, causing bloody urine. The liver stores the blood. If there is dysfunction in the storage of blood, this blood can leak into the urine passage [urethra] and cause bloody urine.

Bloody urine can be acute or chronic. Acute bloody urine is usually caused by heat or trauma (knocks and falls or crushing). Chronic bloody urine can be replete or vacuous. Replete chronic bloody urine is usually caused by heat or blood stasis.[1] Symptoms include bright red or purple blood in the urine, purple tongue, strong pulse, etc. Vacuous chronic bloody urine is usually caused by visceral vacuity. Symptoms include pale, pink blood in the urine, a pale facial complexion, a pale tongue, a forceless pulse, etc. (See Chart 4.2.)

TREATMENT BASED ON PATTERN IDENTIFICATION

REPLETE BLOODY URINE

1. DAMP HEAT POURING DOWNWARD

SIGNS & SYMPTOMS: Acute onset of the disease, fresh red blood in the urine, hot urination, urinary frequency, possible low-grade fever, and lower abdominal distention and pain. The tongue fur is thin and slimy or slimy and yellow, while the pulse is slippery and rapid.

TREATMENT PRINCIPLES: Clear heat and disinhibit dampness, cool the blood and stop bleeding

REPRESENTATIVE FORMULA: Modified *Xiao Ji Yin Zi* (Cephalanoplos Beverage)

Xiao Ji (Cephalanoplos Segeti, Herba), 30g
Ou Jie (Nelumbinis Nuciferae, Nodus Rhizomatis), 9-15g
Pu Huang (Typhae, Pollen), 6-9g
Sheng Di Huang (Rehmanniae Glutinosae, uncooked Radix), 15-30g
Dan Zhu Ye (Lophatheri Gracilis, Herba), 3-9g
Mu Dan Pi (Moutan, Cortex Radicis), 6g
stir-fried *Zhi Zi* (Gardeniae Jasminoidis, Fructus), 9-15g
stir-fried *Dang Gui* (Angelicae Sinensis, Radix), 9g
Che Qian Zi (Plantaginis, Semen), 30g
Gan Cao Xiao (Glycyrrhizae Uralensis, Radix Tenuis), 3-6g
Tong Cao (Tetrapanacis Papyriferi, Medulla), 30g

MODIFICATIONS: If there is aversion to cold and fever, add *Jin Yin Hua* (Lonicerae Japonicae, Flos) and *Lian Qiao* (Forsythiae Suspensae, Fructus). If there is

	TIME	TYPES	CAUSES	SYMPTOMS
Bloody Urine	**Acute**	Replete	Heat Knocks and falls Crushing	Bright red or purple blood, purple tongue, forceful pulse, etc.
	Chronic	Replete	Heat Knocks and falls Crushing Blood stasis	Bright red or purple blood, purple tongue, forceful pulse, etc.
		Vacuous	Visceral Vacuity	Pale pink blood, pale tongue, forceless pulse, etc.

Chart 4.2. Types of bloody urine

a somber facial complexion and lack of strength, add *Shan Yao* (Dioscoreae Oppositae, Radix), *Fu Ling* (Poriae Cocos, Sclerotium), *Xian He Cao* (Agrimoniae Pilosae, Herba), and *Da Zao* (Zizyphi Jujubae, Fructus) to fortify the spleen and supplement the qi. If the tongue is red, the mouth is dry, and the lips are parched, add *Xuan Shen* (Scrophulariae Ningpoensis, Radix), *Han Lian Cao* (Ecliptae Prostratae, Herba), and *Shi Hu* (Dendrobii, Herba) to clear heat and enrich yin. If there are blood clots in the urine, add *Chuan Niu Xi* (Cyathulae Officinalis, Radix) and *Chi Shao* (Paeoniae Lactiflorae, Radix Rubrus). If hematuria is relatively profuse and bleeding will not stop, add *Hua Rui Shi* (Dolomitum), *Shan Cha Hua* (Camelliae Theae, Flos), and *Xue Yu Tan* (Crinis Carbonisatus). If the urination is severely painful, add *Qu Mai* (Dianthi, Herba) and *Bian Xu* (Polygoni Avicularis, Herba). If there is constipation, add *Da Huang* (Rhei, Radix Et Rhizoma).

ACUMOXIBUSTION: Needle *Zhong Ji* (CV 3), *Zu Tong Gu* (Bl 66), *Pang Guang Shu* (Bl 28), *Jin Men* (Bl 63), and *Yin Xi* (Ht 6).

MODIFICATIONS: If there is fever, add *Da Zhui* (GV 14). If there is constipation, add *Shang Ju Xu* (St 37). For painful urination, add *Zhong Feng* (Liv 4).

2. HEART FIRE SHIFTED DOWNWARD

SIGNS & SYMPTOMS: Fresh red blood in the urine or reddish urine, heart vexation, restlessness, and sores in the mouth and on the tongue. The pulse is fine and rapid, the tip of the tongue is red or the sides of the tongue are red and cracked.

TREATMENT PRINCIPLES: Clear the heart and drain fire, cool the blood and stop bleeding

REPRESENTATIVE FORMULA: Modified *Dao Chi San* (Abduct the Red Powder)

Sheng Di Huang (Rehmanniae Glutinosae, uncooked Radix), 15-30g
Dan Zhu Ye (Lophatheri Gracilis, Herba), 6-9g
Mu Tong (Akebiae Mutong, Caulis), 3-6g
Gan Cao Xiao (Glycyrrhizae Uralensis, Radix Tenuis), 3-6g

Huang Lian (Coptidis Chinensis, Rhizoma), 3-6g
Huang Qin (Scutellariae Baicalensis, Radix), 9-15g
processed *Da Huang* (Rhei, Radix Et Rhizoma), 6-9g
Che Qian Zi (Plantaginis, Semen), 30g
Mu Dan Pi (Moutan, Cortex Radicis), 6g
Chi Fu Ling (Poriae Cocos, Sclerotium Rubrum), 9-15g
Ze Xie (Alismatis Orientalis, Rhizoma), 9g

MODIFICATIONS: For sores on the mouth and tongue, add *Lian Qiao* (Forsythiae Suspensae, Fructus) and *Huang Lian* (Coptidis Chinensis, Rhizoma). If liver fire tends to be hyperactive with red eyes and a bitter taste in the mouth, add *Long Dan Cao* (Gentianae Longdancao, Radix), *Zhi Zi* (Gardeniae Jasminoidis, Fructus), and *Chai Hu* (Bupleuri, Radix). For insomnia, profuse dreams, and heart vexation, add *Bai Zi Ren* (Biotae Orientalis, Semen) and *Suan Zao Ren* (Zizyphi Spinosae, Semen). For thirst, add *Mai Men Dong* (Ophiopogonis Japonici, Tuber) and *Zhi Mu* (Anemarrhenae Aspheloidis, Rhizoma). If the urine is turbid as well as red due to the small intestine's inability to divide clear from turbid, add *Bei Xie* (Dioscoreae Hypoglaucae, Rhizoma), *Wu Yao* (Linderae Strychnifoliae, Radix), and *Yi Zhi Ren* (Alpiniae Oxyphyllae, Fructus).

ACUMOXIBUSTION: Needle *Zhong Ji* (CV 3), *Shen Men* (Ht 7), *Da Ling* (Per 7), and *San Yin Jiao* (Sp 6).

MODIFICATIONS: For insomnia, add *An Mian* (N-HN-54). For heart vexation, add *Nei Guan* (Per 6).

3. STATIC BLOOD BINDING INTERNALLY

SIGNS & SYMPTOMS: Blood clots in the urine which are colored either red or purple and dark, possible severe low back pain, and a dark facial complexion. The tongue has static speckles or macules and its substance is dark, while its fur is thin.

TREATMENT PRINCIPLES: Attack, precipitate, and expel stasis, quicken the blood and stop bleeding

REPRESENTATIVE FORMULA: Modified *Shao Fu Zhu Yu Tang* (Lower Abdomen Dispel Stasis Decoction)

Pu Huang (Typhae, Pollen), 6-9g

Wu Ling Zhi (Trogopterori Seu Pteromi, Excrementum), 6-9g

Dang Gui (Angelicae Sinensis, Radix), 9g

Chuan Xiong (Ligustici Wallichii, Radix), 30g

Chi Shao (Paeoniae Lactiflorae, Radix Rubrus), 6-9g

Xiao Hui Xiang (Foeniculi Vulgaris, Fructus), 3-6g

Yan Hu Suo (Corydalis Yanhusuo, Rhizoma), 9-15g

Zhi Ke (Citri Aurantii, Fructus), 6-9g

processed *Da Huang* (Rhei, Radix Et Rhizoma), 6-9g

Hua Rui Shi (Dolomitum), 30g

Shan Cha Hua (Camelliae Theae, Flos), 4.5-6g

MODIFICATIONS: If there is low back chill and limb reversal, add *Fu Zi* (Aconiti Carmichaeli, Radix Lateralis Praeparatus), *Gan Jiang* (Zingiberis Officinalis, dry Rhizoma), and/or *Rou Gui* (Cinnamomi Cassiae, Cortex). If one can feel enlargement of the kidney organ by pressing the abdomen, one can add *San Leng* (Sparganii Stoloniferi, Rhizoma) and *E Zhu* (Curcumae Zedoariae, Rhizoma). If low back pain radiates to the genitalia and thighs, one can add *Jin Qian Cao* (Lysimachiae, Herba), *Hai Jin Cao* (Lygodii Japonici, Spora), and *Ji Nei Jin* (Gigeriae Galli, Endothelium Corneum) or *Shi Wei* (Pyrrosiae, Herba), *Qu Mai* (Dianthi, Herba), and *Dong Gua Zi* (Benincasae Hispidae, Semen).

ACUMOXIBUSTION: Needle *Zhong Ji* (CV 3), *Pang Guang Shu* (Bl 28), *He Gu* (LI 4), *Xue Hai* (Sp 10), and *San Yin Jiao* (Sp 6).

MODIFICATIONS: For fatigue and lack of strength, add *Qi Hai* (CV 6) and *Zu San Li* (St 36). For chest and rib-side distention and fullness, add *Tai Chong* (Liv 3) and *Zhang Men* (Liv 13). If there is simultaneous uterine bleeding, add *Gui Lai* (St 29). If there is cold congelation, add moxibustion at *Ming Men* (GV 4).

VACUITY BLOODY URINE

1. LIVER-KIDNEY YIN VACUITY

SIGNS & SYMPTOMS: Bloody urine accompanied by dizziness, blurred vision, low back and knee soreness and limpness, tinnitus, and malar flushing. The tongue is red and the pulse is fine and rapid.

TREATMENT PRINCIPLES: Nourish the liver and boost the kidney, enrich yin and clear fire

REPRESENTATIVE FORMULA: Modified *Zhi Bai Di Huang Wan* (Anemarrhena & Phellodendron Rehmannia Pills) plus *Er Zhi Wan* (Two Ultimates Pills)

Huang Bai (Phellodendri, Cortex), 9g

Zhi Mu (Anemarrhenae Aspheloidis, Rhizoma), 9-15g

Sheng Di Huang (Rehmanniae Glutinosae, uncooked Radix), 15-30g

Shan Yao (Dioscoreae Oppositae, Radix), 9-15g

Mu Dan Pi (Moutan, Cortex Radicis), 6-9g

Ze Xie (Alismatis Orientalis, Rhizoma), 9g

Nu Zhen Zi (Ligustri Lucidi, Fructus), 9-15g

Han Lian Cao (Ecliptae Prostratae, Herba), 15-30g

Gou Qi Zi (Lycii Chinensis, Fructus), 9g

Shan Zhu Yu (Corni Officinalis, Fructus), 6g

MODIFICATIONS: If there is low-grade fever, add *Yin Chai Hu* (Stellariae Dichotomae, Radix) and *Di Gu Pi* (Lycii Chinensis, Cortex Radicis). If liver yang tends to be hyperactive, add *Gou Teng* (Uncariae Cum Uncis, Ramulus), *Shi Jue Ming* (Haliotidis, Concha), and *Ci Shi* (Magnetitum). If there is simultaneous liver fire, add *Dan Zhu Ye* (Lophatheri Gracilis, Herba), *Mu Tong* (Akebiae Mutong, Caulis), and uncooked *Gan Cao* (Glycyrrhizae Uralensis, Radix). If yin vacuity reaches yang and the *chong* and *ren* lose their regulation, add *Yin Yang Huo* (Epimedii, Herba), *Xian Mao* (Curculiginis Orchioidis, Rhizoma), and *Dang Gui* (Angelicae Sinensis, Radix). For scanty, dark-colored urination, add *Fu Ling* (Poriae Cocos, Sclerotium) and *Che Qian Zi* (Plantaginis, Semen). For insomnia, add *Ye Jiao Teng* (Polygoni Multiflori, Caulis), *Suan Zao Ren* (Zizyphi Spinosae, Semen), and *Yuan Zhi* (Polygalae Tenuifoliae, Radix).

ACUMOXIBUSTION: Needle *Guan Yuan* (CV 4), *Tai Xi* (Ki 3), *San Yin Jiao* (Sp 6), and *Yong Quan* (Ki 1).

MODIFICATIONS: If there is low back and knee soreness and limpness, add *Shen Shu* (Bl 23) and *Pang Guang Shu* (Bl 28). If there is seminal emission, add *Zhi Shi* (Bl 52). If there is sore throat, add *Zhao Hai* (Ki 6).

2. CENTRAL QI FALLING DOWNWARD

SIGNS & SYMPTOMS: Enduring hematuria, a somber white facial complexion, lassitude of the spirit, weakness of the extremities, lack of strength, torpid intake, and shortness of breath. The tongue tends to be pale and the fur is thin.

TREATMENT PRINCIPLES: Supplement the center, upbear and lift, boost the qi and stop bleeding

REPRESENTATIVE FORMULA: Modified *Bu Zhong Yi Qi Tang* (Supplement the Center & Boost the Qi Decoction)

mix-fried *Huang Qi* (Astragali Membranacei, Radix), 15-30g
Tai Zi Shen (Pseudostellariae Heterophyllae, Radix), 15-30g
Chai Hu (Bupleuri, Radix), 3-5g
Sheng Ma (Cimicifugae, Rhizoma), 3-5g
Dang Gui (Angelicae Sinensis, Radix), 9g
Bai Zhu (Atractylodis Macrocephalae, Rhizoma), 9g
Chen Pi (Citri Reticulatae, Pericarpium), 6-9g
mix-fried *Gan Cao* (Glycyrrhizae Uralensis, Radix), 3-6g
Shan Yao (Dioscoreae Oppositae, Radix), 9g
Sheng Di Huang (Rehmanniae Glutinosae, uncooked Radix), 9-15g
Da Zao (Ziziphi Jujubae, Fructus), 10 pieces
Xian He Cao (Agrimoniae Pilosae, Herba), 30g

MODIFICATIONS: If spleen vacuity has caused kidney vacuity, add *Tu Si Zi* (Cuscutae Chinensis, Semen), *Wu Wei Zi* (Schisandrae Chinensis, Fructus), *Du Zhong* (Eucommiae Ulmoidis, Cortex), and *Niu Xi* (Achyranthis Bidentatae, Radix). If enduring hematuria is incessant and there are no signs of heat, add *Mu Li* (Ostreae, Concha) and *Long Gu* (Draconis, Os), *Jin Ying Zi* (Rosae Laevigatae, Fructus) and *Qian Shi* (Euryalis Ferocis, Semen), or *Chi Shi Zhi* (Hallyositum Rubrum) and *Wu Wei Zi* (Schisandrae Chinensis, Fructus).

ACUMOXIBUSTION: Needle *Qi Xue* (Ki 13), *Qi Hai* (CV 6), *Zhong Ji* (CV 3), *Xue Hai* (Sp 10), and *San Yin Jiao* (Sp 6).

MODIFICATIONS: For heart palpitations due to simul-

taneous heart blood vacuity, add *Nei Guan* (Per 6) and *Tai Yuan* (Lu 9). For impaired memory, add *Si Shen Cong* (M-HN-1). For insomnia, add *Shen Men* (Ht 7). For shortness of breath and disinclination to speak and/or a weak voice, add *Shan Zhong* (CV 17).

REPRESENTATIVE CASE HISTORIES

Case history 1: Yu, a 12 year-old boy[2]

Yu's first visit with Dr. Qi was on Sept. 13, 1976. A month prior to this visit, he contracted tonsillitis. A short time later, his low back became sore and his urine turned abnormally yellow. A urinalysis was abnormal and the Western medical diagnosis was acute nephritis. He was given antibiotics for a month but failed to improve. His tonsils remained swollen and painful, his low back remained sore, he had heat in the five hearts, and his urine turned deep yellow. His tongue had a red tip with white fur, and his pulse was deep and slippery. His urinalysis showed protein at 2+ and RBCs at 20-30. Based on these signs and symptoms, Dr. Qi's pattern identification was damp heat damaging the bladder channel. His treatment strategy was to clear heat and eliminate dampness, resolve toxins and cool the blood. His prescription consisted of: *Bai Hua She She Cao* (Oldenlandiae Diffusae, Herba Cum Radice), 50g, *Da Huang* (Rhei, Radix Et Rhizoma), 5g, *Xiao Ji* (Cephalanoplos Segeti, Herba), 50g, *Sheng Di* (Rehmanniae Glutinosae, uncooked Radix), 20g, *Bian Xu* (Polygoni Avicularis, Herba), 20g, *Qu Mai* (Dianthi, Herba), 20g, *Mu Tong* (Akebiae Mutong, Caulis), 10g, *Che Qian Zi* (Plantaginis, Semen), 15g, *Bai Mao Gen* (Imperatae Cylindricae, Rhizoma), 50g, and *Gan Cao* (Glycyrrhizae Uralensis, Radix), 10g. Yu took this formula for 12 days. His tonsils returned to normal and his urinalysis improved to protein 1+ and RBCs 1-2. Everything else was normal and all his other tests were negative. Yu continued on this formula for a few more days to consolidate the therapeutic results.

Case history 2: Tom, a 59 year-old male worker[3]

Tom's first visit to Dr. Qi was on Nov. 29, 1973. He was diagnosed with chronic nephritis. When this was treated, he felt better but his urine often had a slight amount of protein in it. Three days before Tom's first visit, he overexerted himself. His low back became sore, he became fatigued, his lower abdomen became painful, and he had bloody urine. Sometimes he would have purple blood clots passing through his urethra. Often these would obstruct his urethra before entirely passing through, but he had no stones. Examination found Tom's left lower abdomen mildly painful and worse with pressure. He had lower back pain, heat in the five hearts, a dry mouth, and lack of appetite. His tongue was purple with no fur, and his pulse was slippery, deep, and strong. Urinalysis showed protein at 3+, while the RBCs filled the microscopic field.

Based on all this, Dr. Qi thought stagnant heat in the lower burner was forcing blood out of the channels resulting in bloody urine. Therefore, he prescribed the following formula: *Tao Ren* (Pruni Persicae, Semen), 20g, *Da Huang* (Rhei, Radix Et Rhizoma), 10g, *Gui Zhi* (Cinnamomi Cassiae, Ramulus), 15g, *Chi Shao* (Paeoniae Lactiflorae, Radix Rubrus), 20g, *Gan Cao* (Glycyrrhizae Uralensis, Radix), 10g, *Sheng Di* (Rehmanniae Glutinosae, uncooked Radix), 30g, *Bai Mao Gen* (Imperatae Cylindricae, Rhizoma), 50g, *Xiao Ji* (Cephalanoplos Segeti, Herba), 30g, and carbonized *Ce Bai Ye* (Biotae Orientalis, Cacumen), 20g.

On Dec. 3, Tom's second visit, he had taken the formula for three days. There was no more visible blood in his urine, his urinary tract was not obstructed, and he had two formed bowel movements per day. Urinalysis showed RBCs at about 50 and protein at 3+. Tom still had heat in the five hearts and low back soreness. His left lower abdomen was also still mildly painful. His tongue was purple and moist and his pulse was deep and slippery but less forceful. These signs indicated that the heat, though still present, had reduced. Dr. Qi then modified the formula as follows: *Tao Ren* (Pruni Persicae, Semen), 20g, *Da Huang* (Rhei, Radix Et Rhizoma), 7.5g, *Gui Zhi* (Cinnamomi Cassiae, Ramulus), 15g, *Sheng Di* (Rehmanniae Glutinosae, uncooked Radix), 30g, carbonized *Ce Bai Ye* (Biotae Orientalis, Cacumen), 20g, *Bai Mao Gen* (Imperatae Cylindricae, Rhizoma), 50g, *Xiao Ji* (Cephalanoplos Segetis, Herba), 30g, carbonized *Pu Huang* (Typhae, Pollen),

15g, and *Gan Cao* (Glycyrrhizae Uralensis, Radix), 10g.

On Dec. 17, Tom's third visit, he had taken the modified formula for three days. His urine was pale yellow, his lower abdominal pain was gone, and his stool had returned to normal. Urinalysis showed protein at 2+ and RBCs at 15-20. His tongue was red with thin, white fur, and his pulse was deep and slippery. This indicated that the heat was clearing. Dr. Qi then removed *Gui Zhi* and added *Gou Qi Zi* (Lycii Chinensis, Fructus) to supplement kidney yin. The new formula consisted of: *Tao Ren* (Pruni Persicae, Semen), 20g, *Da Huang* (Rhei, Radix Et Rhizoma), 7.5g, carbonized *Ce Bai Ye* (Biotae Orientalis, Cacumen), 15g, carbonized *Pu Huang* (Typhae, Pollen), 15g, *Bai Mao Gen* (Imperatae Cylindricae, Rhizoma), 50g, *Sheng Di* (Rehmanniae Glutinosae, uncooked Radix), 30g, *Xiao Ji* (Cephalanoplos Segeti, Herba), 20g, *Gou Qi Zi* (Lycii Chinensis, Fructus), 20g, and *Gan Cao* (Glycyrrhizae Uralensis, Radix), 10g.

On Dec. 24, Tom's fourth visit, he had taken this formula for nine days. His stools were slightly loose but he had only minimal abdominal discomfort. Urinalysis showed protein +/- and RBCs negative. The patient's tongue color was normal with thin fur, and his pulse was deep. Dr. Qi decided to discontinue the use of medicinals and simply monitor him. On Tom's follow-up visit, there was no recurrence.

Case history 3: Du, a 12 year-old girl[4]

Dr. Qi first saw Du on Oct. 14, 1972 after she was confined to a hospital. One month previous to this, both her lower legs broke out in purple spots. After the spots dissipated, she had abdominal pain and distention, bloody stools a few times, and even vomited blood a few times. The doctors gave her *Yun Nan Bai Yao* (Yunnan White Medicine, a ready-made hemostatic medicine) and the bleeding stopped. But then her low back became painful and she had bloody urine. The Western medical diagnosis was Henoch-Schonlein purpura (*i.e.*, allergic or anaphylactoid purpura). Doctors tried a combination of Chinese medicinals and Western pharmaceuticals but had no success. When Du saw Dr. Qi, she had a pale face with swollen eyelids. She had low back pain, fatigue, heat in the five hearts, and her urine was pink. Her tongue was pale red, and her pulse was bowstring and slippery. Urinalysis showed protein at 2+, with RBCs filling the microscopic field, and WBCs at 10. The pattern identification was heat in the blood aspect. Therefore, the treatment principles were to clear heat, cool the blood, and stop bleeding. Dr. Qi's formula consisted of: *Xiao Ji* (Herba Cephalanoplos Segeti, Herba), 30g, *Pu Huang* (Typhae, Pollen), 15g, *Ou Jie* (Nelumbinis Nuciferae, Nodus Rhizomatis), 20g, *Mu Tong* (Akebiae Mutong, Caulis), 15g, *Hua Shi* (Talcum), 20g, *Sheng Di* (Rehmanniae Glutinosae, uncooked Radix), 30g, *Ce Bai Ye* (Biotae Orientalis, Cacumen), 20g, *Bai Mao Gen* (Imperatae Cylindricae, Rhizoma), 30g, and *Gan Cao* (Glycyrrhizae Uralensis, Radix), 10g.

After taking the formula for six days, Du came back on Oct. 22 with no improvement. Her face was pale, her low back was sore, and her body was weak. Her pulse was bowstring, slippery, deep, and weak. Urinalysis showed protein at 2+, RBCs filling the microscopic field, and WBCs at 2-3. Dr. Qi thought that the strategy of clearing heat and cooling the blood had not succeeded because of Du's extreme qi and yin vacuity. Therefore, he decided to focus on supporting the righteous by supplementing qi and yin with cooling the blood and stanching bleeding only assisting the main strategy. He decided to combine strategies and treat the root and tip at the same time. His formula consisted of: *Huang Qi* (Astragali Membranacei, Radix), 30g, *Shu Di* (Rehmanniae Glutinosae, cooked Radix), 25g, *E Jiao* (Asini, Gelatinum Corii), 15g, *Han Lian Cao* (Ecliptae Prostratae, Herba), 20g, carbonized *Sheng Di* (Rehmanniae Glutinosae, uncooked Radix), 20g, *Xue Yu Tan* (Crinis Carbonisatus), 15g, carbonized *Da Huang* (Rhei, Radix Et Rhizoma), 10g, carbonized *Ce Bai Ye* (Biotae Orientalis, Cacumen), 20g, *Bai Mao Gen* (Imperatae Cylindricae, Rhizoma), 50g, *Xiao Ji* (Cephalanoplos Segeti, Herba), 30g, carbonized *Pu Huang* (Typhae, Pollen), 15g, *Huang Qin* (Scutellariae Baicalensis, Radix), 15g, and *Gan Cao* (Glycyrrhizae Uralensis, Radix), 10g. Du took this formula for six days and her bloody urine improved significantly. Urinalysis showed protein at 1+, RBCs at 2-3, with negative WBCs. Du

continued on this formula for 60 days and had a complete recovery. A follow-up four years later found no recurrence.

Case history 4: Qu, a 25 year-old female[5]

Qu had chronic nephritis for five years. While she frequently had both blood and protein in her urine, typically she had only blood. She tried Western medications with no success. After these, she tried *Lui Wei Di Huang Wan* (Six Flavors Rehmannia Pills) and *Xiao Ji Yin Zi* (Cephalanoplos Drink) to nourish yin and cool blood. This improved her condition for a while, but then there was a recurrence. She tried the same combination again, but it did not work the second time. On the contrary, it seemed to cause difficult urination. Qu was skinny with a dark face. She had dizziness and low back soreness. Her mouth was dry, and she was thirsty without the desire to drink. She also had purple spots on her body. Her tongue was dark red with purple spots, and her pulse was bowstring, thin, and choppy. Urinalysis showed RBCs at 3+ and protein at 1+. Based on these signs and symptoms, Dr. Hou's pattern identification was yin vacuity heat with obstruction in the kidney channel. He thought that the use of *Liu Wei Di Huang Wan* and *Xiao Ji Yin Zi* had relied too heavily on supplementing yin and stanching bleeding without attending to blood stasis. His treatment strategy was to nourish kidney yin, clear heat, and dispel blood stasis. Dr. Hou's formula consisted of: *Sheng Di* (Rehmanniae Glutinosae, uncooked Radix), 12g, *Shu Di* (Rehmanniae Glutinosae, cooked Radix), 12g, *Han Lian Cao* (Ecliptae Prostratae, Herba), 15g, *He Shou Wu* (Polygoni Multiflori, Radix), 9g, *Huang Bai* (Phellodendri, Cortex), 9g, *Da Ji* (Cirsii Japonici, Herba Seu Radix), 15g, *Xiao Ji* (Cephalanoplos Segeti, Herba), 15g, *Chi Shao* (Paeoniae Lactiflorae, Radix Rubrus), 9g, *Mu Dan Pi* (Moutan, Cortex Radicis), 6g, *Tao Ren* (Pruni Persicae, Semen), 9g, *Dang Gui* (Angelicae Sinensis, Radix), 9g, *Hong Hua* (Carthami Tinctorii, Flos), 4.5g, *Bie Jia* (Amydae Sinensis, Carapax), 15g, *Niu Xi* (Achyranthis Bidentatae, Radix), 15g, uncooked *Gan Cao* (Glycyrrhizae Uralensis, Radix), 6g, and *Yi Mu Cao* (Leonuri Heterophylli, Herba), 12g. Qu took this prescription for seven days and her urine became disinhibited. Her urinalysis showed RBCs at

1+ with negative protein. Hence, Dr. Hou removed *Mu Dan Pi* and Qu continued on the modified formula for 14 more days, after which her urine returned to normal.

ENDNOTES

[1] This is often a tumor.
[2] Qing He-chen, *op. cit.*, p. 46
[3] *Ibid.*, p. 47
[4] *Ibid.*, p. 49
[5] *Ibid.*, p. 363

CHAPTER 5
WATER SWELLING

Water swelling refers to edema, and many kidney diseases are accompanied by edema. *Ling Shu*, Chapter 57, "*Shui Zhang* (Water Distention)" states:

> In the initiation of water distention, it appears on the eyelids as if one has just awoken from sleep, the *Ren Ying* pulse on the neck pulsates rapidly, the patient coughs frequently, feels cold in the inner side of the thigh, and has water swelling in the leg. If the abdomen expands, then water swelling has been formed. When one presses the swelling site with one's hand and then releases one's hand, the abdomen swells up in the wake of it as if water is trapped inside. These are the symptoms of water swelling.

In the *Jin Gui Yao Lue*, Chapter 14, "On the Pulse, Patterns & Treatment of Water Swelling," it states:

> . . . water swelling can be classified into five categories: wind water,[1] skin water, regular water, stone water, and yellow sweat. Skin water has symptoms of a floating pulse and acute water distention wherein the doctor's finger will disappear in a fold of skin when the skin is pressed. The abdomen is distended as tight as a drum. The patient is not thirsty and has no aversion to cold. Treatment should be diaphoresis. In regular water, there is a deep, slow pulse and wheezing.

In stone water, there is a deep pulse and abdominal distention without wheezing. In yellow sweat, there is a deep, slow pulse, fever, fullness in the chest, and edema in the extremities, head and face. Welling abscesses may appear if the condition lasts a long time.

DISEASE CAUSES & MECHANISMS

Any of the three causes may produce water swelling. These most commonly affect and disrupt the functions of the kidney, spleen, and lung. The kidney is the source of the body's water. The spleen governs the movement and transformation of water in the triple burner, the body's canal system. The lung is the floodgate to these canals. These viscera must work in a harmonious and coordinated way to control water. When there is kidney yang vacuity, the kidney's qi transformation is inhibited, water is not transformed, and thus accumulates. If there is spleen yang vacuity, water is not governed. Instead, it may flow randomly and also accumulate. Since the lung is the canal's floodgate, if the lung is open, the canal's water passageways (*i.e.*, the triple burner) are open and water can flow properly. If external evils such as cold and dampness block the lung, this compromises the triple burner. In that case, evils close the floodgate, water becomes uncontrolled and flows out of the canals, and, therefore, floods. In fact, water swelling is also called flooding.

Treatment based on pattern identification

1. Wind cold invading the lungs

Signs & symptoms: Sudden onset of edema which first appears on the eyelids and then spreads to the rest of the body, aversion to wind and chill, possible fever, aching joints, and scanty urination. There is white tongue fur and a floating pulse.

Treatment principles: Course and dispel wind cold, diffuse the lung and disinhibit water

Representative formula: *Ma Huang Jia Zhu Tang* (Ephedra Plus Atractylodis Decoction)

Ma Huang (Ephedrae, Herba), 9g
Gui Zhi (Cinnamomi Cassiae, Ramulus), 6g
Xing Ren (Pruni Armeniacae, Semen), 9g
Bai Zhu (Atractylodis Macrocephalae, Rhizoma), 9g
mix-fried *Gan Cao* (Glycyrrhizae Uralensis, Radix), 3g

Modifications: For severe edema, add *Fu Ling Pi* (Poriae Cocos, Cortex Sclerotii) and *Da Fu Pi* (Arecae Catechu, Pericarpium). For severe aversion to cold and fever, add *Zi Su Ye* (Perillae Frutescentis, Folium) and *Qiang Huo* (Notopterygii, Rhizoma Et Radix). For coughing and wheezing, add *Ting Li Zi* (Tinglizi, Semen) and *Zi Su Zi* (Perillae Frutescentis, Fructus).

Acumoxibustion: Needle *Lie Que* (Lu 7), *He Gu* (LI 4), *Feng Men* (Bl 12), *Fei Shu* (Bl 13), *San Yin Jiao* (Sp 6), and *Yin Ling Quan* (Sp 9).

Modifications: For aversion to wind with spontaneous perspiration, add *Zu San Li* (St 36) and *Pi Shu* (Bl 20). If exterior evils have been resolved and dispelled and edema remains, add *Shui Fen* (CV 9) and *Shui Dao* (St 28). For fever, add *Da Zhui* (GV 14).

2. Wind heat harassing the lungs

Signs & symptoms: Sudden onset of edema in the eyelids and face, fever, aversion to wind, sweating, thirst, cough, red, sore throat, and scanty urination. The tongue has a red tip and edges with thin, yellow fur, and the pulse is floating and fast.

Treatment principles: Diffuse the lung, clear heat, and disinhibit water

Representative formula: *Yue Bi Jia Zhu Tang* (Maidservant from Yue Plus Atractylodes Decoction)

Ma Huang (Ephedrae, Herba), 9g
Bai Zhu (Atractylodis Macrocephalae, Rhizoma), 12g
Shi Gao (Gypsum Fibrosum), 24g
Sheng Jiang (Zingiberis Officinalis, uncooked Rhizoma), 6g
Gan Cao (Glycyrrhizae Uralensis, Radix), 3-6g
Da Zao (Zizyphi Jujubae, Fructus), 4 pieces

Modifications: For severe heat, add *Lian Qiao* (Forsythiae Suspensae, Fructus), *Bai Mao Gen* (Imperatae Cylindricae, Rhizoma), and *Chi Xiao Dou* (Phaseoli Calcarati, Semen). For sore throat, add *Ban Lan Gen* (Isatidis Seu Baphicacanthi, Radix), *She Gan* (Belamcandae Chinensis, Rhizoma), and *Niu Bang Zi* (Arctii Lappae, Fructus). For exuberant heat damaging fluids, add *Lu Gen* (Phragmitis Communis, Rhizoma) and *Zhi Mu* (Anemarrhenae Aspheloidis, Rhizoma).

Acumoxibustion: *Feng Men* (Bl 12), *Fei Shu* (Bl 13), *He Gu* (LI 4), *Chi Ze* (Lu 5), *Wei Yang* (Bl 39), and *Yu Ji* (Lu 10).

Modifications: For high fever, add *Da Zhui* (GV 14). For sore throat, prick *Shao Shang* (Lu 11) to bleed. For vexatious heat and scanty urination, add *San Jiao Shu* (Bl 22).

3. Water dampness encumbering the spleen

Signs & symptoms: Edema starting from the limbs

with a slow onset and long course, more severe edema in the abdominal region and limbs, heavy body, fatigue, chest oppression, nausea, a bland taste in the mouth, and scanty urination. There is slimy, white tongue fur and a deep, moderate (*i.e.*, slightly slow) or deep, slow pulse.

TREATMENT PRINCIPLES: Fortify the spleen and transform dampness, free the flow of yang and disinhibit water

REPRESENTATIVE FORMULA: Modified *Wei Ling Tang* (Stomach Poria Decoction) plus *Wu Pi Yin* (Five Peels Beverage)

Cang Zhu (Atractylodis, Rhizoma), 6g
Hou Po (Magnoliae Officinalis, Cortex), 6g
Chen Pi (Citri Reticulatae, Pericarpium), 9g
mix-fried *Gan Cao* (Glycyrrhizae Uralensis, Radix), 3g
Sheng Jiang Pi (Zingiberis Officinalis, Cortex Rhizomatis), 9g
Sang Bai Pi (Mori Albi, Cortex Radicis), 9g
Da Fu Pi (Arecae Catechu, Pericarpium), 9g
Fu Ling Pi (Poriae Cocos, Cortex Sclerotii), 9g
Ze Xie (Alismatis Orientalis, Rhizoma), 9g

MODIFICATIONS: In case of severe edema accompanied by coughing and panting, add *Ma Huang* (Ephedrae, Herba), *Xing Ren* (Pruni Armeniacae, Semen), and *Ting Li Zi* (Tinglizi, Semen). If there is diarrhea, add *Zhu Ling* (Polypori Umbellati, Sclerotium). For abdominal distention, add *Bai Dou Kou* (Cardamomi, Fructus). For a cold sensation in the abdomen, add *Gan Jiang* (Zingiberis Officinalis, dry Rhizoma) and *Rou Dou Kou* (Myristicae Fragrantis, Semen). If there is nausea and vomiting, add *Huo Xiang* (Agastachis Seu Pogostemi, Herba) and *Ban Xia* (Pinelliae Ternatae, Rhizoma).

ACUMOXIBUSTION: Needle *Pi Shu* (Bl 20), *Yin Ling Quan* (Sp 9), *Zhong Wan* (CV 12), *Shui Fen* (CV 9), *Zu San Li* (St 36), and *San Jiao Shu* (Bl 22).

MODIFICATIONS: If there is severe edema accompanied by coughing and panting or hasty breathing, add *Fei Shu* (Bl 13) and *Lie Que* (Lu 7). If there is torpid intake, add *Jian Li* (CV 11).

4. DAMP HEAT ACCUMULATION

SIGNS & SYMPTOMS: Edema of the face and feet or generalized edema in severe cases, moist, shiny skin, chest oppression, epigastric glomus and fullness, reduced food intake, irritability, thirst, dark, scanty urination, and constipation. There is slimy, yellow tongue fur and a soft, rapid, deep, rapid, or slippery, rapid pulse.

TREATMENT PRINCIPLES: Clear heat and eliminate dampness, disinhibit water and disperse swelling

REPRESENTATIVE FORMULA: Modified *Tong Ling San* (Akebia & Poria Powder)

Mu Tong (Akebiae Mutong, Caulis), 5g
Fu Ling (Poriae Cocos, Sclerotium), 9g
Zhu Ling (Polypori Umbellati, Sclerotium), 9g
Bai Zhu (Atractylodis Macrocephalae, Rhizoma), 6g
Ze Xie (Alismatis Orientalis, Rhizoma), 9g
Che Qian Zi (Plantaginis, Semen), 9g
Yin Chen Hao (Artemsiae Yinchenhao, Herba), 6g
Huang Bai (Phellodendri, Cortex), 6g

MODIFICATIONS: If there is turbid urine and low back pain, subtract *Bai Zhu* and add *Bei Xie* (Dioscoreae Hypoglaucae, Rhizoma) and *Ku Shen* (Sophorae Flavescentis, Radix). For heat damaging the network vessels with bloody urine, add *Bai Mao Gen* (Imperatae Cylindricae, Rhizoma), *Sheng Di Huang* (Rehmanniae Glutinosae, uncooked Radix), and *Xiao Ji* (Cephalanoplos Segeti, Herba).

ACUMOXIBUSTION: Needle *Yin Ling Quan* (Sp 9), *Shui Fen* (CV 9), *Wei Yang* (Bl 39), *He Gu* (LI 4), *Qu Chi* (LI 11), and *San Jiao Shu* (Bl 22).

MODIFICATIONS: For hematuria, add *Xue Hai* (Sp 10) and *San Yin Jiao* (Sp 6).

5. SPLEEN QI VACUITY

SIGNS & SYMPTOMS: Facial edema or edema of the four extremities which comes and goes for no apparent reason, a sallow yellow or somber white facial complexion, reduced appetite, fatigue, lack of strength, possible shortness of breath, abdominal distention and fullness, lack of warmth in the four limbs, and loose stools. The tongue is pale with glossy, white fur and the pulse is deep and slow or deep and weak.

TREATMENT PRINCIPLES: Fortify the spleen and supplement the qi, transform dampness and disperse swelling

REPRESENTATIVE FORMULA: Modified *Shen Ling Bai Zhu San* (Ginseng, Poria & Atractylodes Powder)

Bai Bian Dou (Dolichoris Lablab, Semen), 9g
Shan Yao (Dioscoreae Oppositae, Radix), 9g
Bai Zhu (Atractylodis Macrocephalae, Rhizoma), 12g
Fu Ling (Poriae Cocos, Sclerotium), 12g
Dang Shen (Codonopsitis Pilosulae, Radix), 6g
Lian Zi (Nelumbinis Nuciferae, Semen), 6g
Jie Geng (Platycodi Grandiflori, Radix), 3g
Yi Yi Ren (Coicis Lachryma-jobi, Semen), 12g
Sha Ren (Amomi, Fructus), 6g
mix-fried *Gan Cao* (Glycyrrhizae Uralensis, Radix), 3g

MODIFICATIONS: For severe edema, subtract *Jie Geng* and *Gan Cao* and add *Huang Qi* (Astragali Membranacei, Radix) and *Zhu Ling* (Polypori Umbellati, Sclerotium). For severe damp encumbrance, add *Hou Po* (Magnoliae Officinalis, Cortex) and *Cang Zhu* (Atractylodis, Rhizoma). For abdominal distention, add *Mu Xiang* (Auklandiae Lappae, Radix) and *Chen Pi* (Citri Reticulatae, Pericarpium).

ACUMOXIBUSTION: Needle *Pi Shu* (Bl 20), *Wei Shu* (Bl 21), *Zu San Li* (St 36), *Yin Ling Quan* (Sp 9), and *San Yin Jiao* (Sp 6).

MODIFICATIONS: If there is abdominal distention, add *Zhong Wan* (CV 12). If there are loose stools, add *Tian Shu* (St 25) and *Da Chang Shu* (Bl 25).

6. SPLEEN YANG VACUITY

SIGNS & SYMPTOMS: Enduring edema which is worse below the waist, pitting edema, lassitude of the spirit, lack of strength, fear of cold, chilled limbs, torpid intake, a preference for warm drinks and foods,

no thirst, loose stools, and scanty but clear urination. The tongue is pale with thin, white, watery, glossy fur and a deep, slow pulse.

TREATMENT PRINCIPLES: Warm and move spleen yang, transform dampness and disinhibit water

REPRESENTATIVE FORMULA: *Shi Pi Yin* (Bolster the Spleen Beverage)

Hou Po (Magnoliae Officinalis, Cortex), 6g
Bai Zhu (Atractylodis Macrocephalae, Rhizoma), 9g
Mu Gua (Chaenomlis Lagenariae, Fructus), 6g
Mu Xiang (Auklandiae Lappae, Radix), 3g
Cao Dou Kou (Alpiniae Katsumadai, Semen), 9g
Bin Lan (Arecae Catechu, Semen), 9g
Fu Zi (Aconiti Carmichaeli, Radix Lateralis Praeparatus), 3g
Fu Ling (Poriae Cocos, Sclerotium), 12g
Gan Jiang (Zingiberis Officinalis, dry Rhizoma), 3g
mix-fried *Gan Cao* (Glycyrrhizae Uralensis, Radix), 3g

MODIFICATIONS: If there is severe edema, add *Ze Xie* (Alismatis Orientalis, Rhizoma), *Zhu Ling* (Polypori Umbellati, Sclerotium), and *Gui Zhi* (Cinnamomi Cassiae, Ramulus). For fatigue and lack of strength, add *Huang Qi* (Astragali Membranacei, Radix) and *Dang Shen* (Codonopsitis Pilosulae, Radix).

ACUMOXIBUSTION: Moxibustion *Pi Shu* (Bl 20), *Wei Shu* (Bl 21), *Shen Shu* (Bl 23), *Ming Men* (GV 4), and *San Jiao Shu* (Bl 22), and needle *Yin Ling Quan* (Sp 9) and *Zu San Li* (St 36).

MODIFICATIONS: If there is dizziness and vertigo and vomiting of clear, thin drool, moxibustion *Guan Yuan* (CV 4). For heart palpitations and panting, add *Xin Shu* (Bl 15) and *Fei Shu* (Bl 13). For profuse, clear, thin abnormal vaginal discharge, add *Dai Mai* (GB 26). For abdominal distention, add *Gong Sun* (Sp 4) and *Zhong Wan* (CV 12).

7. KIDNEY YANG VACUITY

SIGNS & SYMPTOMS: Generalized pitting edema which is more severe below the waist, tinnitus, dizziness, a pale or somber white facial complexion, heart palpitations, shortness of breath, low back and knee aching and chilliness, clear, scanty urination, nocturia, chilled limbs, fatigue, aversion to cold, and decreased sexual desire. The tongue is pale and swollen with white fur and the pulse is deep and fine or deep, slow, and forceless.

TREATMENT PRINCIPLES: Warm the kidney and transform the qi, disinhibit water and disperse swelling

REPRESENTATIVE FORMULA: *Zhen Wu Tang* (True Warrior Decoction)

Fu Zi (Aconiti Carmichaeli, Radix Lateralis Praeparatus), 3g
Fu Ling (Poriae Cocos, Sclerotium), 9g
Bai Shao (Paeoniae Lactiflorae, Radix Albus), 6g
Bai Zhu (Atractylodis Macrocephalae, Rhizoma), 9g
Sheng Jiang (Zingiberis Officinalis, uncooked Rhizoma), 9g

MODIFICATIONS: To strengthen this formula's warming and invigoration of yang, add *Hu Lu Ba* (Trigonellae Foeni-graeci, Semen), *Ba Ji Tian* (Morindae Officinalis, Radix), and *Rou Gui* (Cinnamomi Cassiae, Cortex). If there is panting and wheezing and hasty breathing, add *Ting Li Zi* (Tinglizi, Semen). If there is concomitant blood stasis, add *Dan Shen* (Salviae Miltiorrhizae, Radix), *Yi Mu Cao* (Leonuri Heterophylli, Herba), *Hong Hua* (Carthami Tinctorii, Flos), mix-fried *Gan Cao* (Glycyrrhizae Uralensis, Radix), and *Gui Zhi* (Cinnamomi Cassiae, Ramulus). If there is somnolence, decreased awareness, nausea, and the taste or furine in the mouth (a serious, acute condition), add *Da Huang* (Rhei, Radix Et Rhizoma), processed *Ban Xia* (Pinelliae Ternatae, Rhizoma), and *Huang Lian* (Coptidis Chinensis, Rhizoma). If there is simultaneous contraction of external evils, subtract *Bai Shao* and add *Ma Huang* (Ephedrae, Herba), *Xi Xin* (Asari, Herba Cum Radice), and *Gan Cao* (Glycyrrhizae Uralensis, Radix).

ACUMOXIBUSTION: Moxibustion *Shen Shu* (Bl 23), *Pi Shu* (Bl 20), *Guan Yuan* (CV 4), *Qi Hai* (CV 6), *Shui Fen* (CV 9), and *Fu Liu* (Ki 7).

MODIFICATIONS: For edematous swelling of the feet, add needling at *Zu Lin Qi* (GB 41) and *Shang Qiu* (Sp 5).

REPRESENTATIVE CASE HISTORIES

Case history of Dr. He Ren-chen: Zuo, a 20 year-old male[2]

Zuo's first visit was on Sept. 19, 1963. He had severe water swelling (*i.e.*, pitting edema). His abdomen was as big as a pregnant woman's, his face was so swollen his cheeks drooped, and his weight had gone up to 80.5 kilograms. He could only urinate once or twice a day with very scanty urine. Zuo was in a lethargic state, his skin was pale, he had loose stools, he had no desire to drink water, and he had insomnia. His tongue fur was glossy and slimy, and his pulse was deep and slow. Dr. He used a formula containing the following: *Fu Ling* (Poriae Cocos, Sclerotium), 12g, *Da Fu Pi* (Arecae Catechu, Pericarpium), 12g, *Bai Zhu* (Atractylodis Macrocephalae, Rhizoma), 12g, *Mu Gua* (Chaenomelis Lagenariae, Fructus), 12g, *Hou Po* (Magnoliae Officinalis, Cortex), 12g, *Zhu Ling* (Polypori Umbellati, Sclerotium), 12g, *Ze Xie* (Alismatis Orientalis, Rhizoma), 12g, *Che Qian Zi* (Plantaginis, Semen), 12g, *Chen Pi* (Citri Reticulatae, Pericarpium), 12g, *Qian Niu Zi* (Pharbitidis, Semen), 9g, *Mu Xiang* (Aucklandiae Lappae, Radix), 9g, *Shu Fu Zi* (Aconiti Carmichaeli, processed Radix Lateralis Praeparatus), 6g, *Cao Dou Kou* (Alpiniae Katsumadai, Semen), 6g, *Gan Jiang* (Zingiberis Officinalis, dry Rhizoma), 6g, *Gan Cao* (Glycyrrhizae Uralensis, Radix), 3g, and *Dong Gua Pi* (Benincasae Hispidae, Pericarpium), 30g. Along with the above, Dr. He prescribed three pills of *Jin Gui Shen Qi Wan* (*Golden Cabinet* Kidney Qi Pills), twice a day. Zuo was in the hospital for 105 days. All his edema dissipated, his weight dropped to 55 kilograms, his urination and defecation returned to normal, his insomnia disappeared, and his appetite and spirits were good. He was discharged, and a checkup one year later showed no recurrence.

Case history of Dr. He Ren-chen: Jiao, a 45 year-old male[3]

Jiao's first visit was on June 21, 1963. He had blood in his stool and was admitted to a hospital. In the hospital, he was given Western medical treatment that had stopped the bleeding, but then Jiao's abdomen, legs, and feet started to swell. He could only urinate 2-3 times a day with yellow and very scanty urination. He was given additional Western medical treatment for 19 days, but his swelling increased day by day. On July 11, he was diagnosed with ascites caused by cirrhosis of the liver. On July 13, he went to Dr. He in the Chinese medical department. At that point in time, Jiao's abdomen and four extremities were very swollen. He had a pale facial complexion, lack of appetite, very scanty urination, and difficulty walking. His pulse was deep, fine, and weak. Dr. He's principal pattern identification was spleen-kidney yang vacuity. He reasoned that, since the liver stores the blood and the kidney is the mother of the liver, this was a case of a disease of the mother affecting the child. Furthermore, concurrent liver depression qi stagnation resulted in the liver invading the spleen, thus compromising spleen yang and its ability to govern the blood. Spleen yang vacuity had resulted first in bleeding and then in water swelling. Therefore, Dr. He's treatment strategy was to warm and supplement the spleen and kidney, course the liver and resolve depression, move the qi and eliminate dampness. His prescription consisted of: *Fu Ling* (Poriae Cocos, Sclerotium), 12g, *Mu Gua* (Chaenomelis Lagenariae, Fructus), 12g, *Bai Zhu* (Atractylodis Macrocephalae, Rhizoma), 12g, *Hou Po* (Magnoliac Officinalis, Cortex), 12g, *Ze Xie* (Alismatis Orientalis, Rhizoma), 12g, *Zhu Ling* (Polypori Umbellati, Sclerotium), 12g, *Chen Pi* (Citri Reticulatae, Pericarpium), 9g, *Cao Dou Kou* (Alpiniae Katsumadai, Semen), 9g, *Gan Jiang* (Zingiberis Officinalis, dry Rhizoma), 9g, *Gan Cao* (Glycyrrhizae Uralensis, Radix), 3g, *Shu Fu Zi* (Aconiti Carmichaeli, processed Radix Lateralis Praeparatus), 3g, *Hong Ren Shen* (Panacis Ginseng, Radix Rubrus), 6g, *Huang Qi* (Astragali Membranacei, Radix), 30g, *Dong Gua Pi* (Benincasae Hispidae, Pericarpium), 30g, and *Bai Shao* (Paeoniae Lactiflorae, Radix Albus), 15g. Along with this formula, Dr. He prescribed two pills of *Jin Gui Shen Qi Wan* (*Golden Cabinet* Kidney Qi Pills) three times a day. In the evening, after Jiao's first dose of the formula, he passed a large amount of urine five times. His abdominal swelling and the edema in his legs reduced. Jiao took the formula for 30 days, and reported that he felt better every day. After taking 216 pills of *Jin Gui Shen Qi Wan*, Jiao's water swelling completely dissipated. His appetite and energy were good, and after a few months with no recurrence, he went back to his job.

Case history of Dr. He Ren-chen: Wang, a 46 year-old female[4]

Wang was diagnosed with chronic nephritis on Nov. 12, 1974. She received Western medical treatment in a hospital for three months but her condition only worsened. By Feb. 17, 1975, her face, legs, and feet were severely swollen. Her abdomen looked like a drum and felt like a stone. It was so big that she could not sit up. She had difficulty urinating and was constipated. Her pulse was fine, deep, and weak. Dr. He identified this patient's pattern as spleen-kidney vacuity with cold. He thought that Wang had been sick for so long her true qi was consumed and there was an urgent need to warm and supplement the spleen and kidney, expel cold and eliminate dampness. Her case was very serious, she was near death, and even Dr. He felt there was little hope. However, he decided to try the following prescription: *Fu Ling* (Poriae Cocos, Sclerotium), 24g, *Che Qian Zi* (Plantaginis, Semen), 24g, *Bai Zhu* (Atractylodis Macrocephalae, Rhizoma), 9g, *Mu Xiang* (Aucklandiae Lappae, Radix), 9g, *Hou Po* (Magnoliae Officinalis, Cortex), 9g, *Ze Xie* (Alismatis Orientalis, Rhizoma), 9g, *Cao Dou Kou* (Alpiniae Katsumadai, Semen), 6g, *Gan Jiang* (Zingiberis Officinalis, dry Rhizoma), 6g, *Shu Fu Zi* (Aconiti Carmichaeli, processed Radix Lateralis Praeparatus), 6g, *Gan Cao* (Glycyrrhizae Uralensis, Radix), 6g, *Da Fu Pi* (Arecae Catechu, Pericarpium), 12g, and *Bai Tong Shen* (Panacis Ginseng, Radix) prepared with white sugar, 12g. After two doses of these medicinals, the water swelling and all of her other symptoms were much improved. After four doses, Wang could sit up and had more of an appetite. After one week, the edema had completely dissipated and Wang resumed her normal activities. Although her appetite was back to normal, she still had slight pain in her epigastrium. So Dr. He added nine grams of *Ban Xia* (Pinelliae Ternatae, Rhizoma) to the prescription.[5]

Case history from Dr. Wei Li's private practice:
Bob, a 44 year-old male

Bob had been diagnosed with chronic renal failure. For two years prior to visiting Dr. Li, he had edema in both legs. Bob took Western diuretics, but these did not help. He also had severe insomnia and fatigue. His tongue was pale and puffy with thin, white fur, and his pulse was slippery, deep, and weak. Based on this, Dr. Li's pattern identification was spleen-kidney yang vacuity with heart blood vacuity. Her treatment strategy was to warm and strengthen the spleen and kidney, transform water, nourish heart blood, and quiet the spirit. She used modified *Wu Ling San* (Five [Ingredients] Poria Powder): *Fu Ling* (Poriae Cocos, Sclerotium), 9g, *Zhu Ling* (Polypori Umbellati, Sclerotium), 9g, *Ze Xie* (Alismatis Orientalis, Rhizoma), 9g, *Gui Zhi* (Cinnamomi Cassiae, Ramulus), 9g, *Bai Zhu* (Atractylodis Macrocephalae, Rhizoma), 9g, *Yi Mu Cao* (Leonuri Heterophylli, Herba), 9g, *He Huan Pi* (Albizziae Julibrissinis, Cortex), 9g, *Ye Jiao Teng* (Polygoni Multiflori, Caulis), 9g, *Suan Sao Ren* (Zizyphi Spinosae, Semen), 9g, *Sheng Jiang* (Zingiberis Officinalis, uncooked Rhizoma), 5g, *Shan Zha* (Crataegi, Fructus), 6g, *Che Qian Zi* (Plantaginis, Semen), 9g, and *Dong Chong Xia Cao* (Cordyceps Sinensis), 5g. Bob took this formula and quickly felt improvement in his energy and sleep. His edema went down by half in the first week. After three weeks, his edema was almost completely dissipated.

Case history from Dr. Wei Li's private practice:
Jane, a 67 year-old female

Jane's first visit was in June 1993. Her left leg below the knee had been swollen, red, and painful for two months, but she had no fever. Her Western doctor thought it might be phlebitis, but an MRI proved negative. The doctor prescribed antibiotics, but these had no effect. Jane usually felt hot. At her first visit, her tongue was red and cracked with thick, gray fur. Her pulse was slippery and fast. Dr. Li identified this disease as yang water. Jane had a yin vacuous constitution and tended to feel hot. When heat evils attacked, they joined with internal heat to affect the water passageways, thus creating yang water. The pattern identification was liver-kidney yin vacuity with damp heat in the lower burner and heat in the constructive. Dr. Li used one of her own formulas consisting of: *Chai Hu* (Bupleuri, Radix), 3g, *Zi Cao* (Arnebiae Seu Lithospermi, Radix), 9g, *Mu Dan Pi* (Moutan, Cortex Radicis), 9g, *Chi Shao* (Paeoniae Lactiflorae, Radix Rubrus), 9g, *Dan Shen* (Salviae Miltiorrhizae, Radix), 6g, *Yi Mu Cao* (Leonuri Heterophylli, Herba), 9g, *Ze Lan* (Lycopi Lucidi, Herba), 9g, *Che Qian Zi* (Plantaginis, Semen), 9g, *Qu Mai* (Dianthi, Herba), 9g, *Jin Yin Hua* (Lonicerae Japonicae, Flos), 15g, *Huang Qin* (Scutellariae Baicalensis, Radix), 9g, *Xuan Shen* (Scrophulariae Ningpoensis, Radix), 9g, *Fu Ping* (Lemnae Seu Spirodelae, Herba), 9g, and *Sheng Di Huang* (Rehmanniae Glutinosae, uncooked Radix), 9g. After one week, the edema was 80% reduced. After two weeks, the edema, redness, and pain completely disappeared.

COMMENTARY: When clearing heat, one must always consider the four aspects. In this case, Dr. Li decided the heat was in the constructive because Jane had a red tongue and skin redness. When clearing heat from the constructive, one should also use medicinals to clear the defensive and qi aspects, and one must make sure that the heat does not penetrate into the deeper blood aspect. Clearing the defensive and qi aspects is like opening the lid of a bottle to let heat out. For this purpose, Dr. Li chose *Jin Yin Hua* and *Huang Qin*. One must also use medicinals that clear blood aspect heat to prevent the heat from penetrating the blood aspect. For this, Dr. Li chose *Zi Cao, Xuan Shen, Dan Shen, Mu Dan Pi, Chi Shao,* and *Sheng Di Huang. Xuan Shen* and *Sheng Di Huang* nourish liver and kidney yin as well as clear heat, thus serving two functions. A small dosage of *Chai Hu* was used to course the liver and resolve depression. *Chai Hu* courses the liver, but when there is concomitant yin vacuity, one should not use a large dose of it as it may plunder the yin. *Yi Mu Cao* and *Ze Lan* quicken the blood and dispel stasis as well as disinhibit urination. *Che Qian Zi* and *Qu Mai* disperse water swelling by precolating dampness. *Fu Ping* is an acrid, cool, exterior-resolving medicinal. In this case, yin vacuity was the root. Therefore, Dr. Li nourished yin as well as cleared heat to consolidate the treatment and prevent a recurrence.

CLINICAL TIPS

1. When water swelling is below the waist, one may use medicinals such as *Chi Xiao Dou* (Phaseoli Calcarati, Semen), *Chi Fu Ling* (Poriae Cocos, Sclerotium Rubrum), *Ze Xie* (Alismatis Orientalis, Rhizoma), *Che Qian Zi* (Plantaginis, Semen), *Bei Xie* (Dioscoreae Hypolagucae, Rhizoma), and *Fang Ji* (Stephaniae Tetrandrae, Radix). When water swelling is above the waist, one may use medicinals such as *Zi Su Ye* (Perillae Frutescentis, Folium), *Jing Jie* (Schizonepetae Tenuifoliae, Herba Seu Flos), *Fang Feng* (Ledebouriellae Divaricatae, Radix), and *Qin Jiao* (Gentianae Qinjiao, Radix). If there is yin water swelling, add *Fu Zi* (Aconiti Carmichaeli, Radix Lateralis Praeparatus), *Gan Jiang* (Zingiberis Officinalis, dry Rhizoma), and *Rou Gui* (Cinnamomi Casiae, Cortex). If there is yang water swelling, add *Lian Qiao* (Forsythiae Suspensae, Fructus), *Huang Bai* (Phellodendri, Cortex), and *Huang Qin* (Scutellariae Baicalensis, Radix). After the water swelling has dissipated, one may use *Li Zhong Wan* (Rectify the Center Pills) to supplement the spleen and stomach or *Jin Gui Shen Qi Wan* to warm the life-gate.

2. As stated previously, ancient potters found that a teapot's lid must be made with a hole in it to allow the tea to flow out of the spout unobstructed.[6] The lung is like the hole in the teapot's lid. The true qi consists of the lung's gathering or ancestral qi combined with the grain qi. It is the basic qi of the body and maintains life activity. Lung blockage impedes the production and circulation of this true qi. This is like blocking the hole in the teapot's lid. The tea cannot pour out in an orderly way but spurts at random. In other words, the blockage of true qi in the lung disrupts the orderly circulation of qi and water in the triple burner.

One conception of the triple burner is that it corresponds to areas of the body. The upper burner includes the thoracic cavity and the head, the middle burner generally corresponds to the abdominal cavity, and the lower burner includes lower abdomen, the pelvic cavity, and the legs. Therefore, if water accumulates in the upper burner, there may be swelling of the head and face. If it accumulates in the middle burner, there may be abdominal bloating and distention as well as water swelling. If it accumulates in the lower burner, there may be water swelling of the legs and feet along with problems with the urine and stool.

The initial location of water swelling varies from case to case depending on where the movement and transportation water begins to be disrupted. In some cases, water swelling starts around the eyes first. In others, the abdomen swells first, especially when patients have liver disease. Sometimes, the lower extremities swell first. However, the whole body might also swell at once.

3. Although the lung, spleen, and kidney are the most commonly affected viscera in the case of water swelling, one must pay special attention to the overall yin and yang pattern. *Su Wen*, Chapter 5, "*Yin Yang Ying Xiang Da Lun* (The Great Treatise on the Corresponding Manifestation of Yin and Yang)" states, "Proper diagnosis involves inspecting the appearance and feeling the pulse and first differentiating yin and yang." When differentiating water swelling, one should first distinguish whether the swelling is yin water or yang water, cold or heat, repletion or vacuity in order to choose the appropriate strategies of supplementing or reducing, warming or clearing heat. The importance of this fundamental Chinese medical concept to water swelling cannot be overemphasized.

Zhu Dan-xi described yang water and yin water swelling in the *Dan Xi Xin Fa* (*Dan-xi's Heart Methods*). Yang water is replete and has the following signs and symptoms: edema beginning on the face, fever and chills, cough, sore throat, rough urine with blood, constipation, and abdominal distention. The tongue has slimy fur, and the pulse is rapid. Yang water is a result of internal water dampness and external evils blocking the lung qi. This compromises the water passageways (*i.e.*, the triple burner) and water accumulates.

Yin water is vacuous and has the following signs and

symptoms: edema of the face and instep or edema in the lower extremities first (with pitting), chest oppression, lack of appetite, cold limbs, lassitude, loose stools, scanty urination, a heavy body, and achy lower back. The tongue is swollen with white fur, and the pulse is deep, slow, and weak. Yin water is a result of spleen-kidney qi and yang vacuity. When these viscera are vacuous, their ability to move and transform water is compromised.

Chart 5.1 provides the basic formulas for yin and yang water swelling. Yang water is usually due to an invasion of wind cold, wind heat, or damp heat. However, all of these generate heat. Even yang water wind cold will transform to heat. The root of this condition is the evils present and the focus of the treatment must be on expelling and clearing these evils. In the case of wind heat and wind cold, the wind constrains the lung, compromising lung's func-

tion of diffusing and downbearing. The water passageways are impeded, water accumulates, and this dampness inhibits kidney qi transformation. (Thus both the lung and kidney are involved.) Furthermore, these evils inhibit the triple burner, causing further water accumulation and water swelling. In this case, the water or dampness is secondary to the evils that caused them. Heat is the most important of the evils. Even when external damp heat invades, the key to successful treatment is clearing heat. Wind is second in importance and dampness third in importance.

When wind and heat combine, one must focus on heat. One must stay ahead of the penetration of heat into the four aspects. Heat can move into the deeper aspects quickly, causing toxins and becoming serious. When using medicinals that clear heat, first one must discern the aspect of the heat. For the defensive

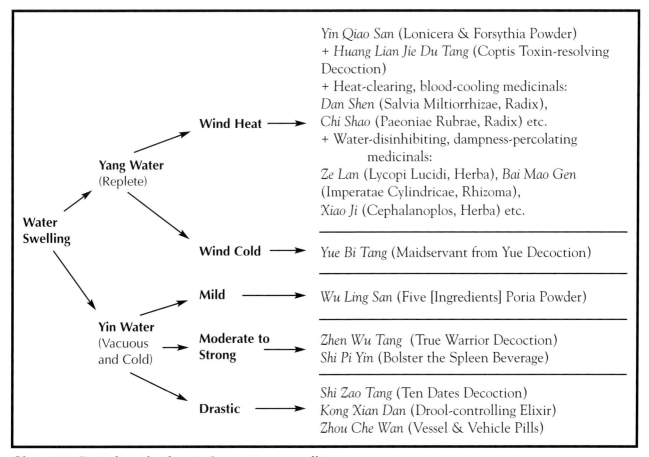

Chart 5.1. Basic formulas for yin & yang water swelling

aspect, one should employ cool, acrid, exterior-resolving medicinals plus certain heat-clearing medicinals, such as *Jin Yin Hua* (Lonicerae Japonicae, Flos), *Lian Qiao* (Forsythiae Suspensae, Fructus), *Ban Lan Gen* (Isatidis Seu Baphicacanthi, Radix), *Da Qing Ye* (Daqingye, Folium), *Niu Bang Zi* (Arctii Lappae, Fructus), etc. For the qi aspect with symptoms and signs such as a big pulse, high fever, profuse sweating, and great thirst, one should use heat-clearing medicinals, such as *Huang Lian* (Coptidis Chinensis, Rhizoma), *Huang Qin* (Scutellariae Baicalensis, Radix), *Huang Bai* (Phellodendri, Cortex), etc. For the yin or blood aspect, when there is blood in the urine, one should add medicinals such as *Mu Dan Pi* (Moutan, Cortex Radicis), *Sheng Di Huang* (Rehmanniae Glutinosae, uncooked Radix), *Chi Shao* (Paeoniae Lactiflorae, Radix Rubrus), and *Dan Shen* (Salviae Miltiorrhizae, Radix).

When dealing with blood in the urine or other bleeding in blood aspect heat, one must be careful to quicken blood and dispel stasis as well as stanching bleeding. Stanching bleeding alone may cause more blood stasis, thus leading to more bleeding. One must also carefully choose medicinals with the proper qi or temperature. In this instance, since one is treating heat, one should use cool blood-stanching medicinals.

Some scholars contend that one should only treat the aspect the heat is in, but, from Dr. Li's clinical experience, heat hardly ever occurs in one aspect alone. By the time the patient is able to buy, prepare, and consume a formula, heat has already penetrated to deeper aspects. Therefore, she feels the best strategy is to treat the next deepest or even two deeper aspects. In other words, if heat is in the defensive, one should clear the qi aspect as well as the defensive aspect. If heat is in the qi aspect, one should clear the constructive and blood aspects as well as qi and defensive aspects. If one can completely and quickly clear heat, the patient can completely recover. If one cannot completely clear heat, the disease may become chronic.

Heat can also stir up wind, and wind can fan heat, causing it to flare up. Thus, while one must focus on heat, one must also address wind to prevent it from fanning the heat. Wind can fan heat even if there is only slight heat or depressive heat, making the heat harder to deal with and even causing the slight heat to flare up. Therefore, one should employ some warm, acrid, exterior-resolving medicinals when coursing wind in water swelling (even in the case of wind heat). Dampness and water are both yin evils associated with cold. Thus when wind constrains the lung, resulting in dampness or water, one must use warm medicinals to overcome the cool nature of the resulting water dampness. When opening the lung to reduce water swelling, one must employ some warm medicinals to overcome the cool nature of water.

This strategy of employing warm medicinals becomes especially important when one is employing many cool or cold medicinals to clear heat. It is necessary to add some warming medicinals to overcome the congealing effects of the cooling medicinals that may reinforce water's cool and congealing tendency. Two strategies are needed here: 1) to get rid of heat and wind, and 2) to get rid of dampness.

Properly used, warming medicinals need not compromise the cooling medicinals' functions. In fact, each may balance the effects of each other. An example of this strategy is in the ancient formula *Ma Huang Lian Qiao Chi Xiao Dou Tang* (Ephedra, Forsythia & Red Bean Decoction): *Ma Huang* (Ephedrae, Herba), *Lian Qiao* (Forsythiae Suspensae, Fructus), *Chi Xiao Dou* (Phaseoli Calcarati, Semen), *Sang Bai Pi* (Mori Albi, Cortex Radicis), *Xing Ren* (Pruni Armeniacae, Semen), *Da Zao* (Zizyphi Jujubae, Fructus), *Sheng Jiang* (Zingiberis Officinalis, uncooked Rhizoma), and *Gan Cao* (Glycyrrhizae Uralensis, Radix). In this formula warm *Ma Huang* balances the effects of cold *Lian Qiao*.

After the water swelling and attendant symptoms have subsided, and one is sure the wind heat is gone, one must harmonize the lung, spleen, and kidney. One should employ some supplementing medicinals to reestablish these viscera's water transforming functions. One should also harmonize the spleen and stomach. This will enable them to more efficiently produce latter heaven qi. Finally, one should secure the kidney's former heaven qi.

In wind cold yang water, cold transforms to heat.

While expelling wind cold, one must still emphasize clearing heat. The representative formula is *Yue Bi Tang* (Maidservant from Yue Decoction). This formula is another example of medicinals balancing each other's effects. The dosage of *Shi Gao* (Gypsum Fibrosum) and *Ma Huang* (Ephedrae, Herba) can be adjusted according to the amount of heat. One should also keep in mind the caveats about heat mentioned above.

Yin water is due to internal damage and has spleen-kidney qi and yang vacuity at the root. With yin water, one usually starts with a mildly draining formula such as *Wu Ling San* (Five [Ingredients] Poria Powder). If this does not work well, one then can use the second level, moderate to strongly draining formulas *Zhen Wu Tang* (True Warrior Decoction) and *Shi Pi Yin* (Bolster the Spleen Beverage). If these are not strong enough, one may add one of the drastic formulas, *Shi Zao Tang* (Ten Dates Decoction), *Kong Xian Dan* (Drool-controlling Elixir), or *Zhou Che Wan* (Vessel & Vehicle Pills) to the moderate formulas.

When using such drastic formulas, one must use them cautiously, observing the following caveats:

A. One should not use these formulas alone. These drastic formulas are so draining that one must support the righteous at the same time. Therefore, one should combine such harsh, attacking formulas with a formula that fortifies the spleen and invigorates the kidney, such as *Zhen Wu Tang* (True Warrior Decoction), *Shi Pi Yin* (Bolster the Spleen Beverage), etc.

B. One should start with a small dosage of these formulas and be careful with the toxic medicinals.

C. What has been described in the ancient literature as stone water is probably not a kidney disease. In all likelihood, stone water describes liver cirrhosis or the effects of an abdominal tumor. In kidney diseases, edema starts on the extremities and the face. Stone water starts in the abdomen or only affects the abdomen because it is due to portal vein obstruction (caused by the cirrhosis or a tumor). When treating stone water, one must be careful using the moderate to strongly draining formulas, and one should not use

the drastic formulas unless one has had vast experience using them. The danger lies in draining the abdominal water too quickly. This may reduce blood pressure suddenly, leading to heart failure and death. Even if this does not lead to heart failure, the patient can still be at risk from the drastic draining. One must be especially careful using the draining method with stone water.

D. Water swelling may also be due to heart failure. For patients with heart disease who are edematous, one should use the mildly draining formulas only. The second level formulas contain *Fu Zi* (Aconiti Carmichaeli, Radix Lateralis Praeparatus). *Fu Zi* can increase the strength of the heartbeat and may conflict with Western cardiotonic drugs. *Fu Zi* may also cause toxic reactions or make it difficult to weigh the dosages of other medicinals. Mildly draining formulas do not cause these problems. Drastic formulas are absolutely forbidden.

E. Even when water swelling is due to a kidney disease, one must be especially careful if there is renal failure. All the formulas listed above are popularly used for kidney diseases, but, in renal failure, the kidney function is especially low. Normally, there are two ways medicinals and drugs are metabolized and excreted: 1) via the liver through the stool, and 2) via the kidney through urination. In renal failure, the kidney metabolizes medicinals very slowly. If medicinals are metabolized in the liver, they can still exit normally via defecation. But if they have to be metabolized and excreted via the kidney and urine, they will build up quickly when the kidney function is low. In that case, normal dosages of medicinals may become toxic since they are not metabolized and excreted.

4. Although water swelling is categorized as yin water and yang water, in the clinic, yin water is much more commonly encountered. As Ye Tian-shi has said, "When dampness prevails, yang is debilitated." Yin water is usually related to spleen-kidney yang vacuity. The kidney stores the former heaven essence and life-gate fire and governs water. The spleen governs movement and transformation. If kidney yang is vacuous, it cannot govern water which may then flood.

An example is kidney vacuity water flooding, a type of water swelling. If spleen yang is vacuous, earth is not solid and cannot "dam" water. This may also result in accumulation of water and dampness. In these patterns, the treatment strategy must include supplementing spleen and kidney yang.

When supplementing spleen-kidney yang in water swelling, one must pay special attention to yin. The *Huang Di Nei Jing* (*Yellow Emperor's Inner Classic*) states, "The interdependence of yin and yang is reflected in all things and cannot be separated." Again, in Chapter 3, it states, "If yin and yang separate, essence and spirit will also leave each other." In water swelling, the strategy of supplementing spleen and kidney yang strengthens these viscera's function of transforming water. However, one cannot rely solely on transforming water or drain too much water. Yin and yang are interconnected, and if one only transforms water or drains too much water, one will damage kidney yin. If kidney yin is damaged, liver yin will also be damaged since "the kidney and liver share a common source." If liver yin is damaged, the liver's yang qi will become excessive, leading to wood overwhelming earth (*i.e.*, damaging the spleen). In that case, weak earth will be incapable of restraining water, and water will then overflow and flood again. Typically, the main reason for recurrences in water swelling is that the importance of supplementing kidney yin was ignored or underestimated. The treatment principles must include supplementing and nourishing kidney yin as well as supplementing and invigorating spleen-kidney yang. The three most commonly used formulas that supplement and invigorate spleen-kidney yang to transform water are *Wu Ling San*, *Shi Pi Yin*, and *Zhen Wu Tang*.

One should also add a formula that protects and nourishes kidney yin while invigorating kidney yang. The most popular one is *Jin Gui Shen Qi Wan* (*Golden Cabinet* Kidney Qi Pills). This formula includes *Liu Wei Di Huang Wan* (Six Flavors Rehmannia Pills) to nourish yin plus *Shu Fu Zi* (Aconiti Carmichaeli, processed Radix Lateralis Praeparatus) and *Rou Gui* (Cinnamonmi Casiae, Cortex) to invigorate yang. While formulas that warm the spleen and kidney yang may drain water

quickly, one must be careful to nourish yin at the same time. Adding *Jin Gui Shen Qi Wan* builds up yin to achieve solid results, and it dispels water without fear of recurrences.

5. As stated above, the most fundamental differentiation of water swelling is into yin water and yang water. When one studies the theories of ancient doctors, one must grasp the essential idea and not slavishly follow their prescriptions. For example, Guo Pong-cheng, mentioned above, categorized water swelling into the following three pairs: exterior or interior, cold or heat, stomach or kidney. In the *Yi Xue Xin Wu* (*New Materials in the Study of Medicine*), he advises the reader:

> If the extremities are swollen but the abdomen is not swollen, this pertains to the exterior . . . If there is serious damp heat, add *Huang Bai* (Phellodendri, Cortex).

Even though Guo specifically recommends *Huang Bai* for damp heat yang water, one must be flexible. One must determine the severity of the problem, the organs involved, and the aspect the heat has penetrated. In the last case, Dr. Li chose *Huang Qin* (Scutellariae Baicalensis, Radix) instead of *Huang Bai*. However, one can also choose from among *Huang Lian* (Coptidis Chinensis, Rhizoma), *Lian Qiao* (Forsythiae Suspensae, Fructus), *Jin Yin Hua* (Lonicerae Japonicae, Flos), etc., if these are more appropriate to the pattern identification and treatment principles.

ENDNOTES

[1] In the modern clinical practice of Chinese medicine, wind water is usually divided into five patterns: wind water wind cold, wind water wind heat, wind water kidney heat, wind water yang vacuity, and wind water yin vacuity. These are discussed with case histories in this chapter.
[2] Qing He-chen, *op. cit.*, p. 348
[3] *Ibid.*, p. 348
[4] *Ibid.*, p. 349
[5] In the *Shen Nong Ben Cao Jing* (*Divine Farmer's Materia Medica Classic*) it states that *Ban Xia* (Pinelliae Ternatae, Rhizoma) can "drain water qi," *i.e.*, transform stagnant water and qi in the epigastrium.
[6] The treatment strategy of diffusing the lung to free the urine is also called "raising the pot and removing the lid."

CHAPTER 6
KIDNEY TAXATION & TAXATION WIND

Kidney taxation and taxation wind are two lesser known Chinese medical diagnostic categories that do not typically appear in Chinese internal medicine texts but are important in nephrology. Kidney taxation refers to exhaustion and damage of the original qi. Thus this condition is synonymous with kidney qi vacuity. Taxation wind is an acute disease associated with or superimposed on kidney taxation. *Su Wen*, Chapter 33, "*Ping Re Bing Lun* (Treatise on the Appraisal of Heat Diseases)" describes it as follows:

> Taxation wind is an attack of wind while the body is already taxed. It occurs in the lower part of the lungs. The patient suffers from a cough so severe it appears as if the eyeballs will pop out, blurred vision, chest fullness and pain, thick, tenacious phlegm, difficulty lying in a supine position, insomnia, chills, aversion to wind, and fever. The mechanism here is exhaustion, vacuity, and taxation rendering the righteous qi vulnerable. This allows wind heat to attack, stagnate, and congest in the lower part of the lungs.

DISEASE CAUSES & MECHANISMS

Although any of the three causes can be a factor in this disease, internal and neither external nor internal causes predominate. When these damage the kidney, the righteous qi is also damaged. With the kidney and righteous qi weakened, any of the six evils may invade with symptoms of fever and chills, aversion to wind, etc. The primary cause of kidney taxation is kidney essence vacuity. Of the three treasures – essence, qi and spirit—essence is the most primordial. Essence, stored in the kidney, is the basis for qi, and qi is the basis for spirit. If essence is damaged, qi will become vacuous and spirit will become ungrounded.

Kidney essence is naturally depleted through the normal course of life as described in *Su Wen*, Chapter 1, "*Shang Gu Tian Zhen Lun* (Preceding Ancients' Heavenly Truth)" where the stages of both male and female growth, maturation, and decline are related to the waxing and waning of the kidney. Kidney essence may also be damaged by overindulgence in sex or what is called bedroom taxation in Chinese. This neither external nor internal cause of disease is a very important factor leading to kidney taxation. Finally, kidney essence and qi may be damaged by toxins or by disharmonies of other viscera and bowels. For instance, the liver stores blood and kidney stores essence, blood and essence are mutually con-

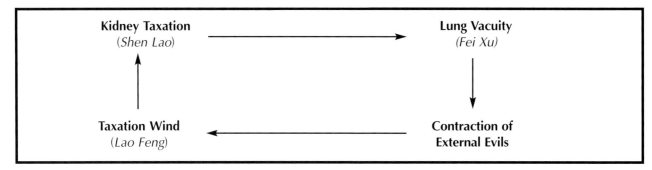

Figure 6.1. Kidney taxation & taxation wind vicious cycle

vertible, and liver blood vacuity may cause kidney vacuity. This example can also be seen as a disease of the child draining the mother according to the five phase generation cycle. However, any of the viscera, especially the spleen, lung, liver, and heart, can damage the kidney through the generating and controlling cycles of the five phases.

Most Chinese medical scholars believe that kidney taxation is the precursor to taxation wind. The kidney channel travels from the kidney through the diaphragm into the lung. Kidney taxation causes general exhaustion, including a weakening of lung qi and a depletion of righteous qi. Such a lung and righteous qi vacuity allows wind to invade, with the resulting taxation wind. Although kidney taxation can occur without a concomitant lung pattern, taxation wind always includes kidney taxation. Taxation wind can also exacerbate kidney taxation, thus leading to a vicious cycle. (See Figure 6.1.)

TREATMENT BASED ON PATTERN IDENTIFICATION

KIDNEY TAXATION

1. SPLEEN-KIDNEY YANG VACUITY

SIGNS & SYMPTOMS: Lassitude of the spirit, bodily fatigue, scanty qi, disinclination to speak and/or a weak voice, a somber white facial complexion, fear of cold, chilled limbs, poor appetite, loose stools, if severe, cockcrow diarrhea, low back and knee soreness and limpness, and possible lower limb superficial edema. The tongue is pale and swollen with white fur, and the pulse is deep and fine.

TREATMENT PRINCIPLES: Warm and supplement the spleen and kidney

REPRESENTATIVE FORMULA: Modified *Fu Zi Li Zhong Tang* (Aconite Rectify the Center Decoction) plus *Si Shen Wan* (Four Spirits Pills)

Fu Zi (Aconiti Carmichaeli, Radix Lateralis Praeparatus), 9g
Dang Shen (Codonopsitis Pilosulae, Radix), 12g
Bai Zhu (Atractylodis Macrocephalae, Rhizoma), 9g
Fu Ling (Poriae Cocos, Sclerotium), 9g
Gan Jiang (Zingiberis Officinalis, dry Rhizoma), 6g
Gan Cao (Glycyrrhizae Uralensis, Radix), 6g
Bu Gu Zhi (Psoraleae Corylifoliae, Fructus), 12g
Wu Zhu Yu (Evodiae Rutecarpae, Fructus), 9g
Rou Dou Kou (Myristicae Fragranthis, Semen), 9g
Wu Wei Zi (Schisandrae Chinensis, Fructus), 6g

MODIFICATIONS: If there is simultaneous abdominal pain, add *Xiao Hui Xiang* (Foeniculi Vulgaris, Fructus) and *Mu Xiang* (Auklandiae Lappae, Radix) to rectify the qi and stop pain. If there is seminal emission, add *Jin Ying Zi* (Rosae Laevigatae, Fructus) and *Lian Xu* (Nelumbinis Nuciferae, Plumula) to secure the kidney and astringe the essence.

If urination is short and scanty and there is generalized edema, use modified *Zhen Wu Tang* (True Warrior Decoction) instead of *Fu Zi Li Zhong Tang* and *Si Shen Wan: Fu Zi* (Aconiti Carmichaeli, Radix Lateralis Praeparatus), 9g, *Bai Zhu* (Atractylodis Macrocephalae, Rhizoma), 9g, *Fu Ling* (Poriae Cocos, Sclerotium), 10g, *Bai Shao* (Paeoniae Lactiflorae, Radix Albus), 6g, *Sheng Jiang* (Zingiberis Officinalis, uncooked Rhizoma), 6g, *Ze Xie*

(Alismatis Orientalis, Rhizoma), 9g, *Yi Yi Ren* (Coicis Lachryma-jobi, Semen), 15g, and *Che Qian Zi* (Plantaginis, Semen), 9g.

ACUMOXIBUSTION: Moxibustion *Guan Yuan* (CV 4), *Qi Hai* (CV 6), *Pi Shu* (Bl 20), *Shen Shu* (Bl 23), and *Zu San Li* (St 36).

MODIFICATIONS: If there is severe edema, add *San Yin Jiao* (Sp 6) and *Yin Ling Quan* (Sp 9).

2. HEART-KIDNEY YANG VACUITY

SIGNS & SYMPTOMS: Heart palpitations, easy fright, shortness of breath and hasty breathing, precordial chest oppression or heart pain, if severe, cyanotic lips, a cold body and fear of chill, lower and upper back pain, a somber white facial complexion, and possible superficial edema of the face. The tongue is pale with white fur and the pulse is fine and weak, bound, or regularly intermittent.

TREATMENT PRINCIPLES: Warm and promote the communication of the heart and kidney

REPRESENTATIVE FORMULA: Modified *Bao Yuan Tang* (Protect the Origin Decoction) plus *Gua Lou Xie Bai Bai Jiu Tang* (Trichosanthes, Allium & Alcohol Decoction)

Fu Zi (Aconiti Carmichaeli, Radix Lateralis Praeparatus), 9g
Rou Gui (Cinnamomi Cassiae, Cortex), 6g
Huang Qi (Astragali Membranacei, Radix), 15g
Dang Shen (Codonopsitis Pilosulae, Radix), 12g
Dang Gui (Angelicae Sinensis, Radix), 9g
Bai Shao (Paeoniae Lactiflorae, Radix Albus), 12g
mix-fried *Gan Cao* (Glycyrrhizae Uralensis, Radix), 9g
Gua Lou Pi (Trichosanthis Kirlowii, Pericarpium), 15-30g
Xie Bai (Allii, Bulbus), 9g
Yu Jin (Curcumae, Tuber), 9g

MODIFICATIONS: If there is heart pain, add powdered *San Qi* (Notoginseng, Radix) and *Dan Shen* (Salviae Miltiorrhizae, Radix). If water rheum has collected internally with superficial edema of the face, add *Bai Zhu* (Atractylodis Macrocephalae, Rhizoma), *Fu Ling* (Poriae Cocos, Sclerotium), and *Sheng Jiang* (Zingiberis Officinalis, uncooked Rhizoma) to warm yang and disinhibit water. If there is reversal chilling of the four limbs and great sweating suggesting that yang is on the verge of expiry, add *Ren Shen* (Panacis Ginseng, Radix).

ACUMOXIBUSTION: Moxibustion *Shan Zhong* (CV 17), *Guan Yuan* (CV 4), *Jue Yin Shu* (Bl 14), *Xin Shu* (Bl 15), *Pi Shu* (Bl 20), *Shen Shu* (Bl 23), and *Zu San Li* (St 36).

MODIFICATIONS: If there is shortness of breath and hasty breathing, add *Fei Shu* (Bl 13) and needle *Tai Yuan* (Lu 9).

3. LIVER-KIDNEY YIN VACUITY

SIGNS & SYMPTOMS: Dizziness, tinnitus, bilaterally dry, rough eyes, malar flushing, heat in the five hearts, seminal emission, night sweats, low back and knee soreness and limpness, dry mouth and parched throat. There is a red tongue with no fur and the pulse is fine, bowstring, and rapid.

TREATMENT PRINCIPLES: Enrich and supplement the liver and kidney

REPRESENTATIVE FORMULA: Modified *Qi Ju Di Huang Wan* (Lycium & Chrysanthemum Rehmannia Pills)

Gou Qi Zi (Lycii Chinensis, Fructus), 12g
Ju Hua (Chrysanthemi Morifolii, Flos), 9g
Sheng Di Huang (Rehmanniae Glutinosae, uncooked Radix), 15g
Shan Yao (Dioscoreae Oppositae, Radix), 9g
Shan Zhu Yu (Corni Officinalis, Fructus), 9g
Mai Men Dong (Ophiopogonis Japonici, Tuber), 12g
Nu Zhen Zi (Ligustri Lucidi, Fructus), 9g
Han Lian Cao (Ecliptae Prostratae, Herba), 15g
Mu Dan Pi (Moutan, Cortex Radicis), 9g
Fu Ling (Poriae Cocos, Sclerotium), 12g

MODIFICATIONS: If there is dizziness and numbness of the extremities, add *Tian Ma* (Gastrodiae Elatae, Rhizoma) and *Gou Teng* (Uncariae Cum Uncis,

Ramulus) to level the liver and extinguish wind. If vacuity heat is egregious, add *Bie Jia* (Amydae Sinensis, Carapax) and *Zhi Mu* (Anemarrhenae Aspheloidis, Rhizoma). If there is seminal emission, add *Jin Ying Zi* (Rosae Laevigatae, Fructus) and *Lian Xu* (Nelumbinis Nuciferae, Plumula).

Acumoxibustion: Needle *Tai Xi* (Ki 3), *San Yin Jiao* (Sp 6), *Qu Quan* (Liv 8), *Guan Yuan* (CV 4), *Ge Shu* (Bl 17), *Gan Shu* (Bl 18), and *Shen Shu* (Bl 23).

Modifications: If there is seminal emission, add *Zhi Shi* (Bl 52). If there is dizziness, add *Feng Chi* (GB 20), *Bai Hui* (GV 20), and *Yin Tang* (M-HN-3). If there is tinnitus, add *Tong Gong* (SI 19).

4. Lung-kidney yin vacuity

Signs & symptoms: Dry cough with scanty phlegm or possible blood within the phlegm, stirring causing qi panting which is worse at night, bone steaming and tidal heat, night sweats, seminal emission, heat in the hands and feet, lower and upper back aching and pain, and a thin body. There is a red tongue with scanty fur and the pulse is fine and fast.

Treatment principles: Enrich the kidney and nourish the lung

Representative formula: Modified *Bai He Gu Jin Tang* (Lily Secure Metal Decoction)

Bai He (Lilii, Bulbus), 30g
Sheng Di Huang (Rehmanniae Glutinosae, uncooked Radix), 15g
Shu Di Huang (Rehmanniae Glutinosae, cooked Radix), 12g
Mai Men Dong (Ophiopogonis Japonici, Tuber), 12g
Xuan Shen (Scrophulariae Ningpoensis, Radix), 12g
Sha Shen (Glehniae Littoralis, Radix), 12g
Chi Shao (Paeoniae Lactiflorae, Radix Rubrus), 9g
Bai Bu (Stemonae, Radix), 15g
Chuan Bei Mu (Fritillariae Cirrhosae, Bulbus), 9g
Zhi Mu (Anemarrhenae Aspheloidis, Rhizoma), 9g

Modifications: If panting prevents lying down (and sleeping), add *Hu Tao Rou* (Juglandis Regiae, Semen) and *Wu Wei Zi* (Schisandrae Chinensis,

Fructus) to supplement the kidney and grasp or absorb the qi. If hacking of blood is severe, add *Ce Bai Ye* (Biotae Orientalis, Cacumen), *Qian Cao Gen* (Rubiae Cordifoliae, Radix), and powdered *San Qi* (Notoginseng, Radix) to cool the blood and stop bleeding.

Acumoxibustion: Needle *Lie Que* (Lu 7), *Zhao Hai* (Ki 6), *San Yin Jiao* (Sp 6), *Shan Zhong* (CV 17), *Guan Yuan* (CV 4), *Fei Shu* (Bl 13), and *Shen Shu* (Bl 23).

Modifications: For qi panting, add *Ding Chuan* (M-BW-1) and *Feng Long* (St 40). For night sweats, add *Yin Xi* (Ht 6). For seminal emission, add *Zhi Shi* (Bl 52).

Taxation wind

Signs & symptoms: Chills, aversion to wind, fever, severe cough, blurred vision, chest fullness and pain, thick, sticky, hard-to-expectorate phlegm, difficulty lying down on one's back, insomnia

Treatment principles: Resolve the exterior and clear heat, clear heat and resolve toxins, transform phlegm

Representative formula: *Yin Qiao San* (Lonicera & Forsythia Powder), *Chai Ge Jie Ji Tang* (Bupleurum & Pueraria Resolve the Muscles Decoction), and *Qing Qi Hua Tan Tang* (Clear the Qi & Transform Phlegm Decoction)

Jin Yin Hua (Lonicerae Japonicae, Flos), 9-15g
Lian Qiao (Forsythiae Suspensae, Fructus), 9-15g
Jie Geng (Platycodi Grandiflori, Radix), 3-6g
Niu Bang Zi (Arctii Lappae, Fructus), 9-12g
Bo He (Menthae Haplocalycis, Herba), 3-6g
Dan Dou Chi (Sojae, Semen Praeparatum), 3-6g
Jing Jie Sui (Schizonepetae Tenuoifoliae, Herba Seu Flos), 6-9g
Dan Zhu Ye (Lophatheri Gracilis, Herba), 3-6g
fresh *Lu Gen* (Phragmitis Communis, Rhizoma), 15-30g
Gan Cao (Glycyrrhizae Uralensis, Radix), 3-6g
Chai Hu (Bupleuri, Radix), 6-9g
Ge Gen (Puerariae, Radix), 9g

Qiang Huo (Notopterygii, Rhizoma Et Radix), 9g

Huang Qin (Scutellariae Baicalensis, Radix), 9g

Shi Gao (Gypsum Fibrosum), 9-15g

Bai Shao (Paeoniae Lactiflorae, Radix Albus), 6g

Sheng Jiang (Zingiberis Officinalis, uncooked Rhizoma), 6g

Da Zao (Zizyphi Jujubae, Fructus), 3 pieces

Dan Nan Xing (Arisaematis, bile-processed Rhizoma), 6-9g

Ban Xia (Pinelliae Ternatae, Rhizoma), 6-9g

Gua Lou Ren (Trichosanthis Kirlowii, Semen), 6-9g

Xing Ren (Pruni Armeniacae, Semen), 6g

Chen Pi (Citri Reticulatae, Pericarpium), 6g

Fu Ling (Poriae Cocos, Sclerotium), 9-12g

Modifications: If the patient has a vacuous pulse, add *Ren Shen* (Panacis Ginseng, Radix), *Xi Yang Shen* (Panacis Quiquefolii, Radix), or *Dang Shen* (Codonopsitis Pilosulae, Radix). If the patient experiences more severe chills and muscle aches, add *Fang Feng* (Ledebouriellae Divaricatae, Radix). If the patient has a severe sore throat, add *Huang Lian* (Coptidis Chinensis, Rhizoma), *Huang Bai* (Phellodendri, Cortex), and *Zhi Zi* (Gardeniae Jasminoidis, Fructus). If heat has damaged yin causing night sweats, add *Sheng Di Huang* (Rehmanniae Glutinosae, uncooked Radix) and *Xuan Shen* (Scrophulariae Ningpoensis, Radix). For insomnia, add *He Huan Pi* (Albizziae Julibrissinis, Cortex), *Ye Jiao Teng* (Polygoni Multiflori, Caulis), and *Suan Zao Ren* (Zizyphi Spinosae, Semen).

Acumoxibustion: Choose from *Da Zhui* (GV 14), *Feng Men* (Bl 12), *Fei Shu* (Bl 13), *Wai Guan* (TB 5), *Qu Chi* (LI 11), *Chi Ze* (Lu 5), *Lie Que* (Lu 7), *Fu Liu* (Ki 7), and *Feng Long* (St 40).

Representative case histories

Case history of Dr. Ji Ma: Liu, a 50 year-old male[1]

Liu was an officer in the army. During World War II, he spent considerable time outdoors and had contracted cold dampness. He subsequently developed low back and knee soreness and weakness. So much so that it was difficult for him to walk. When he came to see Dr. Ji, his lower abdomen was ice cold and numb and he had very frequent urination, more than 10 times during the day and even more at night. He could not sleep because of the frequent night-time urination. His cheeks were red, his tongue was pale with glossy fur, and his pulse was deep, weak, and slow. Upon palpation, his abdomen felt like a cotton ball. There was no strength in it, and, if one scratched Liu's lower abdomen with a fingernail, he was unable to feel it. Based on these signs and symptoms, Dr. Ji believed a cold external evil had invaded Liu's *shao yin* channel and descended to the kidney and bladder organs. His treatment strategy was to warm the life-gate fire, stabilize the kidney, and secure and astringe urination. The prescription was *Jin Gui Shen Qi Wan* (*Golden Cabinet* Kidney Qi Pills) plus additions: *Shu Fu Zi* (Aconiti Carmichaeli, processed Radix Lateralis Praeparatus), *Rou Gui* (Cinnamonmi Casiae, Cortex), *Shu Di Huang* (Rehmanniae Glutinosae, cooked Radix), *Shan Zhu Yu* (Corni Officinalis, Fructus), *Shan Yao* (Dioscoreae Oppositae, Radix), *Ze Xie* (Alismatis Orientalis, Rhizoma), *Mu Dan Pi* (Moutan, Cortex Radicis), *Fu Ling* (Poriae Cocos, Sclerotium), *Sang Piao Xiao* (Mantidis, Ootheca), *Wu Wei Zi* (Schisandrae Chinensis, Fructus), *Yi Zhi Ren* (Alpiniae Oxyphyllae, Fructus), and *Ba Ji Tian* (Morindae Officinalis, Radix) (dosages not given). After one week of taking this formula, the cold in Liu's abdomen dissipated and he urinated much less frequently. After one month, his low back and knees were strong, his movements were faster and stronger, and all of his other symptoms disappeared.

Case history of Dr. Ji Tong: A male military officer (age not ngiven)[2]

Every summer this patient became exhausted, his mind became cloudy, and he lost his balance. He did not want to talk and would sleep all day long. He experienced spermatorrhea and felt hot in the evenings. Dr. Ji analyzed the case as follows: Because this man had not taken care of his health, his kidney was weak and unable to store essence properly in the winter. In summer, when yang becomes very strong, his kidney yin was too weak to counteract the extreme yang of the season. Dr. Ji's strategy was to supplement this patient's kidney essence, reasoning that when his kidney essence was full, his bones would be strong and his qi and spirit would return to normal. Therefore, Dr. Ji prescribed the following: *Shu Di Huang* (Rehmanniae Glutinosae, cooked Radix), 30g, *Shan Zhu Yu* (Corni Officinalis, Fructus), 12g, *Dang Gui* (Angelicae Sinensis, Radix), 9g, *Bai Shao* (Paeoniae Lactiflorae, Radix Albus), 9g, *Mai Men Dong* (Ophiopogonis Japonici, Tuber), 9g, *Bai Zhu* (Atractylodis Macrocephalae, Rhizoma), 9g, *Qian Shi* (Euryalis Ferocis, Semen), 9g, *Suan Sao Ren* (Zizyphi Spinosae, Semen), 9g, *Fu Ling* (Poriae Cocos, Sclerotium), 3g, *Chen Pi* (Citri Reticulatae, Pericarpium), 3g, and *Wu Wei Zi* (Schisandrae Chinensis, Fructus), 3g. The formula was successful, and the military official completely recovered.

Case history of Dr. Yu Tang-qi: A male state official (age not given)[3]

This patient overindulged in sex. His symptoms included irritability, thirst with desire to drink (he drank water all the time), difficult, scanty, and dark urination, constipation, and a cough with a large amount of phlegm. When he came to see Dr. Yu, this patient's face and eyes were red, his tongue was covered with prickles, he had dry, cracked lips, his whole body was feverish, and the soles of his feet were burning "like an oven." His left pulse was surging and fast. Based on these signs and symptoms, Dr. Yu's pattern identification was severe kidney yin vacuity with yang (having nothing to ground it) floating to the exterior. Therefore, the treatment strategy was to strongly nourish yin. Dr. Yu prescribed modified *Ba Wei Wan* (Eight Flavors Pills): *Shu Di Huang* (Rehmanniae Glutinosae, cooked Radix), 30g, *Shan Zhu Yu* (Corni Officinalis, Fructus), 12g, *Shan Yao* (Radix Dioscoreae Oppositae), 12g, *Mu Dan Pi* (Moutan, Cortex Radicis), 9g, *Ze Xie* (Alismatis Orientalis, Rhizoma), 9g, *Fu Ling* (Poriae Cocos, Sclerotium), 9g, *Mai Men Dong* (Ophiopogonis Japonici, Tuber), 9g, *Wu Wei Zi* (Schisandrae Chinensis, Fructus), 15g, and *Qian Shi* (Euryalis Ferocis, Semen), 15g. Dr. Yu also advised the official to drink a tea made of *Rou Gui* (Cinnamonmi Casiae, Cortex), 30g, divided into several servings. The patient took one bowl of tea, immediately went to sleep, and slept very well for half an hour. At mid-

night, he drank another bowl and all his symptoms disappeared.

Although the official felt much better, in the morning he became chilly with cold extremities. These symptoms indicated that his life-gate fire was vacuous and that the treatment strategy must change to boost yang. To achieve this goal, Dr. Yu prescribed *Jin Gui Shen Qi Wan* (*Golden Cabinet* Kidney Qi Pills). After taking this prescription, all the patient's symptoms disappeared. To consolidate the treatment effects, Dr. Yu gave the official *Gui Lu Di Huang Wan* (Turtle & Deer Rehmannia Pills): *Gui Ban Jiao* (Testudinis, Gelatinum Plastri), 90g, *Lu Jiao Jiao* (Cervi, Gelatinum Cornu), 90g, *Xuan Shen* (Scrophulariae Ningpoensis, Radix), 90g, *Mai Men Dong* (Ophiopogonis Japonici, Tuber), 90g, *Shan Zhu Yu* (Corni Officinalis, Fructus), 120g, *Bai Zhu* (Atractylodis Macrocephalae, Rhizoma), 120g, *Bai Shao* (Paeoniae Lactiflorae, Radix Albus), 120g, *Suan Sao Ren* (Zizyphi Spinosae, Semen), 120g, *Gou Qi Zi* (Lycii Chinensis, Fructus), 120g, and *Shu Di Huang* (Rehmanniae Glutinosae, cooked Radix), 240g. These medicinals were ground into powder, mixed with two bowls of human milk, and made into pills.

Case history of Dr. Yu Shang-zou: Chao, a 38 year-old male[4]

Chao's first visit to Dr. Yu was on Sept. 16, 1966. In 1958, he had been diagnosed with chronic nephritis. After some treatment he was fairly stable, but in May 1966, he began to have symptoms of chills, headache, fatigue, shortness of breath, and swollen eyelids. His abdomen was distended and he had loose stools 5-6 times a day (without blood, pus, or mucus). After this he started to vomit. He went to the hospital with water swelling (ascites). Urinalysis showed protein at 2+, pus cells at 0-1, granular casts at 0-3, and urine gravity at 1.009. His BUN was 72.6 mg/100ml, his blood potassium was 4.28 MOS/L, and his blood sodium was 102.6 MOS/L. The Western medical diagnosis was chronic nephritis and early stage uremia. His blood pressure was 170/100mmHg, and he was dizzy and fatigued. Dr. Yu found Chao's tongue pale and his pulse fine and bowstring. Therefore, he identified the disease as kidney taxation, and the pattern as qi and blood vacuity with liver-kidney vacuity. He gave Chao the following prescription: *Sha Yuan Zi* (Astragali Complanati, Semen), 9g, *Gou Qi Zi* (Lycii Chinensis, Fructus), 12g, calcined *Ci Shi* (Magnititum), 18g, *Niu Xi* (Achyranthis Bidentatae, Radix), 5g, *Dang Gui* (Angelicae Sinensis, Radix), 9g, *Huang Qi* (Astragali Membranacei, Radix), 9g, *Dang Shen* (Codonopsitis Pilosulae, Radix), 9g, *Hong Hua* (Carthami Tinctorii, Flos), 5g, *Gou Ji* (Cibotii Barometsis, Rhizoma), 9g, *Hu Tao Ren* (Juglandis Regiae Semen), 9g, *Tu Si Zi* (Cuscutae Chinensis, Semen), 12g, *Nan Sha Shen* (Adenophorae Strictae, Radix), 9g, and *Hai Ge Ke* (Cyclinae Sinensis, Concha), 9g.

After taking this prescription, Chao's energy was better and, by October, his urinalysis was normal, but he still had abdominal distention and diarrhea occasionally, especially when he ate cold food. Hence, Dr. Yu added *Hu Lu Ba* (Trigonellae Foenigracci, Semen), *Zi He Che* (Hominis, Placenta), and *Fo Shou* (Citri Sarcodactylis, Fructus) to the prescription. Chao's abdominal distention improved, but he was still dizzy and his low back was sore. In April 1967, Dr. Yu prescribed an herbal wine with the following ingredients: *Gou Ji* (Cibotii Barometsis, Rhizoma), 15g, *Ba Ji Tian* (Morindae Officinalis, Radix), 15g, *Niu Xi* (Achyranthis Bidentatae, Radix), 15g, *Xu Duan* (Dipsaci Asperi, Radix), 15g, *Dang Gui* (Angelicae Sinensis, Radix), 24g, *Mai Men Dong* (Ophiopogonis Japonici, Tuber), 12g, *Dang Shen* (Codonopsitis Pilosulae, Radix), 15g, *Shu Di Huang* (Rehmanniae Glutinosae, cooked Radix), 9g, *Hong Hua* (Carthami Tinctorii, Flos), 9g, *Da Zao* (Zizyphi Jujubae, Fructus), 7g, *Chen Pi* (Citri Reticulatae, Pericarpium), 9g, and *Yi Yi Ren* (Coicis Lachryma-jobi, Semen), 9g. These medicinals were soaked in 1.25 liters of yellow wine for one week.

Chao's dizziness improved. So he decided to stop taking the wine and come back for a consultation. Dr. Yu advised him to take the original prescription plus the wine. Then in May 1967, Chao lost his appetite and had loose stools with a lot of gas. Dr. Yu felt that the treatment strategy must be changed to transforming dampness, supplementing the

spleen, and upbearing spleen qi. His prescription consisted of: *Wu Shi Chao* (Midday Tea), 3g, *Shan Yao* (Radix Dioscoreae Oppositae), 12g, *Bai Bian Dou* (Dolichoris Lablab, Semen), 12g, *Dang Shen* (Codonopsitis Pilosulae, Radix), 9g, *Fu Ling* (Poriae Cocos, Sclerotium), 9g, *Shen Qu* (Massa Medica Fermentata), 9g, and *He Ye* (Nelumbinis Nuciferae, Folium), 9g. This was to be taken as a decoction along with five grams of *Hou Xiang Zheng Qi San* (Agastaches Rectify the Qi Powder): *Huo Xiang* (Agastaches Seu Pogostemi, Herba), 90g, *Hou Po* (Magnoliae Officinalis, Cortex), 60g, *Chen Pi* (Citri Reticulatae, Pericarpium), 60g, *Zi Su Ye* (Perillae Frutescentis, Folium), 30g, *Bai Zhi* (Angelicae Dahuricae, Radix), 30g, *Ban Xia* (Pinelliae Ternatae, Rhizoma), 60g, *Da Fu Pi* (Arecae Catechu, Pericarpium), 30g, *Bai Zhu* (Atractylodis Macrocephalae, Rhizoma), 60g, *Fu Ling* (Poriae Cocos, Sclerotium), 30g, *Jie Geng* (Platycodi Grandiflori, Radix), 60g, and mix-fried *Gan Cao* (Glycyrrhizae Uralensis, Radix), 75g. These medicinals were ground into powder and administered in 3-6 gram doses as a draft with 3-6 grams of *Shen Jiang* (Zingiberis Officinalis, uncooked Rhizoma) and one *Da Zao* (Zizyphi Jujubae, Fructus). After taking these formulas for a while, Chao's appetite was better and his stools returned to normal. Chao then went back to taking the original prescription that supplemented the kidney and liver.

In 1967, Chao started back to normal work and, in August 1969, all his blood tests were normal. However, on June 23, 1971, he returned to see Dr. Yu. He had overexerted himself and started to experience low back soreness, dizziness, dry mouth, difficult defecation, and numb extremities with spasms. Urinalysis showed protein at 2+ and RBCs at 3+. His pulse was fine and slow, and his blood pressure was 110/90mmHg. Therefore, Dr. Yu changed the treatment strategy to supplementing the liver and spleen. He prescribed a decoction and an herbal wine. The decoction consisted of: *Huang Qi* (Astragali Membranacei, Radix), 18g, *Dang Shen* (Codonopsitis Pilosulae, Radix), 18g, *Gou Qi Zi* (Lycii Chinensis, Fructus), 15g, *Shi Hu* (Dendrobii, Herba), 12g, *Gong Lao Ye* (Ilicis, Folium), 15g, *Niu Xi* (Achyranthis Bidentatae, Radix), 9g, *Ci Shi* (Magnititum), 9g, *Fo Shou* (Citri Sarcodactylis,

Fructus), 9g, *Bai Shao* (Paeoniae Lactiflorae, Radix Albus), 12g, and *Shan Yao* (Radix Dioscoreae Oppositae), 12g. These were cooked together with *Er Zhi Wan* (Two Ultimates Pills), 9g.[5] The wine was made with: *Gou Ji* (Cibotii Barometsis, Rhizoma), 18g, *Ba Ji Tian* (Morindae Officinalis, Radix), 18g, *He Shou Wu* (Polygoni Multiflori, Radix), 30g, *Gou Qi Zi* (Lycii Chinensis, Fructus), 46g, *Shu Di Huang* (Rehmanniae Glutinosae, cooked Radix), 24g, *Dang Shen* (Codonopsitis Pilosulae, Radix), 30g, *Sha Yuan Zi* (Astragali Complanati, Semen), 30g, *Niu Xi* (Achyranthis Bidentatae, Radix), 30g, *Xu Duan* (Dipsaci Asperi, Radix), 30g, *Bai Shao* (Paeoniae Lactiflorae, Radix Albus), 15g, *Huang Lian* (Coptidis Chinensis, Rhizoma), 9g, *Xuan Shen* (Scrophulariae Ningpoensis, Radix), 24g, *Rou Gui* (Cinnamonmi Casiae, Cortex), 0.9g, *Du Zhong* (Eucommiae Ulmoidis, Cortex), 24g, and *Dang Gui* (Angelicae Sinensis, Radix), 18g. These were soaked in 1.5 liters of yellow wine for one week.

By July 1971, Chao's dizziness, numbness, and spasms were better, and his urinalysis was negative. He decided to stop taking the prescriptions. In August 1977, Chao had a checkup. His blood tests were normal, he had no discomfort, and he felt that everything was back to normal.

COMMENTARY: This case is an example of kidney taxation with vacuity of qi, blood, yin, and yang. The spleen and kidney were collapsing, water was failing to nourish wood, and liver yin could not control liver yang, thus leading to ascendant liver yang hyperactivity. Because of the complications, many treatment strategies and many different types of medicinals had to be used: qi supplements and blood supplements, medicinals to harmonize yin and yang, strong supplements for the spleen and kidney, and medicinals that strongly nourished the liver.

CLINICAL TIPS

1. In clinic, medicinal wines are frequently prescribed for kidney taxation to great effect. In kidney taxation, there is often blood disharmony plus stasis in the kidney channel (suggested by symptoms of low back pain and high blood pressure).

The treatment strategy must include harmonizing the blood and freeing the flow of the channels. Wine overcomes the slimy and enriching effects of the supplementing medicinals as well as freeing the flow of the channels and harmonizing blood. Another advantage of medicinal wines is their long shelf life.

There are two ways to make herbal wine. The first is to soak medicinals in wine in a sealed bottle (for one week in the summer and somewhat longer in the winter), then to remove the medicinals. The wine is then ready for use. The second is to put the medicinals in wine in a ceramic pot and then put the pot in boiling water until the wine boils. The pot is then sealed and stored for a long time. The medicinals are discarded and the herbal wine is ready for use.

2. In taxation wind, heat may be in the exterior, in the muscles, or in the interior (*e.g.*, phlegm heat in the lung). *Yin Qiao San* (Lonicera & Forsythia Powder) treats wind heat in the exterior. *Chai Ge Jie Ji Tang* (Bupleurum & Pueraria Resolve the Muscles Decoction) treats heat in the muscles, and *Qing Qi Hua Tan Tang* (Clear the Qi & Transform Phlegm Decoction) treats heat in the lung. One should focus on where the heat resides. One must resolve the exterior using cool, exterior-resolving medicinals. However, one must also clear heat as needed from any or all of the four aspects. The following chart is a guide to choosing medicinals based on clearing heat, draining fire, discharging heat, and nourishing yin. (See Chart 6.1.)

One must also treat the kidney vacuity according to the stage of the disease. During the acute stage, one may supplement the spleen and kidney qi if there is some heat in the defensive aspect but most of the heat is in the qi aspect. Even here one must be careful of the dosages of the qi supplements and focus on expelling and clearing the evils. If the heat is only in the defensive aspect, supplementing the qi may close the pores, locking the heat in the body. One may supplement the qi, but one must not supplement yang. Yang supplements may exacerbate the heat and toxins. However, after the heat has been cleared, one should supplement both kidney yin and yang. (See Chart 6.2.)

METHOD	STRATEGY	REPRESENTATIVE MEDICINALS
Clearing Heat	Clear heat from the four aspects	**Defensive:** *Lian Qiao* (Forsythiae Suspensae, Fructus), *Jin Yin Hua* (Lonicerae Japonicae, Flos), etc. **Qi:** *Huang Lian* (Coptidis, Rhizoma), *Huang Qin* (Scutellariae Baicalensis, Radix), etc. **Construction:** *Sheng Di Huang* (Rehmanniae Glutinosae, uncooked Radix), *Xuan Shen* (Scrophulariae Ningpoensis, Radix), etc. **Blood:** *Xi Jiao* (Rhinoceri, Cornu), *Sheng Di Huang* (Rehmanniae Glutinosae, uncooked Radix), etc.
	Drain fire	*Shi Gao* (Gypsum), *Zhi Mu* (Anemarrhenae Asphodeloidis, Rhizoma), *Dan Zhu Ye* (Lophatheri Gracilis, Herba), etc.
	Discharge heat	*Dan Zhu Ye* ((Lophatheri Gracilis, Herba), *Che Qian Zi* (Plantaginis, Seman), *Mu Tong* (Akebiae Mutong, Caulis), etc.
	Nourish yin, Safeguard fluids	*Mai Men Dong* (Ophiopogonis Japonici, Tuber), *Zhi Mu* (Anemarrhenae Asphodeloidis, Rhizoma), etc.

Chart 6.1. Clearing heat

STRATEGY	LOCATION	FORMULA OR MEDICINAL	ACTION
Clear heat	Wind heat in exterior	*Yin Qiao San*	1. Resolve the exterior 2. Clear heat from the four aspects 3. Drain fire 4. Clear heat 5. Transform phlegm 6. Nourish yin and safeguard fluids
	Heat in muscle layer	*Chai Ge Jie Ji Tang*	
	Phlegm heat in lungs	*Qing Qi Hua Tan Tang*	
Supplement vacuity	Spleen and kidney (During acute phase, if heat mostly in qi aspect)	*Ren Shen, Dang Shen, Xi Yang Shen*	Supplement spleen qi and kidney qi
	Kidney (After the evil has been eliminated)	*Jin Kui Shen Qi Wan, Liu Wei Di Huang Wan,* etc.	Supplement kidney qi, yin, and/or yang

Chart 6.2. Clearing heat in taxation wind.

Endnotes

1 Qing He-chen, *op. cit.*, p. 400
2 Wu Qing, *Song Yuan Ming Qing* (*Song, Yuan, Ming, Qing* [*Famous Doctors' Case Histories*]) Vol. 111, [this is a Qing dynasty book with no other publishing information], p. 33
3 *Ibid.*, p. 34

4 Yu Guan-shi and Shui Jian-shen, *Dong Dai Ming Yi Lin Zheng Jing Hua* (*A Collection of the Clinical Eperiences of Famous Modern Doctors*), Ancient Chinese Medicine Book Publishing Company, Beijing, 1998, p. 240
5 *Er Zhi Wan* (Two Ultimates Pills) consists of *Nu Zhen Zi* (Ligustri Lucidi, Fructus) and *Han Lian Cao* (Ecliptae Prostratae, Herba).

Phlegm rheum refers to several conditions in which body fluids are not being transformed properly, accumulate, and cause stagnation. In point of fact, phlegm rheum is a compound term. Phlegm denotes thick pathological fluids, and rheum denotes thinner pathological fluids. However, as a compound term, it refers to any type of thin fluid arising as a result of lung, spleen, and/or kidney disturbances preventing the normal movement and transformation of fluid. Symptoms of phlegm rheum include cough, wheezing, heart palpitations, dizziness, shortness of breath, rib-side pain, and hypochondriac pain. Phlegm rheum is commonly divided into four patterns, determined by location, that are originally described in the *Jin Gui Yao Lue*, Chapter 12, "On the Pulse, Patterns & Treatment of Phlegm Rheum & Coughing":

> Fluid retention can be divided into four categories . . . If a plump patient loses weight and a splashing sound can be heard in his intestines, this is phlegm rheum. After drinking water, the fluid flows and collects in the patient's costal region. A dragging pain occurs when the patient coughs or spits. This is suspended rheum. After drinking water, the fluid flows and collects in the extremities. The patient cannot sweat when he should and feels pain and heaviness in his body. This is spillage rheum. Propping rheum may

include symptoms and signs of coughing with adverse ascending gas, labored respiration, and shortness of breath that prevents the patient from lying quietly in bed.

In Chapter 11, this work also states:

> If the patient drinks too much water, he will suffer a sudden attack of wheezing with a sensation of fullness. When a patient eats little but drinks copiously, the water will collect in the epigastrium. An acute case will bring about palpitations, while a mild one will cause shortness of breath.

The last quote describes two disease causes of phlegm rheum. In the first, drinking more water than the spleen is able to transform causes damp stagnation that becomes phlegm rheum. In the second, undereating damages the spleen qi. Therefore, the spleen is unable to transform dampness, leading to phlegm rheum.

Phlegmrheum and water[1] both involve excess fluid accumulation. Phlegm rheum is fluid accumulation in the body cavities, while water is fluid accumulation in the skin and muscles that causes water swelling or edema. Each can transform into or cause the other. (See Chart 7.1.)

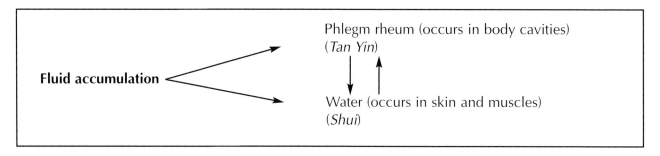

Chart 7.1. Phlegm rheum & water

Disease causes & mechanisms

The causes of phlegm rheum include external contraction of cold dampness, unregulated eating and drinking, and damage due to excessive taxation. For instance, if external cold, damp evils attack the defensive exterior, they first damage the yang qi of the defensive exterior. In that case, the lung loses its diffusion and damp evils spillover into the muscles and flesh. If these evils move from the exterior into the interior, they can encumber the spleen and stomach's qi transformation function. Hence water fluids collect and stagnate, accumulating to produce rheum. Similarly, if one drinks too much water, drinks too many chilled, cold drinks, or eats too much uncooked, chilled food, central yang may be checked and the spleen is not able to move. Once again dampness is engendered internally and fluids and humors collect and produce rheum. Finally, taxation fatigue, excessive indulgence in sex, or bodily vacuity due to enduring disease may damage spleen and stomach yang. Thus water fluids lose their transportation and transformation and collect, producing rheum. If the body is weak and the qi is vacuous, it is easy to be damaged by water dampness which easily collects and amasses to cause disease.

Treatment based on pattern identification

Phlegm rheum

1. Spleen yang vacuity weakness

Signs & symptoms: Chest and rib-side propping fullness, glomus and oppression below the heart, water sloshing in the stomach, a liking for warmth and a fear of chill in the epigastrium, upper back cold, vomiting of clear water and phlegmy drool, vomiting caused by drinking water, thirst but no desire to drink, heart palpitations, shortness of breath, dizziness and vertigo, reduced appetite, possible loose stools, and a body which becomes progressively emaciated. The tongue has slimy, white fur and the pulse is bowstring, fine, and slippery.

Treatment principles: Warm the spleen and transform rheum

Representative formula: *Li Zhong Wan* (Rectify the Center Pills) plus *Wu Ling San* (Five [Ingredients] Poria Powder)

Dang Shen (Codonopsitis Pilosulae, Radix), 9g
Gan Jiang (Zingiberis Officinalis, dry Rhizoma), 9g
Gui Zhi (Cinnamomi Cassiae, Ramulus), 6g
Gan Cao (Glycyrrhizae Uralensis, Radix), 3g
Bai Zhu (Atractylodis Macrocephalae, Rhizoma), 9-12g
Fu Ling (Poriae Cocos, Sclerotium), 9-12g
Ze Xie (Alismatis Orientalis, Rhizoma), 9-12g
Zhu Ling (Polypori Umbellati, Sclerotium), 9g

Modifications: For severe edema, add *Shi Pi Yin* (Bolster the Spleen Beverage). For insomnia, add *Suan Zao Ren* (Zizyphi Spinosae, Semen), *He Huan Pi* (Albizziae Julibrissinis, Cortex), and *Ye Jiao Teng* (Polygoni Multiflori, Caulis). If the patient is very fatigued and feels cold, make a paste from 20-50 grams of powdered *Wu Zhu Yu* (Evodiae Rutecarpae, Fructus) and apply to *Yong Quan* (Ki 1) for 2-4 hours.

For lack of appetite, add *Shan Zha* (Crataegi, Fructus) and *Mai Ya* (Horedi Vulgaris, Fructus Germinatus).

ACUMOXIBUSTION: Moxibustion *Zhong Wan* (CV 12), *Tian Shu* (St 25), *Gao Huang Shu* (Bl 43), *Qi Hai* (CV 6), and *Ming Men* (GV 4).

MODIFICATIONS: If there is nausea and vomiting and/or heart palpitations, add *Nei Guan* (Per 6).

2. RHEUM LODGING IN THE STOMACH & INTESTINES

SIGNS & SYMPTOMS: Hardness and fullness or pain below the heart which spontaneously remits but afterward returns as a lump, possible water sounding within the intestines, abdominal fullness, constipation, and a dry mouth and parched throat. There is slimy white or yellow tongue fur and a deep, bowstring or deep-lying pulse.

TREATMENT PRINCIPLES: Attack and precipitate, dispel rheum

REPRESENTATIVE FORMULA: *Gan Sui Ban Xia Tang* (Euphorbia & Pinellia Decoction)

Gan Sui (Euphorbiae Kansui, Radix), 9g
Ban Xia (Pinelliae Ternatae, Rhizoma), 9g
Bai Shao (Paeoniae Lactiflorae, Radix Albus), 15g
Feng Mi (Mel, honey), 1 tablespoon

MODIFICATIONS: If depressed rheum has transformed heat, use *Ji Jiao Li Huang Wan* (Stephania, Zanthoxylum, Tinglizi & Rhubard Pills) instead: *Da Huang* (Rhei, Radix Et Rhizoma), 6-9g, *Ting Li Zi* (Tinglizi, Semen), 6-9g, *Chuan Jiao* (Zanthoxyli Bungeani, Fructus), 6-9g, and *Han Fang Ji* (Stephaniae Tetrandrae, Radix), 6-9g. If rheum evils counterflow upward with chest fullness, add *Zhi Shi* (Citri Aurantii, Fructus Immaturus) and *Hou Po* (Magnoliae Officinalis, Cortex) to discharge fullness. However, do not attack and dispel too much for fear of damaging the righteous qi.

ACUMOXIBUSTION: Not effective for this pattern of phlegm rheum.

SUSPENDED RHEUM

1. EVILS ASSAILING THE CHEST & LUNG

SIGNS & SYMPTOMS: Alternating fever and chills, scanty perspiration, possible fever with no aversion to cold, fever unresolved by sweating, cough with scanty phlegm, hasty breathing, piercing pain in the chest and rib-side which is worse on inhalation, glomus and hardness below the heart, dry heaves, and a bitter taste in the mouth. The tongue fur is thin and either white or yellow, while the pulse is bowstring and rapid.

TREATMENT PRINCIPLES: Harmonize and resolve, diffuse and disinhibit

REPRESENTATIVE FORMULA: Modified *Chai Zhi Ban Xia Tang* (Bupleurum, Aurantium & Pinellia Decoction)

Chai Hu (Bupleuri, Radix), 9g
Huang Qin (Scutellariae Baicalensis, Radix), 9g
Gua Lou (Trichosanthis Kirlowii, Fructus), 9g
Ban Xia (Pinelliae Ternatae, Rhizoma), 9g
Zhi Ke (Citri Aurantii, Fructus), 6g
Jie Geng (Platycodi Grandiflori, Radix), 6g
Chi Shao (Paeoniae Lactiflorae, Radix Rubrus), 9g

MODIFICATIONS: If there is cough, hasty breathing, and rib-side pain, add *Bai Jie Zi* (Sinapis Albae, Semen) and *Sang Bai Pi* (Mori Albi, Cortex Radicis). If there is glomus and hardness below the heart with a bitter taste in the mouth and dry heaves, add *Huang Lian* (Coptidis Chinensis, Rhizoma). If heat is exuberant with sweating, coughing, and difficulty breathing, subtract *Chai Hu* and add *Ma Huang* (Ephedrae, Herba), *Xing Ren* (Pruni Armeniacae, Semen), *Shi Gao* (Gypsum Fibrosum), and *Gan Cao* (Glycyrrhizae Uralensis, Radix) to clear heat, diffuse the lung, and transform phlegm.

ACUMOXIBUSTION: Moxibustion *Da Zhui* (GV 14), *Tao Dao* (GV 13), *Zhi Yang* (GV 9), and *Ling Tai* (GV 10) and needle *Gan Shu* (Bl 18).

2. RHEUM COLLECTING IN THE CHEST & RIB-SIDE

SIGNS & SYMPTOMS: Coughing when sleeping leading to pain, however only like chest and rib-side pain initially, difficult breathing causing pain to worsen, inability to lie flat due to panting and wheezing or ability to only lie on one side due to distention, pain, and fullness on the other. The tongue fur is thin, white, and slimy, and the pulse is deep and bowstring or bowstring and slippery.

TREATMENT PRINCIPLES: Expel water and dispel rheum

REPRESENTATIVE FORMULA: *Shi Zao Tang* (Ten Date Decoction)

Gan Sui (Euphorbiae Kansui, Radix)
Jing Da Ji (Euphorbiae Seu Knoxiae, Radix)
Yuan Hua (Daphnis Genkwae, Flos)
Da Zao (Zizyphi Jujubae, Fructus)

Grind equal amounts of the first three medicinals into powder and take 0.5-1 gram doses in the early morning on an empty stomach with a warm decoction made from 10 pieces of *Da Zao*.

MODIFICATIONS: After the condition has lessened somewhat, subtract *Yuan Hua* and add *Bai Jie Zi* (Sinapis Albae, Semen).

If this formula causes vomiting, abdominal pain, or excessive diarrhea, reduce the dosage or stop administration. Instead, use *Jiao Mu Gua Lou Tang* (Zanthoxylum & Trichosanthes Decoction): *Ting Li Zi* (Tinglizi, Semen), 6g, *Sang Bai Pi* (Mori Albi, Cortex Radicis), 6g, *Zi Su Zi* (Perillae Frutescentis, Fructus), 9g, *Gua Lou Pi* (Trichosanthis Kirlowii, Pericarpium), 6g, *Chen Pi* (Citri Reticulatae, Pericarpium), 6g, *Ban Xia* (Pinelliae Ternatae, Rhizoma), 9g, *Jiao Mu* (Zanthoxyli Bungeani, Fructus), 3g, *Fu Ling* (Poriae Cocos, Sclerotium), 9g, and *Sheng Jiang* (Zingiberis Officinalis, uncooked Rhizoma), 3g. If phlegm turbidity are exuberant with chest region fullness and oppression and turbid, slimy tongue fur, add *Xing Ren* (Pruni Armeniacae, Semen) and *Xie Bai* (Allii, Bulbus). If water rheum has existed for a long time and is difficult to remove, add *Gui Zhi* (Cinnamomi Cassiae, Ramulus), *Bai Zhu* (Atractylodis Macrocephalae, Rhizoma), and *Gan Cao* (Glycyrrhizae Uralensis, Radix) to free the flow of yang, fortify the spleen, and transform rheum.

ACUMOXIBUSTION: Same as for the preceding pattern.

3. NETWORK VESSEL QI DISHARMONY

SIGNS & SYMPTOMS: Chest and rib-side aching and pain, chest oppression and discomfort, burning chest pain or a sensation of piercing pain, uneasy breathing or oppressive cough. The tongue is dark with thin fur, and the pulse is bowstring.

TREATMENT PRINCIPLES: Rectify the qi and harmonize the network vessels

REPRESENTATIVE FORMULA: Modified *Xiang Fu Xuan Fu Hua Tang* (Cyperus & Inula Decoction)

Xuan Fu Hua (Inulae Racemosae, Flos), 9g
Zi Su Zi (Perillae Frutescentis, Fructus), 12g
Xing Ren (Pruni Armeniacae, Semen), 9g
Ban Xia (Pinelliae Ternatae, Rhizoma), 9g
Yi Yi Ren (Coicis Lachryma-jobi, Semen), 15g
Fu Ling (Poriae Cocos, Sclerotium), 12g
Xiang Fu (Cyperi Rotundi, Rhizoma), 9g
Chen Pi (Citri Reticulatae, Pericarpium), 6g

MODIFICATIONS: If there is phlegm qi depression and obstruction with chest oppression and slimy tongue fur, add *Gua Lou* (Trichosanthis Kirlowii, Fructus) and *Zhi Ke* (Citri Aurantii, Fructus). If the disease has endured for a long time and entered the network vessels with severe piercing pain, add *Dang Gui Wei* (Angelicae Sinensis, Extremitas Radicis), *Chi Shao* (Paeoniae Lactiflorae, Radix Rubrus), *Tao Ren* (Pruni Persicae, Semen), *Hong Hua* (Carthami Tinctorii, Flos), *Ru Xiang* (Olibani, Resina), and *Mo Yao* (Myrrhae, Resina). If water rheum is incessant, add *Tong Cao* (Tetrapanacis Papyriferi, Medulla), *Lu Lu Tong* (Liquidambaris Taiwaniae, Fructus), and *Dong Gua Pi* (Benincasae Hispidae, Epicarpium).

ACUMOXIBUSTION: Same as for evils assailing the chest and lung above. However, add *Xue Hai* (Sp 10) and *He Gu* (LI 4) and prick to bleed and superficial, visibly engorged venules.

4. YIN VACUITY WITH INTERNAL HEAT

SIGNS & SYMPTOMS: Occasional coughing bouts,

hacking and spitting a small amount of thick, sticky phlegm, a dry mouth and parched throat, possible tidal fever in the afternoon, malar flushing, heart vexation, heat in the hearts of the hands and feet (or hands, feet, and heart), night sweats, possible accompanying chest and rib-side oppression and pain, enduring disease with no recovery, and an emaciated, thin body. The tongue tends to be red with scanty fur, while the pulse is small and rapid.

TREATMENT PRINCIPLES: Enrich yin and clear heat

REPRESENTATIVE FORMULA: Modified *Sha Shen Mai Dong Tang* (Glehnia & Ophiopogon Decoction) plus *Xie Bai San* (Drain the White Powder)

Sha Shen (Glehniae Littoralis, Radix), 12g
Mai Men Dong (Ophiopogonis Japonici, Tuber), 12g
Yu Zhu (Polygoni Odorati, Rhizoma), 9g
Tian Hua Fen (Trichosanthis Kirlowii, Radix), 9g
Sang Bai Pi (Mori Albi, Cortex Radicis), 9g
Di Gu Pi (Lycii Chinensis, Cortex Radicis), 9g
Gan Cao (Glycyrrhizae Uralensis, Radix), 3-6g

MODIFICATIONS: If there is tidal fever, add *Bie Jia* (Amydae Sinensis, Carapax) and *Gong Lao Ye* (Ilicis, Folium). If there is cough, add *Bai Bu* (Stemonae, Radix) and *Chuan Bei Mu* (Fritillariae Cirrhosae, Bulbus). If there is chest and rib-side oppression and pain, add *Gua Lou Pi* (Trichosanthis Kirlowii, Pericarpium), *Zhi Ke* (Citri Aurantii, Fructus), *Yu Jin* (Curcumae, Tuber), and *Si Gua Luo* (Luffae Cylindricae, Fasciculus Vascularis). If accumulation of fluids is unremitting, add *Mu Li* (Ostreae, Concha) and *Ze Xie* (Alismatis Orientalis, Rhizoma). For simultaneous qi vacuity, shortness of breath, and easy sweating, add *Tai Zi Shen* (Pseudostellariae Heterophylae, Radix), *Huang Qi* (Astragali Membranacei, Radix), and *Wu Wei Zi* (Schisandrae Chinensis, Fructus).

ACUMOXIBUSTION: Needle *Lie Que* (Lu 7), *Zhao Hai* (Ki 6), *Shan Zhong* (CV 17), *Fei Shu* (Bl 13), and *Feng Long* (St 40).

SPILLAGE RHEUM

SIGNS & SYMPTOMS: Bodily aching, pain, and heaviness, if severe, superficial edema in the extremities, aversion to cold, no sweating, possible coughing and panting, profuse, white, frothy phlegm, chest oppression, dry heaves, no thirst. The tongue fur is white and the pulse is bowstring and tight.

TREATMENT PRINCIPLES: Effuse the exterior and transform rheum

REPRESENTATIVE FORMULA: Modified *Xiao Qing Long Tang* (Minor Blue-green Dragon Decoction)

Ma Huang (Ephedrae, Herba), 9g
Gui Zhi (Cinnamomi Cassiae, Ramulus), 9g
Gan Jiang (Zingiberis Officinalis, dry Rhizoma), 3-6g
Xi Xin (Asari, Herba Cum Radice), 1.5-3g
Ban Xia (Pinelliae Ternatae, Rhizoma), 9g
Gan Cao (Glycyrrhizae Uralensis, Radix), 3-6g
Wu Wei Zi (Schisandrae Chinensis, Fructus), 9g
Bai Shao (Paeoniae Lactiflorae, Radix Albus), 9g

MODIFICATIONS: If there is marked superficial edema and scanty urination, add *Fu Ling* (Poriae Cocos, Sclerotium), *Zhu Ling* (Polypori Umbellati, Sclerotium), and *Ze Xie* (Alismatis Orientalis, Rhizoma). If there is accompanying fever, vexation and agitation, and white and yellow tongue fur showing a combination of exterior cold and interior depressive heat, add *Shi Gao* (Gypsum Fibrosum) to clear internal heat. If cold signs and symptoms are not obvious, delete *Gan Jiang* and *Xi Xin*.

ACUMOXIBUSTION: Moxibustion *Shen Que* (CV 8), *Shui Fen* (CV 9), *Guan Yuan* (CV 4), *Fei Shu* (Bl 13), *Ming Men* (GV 4), *Zhong Wan* (CV 12), and *Zu San Li* (St 36).

PROPPING RHEUM

1. COLD RHEUM DEEP-LYING IN THE LUNGS

SIGNS & SYMPTOMS: Coughing and panting causing an inability to lie down, vomiting of profuse, white, frothy phlegm, prolonged course without healing, worse during chilly weather, if severe, superficial edema of the face and instep. The tongue fur is white and glossy or white and slimy, and the pulse is bowstring and tight.

TREATMENT PRINCIPLES: Warm the lungs and transform rheum

REPRESENTATIVE FORMULA: Modified *Xiao Qing Long Tang* (Minor Blue-green Dragon Decoction)

Ma Huang (Ephedrae, Herba), 9g
Gui Zhi (Cinnamomi Cassiae, Ramulus), 9g
Gan Jiang (Zingiberis Officinalis, dry Rhizoma), 3-6g
Xi Xin (Asari, Herba Cum Radice), 1.5-3g
Ban Xia (Pinelliae Ternatae, Rhizoma), 9g
Gan Cao (Glycyrrhizae Uralensis, Radix), 3-6g
Wu Wei Zi (Schisandrae Chinensis, Fructus), 9g
Bai Shao (Paeoniae Lactiflorae, Radix Albus), 9g

MODIFICATIONS: If there is bodily vacuity and an exterior pattern is apparent, instead of *Xiao Qing Long Tang*, one can use *Ling Gan Jiang Wei Xin Xia Ren Tang* (Poria, Licorice, Ginger, Schisandra, Asarum, Pinellia & Armeniaca Decoction): *Fu Ling* (Poriae Cocos, Sclerotium), 12g, *Gan Cao* (Glycyrrhizae Uralensis, Radix), 3-6g, *Gan Jiang* (Zingiberis Officinalis, dry Rhizoma), 6g, *Wu Wei Zi* (Schisandrae Chinensis, Fructus), 9g, *Xi Xin* (Asari, Herba Cum Radice), 1.5-3g, and *Ban Xia* (Pinelliae Ternatae, Rhizoma), 9g.

If rheum is profuse and cold is less and there is no apparent exterior pattern but there is coughing and panting and exuberant phlegm, one can use *Ting Li Da Zao Xie Fei Tang* (Tinglizi & Red Date Drain the Lung Decoction): *Ting Li Zi* (Tinglizi, Semen), 6g, and *Da Zao* (Zizyphi Jujubae, Fructus), 24g.

ACUMOXIBUSTION: Same as for spillage rheum above.

2. SPLEEN-KIDNEY YANG VACUITY

SIGNS & SYMPTOMS: Panting and hasty breathing which are worse with stirring, shortness of breath, profuse phlegm, reduced appetite, chest oppression, fear of cold and chilled limbs, lassitude of the spirit, lower leg cramping, spasm, and insensitivity, palpitations below the navel, inhibited urination, superficial edema of the feet, possible vomiting of frothy drool, and dizziness and vertigo. The tongue is fat and swollen with wet, white or gray, slimy fur, and

the pulse is deep, fine, and slippery.

TREATMENT PRINCIPLES: Warm and supplement the spleen and kidney in order to transform water rheum

REPRESENTATIVE FORMULA: Modified *Jing Gui Shen Qi Wan* (*Golden Cabinet* Kidney Qi Pills) plus *Ling Gui Zhu Gan Tang* (Poria, Cinnamon, Atractylode & Licorice Decoction)

Shu Fu Zi (Aconiti Carmichaeli, Radix Lateralis Praeparatus), 3g
Gui Zhi (Cinnamomi Cassiae, Ramulus), 9g
Shan Yao (Dioscoreae Oppositae, Radix), 9g
Bai Zhu (Atractylodis Macrocephalae, Rhizoma), 9g
mix-fried *Gan Cao* (Glycyrrhizae Uralensis, Radix), 6-9g
Fu Ling (Poriae Cocos, Sclerotium), 12g
Ze Xie (Alismatis Orientalis, Rhizoma), 9g
Shu Di Huang (Rehmanniae Glutinosae, cooked Radix), 12g
Shan Zhu Yu (Corni Officinalis, Fructus), 6g

MODIFICATIONS: If appetite is reduced and phlegm is profuse, add *Ban Xia* (Pinelliae Ternatae, Rhizoma) and *Chen Pi* (Citri Reticulatae, Pericarpium).

ACUMOXIBUSTION: Moxibustion *Pi Shu* (Bl 20), *Wei Shu* (Bl 21), *Shen Shu* (Bl 23), *Ming Men* (GV 4), *Shan Zhong* (CV 17), *Zhong Wan* (CV 12), *Guan Yuan* (CV 4), and *Zu San Li* (St 36).

REPRESENTATIVE CASE HISTORY

Case history of Dr. Yu Tang-chi: A man of unspecified age[2]

This patient was very boastful. (In China, it is commonly thought that a quiet person keeps their qi inside, but a boastful person dissipates their qi.) One day he suddenly lost his appetite, his mouth became dry, and he spit phlegm. He also experienced abdominal bloating, constipation, and urinary difficulty. The man went to Chinese doctors who gave him phlegm-transforming, qi-rectifying medicinals. These medicinals caused chest oppression with a stifling sensation and exacerbated his other symptoms.

He went to other doctors who gave him phlegm-transforming, qi-rectifying, and food-dispersing medicinals. These caused his abdomen to become so bloated and painful that he could not sit or lie down. He tried other doctors who gave him blood-quickening and qi-rectifying medicinals, but these caused edema in both his feet. Finally, the man came to see Dr. Yu. Upon examination, Dr. Yu found this patient's right inch pulse big and vacuous, his right bar pulse slightly bowstring, and his right cubit pulse coming and going. All three of his left pulses were soft, forceless, and vacuous. Dr. Yu's pattern identification was spleen-kidney dual vacuity. Therefore, he directed the patient to take *Bu Zhong Yi Qi Tang* (Supplement the Center & Boost the Qi Decoction) in the morning and *Jin Gui Shen Qi Wan* (*Golden Cabinet* Kidney Qi Pills) in the morning and evening.

After taking these formulas for a little while, the patient's abdominal distention worsened, but Dr. Yu assured him that if he continued taking the pills he would feel better. The patient was skeptical, but after one month, all his symptoms improved. Then Dr. Yu changed the prescription. He removed *Fu Zi* (Aconiti Carmichaeli, Radix Lateralis Praeparatus) from *Jin Gui Shen Qi Wan* and added *Wu Wei Zi* (Schisandrae Chinensis, Fructus). This was to be taken along with *Gui Pi Tang* (Restore the Spleen Decoction) with *Mu Xiang* (Aucklandiae Lappae, Radix) and mix-fried *Gan Cao* (Glycyrrhizae Uralensis, Radix) removed: *Ren Shen* (Panacis Ginseng, Radix), *Huang Qi* (Astragali Membranacei, Radix), *Bai Zhu* (Atractylodis Macrocephalae, Rhizoma), *Fu Ling* (Poriae Cocos, Sclerotium), *Suan Zao Ren* (Zizyphi Spinosae, Semen), *Long Yan Rou* (Euphoriae Longanae, Arillus), mix-fried *Yuan Zhi* (Polygalae Tenuifoliae, Radix), and *Dang Gui* (Angelicae Sinensis, Radix) (dosages not given). The patient took these for half a year and completely recovered.

CLINICAL TIPS

In general, the treatment of phlegm rheum is accomplished by warming and supplementing the spleen and kidney in order to secure the root and by disinhibiting water and expelling rheum to treat the tip. However, in order to treat phlegm-rheum, we must identify its location. The *Jin Gui Yao Lue* gives some signs and symptoms to aid in this endeavor:

> When water collects in the lung, profuse salivation and thirst will result. When water collects in the spleen, shortness of breath and heaviness or movement will result. When water collects in the liver, the patient will sense distention and fullness in the rib-side regions and a pain in the same area when sneezing. When water collects in the kidney, palpitations beneath the heart will result. When fluid retention occurs in the epigastrium, the patient will feel cold in his back in an area the size of the palm . . . When the phlegm rheum occurs in the chest, the patient feels a shortness of breath and thirst and suffers arthralgia in all the joints of the body. A deep pulse is diagnostic. When phlegm rheum occurs in the cavity above the diaphragm, the following symptoms and signs will be observed: a sensation of fullness, wheezing, coughing, and vomiting. With the onset of the condition, there will be fever and chills, pains in the back and lumbar region, fierce shaking of the body, and spontaneous tears. This is hidden rheum.

ENDNOTES

[1] Fluid exuded by diseased organs is called water rheum. Water is clear and thin, while rheum is sticky. However, rheum (*yin*) is thinner than phlegm (*tan*).
[2] Wu Qing, *op. cit.*, p. 32

CHAPTER 8
LUMBAR PAIN

The defining symptom of lumbar pain is aching, pain, and/or soreness in the lower back on one or both sides. A number of kidney diseases manifest as lumbar pain.

DISEASE CAUSES & MECHANISMS

Su Wen, Chapter 17, "*Mai Yao Jing Wei Lun* (Treatise on the Finest Essence of the Essentials of the Pulse)" states, "The low back is the mansion of the kidney." Therefore, in clinical practice, one often sees kidney disharmonies causing lumbar pain. However, liver disharmonies may also cause lumbar pain as stated in *Su Wen*, Chapter 41, "*Ci Yao Teng* (Needling for Lumbar Pain)," "In lumbar pain of the foot *jue yin* liver origin, the lower back is very stiff, tense, and arched like a bow about to snap." The liver channel winds around the genitals and rises to the lower abdomen. A branch then connects with the *tai yin* and shao yang channels at the lumbar area. Liver disharmonies that cause impediment in the liver channel may also cause impediment in the *tai yin* and *shao yang* channels resulting in low back pain. Injury is another common cause of lumbar pain. In Chapter 4 of the *Ling Shu*, "*Xie Qi Zang Fu Bing Xing* (Evil Qi and Diseases of the Viscera & Bowels)," it states, "High falls may cause blood stasis." In addi-

tion, lumbar pain may be caused by contraction of various evils. For example, *Ling Shu*, Chapter 27, "*Li He Zhen Xie Lun* (Treatise on the Parting & Uniting of True & Evils)" states, "When heaven and earth are cold, the flow of water stagnates." This implies that cold may cause stagnation in the kidney (water) channel and viscus.

TREATMENT BASED ON PATTERN IDENTIFICATION

1. WIND COLD INVASION

SIGNS & SYMPTOMS: Lumbar pain accompanied by hypertonicity and a cold sensation in the low back, difficulty turning from side to side, pain radiating to the upper back, fever, aversion to cold, body aching, and relief on obtaint of warmth but aggravation on exposure to cold. There is thin, white tongue fur, and a floating, tight or bowstring, tight pulse.

TREATMENT PRINCIPLES: Dispel wind and scatter cold

REPRESENTATIVE FORMULA: Modified *Du Huo San* (Angelica Pubescens Powder)

Du Huo (Angelicae Pubescentis, Radix), 12g
Fang Feng (Ledebouriellae Divaricatae, Radix), 9g
Ma Huang(Ephedrae, Herba), 6g
Fu Zi (Aconiti Carmichaeli, Radix Lateralis Praeparatus), 3g
Chuan Xiong (Ligustici Wallichii, Radix), 9g
Chuan Niu Xi (Cyathulae Officinalis, Radix), 6g
wine stir-fried *Dang Gui* (Angelicae Sinensis, Radix), 6g
Ge Gen (Puerariae, Radix), 9g

ACUMOXIBUSTION: Needle *Feng Chi* (GB 20) and *He Gu* (LI 4). Needle and/or moxibustion *Shen Shu* (Bl 23), *Qi Hai Shu* (Bl 24), *Wei Zhong* (Bl 40), and *Kun Lun* (Bl 60).

MODIFICATIONS: Add *Feng Men* (Bl 12) and *Feng Shi* (GB 31) if there is sweating, aversion to wind, pain which moves its location, and a moderate (*i.e.*, relaxed, in this case meaning not bowstring or tight) pulse, all of which suggest predominant wind evils. Moxa *Zhong Wan* (CV 12) to warm the center and scatter cold if there is vomiting and adominal pain. For pain and rigidity of the low back and knees, add *Tai Xi* (Ki 3) and subtract *Feng Chi* (GB 20) and *Kun Lun* (Bl 60). This is in order to strengthen the kidneys. For yang vacuity manifest by spontaneous sweating, add *Ming Men* (GV 4) and subtract *Feng Chi* (GB 20) in order to warm yang and transform dampness.

2. COLD DAMP INVASION

SIGNS & SYMPTOMS: Lumbar pain accompanied by cold and heavy sensations in the low back as if sitting in cold water and carrying some weight, pain worsened by cold, damp weather and improved by warmth, bodily heaviness, numbness, soreness when bending and stretching, and loose stools. There is a pale tongue with slimy, white fur, and a soggy, moderate (*i.e.*, relaxed, in this case meaning slightly slow) pulse.

TREATMENT PRINCIPLES: Scatter cold and transform dampness

REPRESENTATIVE FORMULA: Modified *Shen Zhao Tang* (Affected Kidneys Decoction)

Cang Zhu (Atractylodis, Rhizoma), 9g
Bai Zhu (Atractylodis Macrocephalae, Rhizoma), 9g
Fu Ling (Poriae Cocos, Sclerotium), 6g
Gan Jiang (Zingiberis Officinalis, dry Rhizoma), 3g
Fu Zi (Aconiti Carmichaeli, Radix Lateralis Praeparatus), 3g
Du Zhong (Eucommiae Ulmoidis, Cortex), 9g
mix-fried *Gan Cao* (Glycyrrhizae Uralensis, Radix), 3g

MODIFICATIONS: If there is kidney vacuity, add *Sang Ji Sheng* (Sangjisheng, Ramulus) and *Xu Duan* (Dipsaci Asperi, Radix). If there is a severe cold sensation in the low back, add *Xi Xin* (Asari, Herba Cum Radice). If there is a severe heavy sensation in the low back, add *Mu Gua* (Chaenomelis Lagenariae, Fructus).

ACUMOXIBUSTION: Needle *San Jiao Shu* (Bl 22), *Shen Shu* (Bl 23), *Qi Hai Shu* (Bl 24), *Yin Ling Quan* (Sp 9), and *Yang Fu* (GB 38).

MODIFICATIONS: For severe pain and cold limbs, moxa *Ming Men* (GV 4) to warm the kidneys and help scatter cold. For concomitant lower limb pain, add *Fei Yang* (Bl 58) to warm and free the flow of the channels. For lack of strengh in the low back and knees, add *Fu Liu* (Ki 7) to supplement the kidneys and strengthen the low back. For oppression and distention in the stomach, add *Wei Shu* (Bl 21) to transform dampness and harmonize the center.

3. WIND DAMP INVASION

SIGNS & SYMPTOMS: Lumbar pain often accompanied by heaviness, pain possibly radiating to the lower extremeties, pain worsened by cold, damp weather, fever, aversion to wind, spontaneous perspiration, and bodily heaviness. There is slimy, white tongue fur and a floating, moderate (*i.e.*, relaxed or slightly slow) pulse.

TREATMENT PRINCIPLES: Dispel wind and transform dampness

REPRESENTATIVE FORMULA: Modified *Qiang Huo Sheng Shi Tang* (Notopterygium Overcome Dampness Decoction)

Qiang Huo (Notoptergyii, Rhizoma Et Radix), 9g
Du Huo (Angelicae Pubescentis, Radix), 9g
Gao Ben (Ligustici Chinensis, Radix Et Rhizoma), 6g
Fang Feng (Ledebouriellae Divaricatae, Radix), 6g
Chuan Xiong (Ligustici Wallichii, Radix), 6g
Man Jing Zi (Viticis, Fructus), 6g
Qin Jiao (Gentianae Qinjiao, Radix), 9g
Gan Cao (Glycyrrhizae Uralensis, Radix), 3g

MODIFICATIONS: If there is kidney vacuity, add salt stir-fried *Du Zhong* (Eucommiae Ulmoidis, Cortex) and salt mix-fried *Bu Gu Zhi* (Psoraleae Corylifoliae, Fructus). If there is a severe heavy sensation, add *Cang Zhu* (Atractylodis, Rhizoma) and *Wei Ling Xian* (Clematidis Chinensis, Radix). If there is restriction of mobility, add *Luo Shi Teng* (Trachelospermi Jasminoidis, Caulis) and *Hai Feng Teng* (Piperis Futokadsurae, Caulis).

ACUMOXIBUSTION: Needle *Feng Chi* (GB 20), *He Gu* (LI 4), *Yin Ling Quan* (Sp 9), and *Kun Lun* (Bl 60).

MODIFICATIONS: For a sensation of a bag over the head or a tight band around the head, add *Fu Yang* (Bl 59). For high fever, add *Da Zhui* (GV 14). For lumbar and hip pain, add *Bai Huan Shu* (Bl 30) and *Tian Jing* (TB 10). For lumbosacral and coccygeal pain, add *Yin Bao* (Liv 9). For cold pain in the low back and buttocks, add *Cheng Fu* (Bl 36).

4. DAMP HEAT BREWING & ACCUMULATING

SIGNS & SYMPTOMS: Lumbar pain often accompanied by a hot sensation in the low back, lumbar soreness and heaviness, inability to bend forward and backward, vexatious heat, spontaneous perspiration, thirst, short, dark urination, painful urination, loose stools. There is slimy, yellow tongue fur and a soggy, rapid or slippery, rapid pulse.

TREATMENT PRINCIPLES: Clear heat and disinhibit dampness

REPRESENTATIVE FORMULA: Modified *Si Miao Wan* (Four Marvels Pills)

Huang Bai (Phellodendri, Cortex), 9g

Cang Zhu (Atractylodis, Rhizoma), 12g
Niu Xi (Achyranthis Bidentatae, Radix), 12g
Yi Yi Ren (Coicis Lachryma-jobi, Semen), 30g
Qin Jiao (Gentianae Qinjiao, Radix), 9g

MODIFICATIONS: If there is severe distention and heaviness in the low back, add *Han Fang Ji* (Stephania Tetrandrae, Radix) and steamed *Mu Gua* (Chaenomelis Lagenariae, Fructus). If there is predominant heat with thirst and red urine, add *Lian Qiao* (Forsythiae Suspensae, Fructus), *Zhi Zi* (Gardeniae Jasminoidis, Fructus), and *Mu Tong* (Akebiae Mutong, Caulis). If there is yin vacuity with dry throat and mouth which are worse at night, low back weakness, and vexatious heat in the five hearts, add *Sheng Di Huang* (Rehmanniae Glutinosae, uncooked Radix), *Nu Zhen Zi* (Ligustri Lucidi, Fructus), and *Han Lian Cao* (Ecliptae Prostratae, Herba).

ACUMOXIBUSTION: Needle *Yao Shu* (GV 2), *Wei Zhong* (Bl 40), *Yang Ling Quan* (GB 34), and *Xing Jian* (Liv 2)

MODIFICATIONS: For abdominal distention, add *Tai Bai* (Sp 3) to rectify the qi. For enduring low back and knee aching, add *Shang Liao* (Bl 31).

5. KIDNEY YIN VACUITY

SIGNS & SYMPTOMS: Dull lumbar pain, lack of strength, vexatious heat in the five centers, tidal fever, night sweats, and a dry mouth. There is a red tongue with reduced moisture and a fine, rapid pulse.

TREATMENT PRINCIPLES: Enrich the kidneys, clear heat, and harmonize the network vessels

REPRESENTATIVE FORMULA: Modified *Zuo Gui Wan* (Restore the Left [Kidney] Pills)

Shu Di (Rehmanniae Glutinosae, cooked Radix), 12g
Shan Yao (Dioscoreae Oppositae, Radix), 9g
Shan Zhu Yu (Corni Officinalis, Fructus), 9g
Gou Qi Zi (Lycii Chinensis, Fructus), 9g
Niu Xi (Achyranthis Bidentatae, Radix), 9g
Tu Si Zi (Cuscutae Chinensis, Semen), 9g

Lu Jiao Jiao (Cervi, Gelatinum Cornu), 6g
Gui Ban Jiao (Testudinis, Gelatinum Plastri), 6g
Sang Ji Sheng (Sangjisheng, Ramulus), 9g
Du Zhong (Eucommiae Ulmoidis, Cortex), 12g

MODIFICATIONS: If there is dizziness, tinnitus, heart palpitations, and insomnia, add *Shi Jue Ming* (Haliotidis, Concha), uncooked *Long Gu* (Draconis, Os), and uncooked *Mu Li* (Ostreae, Concha). If there is vacuity heat with dry throat and mouth, vexatious heat, and night sweats, add salt mix-fried *Huang Bai* (Phellodendri, Cortex) and salt mix-fried *Zhi Mu* (Anemarrhenae Aspheloidis, Rhizoma). If there is restriction of mobility, add *Si Gua Luo* (Luffae Cylindricae, Fasciculus Vascularis) and *Luo Shi Teng* (Trachelospermi Jasminoidis, Caulis). If there is concomitant qi stagnation and blood stasis, add *Ru Xiang* (Olibani, Resina) and *Mo Yao* (Myrrhae, Resina).

ACUMOXIBUSTION: Needle *Shen Shu* (Bl 23), *Zhi Shi* (Bl 52), *Tai Xi* (Ki 3), *Fu Liu* (Ki 7), and *San Yin Jiao* (Sp 6).

MODIFICATIONS: For effulgent fire of the heart and kidneys manifest by reduced sleep, seminal emission, and short voidings of dark-colored urine, add *Yong Quan* (Ki 1) and *Xin Shu* (Bl 15) to downbear heart fire. For tinnitus, add *Ting Hui* (GB 2). For sore throat, add *Zhao Hai* (Ki 6).

6. KIDNEY YANG VACUITY

SIGNS & SYMPTOMS: Dull, lingering lumbar pain worsened by overwork, lack of warmth in the hands and feet, fear of cold, especially below the waist, shortness of breath, a bright white facial complexion, long, clear urination, and loose stools. The tongue is pale with white fur, and the pulse is deep, fine, forceless.

TREATMENT PRINCIPLES: Warm the kidneys and scatter cold

REPRESENTATIVE FORMULA: Modified *You Gui Wan* (Restore the Right [Kidney] Pills)

Du Zhong (Eucommiae Ulmoidis, Cortex), 9g

Fu Zi (Aconiti Carmichaeli, Radix Lateralis Praeparatus), 3g
Tu Si Zi (Cuscutae Chinensis, Semen), 9g
Xu Duan (Dipsaci Asperi, Radix), 9g
Lu Jiao Jiao (Cervi, Gelatinum Cornu), 6g
Shan Yao (Disocoreae Oppositae, Radix), 6g
Gou Qi Zi (Lycii Chinensis, Fructus), 9g
Shan Zhu Yu (Corni Officinalis, Fructus), 9g
Shu Di (Rehmanniae Glutinosae, cooked Radix), 12g
Dang Gui (Angelicae Sinensis, Radix), 6g
Gou Ji (Cibotii Barometsis, Rhizoma), 9g

MODIFICATIONS: If there is center qi downward falling with a falling sensation of the lower back and a continuous sensation of hollow pain, subtract *Gou Qi Zi* and *Dang Gui* and add *Dang Shen* (Codonopsitis Pilosulae, Radix), *Huang Qi* (Astragali Membranacei, Radix), *Bai Zhu* (Atractylodis Macrocephalae, Rhizoma), *Chai Hu* (Bupleuri, Radix), and mix-fried *Sheng Ma* (Cimicifugae, Rhizoma). If there is qi stagnation and blood stasis, add *Ru Xiang* (Olibani, Resina) and *Mo Yao* (Myrrhae, Resina) and increase *Dang Gui* up to nine grams.

ACUMOXIBUSTION: Use warm needle technique on *Shen Shu* (Bl 23), *Qi Hai Shu* (Bl 24), and *Guan Yuan Shu* (Bl 26) and needle *Zu San Li* (St 36) and *San Yin Jiao* (Sp 6).

MODIFICATIONS: For severe yang vacuity, use direct moxibustion. For tinnitus, moxibustion *Er Men* (TB 21) indirectly. For dizziness, moxibustion *Bai Hui* (GV 20). For seminal emission, moxibustion *Zhi Shi* (Bl 52). For yang exhaustion, add *Tai Xi* (Ki 3) and *San Yin Jiao* (Sp 6) to supplement yang by nourishing yin. For pain in the lower extremities, add *Cheng Jin* (Bl 56) and *Yang Ling Quan* (GB 34).

7. QI STAGNATION & BLOOD STASIS DUE TO TRAUMATIC INJURY

SIGNS & SYMPTOMS: Lumbar pain with a history of injury, sprain, or strain, pricking, fixed, and/or severe lumbar pain worsened by pressure, effort exertion, and movement, and, in severe cases, even by breathing, and pain which often gets worse at night. Other symptoms may include a dark tongue with static macules, and a deep, choppy pulse.

TREATMENT PRINCIPLES: Move the qi and quicken the blood, dispel stasis and quicken the network vessels to stop pain

REPRESENTATIVE FORMULA: Modified *Shen Tong Zhu Yu Tang* (Body Pain Dispel Stasis Decoction)

Xu Duan (Dipsaci Asperi, Radix), 12g
Gu Sui Bu (Drynariae, Radix), 9g
Chuan Xiong (Ligustici Wallichii, Radix), 9g
Tao Ren (Pruni Persicae, Semen), 9g
Hong Hua (Carthami Tinctorii, Flos), 9g
Qiang Huo (Notopterygii, Rhizoma Et Radix), 9g
Ru Xiang (Olibani, Resina), 9g
Dang Gui (Angelicae Sinensis, Radix), 9g
Xiang Fu (Cyperi Rotundi, Rhizoma), 6g
Chuan Niu Xi (Cyathulae Officinalis, Radix), 9g
Di Long (Lumbricus), 9g
Qin Jiao (Gentianae Qinjiao, Radix), 9g
Gan Cao (Glycyrrhizae Uralensis, Radix), 3g

MODIFICATIONS: If there is qi stagnation and blood stasis due to wind dampness, add *Du Huo* (Angelicae Pubescentis), *Wei Ling Xian* (Clematidis Chinensis, Radix), and *Fang Feng* (Ledebouriellae Divaricatae, Radix). If there has been traumatic injury to the low back, add powdered *San Qi* (Notoginseng, Radix), *Qian Cao* (Rubiae Cordifoliae, Radix), and *Su Mu* (Sappan, Lignum) or *Yun Nan Bai Yao* (Yunnan White Medicine, a Chinese patent medicine).

If there is low back pain with menstrual irregularity, replace *Shen Tong Zhu Yu Tang* with modified *Tao Hong Si Wu Tang* (Persica & Carthamus Four Materials Decoction): *Tao Ren* (Pruni Persciae, Semen), 9g, *Hong Hua* (Carthami Tinctorii, Flos), 9g, wine stir-fried *Dang Gui* (Angelicae Sinensis, Radix), 12g, *Chuan Xiong* (Ligustici Wallichii, Radix), 12g, *Shu Di Huang* (Rehmanniae Glutinosae, cooked Radix), 9g, *Bai Shao* (Paeoniae Lactiflorae, Radix Albus), 9g, *Xu Duan* (Dipsaci Asperi, Radix), 12g, *Xiang Fu* (Cyperi Rotundi, Rhizoma), 9g, and *Chai Hu* (Bupleuri, Radix), 6g.

ACUMOXIBUSTION: Needle any *a shi* points to quicken

the network vessels as well as *Shui Gou* (GV 26) and *Wei Zhong* (Bl 40). Needle the *a shi* points moderately for 20 minutes. Then withdraw the needles. After withdrawal, needle *Shui Gou* and *Wei Zhong* with draining method and ask the patient to do some movement, such as turning, bending, and stretching until the pain is relieved. If three successive treatments fail to achieve an effect, add *San Yin Jiao* (Sp 6) and *He Gu* (LI 4) while subtracting *Shui Gou* and *Wei Zhong*.

MODIFICATIONS: For concomitant menstrual irregularity, add *Xue Hai* (Sp 10) and *Di Ji* (Sp 8). For a fine pulse, add *San Yin Jiao* (Sp 6) and *Zu San Li* (St 36) to nourish the blood. For pain in the rib-side region, add *Dai Mai* (GB 26).

8. LIVER DEPRESSION & QI STAGNATION

SIGNS & SYMPTOMS: Lumbar pain accompanied by distention in the low back and rib-side regions which is worse at dawn but better in the morning after getting up and moving around, hypertonicity in the lower abdomen, enduring standing impossible, depression, and irritability. There is pale tongue with thin fur and a bowstring, choppy pulse.

REPRESENTATIVE FORMULA: Modified *Qi Xiang Wan* (Seven Aromatics Pills)

Chai Hu (Bupleuri, Radix), 6g
Xiang Fu (Cyperi Rotundi, Rhizoma), 9g
E Zhu (Curcumae Zedoariae, Rhizoma), 9g
Sha Ren (Amomi, Fructus), 6g
Ding Xiang (Caryophylli, Flos), 6g
Yi Zhi Ren (Alpiniae Oxyphyllae, Fructus), 9g
Mu Xiang (Auklandiae Lappae, Radix), 9g
Fo Shou (Citri Sacrodactylis, Fructus), 9g
Bai Shao (Paeoniae Lactiflorae, Radix Albus), 9g

MODIFICATIONS: If qi depression transforms into heat, add *Zhi Zi* (Gardeniae Jasminoidis, Fructus) and *Mu Dan Pi* (Moutan, Cortex Radicis). If there is blood stasis, add wine stir-fried *Dang Gui* (Angelicae Sinensis, Radix), *Chuan Xiong* (Ligustici Wallichii, Radix), and *Xu Duan* (Dipsaci Asperi, Radix). If there is concomitant kidney vacuity, add *Sang Ji Sheng* (Sangjisheng, Ramulus) and *Du Zhong* (Eucommiae Ulmoidis, Cortex).

ACUMOXIBUSTION: Needle any *a shi* points as well as *Xing Jian* (Liv 2), *Tai Chong* (Liv 3), and *Li Gou* (Liv 5).

MODIFICATIONS: For blurred vision, add *Tai Xi* (Ki 3) and *San Yin Jiao* (Sp 6). For distending headache, add *Zu Lin Qi* (GB 41). For a bitter taste in the mouth, add *Yang Ling Quan* (GB 34). For lower abdominal pain just before menstruation, add *Qu Quan* (Liv 8) and *Zhong Ji* (CV 3). For frequent sighing, add *Qi Men* (Liv 14). And for lumbar pain and lower abdominal pain, add *Ju Liao* (GB 29).

9. WATER RHEUM COLLECTING INTERNALLY

SIGNS & SYMPTOMS: Heavy lumbar pain, edema, especially below the waist, bodily heaviness, especially in the waist and knees, a bright white facial complexion, lassitude of the spirit, fatigue, and scanty urination. There is a pale tongue with white fur and teeth-marks on its edges and a slow, deep, forceless pulse.

TREATMENT PRINCIPLES: Warm yang and transform water

REPRESENTATIVE FORMULA: Modified *Er Chen Tang* (Two Aged [Ingredients] Decoction)

Chen Pi (Citri Reticulatae, Pericarpium), 9g
Ban Xia (Pinelliae Ternatae, Rhizoma), 9g
Fu Ling (Poriae Cocos, Sclerotium), 9g
mix-fried *Gan Cao* (Glycyrrhizae Uralensis, Radix), 6g
Tian Nan Xing (Arisaematis, Rhizoma), 9g
Cang Zhu (Atractylodis, Rhizoma), 9g
Bai Jie Zi (Sinapis Albae, Semen), 9g
Du Zhong (Eucommiae Ulmoidis, Cortex), 12g

MODIFICATIONS: If there is poor appetite, abdominal distention, and fatigue, add *Bai Zhu* (Atractylodis Macrocephalae, Rhizoma) and *Dang Shen* (Codonopsitis Pilosulae, Radix). If there is nausea and vomiting, add *Sheng Jiang* (Zingiberis Officinalis, uncooked Rhizoma) and *Xuan Fu Hua* (Inulae Racemosae, Flos). If there is severe edema, add *Zhu Ling* (Polypori Umbellati, Sclerotium) and *Ze Xie* (Alismatis Orientalis, Rhizoma). If there is kidney

vacuity, add *Xu Duan* (Dipsaci Asperi, Radix) and *Sang Ji Sheng* (Sangjisheng, Ramulus).

ACUMOXIBUSTION: Use warm needle technique on *Shen Shu* (Bl 23), *Guan Yuan Shu* (Bl 26), *Guan Yuan* (CV 4), and *Qi Hai* (CV 6) and needle *Shui Fen* (CV 9) and *Yin Ling Quan* (Sp 9).

MODIFICATIONS: For long, clear urination or whitish urine, moxibustion *Ming Men* (GV 4) to warm and secure the lower origin. For simultaneous invasion of wind cold, add *Feng Men* (Bl 12). For stomach fullnes and distention and loose stools, add *Zu San Li* (St 36). For scanty urination, add *Pian Li* (LI 16) and *Wen Liu* (LI 17).

10. LOW BACK PAIN IN STONE STRANGURY

SIGNS & SYMPTOMS: Intermittent but unbearable lumbar pain, dark-colored urine with possible sands and stones, painful urination with possible stopping and starting of flow, and profuse sweating when the pain is severe. The tongue can be normal and the pulse is often bowstring.

TREATMENT PRINCIPLES: Disinhibit urination, free the flow of strangury, and stop pain

REPRESENTATIVE FORMULA: Modified *Shi Wei San* (Pyrrosia Powder)

Shi Wei (Pyrrosiae, Folium), 15g
Dong Kui Zi (Abutili Seu Malvae, Semen), 15g
Qu Mai (Dianthi, Herba), 9g
Bian Xu (Polygoni Avicularis, Herba), 9g
Hua Shi (Talcum), 20g
Che Qian Zi (Plantaginis, Semen), 12g
Chuan Niu Xi (Cyathulae Officinalis, Radix), 9g
Ji Nei Jin (Gigeriae Galli, Endothelium Corneum), 9g
Jin Qian Cao (Lysmachiae, Herba), 30g
Hai Jin Sha (Lygodii Japonici, Spora), 12g
powdered *Hu Po* (Succinum), 5g

MODIFICATIONS: In case of bloody strangury, add *Xiao Ji* (Cephalanoplos Segeti, Herba) and *Bai Mao Gen* (Imperatae Cylindricae, Rhizoma). If there is severely painful urination, increase the dosage of *Hai Jin Sha* up to 20 grams.

ACUMOXIBUSTION: Needle *Shen Shu* (Bl 23), *Pang Guang Shu* (Bl 28), *Qu Quan* (Liv 8), *Wei Zhong* (Bl 40), and *Jing Men* (GB 25).

MODIFICATIONS: For bloody urine, add *Xue Hai* (Sp 10). For stones in the upper urinary track, add *Tian Shu* (St 25). For stones in the middle or lower urinary track, add *Shui Dao* (St 28) and *Zhong Ji* (CV 3). For vomiting, add *Nei Guan* (Per 6). For constipation, add *Zhi Gou* (TB 6) and *Tian Shu* (St 25). For severe pain, add *Zhong Feng* (Liv 4).

REPRESENTATIVE CASE HISTORIES

Case history of Dr. Qi Chang: Yu, a 36 year-old female[1]

Yu's first visit was on Dec. 15, 1990. In June 1990, she experienced mild lumbar pain. Then on July 3, she suddenly had bloody urine without pain, frequency, or urgency. That evening, she had right lumbar pain shooting to the right lower abdomen. The pain was so severe that she had to be admitted to a hospital. Urinalysis showed that RBCs filled the microscope field, WBCs were at 3+, and protein was at 1+. Yu had an abdominal x-ray but it was negative (there were no stones). She was given antibiotics and Chinese medicinals to clear heat and disinhibit urination for 10 days. Her urinalysis became normal and she was discharged from the hospital. However, as an outpatient some time later, Yu had an ultrasound and a pyelogram. These showed that her right ureter was inflamed and narrowed and that fluid had accumulated in her left renal pelvis. She began a course of antibiotics and physical therapy, but her condition would improve and worsen without resolving. Yu wanted to avoid surgery and came to the Chinese medical department. When Dr. Qi examined her, Yu was pale and fatigued. She had lumbar discomfort and heat in the five hearts, but her urination was without frequency, urgency, or pain, and her urinalysis was negative. Her tongue was red and moist, and her pulse was deep. Dr. Qi's pattern identification was kidney yang vacuity with inhibited qi transformation, water accumulation in

the kidney, and qi and blood stasis. His treatment strategy was to boost kidney yang, drain dampness, and quicken the blood. His prescription consisted of: *Shu Di Huang* (Rehmanniae Glutinosae, cooked Radix), 25g, *Shan Yao* (Radix Dioscoreae Oppositae), 15g, *Fu Ling* (Poriae Cocos, Sclerotium), 15g, *Mu Dan Pi* (Moutan, Cortex Radicis), 15g, *Ze Xie* (Alismatis Orientalis, Rhizoma), 15g, *Gou Qi Zi* (Lycii Chinensis, Fructus), 15g, *Rou Gui* (Cinnamonmi Casiae, Cortex), 7.5g, *Fu Zi* (Aconiti Carmichaeli, Radix Lateralis Praeparatus), 7.5g, *Che Qian Zi* (Plantaginis, Semen), 15g, *Niu Xi* (Achyranthis Bidentatae, Radix), 15g, *Gan Cao* (Glycyrrhizae Uralensis, Radix), 7.5g, *Dan Shen* (Salviae Miltiorrhizae, Radix), 15g, and *Tu Si Zi* (Cuscutae Chinensis, Semen), 15g. Yu took this formula for 30 days and all her symptoms disappeared. On Mar. 8, 1991, ultrasound showed that her right side ureter was open without any narrowing. The fluid accumulation in the renal pelvis was almost completely gone. She continued on this formula for 20 more days and was considered cured.

COMMENTARY: The *Jin Gui Yao Lue* states that vacuity taxation may cause lumbar pain. This may be accompanied with symptoms of abdominal cramping and inhibition of urination. For this condition, one may use *Ba Wei Shen Qi Wan* (Eight Flavors Kidney Qi Pills): *Fu Zi* (Aconiti Carmichaeli, Radix Lateralis Praeparatus), 9g, *Rou Gui* (Cinnamonmi Casiae, Cortex), 5g, *Shu Di Huang* (Rehmanniae Glutinosae, cooked Radix), 12g, *Shan Yao* (Radix Dioscoreae Oppositae), 12g, *Shan Zhu Yu* (Corni Officinalis, Fructus), 12g, *Ze Xie* (Alismatis Orientalis, Rhizoma), 9g, *Fu Ling* (Poriae Cocos, Sclerotium), 12g, and *Mu Dan Pi* (Moutan, Cortex Radicis), 9g. When the root is kidney yang vacuity with water accumulation, one must employ a treatment strategy that includes boosting the kidney's qi transformation in order to transform water. One must also remember that water accumulation can cause blood stasis, and one will often have better results by adding medicinals that rectify the qi and quicken the blood.

Case history of Dr. Qi Chang: Ding, a 40 year-old male worker[2]

Ding's first visit to Dr. Qi was on Oct. 28, 1993. Ding had lumbar pain for 10 years, but it had intensified in the three years prior to this visit. It was so severe that he could not bend or move and it would shoot all the way to his shoulders and down his legs. The pain was better with heat and worse with cold and sitting. Ding had been treated with Western medication without success. Ding was of a very thin build. He had a pale, red tongue with slimy, white fur, and a deep pulse. Dr. Qi's pattern identification was wind cold invasion of the channels and network vessels with blood stasis. Therefore, the treatment principles were to expel the wind and scatter cold, move the blood and free the flow of the channels. His prescription was: *Wu Tou* (Aconiti Carmichaeli, Radix), 15g, *Chuan Shan Jia* (Manitis Pentadactylis, Squama), 5g, *Di Long* (Lumbricus), 10g, *Tu Bie Chong* (Eupolyphaga Seu Opisthoplatia), 5g, *Quan Xie* (Buthus Martensis), 10g, *Ru Xiang* (Olibani, Resina), 10g, *Mo Yao* (Myrrhae, Resina), 10g, *Dang Gui* (Angelicae Sinensis, Radix), 20g, *Dan Shen* (Salviae Miltiorrhizae, Radix), 20g, *Gou Ji* (Cibotii Barometsis, Rhizoma), 20g, *Qian Nian Jian* (Homalomenae Occultae, Rhizoma), 20g, *Yin Yang Huo* (Epimedii, Herba), 15g, *Qing Feng Teng* (Sinomenii Acuti, Rhizoma), 30g, and *Gan Cao* (Glycyrrhizae Uralensis, Radix), 10g.

Ding took this formula for 20 days and felt much improved, he could bend and move to the left and right, but he still could not sit too long without pain and his lower back still felt cold. Thus, Dr. Qi decided to change the prescription as follows: *Fang Feng* (Ledebouriellae Divaricatae, Radix), 15g, *Qiang Huo* (Notopterygii, Rhizoma Et Radix), 15g, *Qin Jiao* (Gentianae Qinjiao, Radix), 15g, *Wu Tou* (Aconiti Carmichaeli, Radix), 15g, *Chuan Shan Jia* (Manitis Pentadactylis, Squama), 5g, *Quan Xie* (Buthus Martensis), 10g, *Tu Bie Chong* (Eupolyphaga Seu Opisthoplatia), 5g, *Di Long* (Lumbricus), 9g, *Ru Xiang* (Olibani, Resina), 10g, *Mo Yao* (Myrrhae, Resina), 10g, *Shu Di Huang* (Rehmanniae Glutinosae, cooked Radix), 15g, *Gou Ji* (Cibotii Barometsis, Rhizoma), 20g, *Du Zhong* (Eucommiae Ulmoidis, Cortex), 15g, *Qian Nian Jian* (Homalomenae Occultae, Rhizoma), 20g, *Qing Feng Teng* (Sinomenii Acuti, Rhizoma), 30g, *Yin Yang Huo* (Epimedii, Herba), 15g, and *Gan Cao* (Glycyrrhizae Uralensis, Radix), 10g.

Ding took this new formula for 25 days and his lumbar pain almost completely subsided. He could do normal work, but, when he sat too long, his low back still became sore and heavy. His tongue was pale red with thin, white fur, and his pulse was bowstring. Dr. Qi decided to change the treatment strategy to supplement the liver and kidney qi and blood as well as to quicken the blood and free the flow of the channels. His new prescription included: *Shu Di Huang* (Rehmanniae Glutinosae, cooked Radix), 20g, *Rou Cong Rong* (Cistanchis Deserticolae, Herba), 20g, *Ba Ji Tian* (Morindae Officinalis, Radix), 15g, *Gou Ji* (Cibotii Barometsis, Rhizoma), 20g, *Du Zhong* (Eucommiae Ulmoidis, Cortex), 15g, *Huang Qi* (Astragali Membranacei, Radix), 30g, *Dang Gui* (Angelicae Sinensis, Radix), 15g, *Chuan Xiong* (Ligustici Wallichii, Radix), 15g, *Dan Shen* (Salviae Miltiorrhizae, Radix), 20g, *Chuan Shan Jia* (Manitis Pentadactylis, Squama), 5g, *Quan Xie* (Buthus Martensis), 10g, *Tu Bie Chong* (Eupolyphaga Seu Opisthoplatia), 7g, *Di Long* (Lumbricus), 10g, *Tao Ren* (Pruni Persicae, Semen), 15g, *Hong Hua* (Carthami Tinctorii, Flos), 15g, and *Gan Cao* (Glycyrrhizae Uralensis, Radix), 10g. After Ding took this formula for 20 days, his low back was completely without pain. He staged a complete recovery and went back to work. On a follow-up visit a half a year later, Ding reported that there was only a little lumbar discomfort with heavy physical work. Otherwise, everything was normal.

COMMENTARY: Ding presented liver-kidney vacuity with malnourishment of the governing vessel. Therefore, mansion of the kidney was not stabilized. This allowed wind and cold to invade, causing qi and blood stasis and stagnation in the channels and network vessels. This meant that there was repletion at the tip and vacuity at the root. The treatment strategy was to supplement the liver and kidney, strengthen the governing vessel, expel wind and cold, quicken the blood and free the flow of the channels. Because this condition had been chronic for 10 years, Dr. Qi had to use strong stasis-dispelling medicinals, such as the "worm" or "insect" products *Quan Xie*, *Tu Bie Chong*, and *Di Long*.

Case history of Dr. Qi Chang: Wang, a 39 year-old, male cadre[3]

Wang's first visit was on Dec. 8, 1992. He had lumbar pain for one year. The pain was worse at night. In fact, it was so severe at night that he could not turn his body. The pain was also worse in cold and damp weather. Wang's Western physician wanted to perform surgery, but Wang wanted to avoid surgery and came to the Chinese medical department and Dr. Qi. When Dr. Qi saw Wang, he was overweight. His tongue was dark purple on the sides, and his pulse was deep and forceful. Dr. Qi's pattern identification was invasion of the channels and network vessels by wind dampness with blood stasis. His treatment strategy was to expel wind and eliminate dampness, quicken the blood and free the flow of the channels. Therefore, he prescribed the following: *Chuan Niu Xi* (Cyathulae Officinalis, Radix), 15g, *Di Long* (Lumbricus), 15g, *Qiang Huo* (Notopterygii, Rhizoma Et Radix), 10g, *Qin Jiao* (Gentianae Qinjiao, Radix), 15g, *Xiang Fu* (Cyperi Rotundi, Rhizoma), 15g, *Dang Gui* (Angelicae Sinensis, Radix), 15g, *Chuan Xiong* (Ligustici Wallichii, Radix), 15g, *Huang Qi* (Astragali Membranacei, Radix), 30g, *Cang Zhu* (Atractylodis, Rhizoma), 15g, *Huang Bai* (Phellodendri, Cortex), 15g, *Wu Ling Zhi* (Trogopteri Seu Pteromi, Excrementum), 15g, *Tao Ren* (Pruni Persicae, Semen), 15g, *Mo Yao* (Myrrhae, Resina), 10g, *Hong Hua* (Carthami Tinctorii, Flos), 15g, *Dan Shen* (Salviae Miltiorrhizae, Radix), 20g, *Chi Shao* (Paeoniae Lactiflorae, Radix Rubrus), 15g, and *Ru Xiang* (Olibani, Resina), 15g.

On Dec. 14, Wang's second visit, he had taken the medicinals for six days and his lumbar pain was much improved. He was now able to move and turn. However, there was no change in his pulse and tongue. Therefore Dr. Qi changed the prescription to: *Dan Shen* (Salviae Miltiorrhizae, Radix), 20g, *Dang Gui* (Angelicae Sinensis, Radix), 20g, *Ru Xiang* (Olibani, Resina), 10g, *Mo Yao* (Myrrhae, Resina), 10g, *Huang Bai* (Phellodendri, Cortex), 15g, *Zhi Mu* (Anemarrhenae Asphodeloidis, Rhizoma), 15g, *Chi Shao* (Paeoniae Lactiflorae, Radix Rubrus), 20g, *Chuan Niu Xi* (Cyathulae Officinalis, Radix), 15g, *Qiang Huo* (Notopterygii, Rhizoma Et Radix), 15g, *Qin Jiao* (Gentianae Qinjiao, Radix), 15g, *Tian Hua Fen* (Trichosanthis Kirilowii, Radix), 15g, *Hong Hua* (Carthami Tinctorii, Flos), 15g, *Tao Ren* (Pruni

Persicae, Semen), 15g, *Wu Ling Zhi* (Trogopteri Seu Pteromi, Excrementum), 10g, *Cang Zhu* (Atractylodis, Rhizoma), 15g, and *Gan Cao* (Glycyrrhizae Uralensis, Radix), 10g.

On Dec. 22, Wang's third visit, he had taken the new prescription for six days and his lumbar pain continued to improve but he still felt some pain. The pain moved around and even up to his neck. Wang's tongue was moist, and his pulse was deep and slow. Based on these signs and symptoms, Dr. Qi prescribed the following: *Chuan Niu Xi* (Cyathulae Officinalis, Radix), 15g, *Di Long* (Lumbricus), 15g, *Qiang Huo* (Notopterygii, Rhizoma Et Radix), 15g, *Qin Jiao* (Gentianae Qinjiao, Radix), 15g, *Xiang Fu* (Cyperi Rotundi, Rhizoma), 15g, *Dang Gui* (Angelicae Sinensis, Radix), 20g, *Chuan Xiong* (Ligustici Wallichii, Radix), 15g, *Cang Zhu* (Atractylodis, Rhizoma), 15g, *Huang Bai* (Phellodendri, Cortex), 15g, *Wu Ling Zhi* (Trogopteri Seu Pteromi, Excrementum), 15g, *Hong Hua* (Carthami Tinctorii, Flos), 15g, *Mo Yao* (Myrrhae, Resina), 15g, *Ge Gen* (Puerariae, Radix), 15g, *Tao Ren* (Pruni Persicae, Semen), 5g, *Zhi Mu* (Anemarrhenae Asphodeloidis, Rhizoma), 15g, *Huang Qi* (Astragali Membranacei, Radix), 30g, *Tian Hua Fen* (Trichosanthis Kirilowii, Radix), 15g, and *Gan Cao* (Glycyrrhizae Uralensis, Radix), 10g.

On Jan. 6, 1993, Wang's fourth visit, he had taken this last formula for 12 days and his lumbar pain was gone. He now had occasional pain that moved up and down his spine. Dr. Qi changed the prescription to: *Chuan Niu Xi* (Cyathulae Officinalis, Radix), 15g, *Di Long* (Lumbricus), 15g, *Qiang Huo* (Notopterygii, Rhizoma Et Radix), 10g, *Qin Jiao* (Gentianae Qinjiao, Radix), 15g, *Xiang Fu* (Cyperi Rotundi, Rhizoma), 15g, *Dang Gui* (Angelicae Sinensis, Radix), 20g, *Chuan Xiong* (Ligustici Wallichii, Radix), 15g, *Huang Qi* (Astragali Membranacei, Radix), 30g, *Cang Zhu* (Atractylodis, Rhizoma), 15g, *Chuan Shan Jia* (Manitis Pentadactylis, Squama), 5g, *Dan Shen* (Salviae Miltiorrhizae, Radix), 20g, *Zhi Mu* (Anemarrhenae Asphodeloidis, Rhizoma), 15g, *Tian Hua Fen* (Trichosanthis Kirilowii, Radix), 15g, *Ru Xiang* (Olibani, Resina), 10g, *Mo Yao* (Myrrhae, Resina),

10g, *Tao Ren* (Pruni Persicae, Semen), 5g, *Hong Hua* (Carthami Tinctorii, Flos), 15g, and *Gan Cao* (Glycyrrhizae Uralensis, Radix), 10g. After Wang took this formula for 12 days, all his symptoms disappeared and he could move his spine normally. He felt he was completely cured.

COMMENTARY: Wang's case was one of blood stasis. His lumbar pain was worse in the evening and in cold and damp weather, his tongue was dark purple, and his pulse was deep. These signs and symptoms indicate wind cold dampness with blood stasis obstructing the channels. For this pattern, one usually uses *Shen Tong Zhu Yu Tang* (Painful Body Dispel Stasis Decoction) plus *Huo Luo Xiao Ling Dan* (Quicken the Network Vessels Fantastically Effective Pills) with modifications.

Shen Tong Zhu Yu Tang: Qin Jiao (Gentianae Qinjiao, Radix), 3g, *Chuan Xiong* (Ligustici Wallichii, Radix), 15g, *Tao Ren* (Pruni Persicae, Semen), 10g, *Hong Hua* (Carthami Tinctorii, Flos), 7g, *Gan Cao* (Glycyrrhizae Uralensis, Radix), 3g, *Qiang Huo* (Notopterygii, Rhizoma Et Radix), 3g, *Mo Yao* (Myrrhae, Resina), 6g, *Dang Gui* (Angelicae Sinensis, Radix), 10g, *Ling Zhi* (Trogopteri Seu Pteromi, Excrementum), 6g, *Xiang Fu* (Cyperi Rotundi, Rhizoma), 3g, *Chuan Niu Xi* (Cyathulae Officinalis, Radix), 9g, and *Di Long* (Lumbricus), 6g

Huo Luo Xiao Ling Dan: Dang Gui (Angelicae Sinensis, Radix), 15g, *Dan Shen* (Salviae Miltiorrhizae, Radix), 15g, *Ru Xiang* (Olibani, Resina), 15g, and *Mo Yao* (Myrrhae, Resina), 15g

Within this last formula, *Dang Gui* both moves and nourishes the blood, *Dan Shen* quickens the blood and dispels stasis, and *Ru Xiang* and *Mo Yao* quicken the blood, free the flow of the network vessels, and stop pain. The ability of these two formulas to disperse stagnation and stop pain is very strong, especially with the addition of the "worm" or "insect" products.

ENDNOTES

[1] Chang Qi, *Chang Qi Lin Chuang Jin Yen Ji Yao*, (*The Gathered Essentials of the Clinical Experiences of Chang Qi*), China Medical Science Publishing Company, Beijing, 1999, p. 337
[2] *Ibid.*, p. 334
[3] *Ibid.*, p. 335

CHAPTER 9
STRANGURY

Strangury refers to urinary difficulty, pain, frequency, urgency, inhibition, and dribbling. There may be blood or stones in the urine or the urine may be turbid or oily. Strangury generally corresponds to urinary tract infections, kidney infections, and bladder and kidney stones in Western medicine.

DISEASE CAUSES & MECHANISMS

Damp heat is the predominant pattern in the acute phase of strangury. If this is not treated properly and becomes chronic, vacuity replaces repletion, usually with patterns of spleen and kidney vacuity. *Su Wen*, Chapter 71, "*Liu Yuan Zheng Ji Da Lun* (Great Treatise on the Six Origins & Correct Periods)", states:

> When humans are invaded by evils, they will contract diseases of internal heat. The symptoms include . . . water swelling of the face and eyes…yellowish, red urine, frequency, urgency, pain, and dripping of urine . . .

In *Su Wen*, Chapter 74, "*Zhi Zheng Yao Da Lun* (Great Treatise on the Arriving at the Truth of the Essentials)," it states, ". . . all turbid excretions pertain to heat . . . " In the Ming dynasty work, *Jing Yue Quan Shu* (*Jing-yue's Complete Book*) is the following:

In strangury, the urination is difficult, painful, dribbling, urgent, and incomplete. This is usually due to the heart and kidney not communicating, heat and toxin stagnation, engaging in sex while drunk, overeating fried, baked, or other dry and heating foods, or liver qi depression. For heat diseases, one must clear heat. For urinary difficulty, one should smooth the flow of the urine. For sinking qi, one must lift the spleen qi. For vacuity of the life-gate fire, one should warm and supplement the life-gate.

This passage indicates the complexity of strangury. It follows that one must carefully identify the presenting pattern before attempting to treat this condition.

TREATMENT BASED ON PATTERN IDENTIFICATION

The *Zhong Zang Jing* (*Classic of the Central Treasury*) attributed to Hua Tuo classifies strangury into patterns of cold, heat, qi, taxation, turbidity, stones, vacuity, and repletion. The *Ji Yan Fang* (*A Collection of Empirical Formulas*) mentions five types that are still recognized: stone, qi, unctuous, taxation, and heat. Today strangury is divided into six patterns: 1) heat strangury, 2) blood strangury, 3) stone strangury,

TYPE OF STRANGURY		PATTERN IDENTIFICATION
Heat Strangury	**Replete**	1. Damp heat
	Vacuous	2. Heat damages the yin
Blood Strangury	**Replete**	3. Damp heat stagnation 4. Heart fire shifting heat to the small intestine
	Vacuous	5. Yin vacuity heat 6. Kidney yin vacuity 7. Spleen and kidney qi vacuity
Stone Strangury	**Replete**	*8. Damp heat (dampness more than heat)* *9. Damp heat (heat more than dampness)* *10. Qi stagnation*
	Vacuous	*11. Qi vacuity: inhibited kidney and bladder qi transformation* *12. Kidney yin vacuity* *13. Kidney qi vacuity*
Qi Strangury	**Replete**	*14. Liver qi depression and binding*
	Vacuous	*15. Center qi fall*
Taxation Strangury	**Vacuous**	*16. Spleen vacuity* *17. Kidney yang vacuity* *18. Kidney yin vacuity*
Unctuous Strangury	**Replete**	*19. Damp heat in the lower burner*
	Vacuous	*20. Kidney qi vacuity*

Chart 9.1. Types of strangury & their patterns

4) qi strangury, 5) taxation strangury, and 6) unctuous strangury. These six types of strangury are outlined in Chart 9.1.

1. HEAT STRANGURY FROM DAMP HEAT IN THE BLADDER

SIGNS & SYMPTOMS: Painful, urgent, frequent, short, hot, dark yellowish urination, lower abdominal cramping and distention, pain possibly radiating to the umbilicus and low back, possible dribbling urination, possible alternating fever and chills with nausea, vomiting, and a bitter taste in the mouth, and constipation. There is slimy, yellow tongue fur and a slippery, rapid pulse.

TREATMENT PRINCIPLES: Clear heat, disinhibit dampness, and stop pain

REPRESENTATIVE FORMULA: *Ba Zheng San* (Eight [Ingredients] Rectification Powder)

Mu Tong (Akebiae Mutong, Caulis), 6g
Qu Mai (Dianthi, Herba), 9g
Da Huang (Rhei, Radix Et Rhizoma), 9g
Che Qian Zi (Plantaginis, Semen), 12g
Hua Shi (Talcum), 18g
Zhi Zi (Gardeniae Jasminoidis, Fructus), 9g
Bian Xu (Polygoni Avicularis, Herba), 9g
Gan Cao Shao (Glycyrrhizae Uralensis, Radix Tenuis), 6g

MODIFICATIONS: For alternating fever and chills, a bitter taste in the mouth, dry throat, and nausea, add *Xiao Chai Hu Tang* (Minor Bupleurum Decoction): *Chai Hu* (Bupleuri, Radix), 9g, *Huang Qin* (Scutellariae Baicalensis, Radix), 9g, ginger stir-fried *Ban Xia*

(Pinelliae Ternatae, Rhizoma), 9g, *Dang Shen* (Codonopsitis Pilosulae, Radix), 6g, *Sheng Jiang* (Zingiberis Officinalis, uncooked Rhizoma), 6g, and *Da Zao* (Zizyphi Jujubae, Fructus), 4 pieces. For concomitant spleen vacuity, subtract *Da Huang, Mu Tong,* and *Zhi Zi* and add *Fu Ling* (Poriae Cocos, Sclerotium), *Zhu Ling* (Polypori Umbellati, Sclerotium), and *Deng Xin Cao* (Junci Effusi, Medulla). For nausea and vomiting, subtract *Mu Tong,* replace uncooked *Zhi Zi* with stir-fried *Zhi Zi,* and add ginger-processed *Ban Xia* (Pinelliae Ternatae, Rhizoma) and *Sheng Jiang* (Zingiberis Officinalis, uncooked Rhizoma). For low back pain, add *Chuan Niu Xi* (Cyathulae Officinalis, Radix). For constipation, replace cooked with uncooked *Da Huang* and add *Zhi Shi* (Citri Aurantii, Fructus Immaturus). For damp heat damaging yin with thirst and dry, yellow tongue fur, subtract *Da Huang, Mu Tong,* and *Zhi Zi* while adding *Bai Mao Gen* (Imperatae Cylindricae, Rhizoma), *Zhi Mu* (Anemarrhenae Aspheloidis, Rhizoma), and *Sheng Di Huang* (Rehamnniae Glutinosae, uncooked Radix).

ACUMOXIBUSTION: Needle *Zhong Ji* (CV 3), *Pang Guang Shu* (Bl 28), *San Yin Jiao* (5p 6), and *Qu Quan* (Liv 8).

MODIFICATIONS: For fever, a bitter taste in the mouth, nausea, and vomiting, add *San Jiao Shu* (Bl 22) and *Ye Men* (TB 3). For constipation, add *Zhao Hai* (Ki 6) and *Zhi Gou* (TB 6). For fever, add *Qu Chi* (LI 11). For colicky pain in the abdomen and low back, add *Xiao Chang Shu* (Bl 27). For severely painful and/or burning urination, add *Shui Quan* (Ki 5).

2. BLOOD STRANGURY—REPLETE PATTERN FROM DAMP HEAT IN THE BLADDER OR FROM HEART FIRE

SIGNS & SYMPTOMS: Painful, urgent, frequent, astringent, short voidings of hot, reddish urine, sometimes bloody clots in the urine, inhibited urination, sometimes contracting pain in the urethra that radiates to the umbilicus, and heart vexation. There is a red tongue with thin, yellow fur and a slippery, rapid, forceful pulse.

TREATMENT PRINCIPLES: Clear heat and free the flow of strangury, cool the blood and stop bleeding

REPRESENTATIVE FORMULA: Modified *Xiao Ji Yin Zi* (Cephalanoplos Beverage)

Xiao Ji (Cephalanoplos Segeti, Herba), 24g
Sheng Di Huang (Rehmanniae Glutinosae, uncooked Radix), 12g
Hua Shi (Talcum), 18g
Pu Huang (Typhae, Pollen), 9g
Dan Zhu Ye (Lophatheri Gracilis, Herba), 12g
Ou Jie (Nelumbinis Nuciferae, Nodus Rhizomatis), 24g
Zhi Zi (Gardeniae Jasminoidis, Fructus), 9g
Qu Mai (Dianthi, Herba), 9g
Shi Wei (Pyrrosiae, Folium), 9g
Gan Cao Shao (Glycyrrhizae Uralensis, Radix Tenuis), 9g

MODIFICATIONS: For profuse hematuria, add powdered *San Qi* (Notoginseng, Radix) and powdered *Hu Po* (Succinum) taken with the strained decoction. For blood clots in the urine, add *Chuan Niu Xi* (Cyathulae Officinalis, Radix) and *Chi Shao* (Paeoniae Lactiflorae, Radix Rubrus). For severely painful urination, add stir-fried *Ru Xiang* (Olibani, Resina), stir-fried *Mo Yao* (Myrrhae, Resina), and *Yan Hu Suo* (Corydalis Yanhusuo, Rhizoma). For low back pain, add *Chuan Niu Xi* (Cyathulae Officinalis, Radix). For damp heat or heat damaging yin with a red tongue and thin fur, a dry throat and mouth, and a fine, rapid pulse, add *E Jiao* (Asini, Gelatinum Corii), *Han Lian Cao* (Ecliptae Prostratae, Herba), and *Nu Zhen Zi* (Ligustri Lucidi, Fructus). For heart vexation, insomnia, and sores on the tongue, add *Dan Zhu Ye* (Lophatheri Gracilis, Herba), *Deng Xin Cao* (Junci Effusi, Medulla), *Mu Tong* (Akebiae Mutong, Caulis), and powdered *Hu Po* (Succinum) taken with the strained decoction.

ACUMOXIBUSTION: Needle *Zhong Ji* (CV 3), *Pang Guang Shu* (Bl 28), *San Yin Jiao* (Sp 6), and *Xue Hai* (Sp 10).

MODIFICATIONS: For lower abdominal distention and pain, add *Qu Quan* (Liv 8). For severely painful and/or burning urination, add *Shui Quan* (Ki 5). For heart vexation, insomnia, and sores on the tongue, add *Tong Li* (Ht 5). For fever, a bitter taste in the mouth, nausea, and vomiting, add *San Jiao Shu* (Bl 22) and *Ye Men* (TB 3). For fever, add *Qu Chi* (LI 11). For colicky pain in the abdomen and low back, add *Xiao Chang Shu* (Bl 27).

3. BLOOD STRANGURY—VACUITY PATTERN FROM DAMP HEAT OR HEAT DAMAGING KIDNEY YIN

SIGNS & SYMPTOMS: Enduring, slightly painful urination, pale red urination which is worse with taxation, low back and knee soreness and limpness, heart vexation, vexatious heat of the five hearts, possible night sweats, and lassitude of the spirit. There is a pale red tongue with scanty fur and a fine, forceless, rapid pulse.

TREATMENT PRINCIPLES: Enrich yin, clear heat, and stop bleeding

REPRESENTATIVE FORMULA: Modified *Liu Wei Di Huang Wan* (Six Flavors Rehmannia Pills)

Shu Di (Rehmanniae Glutinosae, cooked Radix), 15g
Shan Zhu Yu (Corni Officinalis, Fructus), 9g
Shan Yao (Disocoreae Oppositae, Radix), 9g
Fu Ling (Poriae Cocos, Sclerotium), 9g
Mu Dan Pi (Moutan, Cortex Radicis), 12g
Ze Xie (Alismatis Orientalis, Rhizoma), 9g
E Jiao (Asini, Gelatinum Corii), 9g
Xiao Ji (Cephalanoplos Segeti, Herba), 12g
Han Lian Cao (Ecliptae Prostratae, Herba), 9g
Huang Bai (Phellodendri, Cortex), 9g

MODIFICATIONS: For concomitant qi vacuity with shortness of breath, fatigue, and a pale tongue, add *Dang Shen* (Codonopsitis Pilosulae, Radix) and mix-fried *Huang Qi* (Astragali Membranacei, Radix). For concomitant kidney yang vacuity with cold limbs, aversion to cold, and impotence, add *Fu Zi* (Aconiti Carmichaeli, Radix Lateralis Praeparatus), *Rou Gui* (Cinnamomi Cassiae, Cortex), and *Ba Ji Tian* (Morindae Officinalis, Radix).

For damaged yin from enduring damp heat remaining in the yin aspect, replace *Liu Wei Di Huang Wan* with modified *E Jiao San* (Donkey Skin Glue Powder): *E Jiao* (Asini, Gelatinum Corii), 9g, *Sheng Di Huang* (Rehmanniae Glutinosae, uncooked Radix), 15g, *Zhu Ling* (Polypori Umbellati, Sclerotium), 9g, *Ze Xie* (Alismatis Orientalis, Rhizoma), 9g, *Chi Fu Ling* (Poriae Cocos, Sclerotium Rubrum), 9g, *Hua Shi* (Talcum), 15g, *Che Qian Zi* (Plantaginis, Semen), 12g, *Xiao Ji* (Cephalanoplos Segeti, Herba), 12g, and *Han Lian Cao* (Ecliptae Prostratae, Herba), 9g.

ACUMOXIBUSTION: Needle *Zhong Ji* (CV 3), *Xue Hai* (Sp 10), *Pang Guang Shu* (Bl 28), *Fu Liu* (Ki 7), and *San Yin Jiao* (Sp 6).

MODIFICATIONS: For low back and knee soreness and weakness, add *Shen Shu* (Bl 23). For insomnia, heart vexation, vexatious heat of the five hearts, and night sweats, add *Yin Xi* (Ht 6). For severe kidney yin vacuity with exuberant fire, add *Yin Gu* (Ki 10), *Zhao Hai* (Ki 6), and *Jiao Xing* (Ki 8) to enrich yin, down-bear fire, and free the flow of urination.

4. STONE STRANGURY—REPLETION PATTERN FROM DAMP HEAT IN THE BLADDER

SIGNS & SYMPTOMS: Painful urination with possible stops and starts in the flow of urine, profuse sweating when the pain is severe, inhibited urination, dark-colored urination with possible sand and stones or sometimes bloody clots, intermittent but unbearable low back pain when it attacks radiating to genitals or lower abdomen, lower abdominal cramping, distention, and pain. There is a red tongue with thin, yellow fur, and a bowstring, rapid pulse. In addition, severe, unbearable pain may also cause sweating, vomiting, a pale facial complexion, and a cold form or body. However, this is false cold.

TREATMENT PRINCIPLES: Clear heat and disinhibit urination, expel stones and stop pain

REPRESENTATIVE FORMULA: Modified *Shi Wei San* (Pyrrosia Powder)

Shi Wei (Pyrrosiae, Folium), 15g
Dong Kui Zi (Abutili Seu Malvae, Semen), 15g
Qu Mai (Dianthi, Herba), 9g
Bian Xu (Polygoni Avicularis, Herba), 9g
Hua Shi (Talcum), 15g

Che Qian Zi (Plantaginis, Semen), 15g
Ji Nei Jin (Gigeriae Galli, Endothelium Corneum), 9g
Jin Qian Cao (Lysimachiae, Herba), 15g
Hai Jin Sha (Lygodii Japonici, Spora), 15g

MODIFICATIONS: For severe, spasmodic pain, add *Bai Shao* (Paeoniae Lactiflorae, Radix Albus) and *Gan Cao* (Glycyrrhizae Uralensis, Radix). For blood strangury, add *Xiao Ji* (Cephalanoplos Segeti, Herba), and *Bai Mao Gen* (Imperatae Cylindricae, Rhizoma). For low back pain, add *Chuan Niu Xi* (Cyathulae Officinalis, Radix). For burning urination, add *Mu Tong* (Akebiae Mutong, Caulis), and *Zhi Zi* (Gardeniae Jasminoidis, Fructus). For fever, add *Pu Gong Ying* (Taraxaci Mongolici, Herba Cum Radice), *Huang Bai* (Phellodendri, Cortex), and *Da Huang* (Rhei, Radix Et Rhizoma).

ACUMOXIBUSTION: Needle *Zhong Ji* (CV 3), *Pang Guang Shu* (Bl 28), *Zhong Feng* (Liv 4), *Ran Gu* (Ki 2), and *Wei Yang* (Bl 39).

MODIFICATIONS: For low back pain, add *Shen Shu* (Bl 23). For lower abdominal pain, add *Qu Quan* (Liv 8). For stones in the upper urinary track, add *Tian Shu* (St 25). For stones in the middle or lower track, add *Shui Dao* (St 28). For hematuria, add *Xue Hai* (Sp 10). For vomiting, add *Nei Guan* (Per 6). For constipation, add *Zhi Gou* (TB 6) and *Tian Shu* (St 25).

5. STONE STRANGURY—VACUITY PATTERN FROM KIDNEY VACUITY

SIGNS & SYMPTOMS: Enduring stone strangury, slightly painful urination with possible stops and starts in the flow of urine, inhibited urination, dark-colored urination with frequent sand, dull low back pain, hollow lower abdominal pain, and vexatious heat of the five hearts. There is a red tongue with scanty fur and a fine, weak pulse.

TREATMENT PRINCIPLES: Enrich the kidneys, down-bear fire, and dispel stones

REPRESENTATIVE FORMULA: Modified *Zhi Bai Di Huang Wan* (Anemarrhena & Phellodendron Rehmannia Pills)

Shu Di Huang (Rehmanniae Glutinosae, cooked Radix), 24g
Shan Zhu Yu (Corni Officinalis, Fructus), 9g
Shan Yao (Dioscoreae Oppositae, Radix), 9g
Fu Ling (Poriae Cocos, Sclerotium), 9g
Mu Dan Pi (Moutan, Cortex Radicis), 9g
Ze Xie (Alismatis Orientalis, Rhizoma), 12g
Zhi Mu (Anemarrhenae Aspheloidis, Rhizoma), 9g
Huang Bai (Phellodendri, Cortex), 9g
Hua Shi (Talcum), 12g
Hai Jin Sha (Lygodii Japonici, Spora), 12g

MODIFICATIONS: For enduring stone strangury from kidney qi vacuity with shortness of breath, fatigue, a pale facial complexion, impotence, a tender, enlarged tongue with teeth-marks on its edges and white fur, and a fine, forceless pulse, replace *Zhi Bai Di Huang Wan* with *Niao Lu Pai Shi Tang* (Urethra Expel Stones Decoction): *Jin Qian Cao* (Lysimachiae, Herba), 12g, *Hai Jin Sha* (Lygodii Japonici, Spora), 12g, *Ji Nei Jin* (Gigeriae Galli, Endothelium Corneum), 9g, *Hua Shi* (Talcum), 12g, *Fu Ling* (Poriae Cocos, Sclerotium), 9g, *Chuan Niu Xi* (Cyathulae Officinalis, Radix), 9g, *Tu Si Zi* (Cuscutae Chinensis, Semen), 9g, *Dang Shen* (Codonopsitis Pilosulae, Radix), 9g, *Huang Qi* (Astragali Membranacei, Radix), 15g, *Bu Gu Zhi* (Psoraleae Corylifoliae, Fructus), 9g, and mix-fried *Gan Cao* (Glycyrrhizae Uralensis, Radix), 6g. For enduring stone strangury from both kidney qi and yin vacuity, add to the preceding formula *Shu Di* (Rehmanniae Glutinosae, cooked Radix), 15g, and *Han Lian Cao* (Ecliptae Prostratae, Herba), 9g.

For enduring stone strangury from qi and blood insufficiency, replace *Zhi Bai Di Huang Wan* with *Ba Zhen Tang* (Eight Pearls Decoction) plus *Er Shen San* (Two Spirits Powder): *Shu Di Huang* (Rehmanniae Glutinosae, cooked Radix), 12g, *Bai Shao* (Paeoniae Lactiflorae, Radix Albus), 9g, wine stir-fried *Dang Gui* (Angelicae Sinensis, Radix), 9g, wine stir-fried *Chuan Xiong* (Ligustici Wallichii, Radix), 6g, *Dang Shen* (Codonopsitis Pilosulae, Radix), 12g, *Bai Zhu* (Atractylodis Macrocephalae, Rhizoma), 9g, *Fu Ling* (Poriae Cocos, Sclerotium), 12g, mix-fried *Gan Cao* (Glycyrrhizae Uralensis, Radix), 6g, *Hua Shi* (Talcum), 12g, and *Hai Jin Sha* (Lygodii Japonici, Spora), 12g.

ACUMOXIBUSTION: Needle *Zhong Ji* (CV 3), *Ran Gu* (Ki 2), *Pang Guang Shu* (Bl 28), *Fu Liu* (Ki 7), and *Shen Shu* (Bl 23).

MODIFICATIONS: For severe kidney yin vacuity with exuberant fire, add *Yin Gu* (Ki 10), *Zhao Hai* (Ki 6), and *Jiao Xing* (Ki 8) to enrich yin, downbear fire, and free the flow of urination. For stones in the upper urinary track, add *Tian Shu* (St 25). For stones in the middle or lower track, add *Shui Dao* (St 28). For hematuria, add *Xue Hai* (Sp 10). For insomnia, heart vexation, vexatious heat of the five hearts, and night sweats, add *Yin Xi* (Ht 6).

6. UNCTUOUS STRANGURY—REPLETE PATTERN FROM DAMP HEAT IN THE BLADDER

SIGNS & SYMPTOMS: Frequent, painful, short voidings of hot urine, turbid urination like rice-washing water with a possible floating oily scum, possible clots in the urine, inhibited urination, chest and stomach fullness and oppression, and thirst without large fluid intake. There is a red tongue with slimy, yellow fur and a slippery, rapid pulse.

TREATMENT PRINCIPLES: Clear heat and disinhibit dampness, divide the clear from the turbid

REPRESENTATIVE FORMULA: *Bei Xie Fen Qing Yin* (Dioscorea Hypoglauca Divide the Clear Beverage)

Bei Xie (Dioscoreae Hypoglaucae, Rhizoma), 15g
Huang Bai (Phellodendri, Cortex), 9g
Fu Ling (Poriae Cocos, Sclerotium), 9g
Lian Zi (Nelumbinis Nuciferae, Semen), 9g
Bai Zhu (Atractylodis Macrocephalae, Rhizoma), 9g
Dan Shen (Codonopsitis Pilosulae, Radix), 6g
Che Qian Zi (Plantaginis, Semen), 15g
Pu Huang (Typhae, Pollen), 9g

MODIFICATIONS: For severe turbid urination, add *Shi Chang Pu* (Acori Graminei, Rhizoma) and *Hai Jin Sha* (Lygodii Japonici, Spora). For severely burning urination, add *Hua Shi* (Talcum) and *Shi Wei* (Pyrrosiae, Folium). For hematuria, add *Hai Jin Sha* (Lygodii Japonici, Spora). For lower abdominal distention and rough, inhibited urination, add *Wu Yao*

(Linderae Strychifoliae, Radix) and *Qing Pi* (Citri Reticulatae Viride, Pericarpium). For blood clots in the urine, add *Xiao Ji* (Cephalanoplos Segeti, Herba) and *Bai Mao Gen* (Imperatae Cylindricae, Rhizoma).

ACUMOXIBUSTION: Needle *Zhong Ji* (CV 3), *Pang Guang Shu* (Bl 28), *San Yin Jiao* (Sp 6), and *Yin Ling Quan* (Sp 9) and moxibustion *Bai Hui* (GV 20).

MODIFICATIONS: For hematuria or blood clots in turbid urination, add *Xue Hai* (Sp 10). For lumbar pain, add *Shen Shu* (Bl 23). For lower abdominal pain, add *Qu Quan* (Liv 8). For severely painful and/or burning urination, add *Shui Quan* (Ki 5).

7. UNCTUOUS STRANGURY—VACUOUS PATTERN FROM KIDNEY VACUITY

SIGNS & SYMPTOMS: Enduring turbid strangury which sometimes is better and sometimes worse, slightly painful urination, urine as turbid as fat which is worse with taxation, emaciation, low back and knee soreness and limpness, dizziness, and lassitude of the spirit. There is a pale tongue with slimy fur and a fine, forceless pulse.

TREATMENT PRINCIPLES: Supplement the kidneys, secure and astringe

REPRESENTATIVE FORMULAS: For kidney qi vacuity, use modified *Jin Suo Gu Jing Wan* (Golden Lock Secure the Essence Pills)

Sha Yuan Zi (Astragali Complanati, Semen), 9g
Qian Shi (Euryalis Ferocis, Semen), 9g
Jin Ying Zi (Rosae Laevigatae, Fructus), 9g
Lian Xu (Nelumbinis Nuciferae, Plumula), 9g
calcined *Mu Li* (Ostreae, Concha), 20g
Fu Pen Zi (Rubi Chingii, Fructus), 9g
Wu Wei Zi (Schisandrae Chinensis, Fructus), 9g
Yi Zhi Ren (Alpiniae Oxyphyllae, Fructus), 12g
Shi Chang Pu (Acori Graminei, Rhizoma), 9g

For kidney yin vacuity, use modified *Zhi Bai Di Huang Wan* (Anemarrhena & Phellodendron Rehmannia Pills)

Shu Di Huang (Rehmanniae Glutinosae, cooked Radix), 18g
Shan Zhu Yu (Corni Officinalis, Fructus), 9g
Shan Yao (Dioscoreae Oppositae, Radix), 12g
Fu Ling (Poriae Cocos, Sclerotium), 12g
Mu Dan Pi (Moutan, Cortex Radicis), 9g
Ze Xie (Alismatis Orientalis, Rhizoma), 9g
Zhi Mu (Anemarrhenae Aspheloidis, Rhizoma), 6g
Huang Bai (Phellodendri, Cortex), 9g
Shi Chang Pu (Acori Graminei, Rhizoma), 9g
Bei Xie (Dioscoreae Hypoglaucae, Rhizoma), 9g

MODIFICATIONS: For low back pain, add *Du Zhong* (Eucommiae Ulmoidis, Cortex) and *Gou Ji* (Cibotii Barometsis, Rhizoma). For impotence, add *Ba Ji Tian* (Morindae Officinalis, Radix). For profuse vaginal discharge, add stir-fried *Shan Yao* (Dioscoreae Oppositae, Radix). For concomitant spleen qi vacuity, add *Dang Shen* (Codonopsitis Pilosulae, Radix), *Huang Qi* (Astragali Membranacei, Radix), and *Bai Zhu* (Atractylodis Macrocephalae, Rhizoma). For seminal emission, add wine-steamed *Wu Wei Zi* (Schisandrae Chinensis, Fructus) and *Jin Ying Zi* (Rosae Laevigatae, Fructus). For severe yin vacuity, add *Er Zhi Wan* (Two Ultimates Pills), *i.e.*, *Nu Zhen Zi* (Ligustri Lucidi, Fructus) and *Han Lian Cao* (Ecliptae Prostratae, Herba). For thirst and a dry mouth and throat at night, add *Xuan Shen* (Scrophulariae Ningpoensis, Radix), and *Mai Men Dong* (Ophiopogonis Japonici, Tuber) and increase the dosage of *Zhi Mu* up to nine grams. For night sweats, add *Wu Wei Zi* (Schisandrae Chinensis, Fructus) and *Suan Zao Ren* (Zizyphi Spinosae, Semen).

ACUMOXIBUSTION: For kidney qi vacuity with frequent voiding of turbid, light-colored urine, aversion to cold, cold limbs, nocturia, and dribbling urination, moxibustion *Guan Yuan* (CV 4), *Qi Hai* (CV 6), *Shen Shu* (Bl 23), and *Bai Hui* (GV 20).

For kidney yin vacuity with short voiding of turbid, dark urine, possibly slightly hot urine, vexatious heat of the five hearts, night sweats, night-time thirst, a dry throat and mouth, and hot flashes in the face, needle *Zhong Ji* (CV 3), *Tai Xi* (Ki 3), *San Yin Jiao* (Sp 6), *Shen Shu* (Bl 23), and *Pi Shu* (Bl 20).

MODIFICATIONS: For impotence, add *Qu Gu* (CV 2). For seminal emission, add *Zhi Shi* (Bl 52). For enduring diarrhea, moxa *Shen Que* (CV 8). For constipation, add *Zhao Hai* (Ki 6). For scanty menstruation, add *Xue Hai* (Sp 10). For painful menstruation, add *San Yin Jiao* (Sp 6) and *Xue Hai* (Sp 10). For profuse, clear vaginal discharge, add *Dai Mai* (GB 26) and *Yin Ling Quan* (Sp 9). For dizziness and somnolence, moxa *Ming Men* (GV 4). For insomnia, add *Shen Men* (Ht 7). For vexatious heat of the five hearts, add *Da Ling* (Per 7) and *Fu Liu* (Ki 7).

8. QI STRANGURY—REPLETE PATTERN FROM LIVER DEPRESSION QI STAGNATION

SIGNS & SYMPTOMS: Distention and pain in the urethra during urination, astringent, inhibited urination, dribbling urination or incomplete urination, umbilical and lower abdominal distention and pain, headache, dizziness, chest and rib-side distention, and menstrual irregularities. There is a possibly greenish blue tongue and a deep, bowstring pulse.

TREATMENT PRINCIPLES: Course the liver and rectify the qi

REPRESENTATIVE FORMULA: Modified *Chen Xiang San* (Aquilaria Powder)

powdered *Chen Xiang* (Aquilariae Agallochae, Lignum), 3g taken with the strained decoction
Qing Pi (Citri Reticulatae Viride, Pericarpium), 6g
Xiao Hui Xiang (Foeniculi Vulgaris, Fructus), 6g
Hua Shi (Talcum), 15g
Shi Wei (Pyrrosiae, Folium), 9g
Chen Pi (Citri Reticulatae, Pericarpium), 6g
Bai Shao (Paeoniae Lactiflorae, Radix Albus), 9g
Dong Kui Zi (Abutili Seu Malvae, Semen), 9g
Gan Cao (Glycyrrhizae Uralensis, Radix), 6g
Hai Jin Sha (Lygodii Japonici, Spora), 12g
Yu Jin (Curcumae, Tuber), 9g

MODIFICATIONS: For stabbing pain due to blood stasis, add *Chuan Niu Xi* (Cyathulae Officinalis, Radix). For severe lower abdominal distention and pain, add stir-fried till scorched *Chuan Lian Zi* (Meliae Toosendam, Fructus) and *Yan Hu Suo* (Corydalis

Yanhusuo, Rhizoma). For painful urination which gets worse with emotional disturbance, such as anger, frustration, and depression, add *Suan Zao Ren* (Zizyphi Spinosae, Semen), *He Huan Pi* (Albizziae Julibrissinis, Cortex), and *Ye Jiao Teng* (Polygoni Multiflori, Caulis). For a bitter taste in the mouth and thin, yellow tongue fur, subtract *Xiao Hui Xiang* and add *Zhi Zi* (Gardeniae Jasminoidis, Fructus) and *Mu Dan Pi* (Moutan, Cortex Radicis).

ACUMOXIBUSTION: Needle *Tai Chong* (Liv 3), *Qu Quan* (Liv 8), *Zhong Feng* (Liv 4), *Zhong Ji* (CV 3), *Gui Lai* (St 29), and *Pang Guang Shu* (Bl 28).

MODIFICATIONS: For headache, join *Si Zhu Kong* (TB 23) to *Shuai Gu* (GB 8). For lower abdominal distention and pain, add *Yin Bao* (Liv 9). For frequent sighing, add *Yang Ling Quan* (GB 34). For chest oppression, add *Dan Zhong* (CV 17). For ribside pain, add *Qi Men* (Liv 14). For a bitter taste in the mouth due to depressive heat, add *Xia Xi* (GB 43).

9. QI STRANGURY—VACUOUS PATTERN FROM SPLEEN VACUITY

SIGNS & SYMPTOMS: Slightly painful urination, a sensation of hollow pain which is better with pressure and worse with exertion and taxation, frequent, clear urination, dribbling urination, lower abdominal sagging and distention, a bright white facial complexion, shortness of breath, fatigue, and lassitude of the spirit. There is a pale tongue with thin, white fur and a fine, forceless pulse.

TREATMENT PRINCIPLES: Supplement the center and fortify the spleen, boost the qi and upbear the clear

REPRESENTATIVE FORMULA: Modified *Bu Zhong Yi Qi Tang* (Supplement the Center & Boost the Qi Decoction)

Huang Qi (Astragali Membranacei, Radix), 15g
Dang Shen (Codonopsitis Pilosulae, Radix), 12g
Bai Zhu (Atractylodis Macrocephalae, Rhizoma), 12g

Chen Pi (Citri Reticulatae, Pericarpium), 6g
Chai Hu (Bupleuri, Radix), 6g
Sheng Ma (Cimicifugae, Rhizoma), 6g
Fu Ling (Poriae Cocos, Sclerotium), 9g
Zhi Ke (Citri Aurantii, Fructus), 6g

MODIFICATIONS: For concomitant kidney qi vacuity, add *Yi Zhi Ren* (Alpiniae Oxyphllae, Fructus) and *Ba Ji Tian* (Morindae Officinalis, Radix) or use *Bu Zhong Yi Qi Tang* in the morning and *Jin Gui Shen Qi Wan* (*Golden Cabinet* Kidney Qi Pills) plus *Yi Zhi Ren* and *Ba Ji Tian* in the late afternoon. For concomitant lung qi vacuity, add *Wu Wei Zi* (Schisandrae Chinensis, Fructus).

For heart-spleen dual vacuity, replace *Bu Zhong Yi Qi Tang* with modified *Gui Pi Tang* (Restore the Spleen Decoction): *Huang Qi* (Astragali Membranacei, Radix), 15g, *Bai Zhu* (Atractylodis Macrocephalae, Rhizoma), 12g, *Dang Gui* (Angelicae Sinensis, Radix), 9g, *Long Yan Rou* (Euphoriae Longanae, Arillus), 9g, *Fu Ling* (Poriae Cocos, Sclerotium), 9g, *Mu Xiang* (Auklandiae Lappae, Radix), 6g, *Dang Shen* (Codonopsitis Pilosulae, Radix), 9g, *Suan Zao Ren* (Zizyphi Spinosae, Semen), 6g, mix-fried *Gan Cao* (Glycyrrhizae Uralensis, Radix), 3g, processed *Yuan Zhi* (Polygalae Tenuifoliae, Radix), 9g, and *Yi Zhi Ren* (Alpiniae Oxyphyllae, Fructus), 9g.

For both qi and blood vacuity, replace *Bu Zhong Yi Qi Tang* with modified *Ba Zhen Tang* (Eight Pearls Decoction): *Shu Di Huang* (Rehmanniae Glutinosae, cooked Radix), 18g, *Bai Shao* (Paeoniae Lactiflorae, Radix Albus), 9g, wine stir-fried *Dang Gui* (Angelicae Sinensis, Radix), 9g, wine stir-fried *Chuan Xiong* (Ligustici Wallichii, Radix), 6g, *Dang Shen* (Codonopsitis Pilosulae, Radix), 9g, *Bai Zhu* (Atractylodis Macrocephalae, Rhizoma), 15g, *Fu Ling* (Poriae Cocos, Sclerotium), 12g, mix-fried *Gan Cao* (Glycyrrhizae Uralensis, Radix), 6g, *Huang Qi* (Astragali Membranacei, Radix), 15g, and *Gui Zhi* (Cinnamomi Cassiae, Ramulus), 6g.

ACUMOXIBUSTION: Moxibustion *Guan Yuan* (CV 4), *Qi Hai* (CV 6), and *Bai Hui* (GV 20) and needle *Zu San Li* (St 36) and *San Yin Jiao* (Sp 6).

REPRESENTATIVE CASE HISTORY

Case history from Dr. Wei Li's private practice: Joe, a 34 year-old male

When Joe came to Dr. Li he had acute prostatitis for two months. He had taken antibiotics but these were not completely successful. He continued to experience dribbling and painful urination as well as low back pain. His tongue was red with thick, yellow fur, and his pulse was fast, forceful, slippery, and bowstring. Based on these signs and symptoms, Dr. Li's pattern identification was damp heat and phlegm in the lower burner. Her treatment principles were to clear and eliminate dampness and heat and transform phlegm in the lower burner. Thus she prescribed modified *Hai Zao Yu Hu Tang* (Sargassium Jade Flask Decoction):

Fu Hai She (Pumice), 9g, *Xia Ku Cao* (Prunellae Vulgaris, Spica), 9g, *Hai Zao* (Sargassii, Herba), 9g, *Kun Bu* (Algae, Thallus), 7g, *Niu Xi* (Achyranthis Bidentatae, Radix), 12g, *Che Qian Zi* (Plantaginis, Semen), 9g, *Ban Xia* (Pinelliae Ternatae, Rhizoma), 4g, *Huang Bai* (Phellodendri, Cortex), 9g, *Zhi Mu* (Anemarrhenae Asphodeloidis, Rhizoma), 9g, *Chai Hu* (Bupleuri, Radix), 6g, *Xiang Fu* (Cyperi Rotundi, Rhizoma), 9g, *Chuan Xiong* (Ligustici Wallichii, Radix), 9g, and *Mu Dan Pi* (Moutan, Cortex Radicis), 9g. After one week, Joe's condition improved 50-60%. After two weeks, he had almost completely recovered. Joe took the formula for a total of six weeks, after which he felt he no longer needed any therapy—he was cured.

CLINICAL TIP: In general, this condition is easier to treat in younger men than in older men. It is usual for younger men with damp heat for heat to be more prominent than dampness, while the opposite is true in older men. Since dampness is tenacious by nature, conditions with a preponderance of dampness take longer to resolve.

CHAPTER 10
TURBIDITY CONDITION

Turbidity condition is also referred to as excretory turbidity, dripping turbidity, dripping white, and trickling turbidity. This condition includes urinary turbidity and essence turbidity. In urinary turbidity, the urine is not clear. When it is white like "rice-washing water," it is called white turbidity. When the urine is red, it is called red turbidity. Essence turbidity denotes sperm in the urine or leakage of sperm before or after urination. There is also a white and red type of essence turbidity. Please note, however, that the distinction between white and red turbidity does not affect pattern identification or treatment. (Please see Chart 10.1.)

DISEASE CAUSES & MECHANISMS

Several causes for turbidity have been given throughout Chinese medical history. For instance, *Su Wen*, Chapter 74, "*Zhi Zhen Yao Da Lun* (Great Treatise on Arriving at the Truth of the Essentials)" states, "All patterns of turbid excreted fluid belong to heat." *Ling Shu*, Chapter 28, "*Kou Wen* (Oral Questioning)" states, "When there is qi vacuity in the center, feces and urine will be abnormal." Zhu Dan-xi, in the *Dan Xi Xin Fa (Dan-xi's Heart Methods)*, stated that red turbidity is most often caused by damp heat, while white turbidity is usual-

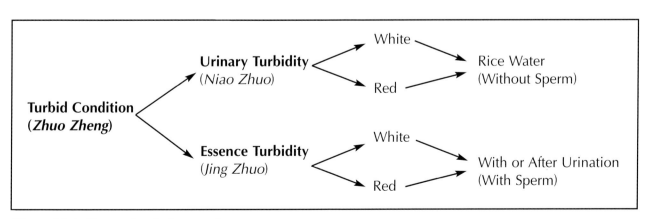

Chart 10.1. Types of turbidity condition

ly kidney qi vacuity cold. He thought that the cause was overindulgence in sex. However, he also stated that red turbidity is due to damp heat in the blood aspect, while white turbidity is due to damp heat in the qi aspect. The *Zhu Bing Yuan Hou Lun (Treatise on the Origins & Symptoms of All Diseases)* states that, when taxation damages the kidney resulting in kidney qi vacuity cold, the urine can be white or turbid.

The kidney governs water. In the bladder, there is a "confluence of waters." This is where the fluids pass out of the body. The qi transformation of both the kidney and bladder is responsible for the return of the clear and the discharge of the turbid, *i.e.*, the manufacture of urine and its excretion from the body. Normal urine should be clear and slightly yellow. If there is kidney-bladder qi transformation failure, the clear cannot be separated from the turbid, thus resulting in turbid urine. Spleen-stomch dysfunction may also cause turbid syndrome. Spleen-stomach dysfunction causes damp accumulation. In that case, the dampness descends to the bladder and inhibits bladder transformation.

TREATMENT BASED ON PATTERN IDENTIFICATION

URINARY TURBIDITY

1. SPLEEN-STOMACH DAMPNESS POURING DOWN TO THE BLADDER

SIGNS & SYMPTOMS: Turbid urine or urine that looks like rice-washing water, inhibited urination, chest oppression, and sticky stools. The tongue is slimy and the pulse is slippery.

TREATMENT PRINCIPLES: Transform the qi and dampness and divide the clear from the turbid

REPRESENTATIVE FORMULA: *Bei Xie Fen Qing Yin* (Dioscorea Hypoglauca Separate the Clear Beverage)

Bei Xie (Dioscoreae Hypoglaucae, Rhizoma), 12g
Yi Zhi Ren (Alpiniae Oxyphyllae, Fructus), 9g

Wu Yao (Linderae Strychnifoliae, Radix), 9g
Shi Chang Pu (Acori Graminei, Rhizoma), 9g

MODIFICATIONS: For lower abdominal distention and inhibited urination, add *Qing Pi* (Citri Reticulatae Viride, Pericarpium). For turbid urine mixed with blood, add *Xiao Ji* (Cephalanoplos Segeti, Herba), *Bai Mao Gen* (Imperatae Cylindricae, Rhizoma), and *Ce Bai Ye* (Biotae Orientalis, Cacumen). For frequent, short urination with a hot, rough sensation and pain in the urethra, delete *Tu Si Zi* and *Shan Zhu Yu*, add *Qu Mai* (Dianthi, Herba), *Shi Wei* (Pyrrosiae, Folium), and *Hai Jin Sha* (Lygodii Japonici, Spora).

ACUMOXIBUSTION: Needle *Zhong Ji* (CV 3), *San Yin Jiao* (Sp 6), *Yin Ling Quan* (Sp 9), *Pi Shu* (Bl 20) and *Wei Shu* (Bl 21).

MODIFICATIONS: For hot, rough urination, add *Ci Liao* (Bl 32). For uneasy defecation or loose stools, add *Tian Shu* (St 25). For constipation, add *Shang Ju Xu* (St 37). For torpid intake, add *Zhong Wan* (CV 12).

2. DAMP HEAT IN THE LOWER BURNER

SIGNS & SYMPTOMS: Turbid urine which may have white clots or strings or blood clots, thirst, chest distention and vexation, dry stools with a bad smell or constipation, and bad breath. The tongue is red with thick, yellow, slimy fur, and the pulse is fast and soggy.

TREATMENT PRINCIPLES: Clear heat and drain dampness from the lower burner, separate the clear from the turbid

REPRESENTATIVE FORMULA: *Bei Xie Fen Qing Yin* (Disocorea Hypoglauca Separate the Clear Beverage) plus *Huang Lian Jie Du Tang* (Coptis Toxin-resolving Decoction)

Bei Xie (Dioscoreae Hypoglaucae, Rhizoma), 12g
Yi Zhi Ren (Alpiniae Oxyphyllae, Fructus), 9g
Wu Yao (Linderae Strychnifoliae, Radix), 9g
Shi Chang Pu (Acori Graminei, Rhizoma), 9g
Huang Lian (Coptidis Chinensis, Rhizoma), 9g

Huang Qin (Scutellariae Baicalensis, Radix), 9g
Huang Bai (Phellodendri, Cortex), 9g
Zhi Zi (Gardeniae Jasminoidis, Fructus), 9g

MODIFICATIONS: If there is constipation, add *Da Huang* (Rhei, Radix Et Rhizoma). If there is severe fatigue, add *Huang Qi* (Astragali Membranacei, Radix), *Dang Shen* (Codonopsitis Pilosulae, Radix), *Shu Di Huang* (Rehmanniae Glutinosae, cooked Radix), and *Shan Zhu Yu* (Corni Officinalis, Fructus). If there is severe hematuria, add carbonized *Ce Bai Ye* (Biotae Orientalis, Cacumen), *Xian He Cao* (Agrimoniae Pilosae, Herba), *Xiao Ji* (Cephalanoplos Segeti, Herba), and *Ou Jie* (Nelumbinis Nuciferae, Nodus Rhizomatis). If there is more dampness than heat (*i.e.*, there is thick, white and yellow or greyish tongue fur), add *Cang Zhu* (Atractylodis, Rhizoma), *Hou Po* (Magnoliae Officinalis, Cortex), *Ban Xia* (Pinelliae Ternatae, Rhizoma), and *Chen Pi* (Citri Reticulatae, Pericarpium).

ACUMOXIBUSTION: Choose from *Wei Zhong* (Bl 40), *Zhong Ji* (CV 3), *Fu Liu* (Ki 7), *Pang Guang Shu* (Bl 28), *Yin Ling Quan* (Sp 9), *San Yin Jiao* (Sp 6), *Guan Yuan* (CV 4), *Shui Dao* (St 28), *Ci Liao* (Bl 32), and *Nei Ting* (St 44).

ESSENCE TURBIDITY

1. KIDNEY YIN VACUITY

SIGNS & SYMPTOMS: Burning urination with dark yellow urine, turbid urine or turbid fluid passing out after urination, heat in the five hearts, insomnia, and dry mouth. The tongue is red and without fur, while the pulse is fine.

TREATMENT PRINCIPLES: Nourish yin and clear heat

REPRESENTATIVE FORMULA: Modified *Zhi Bai Di Huang Wan* (Anemarrhena & Phellodendron Rehmannia Pills)

Zhi Mu (Anemarrhenae Asphodeloidis, Rhizoma), 9g
Huang Bai (Phellodendri, Cortex), 9g

Sheng Di Huang (Rehmanniae Glutinosae, uncooked Radix), 12g
Shan Yao (Dioscoreae Oppositae, Radix), 12g
Shan Zhu Yu (Corni Officinalis, Fructus), 12g
Fu Ling (Poriae Cocos, Sclerotium), 9g
Ze Xie (Alismatis Orientalis, Rhizoma), 9g
Mu Dan Pi (Moutan, Cortex Radicis), 12g
Tu Si Zi (Cuscutae Chinensis, Semen), 9g
Lian Zi (Nelumbinis Nuciferae, Semen), 9g

MODIFICATIONS: For turbid urine mixed with blood, add *Xiao Ji* (Cephalanoplos Segeti, Herba), *Bai Mao Gen* (Imperatae Cylindricae, Rhizoma), and *Ce Bai Ye* (Biotae Orientalis, Cacumen). For severe yin vacuity, add *Nu Zhen Zi* (Ligustri Lucidi, Fructus) and *Han Lian Cao* (Ecliptae Prostratae, Herba). For fire effulgence with tidal fever, add *Bai Wei* (Cynanchi Baiwei, Radix) and *Di Gu Pi* (Lycii Chinensis, Cortex Radicis).

ACUMOXIBUSTION: Needle *Guan Yuan* (CV 4), *San Yin Jiao* (Sp 6), *Tai Xi* (Ki 3), *Shen Shu* (Bl 23), and *Pi Shu* (Bl 20).

MODIFICATIONS: For seminal emission, add *Zhi Shi* (Bl 52). For constipation, add *Tian Shu* (St 25), *Da Chang Shu* (Bl 25), and *Zhao Hai* (Ki 6). For insomnia, add *Shen Men* (Ht 7). For scanty menstruation, add *Xue Hai* (Sp 10). For vexatious heat of the five hearts, add *Da Ling* (Per 7) and *Fu Liu* (Ki 7).

2. KIDNEY QI VACUITY (A.K.A., KIDNEY QI NOT SECURING)

SIGNS & SYMPTOMS: White mucus passing out of the urethra after clear, frequent urination, dizziness, chilliness, low back and knee pain and soreness, seminal emission. The pulse is weak.

TREATMENT PRINCIPLES: Supplement and secure the kidney qi

REPRESENTATIVE FORMULA: Modified *Jin Gui Shen Qi Wan* (*Golden Cabinet* Kidney Qi Pills)

Fu Zi (Aconiti Carmichaeli, Radix Lateralis Praeparatus), 9g

Rou Gui (Cinnamonmi Casiae, Cortex), 9g

Shu Di Huang (Rehmanniae Glutinosae, cooked Radix), 12g

Shan Yao (Dioscoreae Oppositae, Radix), 12g

Shan Zhu Yu (Corni Officinalis, Fructus), 12g

Ze Xie (Alismatis Orientalis, Rhizoma), 9g

Fu Ling (Poriae Cocos, Sclerotium), 9g

Bu Gu Zhi (Psoraleae Corylifoliae, Fructus), 9g

Jing Ying Zi (Rosae Laevigatae, Fructus), 9g

Lian Zi (Nelumbinis Nuciferae, Semen), 9g

MODIFICATIONS: For turbid urine mixed with blood, add *Pao Jiang* (Zingiberis Officinalis, blast-fried Rhizoma) and *Ce Bai Ye* (Biotae Orientalis, Cacumen).

For spleen-kidney yang vacuity, replace *Jin Gui Shen Qi Wan* with modified *Bu Zhong Yi Qi Tang* (Supplement the Center & Boost the Qi Decoction) plus *Wu Bi Shan Yao Wan* (Incomparable Disocorea Pills): *Huang Qi* (Astragali Membranacei, Radix), 12g, mix-fried *Gan Cao* (Glycyrrhizae Uralensis, Radix), 3g, *Dang Shen* (Codonopsitis Pilosulae, Radix), 9g, *Bai Zhu* (Atractylodis Macrocephalae, Rhizoma), 12g, *Shan Yao* (Dioscoreae Oppositae, Radix), 12g, *Shu Di Huang* (Rehmannia Glutinosae, cooked Radix), 6g, *Shan Zhu Yu* (Corni Officinalis, Fructus), 6g, *Fu Ling* (Poriae Cocos, Sclerotium), 12g, *Ze Xie* (Alismatis Orientalis, Rhizoma), 9g, *Rou Cong Rong* (Cistanchis Deserticolae, Herba), 6g, *Tu Si Zi* (Cuscutae Chinensis, Semen), 9g, *Wu Wei Zi* (Schisandrae Chinensis, Fructus), 6g, *Ba Ji Tian* (Morindae Officinalis, Radix), 9g, and *Shi Chang Pu* (Acori Graminei, Rhizoma), 6g.

ACUMOXIBUSTION: Moxibustion *Guan Yuan* (CV 4), *Qi Hai* (CV 6), *Shen Shu* (Bl 23), and *Bai Hui* (GV 20).

MODIFICATIONS: For impotence, add *Qu Gu* (CV 2). For enduring diarrhea due to spleen-kidney yang vacuity, moxibustion *Shen Que* (CV 8). For painful menstruation, add *San Yin Jiao* (Sp 6) and *Xue Hai* (Sp 10). For profuse, clear vaginal discharge, add *Dai Mai* (GB 26) and *Yin Ling Quan* (Sp 9). For dizziness and somnolence, moxibustion *Ming Men* (GV 4).

CLINICAL TIPS

1. As Ye Tian-shi pointed out, pain is associated with strangury, while, in turbidity condition, there is no pain. For instance, in unctuous strangury, the urine is turbid, but this is distinguished from turbidity condition because it is accompanied by pain.

2. It is important to apply eight principle pattern identification when treating turbidity condition in order to determine if it is hot or cold, replete or vacuous. However, this is not always readily apparent because chronic damp heat may damage the qi and cause qi, yang, or yin vacuity. On the other hand, chronic vacuity allows for easy invasion by evils. Therefore, there is often a mixture of hot and cold, repletion and vacuity. Nevertheless, one must try to determine which is more prominent. If there is heat, whether replete or vacuous, one must focus on clearing heat without neglecting to supplement any vacuity. After the heat has been cleared, one may focus on supplementation. Supplementing the kidney usually takes from six months to one year.

CHAPTER 11
ABDOMINAL DISTENTION

Patients with kidney disease often have abdominal distention. *Su Wen*, Chapter 74, "*Zhi Zhen Yao Da Lun* (Great Treatise on Arriving at the Truth of the Essentials)" states, "all the syndromes of water swelling and distention caused by dampness pertain to the spleen . . ." The spleen governs the movement and transformation of water and the kidney governs water. In addition, damage to the spleen easily affects the kidney and vice versa. Kidney disease damages the kidney's ability to govern water. In that case, water dampness accumulates and overwhelms the spleen's ability to govern the movement and transformation of water resulting in abdominal distention. Therefore, when treating kidney disease, we must pay attention to the spleen and digestion as well as the kidney. In kidney disease, abdominal distention is usually seen in patterns of spleen and kidney vacuity and/or water damp repletion. In these patterns, besides supplementing the kidney and draining water, one must supplement the spleen. A strong spleen will move and transform water dampness. Moreover, the spleen is the source of latter heaven qi. Thus, when the spleen is fortified, the patient's righteous qi will be strengthened, helping in the resolution of any disease.

DISEASE CAUSES & MECHANISMS

There are many causes of abdominal distention. These include contraction of external evils, excessive thinking and obsessing, food stagnation, parasites, qi stagnation, and blood stasis. However, pattern identification of abdominal distention can be categorized simply as 1) vacuity, 2) repletion, or 3) vacuity with repletion. In all these cases, it is the non-downbearing of the stomach qi which causes abdominal distention.

TREATMENT BASED ON PATTERN IDENTIFICATION

1. SPLEEN VACUITY

SIGNS & SYMPTOMS: Abdominal distention and pain, low appetite, cold hands and feet. The pulse is slow.

TREATMENT PRINCIPLES: Fortify the spleen, warm the middle, and dispel cold

REPRESENTATIVE FORMULA: *Li Zhong Wan* (Rectify the Center Pills)

Dang Shen (Codonopsitis Pilosulae, Radix), 9g
Gan Jiang (Zingiberis Officinalis, dry Rhizoma), 9g
Bai Zhu (Atractylodis Macrocephalae, Rhizoma), 9g
Gan Cao (Glycyrrhizae Uralensis, Radix), 3g

MODIFICATIONS: If there is simultaneous qi stagnation, one can use *Xiang Sha Liu Jun Si Tang* (Cyperus & Amomum Six Gentlemen Decoction: *Dang Shen* (Codonopsitis Pilosulae, Radix), 9g, *Fu Ling* (Poriae Cocos, Sclerotium), 9g, *Bai Zhu* (Atractylodis Macrocephalae, Rhizoma), 9g, *Sha Ren* (Amomi, Fructus), 6g, *Chen Pi* (Citri Reticulatae, Pericarpium), 9g, *Mu Xiang* (Aucklandiae Lappae, Radix), 6g, *Ban Xia* (Pinelliae Ternatae, Rhizoma), 9g, and mix-fried *Gan Cao* (Glycyrrhizae Uralensis, Radix), 3g.

ACUMOXIBUSTION: Choose from *Pi Shu* (Bl 20), *Zhong Wan* (CV 12), *Qi Hai* (CV 6), *Nei Guan* (Per 6), *Tai Bai* (Sp 3), *Gong Sun* (Sp 4), *San Yin Jiao* (Sp 6), and *Zu San Li* (St 36).

MODIFICATIONS: If there is concomitant qi stagnation, add *Tai Chong* (Liv 3) and *He Gu* (LI 4). If there is concomitant edema, add *Yin Ling Quan* (Sp 9). If there is simultaneous blood stasis, add *Xue Hai* (Sp 10).

2. REPLETION

SIGNS & SYMPTOMS: Abdominal distention and pain, dry stool, dry mouth, fever, and chills. The pulse is fast.

TREATMENT PRINCIPLES: Resolve the exterior and drain the interior

REPRESENTATIVE FORMULA: Modified *Hou Po San Wu Tang* (Magnoliae Three Materials Decoction)

Hou Po (Magnoliae Officinalis, Cortex), 15g
Da Huang (Rhei, Radix Et Rhizoma), 9g
Zhi Shi (Citri Aurantii, Fructus Immaturus), 9g
Gui Zhi (Cinnamomi Cassiae, Ramulus), 9g
Sheng Jiang (Zingiberis Officinalis, uncooked Rhizoma), 6g
Da Zao (Zizyphi Jujubae, Fructus), 2 pieces

Gan Cao (Glycyrrhizae Uralensis, Radix), 3g
Mai Men Dong (Ophiopogonis Japonici, Tuber), 6g
Zhi Mu (Anemarrhenae Asphodeloidis, Rhizoma), 6g

MODIFICATIONS: Since abdominal distention is typically only a complicating symptom of kidney disease, modifications are not generally necessary.

ACUMOXIBUSTION: Choose from *Pi Shu* (Bl 20), *Zhong Wan* (CV 12), *Qi Hai* (CV 6), *Nei Guan* (Per 6), *Tian Shu* (St 25), *Yin Ling Quan* (Sp 9), *Zu San Li* (St 36), *Feng Long* (St 40), and *Nei Ting* (St 44).

3. VACUITY WITH REPLETION

There are three types of vacuity with repletion abdominal distention: A) spleen qi vacuity with damp encumbrance, B) spleen cold with stomach heat, and C) spleen vacuity with food damage.

A. SPLEEN QI VACUITY WITH DAMP ENCUMBRANCE

SIGNS & SYMPTOMS: Abdominal distention, nausea, and vomiting. The tongue is covered with thick, white fur, and the pulse is weak.

TREATMENT PRINCIPLES: Supplement the spleen, harmonize the stomach, and descend the qi

REPRESENTATIVE FORMULA: Modified *Hou Po Wen Zhong Tang* (Magnolia Warm the Center Decoction)

Hou Po (Magnoliae Officinalis, Cortex), 12g
Sheng Jiang (Zingiberis Officinalis, uncooked Rhizoma), 9g
Ban Xia (Pinelliae Ternatae, Rhizoma), 9g
Bai Zhu (Atractylodis Macrocephalae, Rhizoma), 9g
Dang Shen (Codonopsitis Pilosulae, Radix), 9g
mix-fried *Gan Cao* (Glycyrrhizae Uralensis, Radix), 3g
Huo Xiang (Agastaches Seu Pogostemi, Herba), 9g
Shan Yao (Dioscoreae Oppositae, Radix), 15g
Shan Zha (Crataegi, Fructus), 8g

ACUMOXIBUSTION: Choose from *Pi Shu* (Bl 20), *Zhong Wan* (CV 12), *Qi Hai* (CV 6), *Nei Guan* (Per

6), *Tian Shu* (St 25), *Yin Ling Quan* (Sp 9), *Zu San Li* (St 36), *Feng Long* (St 40), and *Nei Ting* (St 44).

B. SPLEEN COLD WITH STOMACH HEAT

SIGNS & SYMPTOMS: Abdominal distention, dry heaves, nausea and vomiting, diarrhea, and borborygmus.

TREATMENT PRINCIPLES: Percolate damp and downbear the stomach qi, dispel stagnation and clear heat

REPRESENTATIVE FORMULA: Modified *Ban Xia Xie Xin Tang* (Pinellia Drain the Heart Decoction)

Ban Xia (Pinelliae Ternatae, Rhizoma), 9g
Huang Qin (Scutellariae Baicalensis, Radix), 9g
Gan Jiang (Zingiberis Officinalis, dry Rhizoma), 9g
mix-fried *Gan Cao* (Glycyrrhizae Uralensis, Radix), 6g
Dang Shen (Codonopsitis Pilosulae, Radix), 9g
Huang Lian (Coptidis Chinensis, Rhizoma), 9g
Da Zao (Ziziphi Jujubae, Fructus), 3 pieces

ACUMOXIBUSTION: Choose from *Pi Shu* (Bl 20), *Wei Shu* (Bl 21), *Zhong Wan* (CV 12), *Qi Hai* (CV 6), *He Gu* (LI 4), *Nei Guan* (Per 6), *Tian Shu* (St 25), *Zu San Li* (St 36), *Nei Ting* (St 44), and *Li Dui* (St 45).

C. SPLEEN QI VACUITY WITH FOOD DAMAGE

SIGNS & SYMPTOMS: Abdominal distention and pain, sour acid regurgitation, rotten belching, and constipation or diarrhea. The tongue has thick, yellow, slimy fur.

TREATMENT PRINCIPLES: Fortify the spleen and boost the qi, abduct food and disperse stagnation

REPRESENTATIVE FORMULA: Modified *Bao He Wan* (Preserve Harmony Pills)

Shan Zha (Crataegi, Fructus), 10g
Shen Qu (Massa Medica Fermentata), 10g
Ban Xia (Pinelliae Ternatae, Rhizoma), 10g
Fu Ling (Poriae Cocos, Sclerotium), 10g
Chen Pi (Citri Reticulatae, Pericarpium), 7g
Lai Fu Zi (Raphani Sativi, Semen), 7g
Lian Qiao (Forsythiae Suspensae, Fructus), 7g
Bai Zhu (Atractylodis Macrocephalae, Rhizoma), 10g
Shan Yao (Dioscoreae Oppositae, Radix), 10g

ACUMOXIBUSTION: Choose from *Pi Shu* (Bl 20), *Wei Shu* (Bl 21), *Zhong Wan* (CV 12), *Qi Hai* (CV 6), *He Gu* (LI 4), *Nei Guan* (Per 6), *Tian Shu* (St 25), *Zu San Li* (St 36), *Nei Ting* (St 44), and *Li Dui* (St 45).

CLINICAL TIPS

1. As stated in the introduction, abdominal distention often accompanies kidney diseases, but this symptom or disease is located in the spleen-stomach, not the kidney.

2. One must seek the root cause of this condition before attempting to treat it. Even though the spleen-stomach is involved, any of the replete or vacuous abdominal distention patterns may have kidney vacuity at the root.

3. Many kidney diseases, including strangury, may disrupt the central qi resulting in abdominal distention. Even though a disease such as strangury is replete, it may lead to kidney vacuity and then to abdominal distention.

CHAPTER 12
DIZZINESS

In Chinese, dizziness is *xuan yun*. *Xuan* means dark, blurry, or dizzy vision. *Yun* means dizziness and things spinning around. Dizziness, a combination of these two symptoms, is often seen in clinic. In mild cases, if the patient closes his or her eyes, the dizziness will stop. In serious cases, there may be nausea, vomiting, and/or syncope.

DISEASE CAUSES & MECHANISMS

Dizziness is usually caused by contraction of external wind evils or internal stirring of liver wind, but it may also be caused by any of the six environmental excesses as well as internal damage to the qi, blood, or viscera. For instance, *Ling Shu,* Chapter 28, *"Kou Wen* (Oral Questioning)" states, "When qi is insufficient in the upper burner, the marrow will not be full in the brain and frequent tinnitus, drooping of the head, and dizzy vision will occur . . ." *Su Wen*, Chapter 74, *"Zhi Zhen Yao Da Lun* (The Great Treatise on Arriving at the Truth of the Essentials)" states:

> When the wind of *jue yin* is replete and invades, people will have tinnitus, dizziness. . . . Symptoms of tremors, shaking of the limbs, and dizziness are caused by wind and pertain to the liver . . .

Emotional depression or anger can damage liver yin and result in ascendancy of liver yang. Similarly, long-term illness, stress, anxiety, overthinking, or worry can damage the heart and spleen qi and blood, while overindulgent sexual activity, chronic illness, or debility due to aging can lead to vacuity of kidney essence. In addition, improper diet may cause damage to the spleen and stomach, leading to obstruction of the middle burner by phlegm and dampness. If depression gives rise to depressive heat, phlegm dampness may transform into phlegm fire.

TREATMENT BASED ON PATTERN IDENTIFICATION

1. WIND FIRE

SIGNS & SYMPTOMS: Dizziness or vertigo with headache and head distention exacerbated by anger, vexation and agitation, irascibility, a red facial complexion, tinnitus, scanty, dream-disturbed sleep, dryness and a bitter taste in the mouth. There is a red tongue with yellow fur and a bowstring, rapid pulse.

TREATMENT PRINCIPLES: Clear heat and extinguish

wind, level the liver and subdue yang, stop dizziness

REPRESENTATIVE FORMULA: Modified *Tian Ma Gou Teng Yin* (Gastrodia & Uncaria Beverage)

Tian Ma (Gastrodiae Elatae, Rhizoma), 9g
Gou Teng (Uncariae Cum Uncis, Ramulus), 12g
Shi Jue Ming (Haliotidis, Concha), 15g
Zhi Zi (Gardeniae Jasminoidis, Fructus), 9g
Huang Qin (Scutellariae Baicalensis, Radix), 9g
Niu Xi (Achyranthis Bidentatae, Radix), 12g
Du Zhong (Eucommiae Ulmoidis, Cortex), 9g
Ju Hua (Chrysanthemi Morifolii, Flos), 9g
Sang Ji Sheng (Sangjisheng, Ramulus), 9g
Ye Jiao Teng (Polygoni Multiflori, Caulus), 9g
Fu Shen (Poriae Cocos, Sclerotium Pararadicis), 9g

MODIFICATIONS: To enhance subduing of the liver, add *Bai Ji Li* (Tribuli Terrestris, Fructus) and *Xia Ku Cao* (Prunellae Vulgaris, Spica). If liver yang transforms into internal wind, add *Long Gu* (Draconis, Os), *Mu Li* (Ostreae, Concha) and/or *Ling Yang Jiao* (Antelopis Saiga-tatarici, Cornu). If there is concomitant constipation, add *Da Huang* (Rhei, Radix Et Rhizoma) and/or *Lu Hui* (Aloes, Herba).

If there is actual liver fire, use modified *Long Dan Xie Gan Tang* (Gentiana Drain the Liver Decoction) instead: *Long Dan Cao* (Gentianae Longdancao, Radix), 6g, *Zhi Zi* (Gardeniae Jasminoidis, Fructus), 9g, *Huang Qin* (Scutellariae Baicalensis, Radix), 9g, *Chai Hu* (Bupleuri, Radix), 6g, *Xia Ku Cao* (Prunellae Vulgaris, Spica), 6g, *Ju Hua* (Chrysanthemi Morifolii, Flos), 9g, *Gou Teng* (Uncariae Cum Uncis, Ramulus), 12g, *Sheng Di Huang* (Rehmanniae Glutinosae, uncooked Radix), 6g, *Dang Gui* (Angelicae Sinensis, Radix), 6g, and *Che Qian Zi* (Plantaginis, Semen), 6g.

ACUMOXIBUSTION: For predominant exuberant yang, needle *Feng Chi* (GB 20), *Tai Chong* (Liv 3), *Wai Guan* (TB 5), *Tai Xi* (Ki 3), and *San Yin Jiao* (Sp 6). For predominant liver fire, needle *Feng Chi* (GB 20), *Xing Jian* (Liv 2), *Zu Qiao Yin* (GB 44), *Ran Gu* (Ki 2), and *San Yin Jiao* (Sp 6).

MODIFICATIONS: For rib-side distention and pain,

add *Yang Ling Quan* (GB 34). For tinnitus, add *Ting Gong* (SI 19).

2. ASCENDANT YANG DUE TO YIN VACUITY

SIGNS & SYMPTOMS: Dizziness or vertigo with rubbing of the eyes, possible distention of the eyes, vexation, insomnia, dream-disturbed sleep, night sweats, heat in the palms of the hands and soles of the feet, dry mouth, and tinnitus. There is a red tongue with scanty fur or even no fur and a fine and rapid or fine and bowstring pulse.

TREATMENT PRINCIPLES: Enrich yin and level the liver, subdue yang and settle vertigo

REPRESENTATIVE FORMULA: Modified *Ju Hua Shao Yao Tang* (Chrysanthemum & Peony Decoction)

Ju Hua (Chrysanthemi Morifolii, Flos), 9g
Bai Shao (Paeoniae Lactiflorae, Radix Albus), 9g
Bai Ji Li (Tribuli Terrestris, Fructus), 6g
Mu Dan Pi (Moutan, Cortex Radicis), 6g
Gou Teng (Uncariae Cum Uncis, Ramulus), 12g
Tian Ma (Gastrodiae Elatae, Rhizoma), 9g
Ye Jiao Teng (Polygoni Multiflori, Caulus), 9g
Sheng Di Huang (Rehmanniae Glutinosae, uncooked Radix), 9g
Gou Qi Zi (Lycii Chinensis, Fructus), 9g

MODIFICATIONS: If there is simultaneous edema, add *Fun Ling* (Poriae Cocos, Sclerotium) and *Ze Xie* (Alismatis Orientalis, Rhizoma). If there is accompanying fatigue and lack of strength, add *Huang Qi* (Astragali Membranacei, Radix) and *Tai Zi Shen* (Pseudostellariae Heterophyllae, Radix) or *Xi Yang Shen* (Panacis Quinquefolii, Radix).

ACUMOXIBUSTION: Needle *Feng Chi* (GB 20), *Gan Shu* (Bl 18), *Xing Jian* (Liv 2), *Shen Shu* (Bl 23), *Tai Xi* (Ki 3), and *San Yin Jiao* (Sp 6).

3. HEART-SPLEEN DUAL VACUITY

SIGNS & SYMPTOMS: Dizziness and vertigo with blurred vision which is exacerbated by overthinking, heart palpitations, lassitude of the spirit, shortness of breath, bodily exhaustion, insomnia, reduced food intake, a somber white or sallow yellow facial complexion, and pale lips. The tongue is pale with thin, white fur and the pulse is fine and forceless.

TREATMENT PRINCIPLES: Supplement the heart and fortify the spleen, boost the qi and nourish the blood

REPRESENTATIVE FORMULA: Modified *Gui Pi Tang* (Restore the Spleen Decoction)

Bai Zhu (Atractylodis Macrocephalae, Rhizoma), 9g
Fu Shen (Poriae Cocos, Sclerotium Pararadicis), 9g
Huang Qi (Astragali Membranacei, Radix), 12g
Long Yan Rou (Euphoriae Longanae, Arillus), 9g
Suan Zao Ren (Zizyphi Spinosae, Semen), 12g
Dang Shen (Codonopsitis Pilosulae, Radix), 9g
Dang Gui (Angelicae Sinensis, Radix), 9g
mix-fried *Gan Cao* (Glycyrrhizae Uralensis, Radix), 3g
Mu Xiang (Auklandia Lappae, Radix), 6g
Yuan Zhi (Polygalae Tenuifoliae, Radix), 3g
Bai Shao (Paeoniae Lactiflorae, Radix Albus), 9g

MODIFICATIONS: If there is simultaneous liver depression, add *Chai Hu* (Bupleuri, Radix) and *Chen Pi* (Citri Reticulatae, Pericarpium). If there is simultaneous blood stasis, add *Dan Shen* (Salviae Miltiorrhizae, Radix). If blood vacuity is severe, add *Shu Di Huang* (Rehmanniae Glutinosae, cooked Radix), *Zi He Che* (Hominis, Placenta), and *E Jiao* (Asini, Gelatinum Corii). If there are loose stools and poor appetite, add *Sha Ren* (Amomi, Fructus), *Shen Qu* (Massa Medica Fermentata), *Ze Xie* (Alismatis Orientalis, Rhizoma), and *Yi Yi Ren* (Coicis Lachryma-jobi, Semen).

ACUMOXIBUSTION: Moxibustion *Bai Hui* (GV 20), *Xin Shu* (Bl 15), and *Ge Shu* (Bl 17) and needle *Zu San Li* (St 36) and *San Yin Jiao* (Sp 6).

MODIFICATIONS: If there is concomitant liver depression, add *Tai Chong* (Liv 3) and *He Gu* (LI 4). If there is concomitant kidney vacuity, add *Shen Shu* (Bl 23) and *Tai Xi* (Ki 3). If there is simultaneous depressive heat, add *Xing Jian* (Liv 2) and *Nei Ting* (St 44). If there are heart palpitations, add *Nei Guan*

(Per 6). If there is insomnia, add *Shen Men* (Ht 7).

4. CENTRAL QI INSUFFICIENCY

SIGNS & SYMPTOMS: Dizziness and vertigo with an inclination to lie down and which is exacerbated by standing up or triggered by overtaxation, lassitude of the spirit, disinclination to talk, shortness of breath, lack of strength, spontaneous perspiration, reduced food intake, and loose stools. There is a pale tongue and a fine, weak pulse.

TREATMENT PRINCIPLES: Supplement the center, boost the qi, and stop vertigo

REPRESENTATIVE FORMULA: *Bu Zhong Yi Qi Tang* (Supplement the Center & Boost the Qi Decoction)

Huang Qi (Astragali Membranacei, Radix), 20g
mix-fried *Gan Cao* (Glycyrrhizae Uralensis, Radix), 6g
Dang Shen (Codonopsitis Pilosulae, Radix), 12g
Dang Gui (Angelicae Sinensis, Radix), 6g
Chen Pi (Citri Reticulatae, Pericarpium), 6g
Sheng Ma (Cimicifugae, Rhizoma), 3g
Chai Hu (Bupleuri, Radix), 3g
Bai Zhu (Atractylodis Macrocephalae, Rhizoma), 9g

ACUMOXIBUSTION: Moxibustion *Bai Hui* (GV 20), *Shang Xing* (GV 23), *Qi Hai* (CV 6), *Guan Yuan* (CV 4), and *Zu San Li* (St 36).

5. KIDNEY ESSENCE VACUITY

SIGNS & SYMPTOMS: Dizziness and vertigo with tinnitus, possibly an empty sensation in the head, lassitude of the spirit, impaired memory, blurred vision, low back and knee pain and weakness, seminal emission, impotence, and premature greying of the hair. There is a thin, pale red tongue and a deep, fine pulse.

TREATMENT PRINCIPLES: Supplement the kidneys, fill the essence, and stop dizziness

REPRESENTATIVE FORMULA: *Zuo Gui Wan* (Restore the Left [Kidney] Pills)

Shu Di Huang (Rehmanniae Glutinosae, cooked Radix), 18g
Shan Yao (Disocroeae Oppositae, Radix), 9g
Gou Qi Zi (Lycii Chinensis, Fructus), 12g
Shan Zhu Yu (Corni Officinalis, Fructus), 12g
Niu Xi (Achyranthis Bidentatae, Radix), 9g
Tu Si Zi (Cuscutae Chinensis, Semen), 9g
Lu Jiao Jiao (Cervi, Gelatinum Cornu), 5g
Gui Ban Jiao (Testudinis, Gelatinum Plastri), 5g

MODIFICATIONS: If there is marked yin vacuity with internal heat, add *Bie Jia* (Amydae Sinensis, Carapax), *Zhi Mu* (Anemarrhenae Aspheloidis, Rhizoma), *Huang Bai* (Phellodendri, Cortex), and *Di Gu Pi* (Lycii Chinensis, Cortex Radicis). If there is severe dizziness and vertigo, add *Long Gu* (Draconis, Os), *Mu Li* (Ostreae, Concha), and *Zhen Zhu Mu* (Margaritiferae, Concha). If there is aversion to cold, chilled limbs, impotence, and a pale tongue due to kidney yang vacuity, add *Xian Mao* (Curculiginis Orchioidis, Rhizoma) and *Yin Yang Huo* (Epimedii, Herba). If there is shortness of breath, lassitude of the spirit, and spontaneous perspiration due to qi vacuity, add *Ren Shen* (Panacis Ginseng, Radix). If there is seminal emission, white vaginal discharge, or diarrhea, add *Bu Gu Zhi* (Psoraleae Corylifoliae, Fructus) and *Qian Shi* (Euryalis Ferocis, Semen). If there is low back and knee pain and limpness, add *Du Zhong* (Eucommiae Ulmoidis, Cortex) and *Xu Duan* (Dipsaci Asperi, Radix).

ACUMOXIBUSTION: Needle *Tong Tian* (Bl 7), *Ting Gong* (SI 19), *Yi Feng* (TB 17), *Tai Xi* (Ki 3), and *Shen Shu* (Bl 23).

MODIFICATIONS: If there is simultaneous liver depression, add *Gan Shu* (Bl 18), *San Yin Jiao* (Sp 6), and *Tai Chong* (Liv 3).

6. PHLEGM DAMPNESS

SIGNS & SYMPTOMS: Vertigo and dizziness with heavy-headedness, chest and diaphragmatic fullness and oppression, nausea, vomiting, poor appetite, possible hypersomnia, possible obesity, and possible heavy body. There is slimy white tongue fur and a soggy, slippery pulse.

TREATMENT PRINCIPLES: Fortify the spleen and transform phlegm, eliminate dampness and settle vertigo

REPRESENTATIVE FORMULA: Modified *Ban Xia Bai Zhu Tian Ma Tang* (Pinellia, Atractylodes & Gastrodia Decoction)

Ban Xia (Pinelliae Ternatae, Rhizoma), 12g
Bai Zhu (Atractylodis Macrocephalae, Rhizoma), 9g
Chen Pi (Citri Reticulatae, Pericarpium), 6g
Tian Ma (Gastrodiae Elatae, Rhizoma), 12g
Fu Ling (Poriae Cocos, Sclerotium), 6g
Tian Nan Xing (Arisaematis, Rhizoma), 6g
Dang Shen (Codonopsitis Pilosulae, Radix), 9g
mix-fried *Gan Cao* (Glycyrrhizae Uralensis, Radix), 3g

MODIFICATIONS: For severe dizziness and vertigo with nausea and vomiting, add *Dai Zhe Shi* (Haemititum) and *Zhu Ru* (Bambusae In Taeniis, Caulis). If there is epigastric fullness and loss of appetite, add *Bai Dou Kou* (Cardamomi, Fructus) and *Sha Ren* (Amomi, Fructus). If there is accompanying tinnitus and deafness, add *Cong Bai* (Allii Fistulosi, Bulbus), *Yu Jin* (Curcumae, Tuber), and *Shi Chang Pu* (Acori Graminei, Rhizoma).

ACUMOXIBUSTION: Needle *Tou Wei* (St 8), *Nei Guan* (Per 6), *Zhong Wan* (CV 12), *Pi Shu* (Bl 20), *Feng Long* (St 40), and *Zu San Li* (St 36).

MODIFICATIONS: For severe dizziness and vertigo, add *Feng Chi* (GB 20) and *Yin Tang* (M-HN-3).

7. PHLEGM FIRE

SIGNS & SYMPTOMS: Dizziness and vertigo, a heavy head as if tightly bound, chest oppression, nausea, headache, a distended sensation in the eyes, irritability, a bitter taste in the mouth, and thirst without desire to drink. There is yellow, slimy tongue fur and a slippery, bowstring, rapid pulse.

TREATMENT PRINCIPLES: Clear heat and transform phlegm

REPRESENTATIVE FORMULA: Modified *Wen Dan Tang* (Warm the Gallbladder Decoction)

Ban Xia (Pinelliae Ternatae, Rhizoma), 9g
Zhu Ru (Bambusae In Taeniis, Caulis), 9g
Zhi Shi (Citri Aurantii, Fructus Immaturus), 6g
Chen Pi (Citri Reticulatae, Pericarpium), 6g
Gan Cao (Glycyrrhizae Uralensis, Radix), 3-6g
Fu Ling (Poriae Cocos, Sclerotium), 12g
Sheng Jiang (Zingiberis Officinalis, uncooked Rhizoma), 2 pieces
Da Zao (Zizyphi Jujubae, Fructus), 3 pieces
Huang Lian (Coptidis Chinensis, Rhizoma), 9g
Huang Qin (Scutellariae Baicalensis, Radix), 9g

ACUMOXIBUSTION: Needle *Tou Wei* (St 8), *Feng Long* (St 40), *Zhong Wan* (CV 12), *Nei Guan* (Per 6), *Xing Jian* (Liv 2), and *Feng Chi* (GB 20).

MODIFICATIONS: If there is vexation and agitation and irascibility, add *Yin Tang* (M-HN-3).

REPRESENTATIVE CASE HISTORIES

Case history of Dr. Li Jin-yong: An unnamed 40 year-old female[1]

This patient's first visit was in the autumn of 1993. Three days prior to this visit, she was standing in a river washing clothes when she became cold. She began to have chills and fever. She had been menstruating, but her menses stopped and did not finish its normal course. After three days, the woman was no longer cold, and her chills and fever were gone, but she became dizzy. She could not even stand up or open her eyes. Her pulse was fine, deep, and choppy. Therefore, Dr. Li's pattern identification was blood stasis with righteous qi vacuity and liver wind harassing the upper burner. His treatment principles were to nourish water and wood, quicken the blood, and extinguish wind, and he prescribed modified *Zuo Gui Yin* (Restore the Left [Kidney] Decoction): *Shu Di Huang* (Rehmanniae Glutinosae, cooked Radix), 15g, *Shan Yao* (Dioscoreae Oppositae, Radix), 12g, *Shan Zhu Yu* (Corni Officinalis, Fructus), 12g, *Fu Ling* (Poriae Cocos, Sclerotium), 12g, mix-fried *Gan Cao* (Glycyrrhizae Uralensis, Radix), 9g, *Gou Qi Zi* (Lycii Chinensis, Fructus), 12g, *Che Qian Zi* (Plantaginis, Semen), 9g, and *Wu Wei Zi* (Schisandrae Chinensis, Fructus), 6g. The patient came back the next day and reported that after she

had blood in her stool, all the symptoms disappeared. She took the formula one more day and completely recovered.

COMMENTARY: The liver pertains to wood, relates to wind, stores the blood, and controls menstruation (through its function of storing the blood). In menstruation, there is bleeding, and blood "likes warmth and hates cold." This patient became cold while in a river. *Su Wen*, Chapter 27, "*Li He Zhen Xie Lun*" (Treatise on the Parting & Uniting of the True & Evils)" states, "When heaven and earth are warm, the flow of water in rivers is calm; when heaven and earth are cold, the flow of water in rivers stagnates." Similarly, the cold caused general qi and blood stasis, thus stopping her menses. It also caused constructive and defensive disharmony with the exterior symptoms of chills and fever. After three days, the cold had penetrated deeper and caused liver depression qi stagnation. The qi stagnation compromised the liver's ability to store blood. Both liver qi and blood were impeded with resultant liver blood vacuity, and liver blood vacuity led to stirring of liver wind. The liver wind caused the dizziness. Water generates wood, and the kidney must be strong for the liver to function well. Thus Dr. Li chose to supplement water, the mother, to nourish the child, wood. He used *Zuo Gui Yin* plus *Wu Wei Zi* and *Che Qian Zi*. After taking these medicinals, improved liver function restored the free flow of qi and blood stasis was dispersed. The stagnant blood exited via the stool. After this, all the symptoms disappeared.

Case history of Dr. Chang Ji: Chang, a 59 year-old male cadre[2]

This patient's first visit was on June 23, 1992. For the previous year, he felt heat rising from his epigastrium, distention in his head, and dizziness. He also had a red facial complexion, irritability, and heart palpitations. His tongue was red with white, slimy fur, and his pulse was slippery and bowstring. A Western doctor diagnosed brain arteriosclerosis, and the man was treated with Chinese and Western medication without success. When the patient came to see Dr. Chang, he was irritable, anxious, and very easily excited and angered. He often had flushing-up and dizziness. Dr. Chang decided to use bitter (flavors) and cold (qi) to clear heat and cool the blood. His prescription consisted of: *Huang Lian* (Coptidis Chinensis, Rhizoma), 10g, *Huang Qin* (Scutellariae Baicalensis, Radix), 15g, *Da Huang* (Rhei, Radix Et Rhizoma), 7g, *Sheng Di Huang* (Rehmanniae Glutinosae, uncooked Radix), 20g, *Mai Men Dong* (Ophiopogonis Japonici, Tuber), 15g, *Chi Shao* (Paeoniae Lactiflorae, Radix Rubrus), 15g, *Shi Hu* (Dendrobii, Herba), 15g, *Yin Chen Hao* (Artemisiae Yinchenhao, Herba), 15g, *Pi Pa Ye* (Eriobotryae Japonicae, Folium), 15g, and *Gan Cao* (Glycyrrhizae Uralensis, Radix), 10g.

On July 2, 1992, the patient's second visit, he had taken the prescription for eight days. His heat and dizziness were much reduced. His tongue was red with thin, white fur, and his pulse was bowstring and slow. Dr. Chang modified the prescription as follows: *Huang Lian* (Coptidis Chinensis, Rhizoma), 10g, *Huang Qin* (Scutellariae Baicalensis, Radix), 15g, *Da Huang* (Rhei, Radix Et Rhizoma), 7g, *Sheng Di Huang* (Rehmanniae Glutinosae, uncooked Radix), 20g, *Mai Men Dong* (Ophiopogonis Japonici, Tuber), 15g, *Bai Shao* (Paeoniae Lactiflorae, Radix Albus), 15g, *Shi Hu* (Dendrobii, Herba), 15g, *Yin Chen Hao* (Artemisiae Yinchenhao, Herba), 15g, *Pi Pa Ye* (Eriobotryae Japonicae, Folium), 15g, *Gan Cao* (Glycyrrhizae Uralensis, Radix), 10g, *Zhi Ke* (Citri Aurantii, Fructus), 15g, *Ju Hua* (Chrysanthemi Morifolii, Flos), 15g, and *Sang Ye* (Mori Albi, Folium), 15g.

On July 10, the patient's third visit, he had taken this modified prescription for six days. All his symptoms were much improved, but he still had some slight attacks. Dr. Chang decided to add some yang-subduing medicinals. The new prescription included: *Dai Zhe Shi* (Haematitum), 30g, *Huang Lian* (Coptidis Chinensis, Rhizoma), 10g, *Huang Qin* (Scutellariae Baicalensis, Radix), 15g, *Da Huang* (Rhei, Radix Et Rhizoma), 7g, *Mu Li* (Ostreae, Concha), 20g, *Zhen Zhu Mu* (Margaritiferae, Concha), 30g, *Sheng Di Huang* (Rehmanniae Glutinosae, uncooked Radix), 20g, *Xuan Shen* (Scrophulariae Ningpoensis, Radix), 20g, *Long Dan Cao* (Gentianae Longdancao, Radix), 10g, *Niu Xi* (Achyranthis Bidentatae, Radix), 15g, and uncooked *Gan Cao* (Glycyrrhizae Uralensis, Radix), 10g.

On July 17, the patient's fourth visit, he had taken this prescription for six days and all his symptoms had disappeared. But then, because of stress, they started to come back, though not as strongly as before. Dr. Chang prescribed the following: *Huang Lian* (Coptidis Chinensis, Rhizoma), 10g, *Huang Qin* (Scutellariae Baicalensis, Radix), 15g, *Da Huang* (Rhei, Radix Et Rhizoma), 10g, *Tao Ren* (Pruni Persicae, Semen), 15g, *Dai Zhe Shi* (Haematitum), 30g, *Zhen Zhu Mu* (Margaritiferae, Concha), 30g, *Long Dan Cao* (Gentianae Longdancao, Radix), 10g, *Zhi Zi* (Gardeniae Jasminoidis, Fructus), 10g, *Mu Dan Pi* (Moutan, Cortex Radicis), 15g, *Sheng Di Huang* (Rehmanniae Glutinosae, uncooked Radix), 20g, *Yin Chen Hao* (Artemisiae Yinchenhao, Herba), 15g, uncooked *Mu Li* (Ostreae, Concha), 20g, *Gan Cao* (Glycyrrhizae Uralensis, Radix), 10g, and *Mai Men Dong* (Ophiopogonis Japonici, Tuber), 15g. The patient took this last formula for six days and all his symptoms completely disappeared.

COMMENTARY: Dr. Chang believed that stirring of the ministerial fire had caused this patient's dizziness. Different scholars have had different opinions about the nature of ministerial fire. Zhao Xian-ke believed that the ministerial fire is stored in the kidney and is the same as life-gate fire. When there is insufficiency of liver-kidney yin, this ministerial fire can become vacuity fire flaming upward in patterns such as ascendant liver yang hyperactivity or kidney vacuity-fire effulgence. Symptoms include dizziness, headache, unclear vision, and irascibility. The proper treatment strategy is to lead vacuity fire back to the kidney. Li Shi-zhen, on the other hand, thought ministerial fire was pericardium fire. He reasoned that, since the heart stores the spirit and is the sovereign fire, the pericardium, adjacent to the heart, must store the ministerial fire. If this ministerial fire is out of control, it is replete in nature and can cause heart palpitations, red face, irritability, and dizziness. In this case the treatment strategy must be to clear and drain replete heat. Dr. Chang thought that both theories applied in Chang's case. Chang had both vacuity and replete fire, *i.e.*, pericardium fire and kidney vacuity with ascendant yang. Therefore, the treatment principles had to include both supplementing yin and subduing yang, bringing the fire back to the kidney, and clearing pericardium fire.

ENDNOTES

[1] *Li Jin Yong Ling Chuan Jing Yen Ji Yao* (*A Collection of the Clinical Experiences of Li Jin-yong*), Beijing Chinese Medical Science Publisher, Beijing, 1998, p. 260
[2] Chang Qi, *op. cit.*, p. 350

CHAPTER 13
BLOOD STASIS

In Chinese medicine, blood stasis is not a disease. Rather, it is a secondary cause of disease as well as a pattern. However, it is such an important part of many kidney diseases that we feel that we must discuss this pattern in more detail. Therefore, we have chosen to append its discussion to the Chinese disease categories which correspond to modern Western kidney diseases. As a secondary cause of disease, one or more of the three categories of primary diseases causes (*i.e.*, external, internal, and neither external nor internal neutral disease causes) must instigate blood stasis. However, once established, blood stasis can cause further disease.

DISEASE CAUSES & MECHANISMS

As stated above, blood stasis is one of the secondary causes of disease. Anything which hinders or impedes the free flow of blood may result in blood stasis as well as anything which hinders or impedes the free flow of the channels and vessels through which the blood flows. For instance, traumatic injury damaging the channels and vessels may result in blood leaving its channels and vessels. However, blood can only flow as long as it abides in the channels and vessels. So traumatic injury may directly cause blood stasis. Because

the qi moves the blood, anything which disturbs or hinders the flow of qi may result in blood stasis. For instance, qi stagnation may eventually result in blood stasis as so may food stagnation, phlegm obstruction, and damp accumulation. Insufficient qi to move the blood may cause blood stasis just as blood vacuity not nourishing the heart and vessels may also cause blood stasis. Since yin is made up of blood and fluids and yang vacuity results in vacuity cold with congelation constriction, yin and/or yang vacuity may both also result in blood stasis. And finally, blood stasis may be due to heat damaging the blood. This can be either replete or vacuity heat, wind heat, dry heat, damp heat, or phlegm heat. Because blood stasis is secondary to other disease causes and mechanisms, in clinic, we rarely see blood stasis all by itself. Most commonly it presents as one element of a complicated, multifaceted pattern presentation. Chart 13.1 on the next page presents some of the most commonly seen patterns involving blood stasis.

TREATMENT BASED ON PATTERN IDENTIFICATION

1. QI VACUITY CAUSING BLOOD STASIS

SIGNS & SYMPTOMS: Fixed, severe, or piercing pain

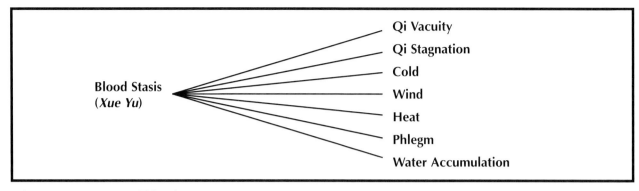

Chart 13.1. Causes of blood stasis

which typically refuses pressure and is worse at night, dry, scaly skin, dry, withered, and/or falling hair, visible varicosities, spider nevi, cherry hemangiomas, easy bruising, fatigue, lack of strength, dizziness when standing up, abdominal distention after meals, possible poor appetite, shortness of breath, and a sooty facial complexion or dark circles around the eyes. The tongue is tender or swollen with thin, white fur and the pulse is fine and weak.

TREATMENT PRINCIPLES: Fortify the spleen and boost the qi, quicken the blood and transform stasis

REPRESENTATIVE FORMULA: *Huang Qi Gui Zhi Wu Wu Tang* (Astragalus & Cinnamon Twig Five Materials Decoction)

Huang Qi (Astragali Membranacei, Radix), 9g
Bai Shao (Paeoniae Lactiflorae, Radix Albus), 9g
Gui Zhi (Cinnamomi Cassiae, Ramulus), 9g
Sheng Jiang (Zingiberis Officinalis, uncooked Rhizoma), 18g
Da Zao (Zizyphi Jujubae, Fructus), 12 pieces

MODIFICATIONS: If qi vacuity is more marked, add *Dang Shen* (Codonopsitis Pilosulae, Radix) and mix-fried *Gan Cao* (Glycyrrhizae Uralensis, Radix). If there is concomitant blood vacuity, add *Dang Gui* (Angelicae Sinensis, Radix) and *Ji Xue Teng* (Jixueteng, Radix Et Caulis).

If blood stasis has entered the network vessels, instead of *Huang Qi Gui Zhi Wu Wu Tang,* use *Bu Yang Huan Wu Tang* (Supplement Yang to Restore

Five [Tenths] Decoction): *Huang Qi* (Astragali Membranacei, Radix), 12g, *Dang Gui Wei* (Angelicae Sinensis, Extremitas Radicis), 9g, *Chuan Xiong* (Ligustici Wallichii, Radix), 3g, *Chi Shao* (Paeoniae Lactiflorae, Radix Rubrus), 4.5g, *Tao Ren* (Pruni Persicae, Semen), 3g, *Hong Hua* (Carthami Tinctorii, Flos), 3g, and *Di Long* (Lumbricus), 3g.

ACUMOXIBUSTION: Needle *Xue Hai* (Sp 10), *Ge Shu* (Bl 17), *Gan Shu* (Bl 18), *Pi Shu* (Bl 20), and *Zu San Li* (St 36).

MODIFICATIONS: Depending on the site of pain or the location of the disease, needle local points. If stasis has entered the network vessels, puncture to bleed any visibly engorged superficial veins.

2. QI STAGNATION CAUSING BLOOD STASIS

SIGNS & SYMPTOMS: Emotional depression, enduring great anger, stress and frustration, unfulfilled desires, irritability, chest and epigastric fullness and oppression, rib-side distention, possible breast distention and pain and/or menstrual pain in women, fixed, severe, or piercing pain which typically refuses pressure and is worse at night, dry, scaly skin, dry, withered, and/or falling hair, visible varicosities, spider nevi, and cherry hemangiomas. The tongue is dark in color with normal fur. There may be static speckles or macules on the tongue, and the pulse is bowstring or bowstring and choppy.

TREATMENT PRINCIPLES: Course the liver and rectify the qi, quicken the blood and transform stasis

REPRESENTATIVE FORMULA: *Han Jiang Tang* (Cold, Downbearing Decoction)

uncooked *Dai Zhe Shi* (Haematitum), 18g
lime-processed *Ban Xia* ((Pinelliae Ternatae, Rhizoma), 9g
Gua Lou ((Trichosanthis Kirlowii, Fructus), 12g
uncooked *Bai Shao* (Paeoniae Lactiflorae, Radix Albus), 12g
Zhu Ru (Bambusae in Taeniis, Caulis), 9g
Niu Bang Zi (Arctii Lappae, Fructus), 9g
Gan Cao (Glycyrrhizae Uralensis, Radix), 4.5g

MODIFICATIONS: If blood stasis is marked, add *Dang Gui* (Angelicae Sinensis, Radix) and *Chi Shao* (Paeoniae Lactiflorae, Radix Rubrus). If qi depression has transformed heat, add *Huang Lian* (Coptidis Chinensis, Rhizoma) and *Huang Qin* (Scutellariae Baicalensis, Radix). If there is concomitant spleen vacuity, add *Bai Zhu* (Atractylodis Macrocephalae, Rhizoma) and *Fu Ling* (Poriae Cocos, Sclerotium).

ACUMOXIBUSTION: Needle *Tai Chong* (Liv 3), *He Gu* (LI 4), *San Yin Jiao* (Sp 6), and *Xue Hai* (Sp 10).

MODIFICATIONS: Add local points depending on the site of pain or the location of the disease.

3. COLD CAUSING BLOOD STASIS

SIGNS & SYMPTOMS: Fixed, severe, or piercing pain which typically refuses pressure and is worse at night and worse on exposure to cold, aversion to cold, chilled extremities, and cyanotic fingertips and lips. There is a blue-purple tongue with thin, white fur and a slow, deep, possibly choppy pulse.

TREATMENT PRINCIPLES: Warm the channels and scatter cold, quicken the blood and transform stasis

REPRESENTATIVE FORMULAS: If cold has caused blood stasis in the *chong mai*, use *Wen Jing Tang* (Warm the Menses Decoction):

Wu Zhu Yu (Evodiae Rutaecarpae, Fructus), 9g
Gui Zhi (Cinnamomi Cassiae, Ramulus), 6g
Dang Gui (Angelicae Sinensis, Radix), 9g
Chuan Xiong (Ligustici Wallichii, Radix), 6g
Bai Shao (Paeoniae Lactiflorae, Radix Albus), 6g
E Jiao (Asini, Gelatinum Corii), 6g
Mai Men Dong (Ophiopogonis Japonici, Tuber), 9g
Mu Dan Pi (Moutan, Cortex Radicis), 6g
Ren Shen (Panacis Ginseng, Radix), 6g
Gan Cao (Glycyrrhizae Uralensis, Radix), 6g
Sheng Jiang (Zingiberis Officinalis, uncooked Rhizoma), 6g
Ban Xia (Pinelliae Ternatae, Rhizoma), 6g

Use *Shao Fu Zhu Yu Tang* (Lower Abdomen Stasis-dispelling Decoction) for cold-type blood stasis in the lower burner:

stir-fried *Xiao Hui Xiang* (Foeniculi Vulgaris, Fructus), 1.5g
Gan Jiang (Zingiberis Officinalis, dry Rhizoma), 6g
Yuan Hu Suo (Corydalis Yanhusuo, Rhizoma), 3g
Dang Gui (Angelicae Sinensis, Radix), 9g
Chuan Xiong (Ligustici Wallichii, Radix), 3g
Mo Yao (Myrrhae, Resina), 3g
Rou Gui (Cinnamomi Cassiae, Cortex), 3g
Chi Shao (Paeoniae Lactiflorae, Radix Rubrus), 6g
Pu Huang (Typhae, Pollen), 9g
stir-fried *Wu Ling Zhi* (Trogopteri Seu Pteromi, Excrementum), 6g

Use *Sheng Hua Tang* (Generation & Transformation Decoction) to treat postpartum cold causing blood stasis:

Dang Gui (Angelicae Sinensis, Radix), 24g
Chuan Xiong (Ligustici Wallichii, Radix), 9g
Tao Ren (Pruni Persicae, Semen), 14 pieces
Pao Jiang (Zingiberis Officinalis, blast-fried Rhizoma), 1.5g
mix-fried *Gan Cao* (Glycyrrhizae Uralensis, Radix), 1.5g

Use *Dang Gui Si Ni Tang* (Dang Gui Four Counterflows Decoction) to treat cold in the channels:

Dang Gui (Angelicae Sinensis, Radix), 9g
Bai Shao (Paeoniae Lactiflorae, Radix Albus), 9g
Gui Zhi (Cinnamomi Cassiae, Ramulus), 9g

Xi Xin (Asari, Herba Cum Radice), 6g
mix-fried *Gan Cao* (Glycyrrhizae Uralensis, Radix), 6g
Da Zao (Zizyphi Jujubae, Fructus), 5 pieces
Mu Tong (Akebiae Mutong, Caulis), 6g

ACUMOXIBUSTION: Moxibustion the affected area or location of the disease.

4. WIND CAUSING BLOOD STASIS

SIGNS & SYMPTOMS: Heavy, painful sensations at fixed locations in the lower back and lower extremities accompanied by weakness and stiffness, aversion to cold, a liking for warmth, possible numbness, possible heart palpitations and shortness of breath. There is a pale tongue with white fur and a fine, weak, slow pulse.

TREATMENT PRINCIPLES: Dispel wind and eliminate dampness, quicken the blood and free the flow of impediment

REPRESENTATIVE FORMULA: *Du Huo Ji Sheng Tang* (Angelica Pubescens & Ramulus Sangjisheng Decoction)

Du Huo (Angelicae Pubescentis, Radix), 9g
Xi Xin (Asari, Herba Cum Radice), 6g
Fang Feng (Ledebouriellae Divaricatae, Radix), 6g
Qin Jiao (Gentianae Qinjiao, Radix), 6g
Sang Ji Sheng (Sangjisheng, Ramulus), 6g
Du Zhong (Eucommiae Ulmoidis, Cortex), 6g
Niu Xi (Achyranthis Bidentatae, Radix), 6g
Rou Gui (Cinnamonmi Cassiae, Cortex), 6g
Dang Gui (Angelicae Sinensis, Radix), 6g
Chuan Xiong (Ligustici Wallichii, Radix), 6g
Sheng Di Huang (Rehmanniae Glutinosae, uncooked Radix), 6g
Bai Shao (Paeoniae Lactiflorae, Radix Albus), 6g
Ren Shen (Panacis Ginseng, Radix), 6g
Fu Ling (Poriae Cocos, Sclerotium), 6g
mix-fried *Gan Cao* (Glycyrrhizae Uralensis, Radix), 6g

MODIFICATIONS: For severe pain, add *Bai Hua She* (Bungarus Multicinctus), *Di Long* (Lumbricus), and *Hong Hua* (Carthami Tinctorii, Flos). For severe

cold, add *Fu Zi* (Aconiti Carmichaeli, Radix Lateralis Praeparatus) and *Gan Jiang* (Zingiberis Officinalis, dry Rhizoma). For severe dampness, add *Cang Zhu* (Atractylodis, Rhizoma) and *Yi Yi Ren* (Coicis Lachryma-jobi, Semen). If there is no concomitant qi and blood vacuity, subtract *Ren Shen* and *Bai Shao*.

ACUMOXIBUSTION: In general, points should be chosen from the yang channels according to the principle, "The course of the channel is amenable to treatment." One usually chooses local, adjacent and distant points to the affected area. For example, for impediment, one might choose *Jian Yu* (LI 15) as a local point, *Jian Liao* (TB 14) as an adjacent point, and *He Gu* (LI 4) as a distant point. To these, one may add points that dispel wind (these generally have *feng* or wind in their name), such as *Feng Fu* (GV 16), *Feng Chi* (GB 20), *Bing Feng* (SI 12), *Yi Feng* (TB 17), *Feng Men* (Bl 12), and *Feng Shi* (GB 31) plus points that quicken the blood, such as *Ge Shu* (Bl 17) and *Xue Hai* (Sp 10). If there is prominent cold and/or dampness, one can also use moxibustion.

5. HEAT CAUSING BLOOD STASIS

SIGNS & SYMPTOMS: Acute lower abdominal pain, incontinence of urine, night fevers, deranged speech, irritability, restlessness, and vexatious thirst. There is a purple-red tongue with yellow fur on its root and a deep-lying, replete, or choppy pulse.

TREATMENT PRINCIPLES: Clear heat and disperse accumulation, quicken the blood and dispel stasis

REPRESENTATIVE FORMULA: *Tao He Cheng Qi Tang* (Persica Order the Qi Decoction)

Tao Ren (Pruni Persicae, Semen), 50 pieces
Da Huang (Rhei, Radix Et Rhizoma), 12g
Gui Zhi (Cinnamomi Cassiae, Ramulus), 6g
Mang Xiao (Mirabilitum), 6g
mix-fried *Gan Cao* (Glycyrrhizae Uralensis, Radix), 6g

MODIFICATIONS: If there is irregular menstruation or dysmenorrhea, add *Dang Gui* (Angelicae Sinensis,

Radix) and *Hong Hua* (Carthami Tinctorii, Flos). If there is simultaneous qi stagnation, add *Xiang Fu* (Cyperi Rotundi, Rhizoma), *Wu Yao* (Linderae Strychnifoliae, Radix), *Qing Pi* (Citri Reticulatae Viride, Pericarpium), and *Mu Xiang* (Auklandiae Lappae, Radix). If blood stasis is egregious, add *Chi Shao* (Paeoniae Lactiflorae, Radix Rubrus) and *San Qi* (Notoginseng, Radix) or *Shui Zhi* (Hirudo Seu Whitmania) and *Meng Chong* (Tabanus).

If heat evils have entered the blood aspect and have caused blood stasis, use modified *Xi Jiao Di Huang Tang* (Rhinoceros Horn & Rehmannia Decoction): *Shui Niu Jiao* (Bubali, Cornu), 20g, *Sheng Di Huang* (Rehmanniae Glutinosae, uncooked Radix), 24g, *Chi Yao* (Paeoniae Lactiflorae, Radix Rubrus), 9g, and *Mu Dan Pi* (Moutan, Cortex Radicis), 6g. If there is manic behavior, add *Huang Qin* (Scutellariae Baicalensis, Radix) and *Da Huang* (Rhei, Radix Et Rhizoma). If there is hematemesis, add *Ce Bai Ye* (Biotae Orientalis, Cacumen) and *Bai Mao Gen* (Imperatae Cylindricae, Rhizoma). For hemafecia, add *Di Yu* (Sanguisorbae Officinalis, Radix) and *Huai Hua Mi* (Sophorae Japonicae, Flos Immaturus). For hematuria, add *Bai Mao Gen* (Imperatae Cylindricae, Rhizoma) and *Xiao Ji* (Cephalanoplos Segeti, Herba). If yin has been severely damaged by heat, subtract *Chi Shao* and replace with *Bai Shao* (Paeoniae Lactiflorae, Radix Albus). If there is concomitant irritability, add *Chai Hu* (Bupleuri, Radix) and *Zhi Zi* (Gardeniae Jasminoidis, Fructus). If there is simultaneous qi vacuity, add *Ren Shen* (Panacis Ginseng, Radix) and *Huang Qi* (Astragali Membranacei, Radix).

ACUMOXIBUSTION: Choose from *Wei Zhong* (Bl 40), *Qu Chi* (LI 11), *He Gu* (LI 4), *Zhong Ji* (CV 3), *Tian Shu* (St 25), *Shang Ju Xu* (St 37), and *Xue Hai* (Sp 10).

6. PHLEGM CAUSING BLOOD STASIS

SIGNS & SYMPTOMS: Recurrent vertigo, weakness, chest oppression, possible sudden loss of consciousness or syncope, upward staring of the eyes, deviation of the mouth, profuse phlegm, the sound of phlegm in the back of the throat, convulsions, incontinence of the bowels or urine. There is slimy,

white tongue fur and a bowstring, slippery pulse.

TREATMENT PRINCIPLES: Wash away phlegm and open the orifices, quicken the blood and extinguish wind

REPRESENTATIVE FORMULA: *Ding Xian Wan* (Stabilize Epilepsy Pills)

Tian Ma (Gastrodia Elatae, Rhizoma), 30g
Chuan Bei Mu (Fritillariae Cirrhosae, Bulbus), 30g
ginger-processed *Ban Xia* (Pinelliae Ternatae, Rhizoma), 30g
Fu Ling (Poriae Cocos, Sclerotium), 30g
Fu Shen (Poriae Cocos, Sclerotium Pararadicis), 30g
Dan Nan Xing (Arisaematis, bile-processed Rhizoma), 15g
Shi Chang Pu (Acori Graminei, Rhizoma), 15g
Quan Xie (Buthus Martensi), 15g
Jian Can (Bombyx Batryticatus), 15g
Hu Po (Succinum), 15g
Deng Xin Cao (Junci Effusi, Medulla), 15g
Chen Pi (Citri Reticulatae, Pericarpium), 21g
Yuan Zhi (Polygalae Tenuifoliae, Radix), 21g
Dan Shen (Salviae Miltiorrhizae, Radix), 60g
Mai Men Dong (Ophiopogonis Japonici, Tuber), 60g
Zhu Sha (Cinnabar), 9g
Gan Cao (Glycyrrhizae Uralensis, Radix), 120g
mix-fried *Gan Cao* (Glycyrrhizae Uralensis, Radix), 100g
Sheng Jiang Zhi (Zingiberis Officinalis, Succus Rhizomatis), 50ml

MODIFICATIONS: For patients who are vacuous and weak, add *Ren Shen* (Panacis Ginseng, Radix).

If there is chest impediment accompanied by phlegm and blood stasis, use *Zhi Shi Gua Lou Gui Zhi Tang* (Immature Aurantium, Trichosanthes & Cinnamon Twig Decoction): *Gua Lou* (Trichosanthis Kirlowii, Fructus), 12g, *Xie Bai* (Allii, Bulbus), 9g, *Zhi Shi* (Citri Aurantii, Fructus Immaturus), 12g, *Hou Po* (Magnoliae Officinalis, Cortex), 12g, and *Gui Zhi* (Cinnamomi Cassiae, Ramulus), 3g. For angina pectoris, add *Dan Shen* (Salviae Miltiorrhizae, Radix), *Chi Shao* (Paeoniae Lactiflorae, Radix Rubrus), *Chuan Xiong* (Ligustici Wallichii, Radix), and *Hong Hua* (Carthami Tinctorii, Flos).

ACUMOXIBUSTION: Choose from *He Gu* (LI 4), *Zhong Ji* (CV 3), *Tian Shu* (St 25), *Feng Long* (St 40), *Zhong Wan* (CV 12), *San Yin Jiao* (Sp 6), and *Xue Hai* (Sp 10)

7. WATER ACCUMULATION CAUSING BLOOD STASIS

SIGNS & SYMPTOMS: Edema, difficult, scanty urination, headache, high blood pressure, low back pain, weakness, and fatigue. The tongue is dark purple with static speckles. The pulse is bowstring and choppy.

TREATMENT PRINCIPLES: Quicken the blood, dispel stasis, and drain dampness

REPRESENTATIVE FORMULA: Modified *Xue Fu Zhu Yu Tang* (Blood Mansion Stasis-dispelling Decoction)

Tao Ren (Pruni Persicae, Semen), 9g
Hong Hua (Carthami Tinctorii, Flos), 6g
Chuan Xiong (Ligustici Wallichii, Radix), 9g
Dang Gui (Angelicae Sinensis, Radix), 9g
Chi Shao (Paeoniae Lactiflorae, Radix Rubrus), 9g
Mu Dan Pi (Moutan, Cortex Radicis), 9g
Niu Xi (Achyranthis Bidentatae, Radix), 6g
Chai Hu (Bupleuri, Radix), 3g
Sheng Di Huang (Rehmanniae Glutinosae, uncooked Radix), 9g
Zhi Ke (Citri Aurantii, Fructus), 6g
Gan Cao (Glycyrrhizae Uralensis, Radix), 3g
Shui Zhi (Hirudo Seu Whitmania), 9g
Ze Lan (Lycopi Lucidi, Herba), 9g
Yi Mu Cao (Leonuri Heterophylli, Herba), 9g
Che Qian Zi (Plantaginis, Semen), 9g

MODIFICATIONS: For pronounced, tenacious dampness, add *Qu Mai* (Dianthi, Herba) and *Shi Wei* (Pyrrosiae, Folium). For headache, add *Fang Feng* (Ledebouriellae Divaricatae, Radix) and *Man Jing Zi* (Viticis, Fructus). However, if the patient has high blood pressure, do not use *Fang Feng* but increase the dose of *Niu Xi* to 12-15 grams. For insomnia, add *Suan Zao Ren* (Zizyphi Spinosae, Semen), *He Huan Pi* (Albizziae Julibrissinis, Cortex), and *Ye Jiao Teng* (Polygoni Multiflori, Caulis). For irascibility or anxiety, add *Xiang Fu* (Cyperi Rotundi, Rhizoma). If there is severe fatigue, add *Ren Shen* (Panacis Ginseng, Radix) or *Xi Yang Shen* (Panacis Quinquefolii, Radix).

NOTE: When there is concurrent water accumulation and blood stasis, it is often impossible to determine which humor preceded or caused the other. Often blood stasis precedes water accumulation, but the resultant water accumulation exacerbates the blood stasis, leading to a vicious cycle.

ACUMOXIBUSTION: Choose from *Ge Shu* (Bl 17), *Pang Guang Shu* (Bl 28), *Shui Fen* (CV 9), *He Gu* (LI 4), *Xue Hai* (Sp 10), *Feng Long* (St 40), *Yin Ling Quan* (Sp 9), *Tai Chong* (Liv 3), and *Tai Xi* (Ki 3).

REPRESENTATIVE CASE HISTORIES

Case history of Dr. Xi Wen-ban: Wang, a 38 year-old female[1]

Wang had low back pain and painful urination with bloody urine. She went to a Western doctor, and, after treatment, her bleeding and painful urination were alleviated, but her low back pain remained. Her back became so painful she could not sit or stand for any length of time. At the time of examination by Dr. Xi, Wang had a dry mouth, thirst without desire to drink, tidal fever, and difficulty falling asleep. Her appetite and stools were normal. Her tongue had a slightly red tip, and her pulse was fine and slightly rapid. Dr. Xi's pattern identification was blood stasis and kidney yin vacuity heat. Therefore, he prescribed *Wu Zi Bu Shen Wan* (Schisandra Supplement the Kidney Pills): *Fu Pen Zi* (Rubi Chingii, Fructus), 9g, *Che Qian Zi* (Plantaginis, Semen), 9g, *Wu Wei Zi* (Schisandrae Chinensis, Fructus), 5g, *Nu Zhen Zi* (Ligustri Lucidi, Fructus), 9g, *Gou Qi Zi* (Lycii Chinensis, Fructus), 12g, *Ji Xue Teng* (Jixueteng, Radix Et Caulis), 8g, *Yi Mu Cao* (Leonuri Heterophylli, Herba), 30g, *Ze Lan* (Lycopi Lucidi, Herba), 6g, *Di Gu Pi* (Lycii Chinensis, Cortex Radicis), 9g, *Han Lian Cao* (Ecliptae Prostratae, Herba), 18g, and *Mu Dan Pi* (Moutan, Cortex Radicis), 9g. Wang took the prescription for 12 days and her low back pain was completely alleviated.

Case history of Dr. He He-ling: Xu, a four year-old boy[2]

Xu had chronic recurring nephritis for over one year. Three months prior to his first visit, he caught cold and had another recurrence. His whole body was edematous, and he had a yellow face, fatigue, abdominal bloating, loose stools, and scanty urination. His tongue was pale with thin, white fur and purple stasis speckles on the sides. His pulse was deep and fine. Based on these signs and symptoms, Dr. He's pattern identification was spleen-kidney yang vacuity water swelling with blood stasis. His first prescription consisted of: *Dang Shen* (Codonopsitis Pilosulae, Radix), 9g, *Bai Zhu* (Atractylodis Macrocephalae, Rhizoma), 9g, *Yi Yi Ren* (Coicis Lachryma-jobi, Semen), 9g, *Chi Xiao Dou* (Phaseoli Calcarati, Semen), 9g, *Huang Qi* (Astragali Membranacei, Radix), 9g, *Dan Shen* (Salviae Miltiorrhizae, Radix), 9g, *Rou Gui* (Cinnamomi Cassiae, Cortex), 3g, *Bai Hua She She Cao* (Hedyotidis Diffusae, Herba), 15g, *Ban Bian Lian* (Lobeliae Chinensis, Herba Cum Radice), 15g, *Pu Gong Ying* (Taraxaci Mongolici, Herba Cum Radice), 5g, and *Gan Cao* (Glycyrrhizae Uralensis, Radix), 2g.

Xu took this prescription for 15 days without any improvement. He still has edema and his urine protein was unchanged at 3+. Dr. He thought his prescription had been unsuccessful because it had not emphasized dispelling stasis. Therefore, he removed *Pu Gong Ying* and *Yi Yi Ren* and added *Fu Zi* (Aconiti Carmichaeli, Radix Lateralis Præparatus), 5g, *Yi Mu Cao* (Leonuri Heterophylli, Herba), 9g, and *Tao Ren* (Pruni Persicae, Semen), 7g. Xu took this new prescription for seven days and his edema dissipated. His urine protein reduced to less than 1+. Dr. He consolidated the results by prescribing modified *Jin Gui Shen Qi Wan* (*Golden Cabinet* Kidney Qi Pills). Xu took this formula for six months and three urinalyses proved negative. A follow-up one and a half years later showed no recurrence.

CLINICAL TIPS

1. The major symptoms of blood stasis are fixed pain that is unrelieved or worse with pressure, pain that is worse at night, and hard, unmovable masses. The tongue tends to be dark red or purple and/or have purple stasis macules or speckles. The pulse tends to be replete and choppy. Other symptoms are location specific. In the upper burner, these include chest pain, coughing up blood, heart palpitations, irritability, forgetfulness, and inability to swallow water. If the middle burner is affected, there may be symptoms of abdominal pain, hypochondriac pain, a swollen abdomen, and a dark or purple color on the extremities. If the lower burner is affected, there may be lower abdominal bloating and sharp pain, dark stools, hard masses, and manic behavior. If the blood stasis is in the extremities, these may be painful, numb, and/or paralyzed. In woman, blood stasis may cause menstrual problems.

2. Even if one rectifies the qi first, one must still use stasis-dispelling, blood-quickening medicinals to treat blood stasis. One must be conscious of the strength of these medicinals which may be grouped into three categories. The blood-quickening (or harmonizing) medicinals are the mildest. They nourish as well as quicken the blood. These include *Dan Shen* (Salviae Miltiorrhizae, Radix), *Dang Gui* (Angelicae Sinensis, Radix), *Chuan Xiong* (Ligustici Wallichii, Radix), *Mu Dan Pi* (Moutan, Cortex Radicis), *Chi Shao* (Paeoniae Lactiflorae, Radix Rubrus), and *Ji Xue Teng* (Jixueteng, Radix Et Caulis). In the second category are the stasis-transforming medicinals. They are stronger in action and do not supplement the blood. These include *Yan Hu Suo* (Corydalis Yanhusuo, Rhizoma), *Tao Ren* (Pruni Persicae, Semen), *Hong Hua* (Carthami Tinctorii, Flos), *Da Huang* (Rhei, Radix Et Rhizoma), *Ze Lan* (Lycopi Lucidi, Herba), *Ru Xiang* (Olibani, Resina), *Mo Yao* (Myrrhae, Resina), *San Qi* (Notoginseng, Radix), *Pu Huang* (Typhae, Pollen), and *Yi Mu Cao* (Leonuri Heterophylli, Herba). The third category, called blood-breaking medicinals, are the strongest and include *San Leng* (Sparganii Stoloniferi, Rhizoma) and *E Zhu* (Curcumae Ezhu, Rhizoma) as well as insect or worm products such as *Shui Zhi* (Hirudo Seu Whitmania), *Tu Bie Chong* (Eupolyphaga Seu Opisthoplatia), and *Meng Chong* (Tabanus).

3. One must also attend to the location of the blood

stasis to properly formulate a treatment strategy. If it occurs in the upper burner, one must free the flow or descend. If it is in the middle burner, one must harmonize and move as well as pay special attention to the protection of the spleen and stomach. If it is in the lower burner, one must warm and free the flow. If the blood stasis is in the muscles and sinews, one should combine blood-quickening medicinals with medicinals or formulas that resolve the exterior.

4. It cannot be overemphasized that, when dealing with blood stasis, one must always be careful of the strength of the medicinals in relation to the patient's constitution. If one uses medicinals that are too strong, one may damage the true qi. Therefore, treatment strategies usually combine dispelling stasis with supplementing the qi and blood.

ENDNOTES

[1] Chang Qi, *op. cit.*, p. 565
[2] Yu Wong-shi, *op. cit.*, p. 183

PART 3
THE CHINESE MEDICAL TREATMENT OF KIDNEY & BLADDER DISEASES

CHAPTER 1
URINARY TRACT INFECTIONS(UTI)

Millions of people every year are afflicted with infections of the urinary tract. In 1997, more than eight million medical office visits were made due to infection-caused symptoms of the genitourinary system. Urinary tract infections (UTI) are one of the most common types of human infection, second only to upper respiratory infections. A variety of etiologies may be found for the disorders comprising UTIs, but all of them either begin with or result in an abnormal overgrowth of bacteria. There are five primary bacterial conditions associated with the upper and lower urinary tracts. These are urethritis, cystitis, prostatitis, and acute and chronic pyelonephritis. Each disorder is associated with bacterial overgrowth and affects distinct regions of the genitourinary system.

NOSOLOGY

Urinary tract infections are classified primarily according to their location within the genitourinary (GU) system. Upper UTIs consist of those conditions that affect the kidneys. Pyelonephritis is a common example. Lower UTIs consist of those conditions extending from the external urethral meatus to, but not including, the kidneys. Lower UTIs are more common in occurrence and tend to be less critical medically. More often than not, lower UTIs are

uncomplicated, albeit bothersome and at times debilitating, but they do have the potential to result in serious infections which can compromise the entire GU system.

Urethritis is an infection and inflammation of the urethra. It is also known as acute urethral syndrome. In males, microbial colonization localizes in the bulbous and pendulous portions of the urethra, and, in females, the entire urethra may become infected. Urethritis is primarily considered a sexually transmitted infection. Gonorrhea and chlamydia are the principal etiological agents. Onset tends to be gradual. Classically, males report purulent urethral discharge. Females classically present with cystitis-type symptoms.

Prostatitis is a hugely significant health problem for older males. Bacteria in the prostate are the most common cause of UTIs in men. Acute and chronic conditions exist. In acute episodes, the symptoms can be severe and systemic.

Cystitis is the term for infection and inflammation of the bladder itself. Urinary tract infections in general are commonly referred to as "bladder infections," though cystitis is the only one which is specific to the bladder. (Numerous texts and articles use the term cystitis interchangeably with lower urinary tract infection.) Cystitis may be further classified with the following five designations: asymptomatic bacteriuria, initial cystitis, reinfection cystitis, chronic cystitis, and recurrent cystitis. Asymptomatic bacteriuria is identified as a condition in which bacteria is detected on laboratory examination but there are no associated signs or symptoms. Initial cystitis is the first diagnosed episode of infection. This may resolve or reoccur. Reinfection cystitis is understood to be an entirely new episode of cystitis after a previous bout of the infection was cured. This is an important category of cystitis because it may help the practitioner to more readily identify the etiological vector. Chronic cystitis refers to an ongoing case of the disease which is not cured with treatment. Onset tends to be gradual. Symptoms tend to linger. Recurrent cystitis is defined as reinfection cystitis occurring three or more times within a one year period. Unfortunately, it is the norm for many people who develop an initial case of lower UTI.

EPIDEMIOLOGY

Lower UTI in general, and cystitis specifically, affect populations differently depending on age and gender. Of the more than eight million medical office visits per year are for UTIs, most for cystitis. Approximately 100,000 hospital admissions are made yearly for UTIs. The majority of these are for acute pyelonephritis, many of which are secondary to lower UTIs. More than $1 billion annually is dedicated from the national healthcare budget for the study and treatment of UTIs. Fifty percent of females report at least one episode of cystitis in their lifetime. Twenty percent of adult females report UTI symptoms annually. Urinary tract infections are most common in sexually active women 20-50 years in age. Urinary tract infections may also occur in young girls and are recognized as increasing in frequency in that age group. Interestingly, newborn males have a higher incidence of UTIs than females. This is thought to be due to the increased incidence of GU abnormalities in boys of that age group. For example, the incidence of vesicoureteral reflux in male neonates translates into a 10 to 30 times greater risk of developing a UTI than for a healthy

male. In older populations, specifically those who are institutionalized, there is a fairly equal ratio between males and females with UTIs. Urinary tract infections for these groups are primarily iatrogenic in origin. Typically, they are due to catheterization. Also, as older males develop more diseases of the prostate, this increases their chances of developing UTIs. As many as 10% of pregnant women have asymptomatic bacteriuria. Almost half of these women will proceed to symptomatic cystitis. Urinary tract infections represent the most common infectious complication of pregnancy. In addition, the risk of developing pyelonephritis is much higher in this population.

ETIOLOGY & PATHOPHYSIOLOGY

The mode of origin and development of UTIs encompasses an intricate exchange between certain microbes and the environment of their host. The primary bacteria responsible for most cases of cystitis are *Escherichia coli*, *E. coli*, a facultative anaerobe. It is implicated in 85% of infections in ambulatory patients and 50% of nosocomial infections. *Proteus mirabilis*, *Klebsiella pneumonia*, and *Enterococcus fecalis*, are the next most frequent isolates. In rare cases *Candida albicans* may be responsible. *E. coli* is most frequently fecal in origin. The majority of infections are termed ascending. *E. coli* enters and ascends the urethra to the bladder. It is conventionally believed that the relatively shorter length of the urethra in females increases their susceptibility to ascending infection. (There is debate on this theory in the literature.) It is believed that fecal microbes, primarily *E. coli*, may have a tendency to colonize the areas surrounding the urethral meatus, the perineum and vaginal opening. This may be true especially in cases of poor hygiene.

In men it is uncommon to experience cystitis before the age of 50. After that age, on average, men begin to experience progressive obstruction of their prostate. This obstruction can compromise the normal flow of urine and predispose them to infection. Additionally, zinc, which is found in healthy prostatic fluid and semen, is considered to be antimicrobial. If the fluid becomes deficient, as may be the case with obstruction, there may not be adequate quantities of zinc to protect the urinary tract from ascending infection.

In general, the most important function for the prevention of ascending infection is healthy and normal flow of urine. Micturition serves to remove unwanted microbes as well as withered epithelial lining cells within the urinary tract. Reluctance to void, *i.e.*, holding urine, is considered unhealthy.

In terms of the bacteria itself, *E. coli* has an ability to produce pili which serve to anchor it to the lining of the urinary tract. The relative virulence of a particular strain of bacteria is associated with the type and effectiveness of its pili. Certain strains are significantly aggressive in their ability to lock on to the mucosal lining and reject attempts both by the body and through medications to let go.

The use of antibiotics and spermicides have a similar effect in that they may change the normal bacterial flora of the GU system and vagina as well as altering the pH. The death of normal, commensal, *i.e.*, good, bacteria may give harmful bacteria the opportunity to grow unchecked. An overgrowth in bacteria in the vagina may then correspond with an increased likelihood of migrating to the urethra. There are a number of studies associating diaphragm use with spermicide and a higher number of UTIs.

There are two additional conditions that may predispose someone to cystitis. These are malposition of the uterus or bladder. An anteverted uterus may complicate an infection because pressure on the bladder may not allow it to drain fully. Malposition of the bladder may be the result of heavy lifting, strain to the lower abdominal ligaments, or hernia. Any situation that causes a slouching or prolapse of the bladder may increase the susceptibility to infection.

RISK FACTORS

It is well documented that sexual intercourse contributes to a higher number of UTIs in women. Celibate women have considerably lower incidences of bacteriuria. Older adults are at high risk for developing cystitis, with the incidence in the elderly being as high as 33 out of 100 people. As previously

mentioned, conditions associated with incomplete voiding of the bladder are more common in the elderly. These include prostatitis, benign prostatic hypertrophy and urethral strictures. Whenever the flow of urine becomes blocked or obstructed there is a higher risk of infection. This is particularly true in the hospital setting with cytoscopic examination and urethral catheterization. Invariably, with prolonged catheterization, infection will occur. Prophylactic use of antibiotics in such settings is the norm. As previously discussed, pregnant women are at higher risk for developing UTIs. Other conditions which pose a risk for developing cystitis include diabetes, analgesic nephropathy, those who have sustained prolonged or chronic intake of analgesic medication, reflux nephropathy, those with compromised structures between the bladder and kidneys allowing back-flow, *i.e.*, vesicoureteral reflux, and sickle-cell anemia. Further, it is important to consider those people who do not have adequate fluid intake and those with bowel incontinence or chronic diarrhea, as potentially at risk for developing UTIs. Cigarette smoking is a major cause of bladder cancer. It also has been implicated in specific changes in the epithelial cell lining of the bladder which may predispose one to an increased risk of cystitis.

SYMPTOMATOLOGY

The classic symptoms of UTI include dysuria (pain with urination), frequency, and urgency. These may be accompanied by nocturia, and suprapubic discomfort. Signs of UTI may include cloudy or dark urine, hematuria, and foul or strong odor to the urine. Fever is not characteristic of lower UTI. Additional symptoms include pain with intercourse, for males or females, flank pain, penis pain, vaginal pain, fatigue, chills or fever, and nausea and/or vomiting. Complaints of confusion or mental changes may occur. This should be considered especially in elderly populations.

DIAGNOSIS

In the past, the Western medical diagnosis of UTIs was determined by urine culture. A culture that generated greater than 100,000 colony-forming units (CFU) was considered to be "significant" for bacterial overgrowth. Laboratory analysis, however, indicates that many people, women especially, who have UTI symptoms have far lower counts than the diagnostic 100,000 CFU/ml. Understanding that *E. coli* is the most active and recognized microbe for uncomplicated UTIs (as much as 90% of the time), it has since become the norm to forego routine urine culture analysis. Since conventional therapeutics are mostly limited to antibiotics, and given the minimal possibility of microbial agents involved other than *E. coli*, nowadays diagnosis is based on an abbreviated laboratory analysis. This consists of a wet-mount microscopic examination of spun urine and/or a urine dipstick test.

In terms of wet-mount analysis, the evidence of pyuria is defined as the visualization of more than eight white blood cells (WBCs) per microscopic field. White blood cells are frequently the aspect of the urine which makes it cloudy, *i.e.*, pus-like. The presence of WBCs indicates bacterial infection. The urine dipstick is considered an equally sensitive test for detecting pyuria. The leukocyte and nitrite markers indicate the presence of WBCs and bacteria respectively.

In addition to laboratory testing, it is important to perform a physical examination. This should include abdominal and flank palpation. Attention should be given to the possibility of suprapubic tenderness and bladder distention. Flank examination and costovertebral angle tenderness may reveal possible kidney involvement and pyelonephritis. A genital examination is occasionally warranted. For boys, circumcision status should be noted. Some in the medical profession consider an uncircumcised penis to be a risk factor for UTIs. Positioning of the meatus should be ascertained to rule out stenosis or phimosis. In men suspected of having urethritis, inspection should be made for the evidence of discharge. A GC/chlamydia swab-culture may also be indicated. Examination for prostatic hypertrophy should be considered. For females, attention should be given to the possibility of labial adhesions as this may create an increased susceptibility to bacterial colonization. Pelvic examination for vaginitis may be indicated. If there are symptoms of voiding dysfunctions, neurological examinations may be indicated. These may include peripheral reflexes, perineal sensation and an examination of the spine for dimpling or other abnormalities.

DIFFERENTIAL DIAGNOSIS

The differential diagnosis for lower UTIs is long and varied. An overview is necessary due to the grave nature of a number of the potential disorders. Though lower UTIs, in general, and cystitis, specifically, are fairly easy to diagnose, attention should be given to the number of other potential causes of urinary symptoms. It should be noted that the diagnosis of UTI does not, in any way, rule out other potential disorders. A differential diagnosis for UTI should include:

Balanitis
Benign prostatic hypertrophy
Bladder cancer
Diabetes mellitus
Diuretic use, including drugs, caffeine and teas
Endometriosis
Estrogen deficiencies causing atrophic changes
Genital herpes
Interstitial cystitis
Kidney disease
Kidney stone
Neurological dysfunction
Papillary necrosis
Pelvic inflammatory disease
Pelvic mass
Pregnancy
Radiation-induced bladder inflammation
Sexually transmitted infections, especially chlamydia
Sickle-cell anemia
Vaginal infection

WESTERN MEDICAL TREATMENT

In modern Western medicine, the treatment strategy is to sterilize the urine and the urinary tract. This is done with antimicrobial, antibiotic medicines. The goal is to eliminate or at least reduce the number of offending agents within the length of the tract. The object is threefold: 1) to prevent continual and local irritation, 2) to halt proliferation of the microbes and 3) to avoid the possible ascent of bacteria into the kidneys. As previously mentioned, diagnosis of cystitis, though sensitive for bacteria, is not specific for which particular bacteria is involved. Current standard of care allows for a presumptive diagnosis of *E. coli* and the use of antibiotic therapy to combat it. Neglecting to diagnose with specifics of the microbial agents involved has led to an epidemic of antimicrobial resistance and a marked increase in ever-worsening and virulent microbes. Conventional treatment regimens also fail to address the unwanted side effect of dysbiosis following antibiotic therapy. It is unusual to find a conventional medical protocol which supplements the vaginal or gastrointestinal regions with "good" flora following antibiotics.

Conventional treatment for lower UTIs is determined by whether the infection is community-acquired or hospital-induced, *i.e.*, nosocomial, and by the sex of the patient. For women experiencing acute cystitis the choice of therapy is a three-day course of trimethoprin-sulfamethoxazole (TMP-SMX). The dosage is 160-800mg every 12 hours. Follow up urinalysis should be done within seven to ten days after treatment. TMP-SMX is considered a broad-spectrum antibiotic, except for the pseudomonas and enterococus species, and works by hindering folate metabolism. It is less expensive than other UTI drugs and is considered to have only minimal negative effect on the gastrointestinal flora. Side effects do include skin rashes and intestinal complaints. It is contraindicated in pregnancy and newborns less than one month of age. Men with acute cystitis are also prescribed TMP-SMX. Their dosage typically extends to seven days. Fluoroquinolones are another, more expensive class of antibiotics that are truly broad-spectrum and work by inhibiting DNA gyrase. They are reserved for cases of recurrent cystitis, patients with sensitivity or allergy to TMP-SMX, and for patients who may have developed bacterial resistance to TMP-SMX. Dosage for men and women is typically the same as TMP-SMX, 160-800mg every 12 hours for seven days. Ampicillin and amoxicillin, examples of aminopenicillins, have been used for years for a vast array of infectious processes, including UTIs. Their use has become significantly reduced due to an abundance of resistant microbes. Aminoglycosides and nitrofuran-

toin are also occasionally used, though more often with complicated cases of UTI. They are associated with more serious complications, including kidney toxicity. Interestingly, nitrofurantoin is considered a legitimate prophylactic therapy. Patients are prescribed a night-time dose of 50mg for six to twelve months. Other prophylactic medications include TMP-SMX, 1/2 tablet nightly, or cephalexin, 250mg nightly. Patients who identify UTI occurrence with sexual intercourse may also be instructed to take a single dosage of the same medication postcoitally.

PROGNOSIS & COMPLICATIONS

For adults, the symptoms of cystitis usually resolve within 24-48 hours after beginning treatment. In general, the prognosis for UTIs is good. Symptoms may be uncomfortable and at times severe, but they do not frequently develop into complications. For boys, even the incidence of one UTI is reason for concern as it is indicative of a possible urinary tract abnormality, such as vesicoureteral reflux. The tendency within the medical profession in recent years is not to be as concerned with young girls who experience UTIs as with boys. There is a belief that the female urethral anatomy is principally to blame. This is a shortsighted diagnosis and neglects the potential for more serious causes such as vesicoureteral reflux. Children, both boys and girls, deserve a complete diagnostic intake to rule out serious complications.

Complications of UTIs are generally defined as kidney infections. This is otherwise known as pyelonephritis. Pyelonephritis is not common but becomes increasingly likely if there is a history of recurrent or chronic cystitis, kidney stones, vesicoureteral reflux, or other obstructive disorders of the urinary tract. Particularly virulent bacteria may also be implicated even in a single, isolated episode of cystitis. Progressive pyelonephritis can potentially result in systemic bacteremia, chronic pyelonephritis, renal failure and death.

CHINESE MEDICAL DISEASE CATEGORIZATION

Urinary tract infections are categorized as strangury in Chinese medicine. Strangury is defined as a disease condition characterized by urinary urgency, fre-

TYPE OF STRANGURY	PATTERN IDENTIFICATION	
Heat Strangury	Replete	1. Damp heat
	Vacuous	2. Heat damages the yin
Blood Strangury	Replete	3. Damp heat stagnation 4. Heart fire shifting heat to the small intestine
	Vacuous	5. Yin vacuity heat 6. Kidney yin vacuity 7. Spleen and kidney qi vacuity
Stone Strangury	Replete	8. Damp heat (dampness more than heat) 9. Damp heat (heat more than dampness) 10. Qi stagnation
	Vacuous	11. Qi vacuity: inhibited kidney and bladder qi transformation 12. Kidney yin vacuity 13. Kidney qi vacuity
Qi Strangury	Replete	14. Liver qi depression & binding
	Vacuous	15. Center qi fall
Taxation Strangury	Vacuous	16. Spleen vacuity 17. Kidney yang vacuity 18. Kidney yin vacuity
Unctuous Strangury	Replete	19. Damp heat in the lower burner
	Vacuous	20. Kidney qi vacuity

Chart 1.1. Types of strangury & their patterns

quent, short, painful, rough voidings, and dribbling incontinence. There are six kinds of strangury: heat strangury, blood strangury, stone strangury, qi strangury, taxation strangury, and unctuous strangury. (See Chart 1.1 above.)

TREATMENT BASED ON PATTERN IDENTIFICATION

HEAT STRANGURY

1. DAMP HEAT

SIGNS & SYMPTOMS: Frequent, urgent, difficult, scanty, and painful urination that is reddish yellow or dark yellow. Fever, thirst, and constipation often accompany this. The tongue is red with yellow, slimy fur, and the pulse is fast.

TREATMENT PRINCIPLES: Clear heat and eliminate dampness

REPRESENTATIVE FORMULA: *Ba Zheng San* (Eight [Ingredients] Rectifying Powder)

Mu Tong (Akebiae, Caulis), 9g
Qu Mai (Dianthi, Herba), 9g
Bian Xu (Polygoni Avicularis, Herba), 9g
Hua Shi (Talcum), 6g
Deng Xin Cao (Junci Effusi, Medulla), 9g
Che Qian Zi (Plantaginis, Semen), 9g
Zhi Zi (Gardeniae Jasminoidis, Fructus), 9g
Da Huang (Rhei, Radix Et Rhizoma), 9g
Gan Cao (Glycyrrhizae Uralensis, Radix), 9g
Huang Bai (Phellodendri, Cortex), 9g
Zhi Mu (Anemarrhenae Asphodeloidis, Rhizoma), 9g

ACUMOXIBUSTION: Choose from *Zhong Ji* (CV 3),

Yun Men (Liv 2), *Chi Ze* (Liv 5), *Shao Fu* (Ht 8), *Yin Ling Quan* (Sp 9), *San Yin Jiao* (Sp 6), *Pang Guang Shu* (Bl 28), *Yang Ling Quan* (GB 34), *Shen Shu* (Bl 23), *Pang Guang Shu* (Bl 28), *Wei Yang* (Bl 53), and *Zhong Ji* (CV 3).

Case history from Dr. Wei Li's private practice: Carol, a 27 year-old female

Carol had three recurrences of burinignurination in one year. She took antibiotics, but these did not stop the recurrences. When she came to Dr. Li, she presented with burning, frequent, scanty urination with urgency and a feeling that her urination was incomplete for one week. She was thirsty, irritable, and anxious. She had a red tongue with yellow fur and a fast, bowstring, slippery pulse. Dr. Li's pattern identification was damp heat in the lower burner with inhibited bladder qi transformation. Her treatment strategy was to clear and eliminate damp heat in the lower burner and harmonize the water passageways. Her prescription was modified *Ba Zheng San* (Eight [Ingredients] Rectifying Powder): *Mu Tong* (Akebiae, Caulis), 6g, *Hua Shi* (Talcum), 6g, *Che Qian Zi* (Plantaginis, Semen), 9g, *Qu Mai* (Dianthi, Herba), 9g, *Bian Xu* (Polygoni Avicularis, Herba), 9g, *Zhi Zi* (Gardeniae Jasminoidis, Fructus), 9g, *Da Huang* (Rhei, Radix Et Rhizoma), 9g, *Deng Xin Cao* (Junci Effusi, Medulla), 9g, *Gan Cao* (Glycyrrhizae Uralensis, Radix), 9g, *Huang Lian* (Coptidis, Rhizoma), 6g, and *Sheng Di Huang* (Rehmanniae Glutinosae, uncooked Radix), 8g. After the first day of taking this formula, Carol felt better. In one week, the symptoms were almost completely gone. Since this condition had recurred, Dr. Li prescribed *Zhi Bai Di Huang Wan* (Anemarrhena & Phellodendron Rehmannia Pills), five pills three times per day, for one month to consolidate the results.

2. HEAT DAMAGING YIN

SIGNS & SYMPTOMS: Frequent, urgent, painful, scanty, dark yellow urination, possible vexation, thirst, and insomnia. The tongue is red with little fur, and the pulse is thin and rapid.

TREATMENT PRINCIPLES: Clear heat, eliminate dampness, and nourish yin

REPRESENTATIVE FORMULA: Modified *Zhi Bai Di Huang Wan* (Anemarrhena & Phellodendron Rehmannia Pills) plus *Zhu Ling Tang* (Polyporus Decoction)

Huang Bai (Phellodendri, Cortex), 9g
Zhi Mu (Anemarrhenae Asphodeloidis, Rhizoma), 9g
Sheng Di Huang (Rehmanniae Glutinosae, uncooked Radix), 12g
Shan Zhu Yu (Corni Officinalis, Fructus), 12g
Shan Yao (Discoreae Opposiate, Radix), 12g
Fu Ling (Poriae Cocos, Sclerotium), 9g
Ze Xie (Alismatis Orientalis, Rhizoma), 9g
Mu Dan Pi (Moutan, Cortex Radicis), 9g
Zhu Ling (Polypori Umbellati, Sclerotium), 9g
E Jiao (Corii Asini, Gelatinum), 9g
Hua Shi (Talcum), 9g

ACUMOXIBUSTION: Choose from *Shen Shu* (Bl 23), *Pang Guang Shu* (Bl 28), *Wei Zhong* (Bl 40), *Wei Yang* (Bl 53), *Tai Xi* (Ki 3), *Zhao Hai* (Ki 6), *Tai Chong* (Liv 3), *Chi Ze* (Liv 5), and *Zhong Ji* (CV 3).

Case history of Dr. Chang Qi: Yang, a 50 year-old female[1]

Yang's first visit to Dr. Chang was on Nov. 19, 1987. Ten years previous to this visit, she had frequent, urgent, painful urination accompanied by fever and low back pain. She took antibiotics and the symptoms disappeared. She continued to take antibiotics for recurring infections, but they could not prevent these recurrences 2-3 times every year. As time went on, the recurrences became more frequent, and she began to have them every month. The antibiotics began to lose effectiveness, and, 20 days before her visit, they completely failed to halt a recurrence.

Yang presented with frequent and burning urination, low back pain, fatigue, heat in the five hearts, and a dry mouth without the desire to drink. Her tongue was pale red, and her pulse was fast, thin, and forceless. Urinalysis showed protein negative, and WBCs 50. A urine culture showed about 10,000/ml of bacteria. The pattern identification was damp heat in the lower burner with damage to qi and yin. Dr. Chang's treatment strategy was to boost the qi and nourish yin, clear and eliminate bladder damp heat.

His formula consisted of: *Huang Qi* (Astragali Membranacei, Radix), 30g, *Dang Shen* (Codonopsitis Pilosulae, Radix), 20g, *Lian Zi* (Nelumbinis Nuciferae, Semen), 15g, *Fu Ling* (Poriae Cocos, Sclerotium), 15g, *Mai Men Dong* (Ophiopogonis Japonici, Tuber), 15g, *Che Qian Zi* (Plantaginis, Semen), 15g, *Di Gu Pi* (Lycii Chinensis, Cortex Radicis), 15g, *Qu Mai* (Dianthi, Herba), 20g, *Bian Xu* (Polygoni Avicularis, Herba), 20g, *Pu Gong Yin* (Taraxaci Mongolici Cum Radice, Herba), 30g, *Bai Hua She She Cao* (Hedyotidis Diffusae, Herba), 50g, and *Gan Cao* (Glycyrrhizae Uralensis, Radix), 10g.

Yang returned for her second visit on Nov. 26. She had taken the prescription for six days and she had less frequent and burning urination. By Dec. 4, all Yang's symptoms had disappeared except for low back soreness and fatigue. Her tongue was pale red with thick, white fur. Her urine culture was negative. Therefore, Yang was administered this formula for another 20 days, after which she became free of urinary symptoms and her low back soreness and fatigue were better. She finished her course of treatment by taking the same prescription 10 more days. A follow up visit a half year later found no recurrence and a urine culture was negative.

BLOOD STRANGURY

1. DAMP HEAT STAGNATION

SIGNS & SYMPTOMS: Fresh blood in the urine that is warmer than normal body temperature, frequent, urgent, and burning urination. The tongue is red with yellow fur, and the pulse is big and forceful.

TREATMENT PRINCIPLES: Clear heat and eliminate dampness, cool the blood and stop bleeding

REPRESENTATIVE FORMULA: *Xiao Ji Yin Zi* (Cephalanoplos Beverage)

Xiao Ji (Cephalanoplos, Herba), 9g
Pu Huang (Typhae, Pollen), 9g
Ou Jie (Nelumbinis Nuciferae, Nodus Rhizomatis), 9g
Hua Shi (Talcum), 3g
Mu Tong (Akebiae, Caulis), 9g

Sheng Di Huang (Rehmanniae Glutinosae, uncooked Radix), 9g
Dang Gui (Angelicae Sinensis, Radix), 6g
Zhi Zi (Gardeniae Jasminoidis, Fructus), 9g
Dan Zhu Ye (Lophatheri Gracilis, Herba), 9g
Gan Cao (Glycyrrhizae Uralensis, Radix), 3g

MODIFICATIONS: If there is thirst, add *Shi Hu* (Dendrobii, Herba) and *Tian Hua Fen* (Trichosanthis Kirlowii, Radix). If the bleeding does not stop, add *Bai Mao Gen* (Imperatae Cylindricae, Rhizoma) and *Di Yu* (Sanguisorbae Officinalis, Radix).

Dr. Li's empirical formula:

Huang Bai (Phellodendri, Cortex), 9g
Zhi Mu (Anemarrhenae Asphodeloidis, Rhizoma), 9g
Shan Zhu Yu (Corni Officinalis, Fructus), 9g
Mu Dan Pi (Moutan, Cortex Radicis), 9g
Shan Yao (Dioscoreae Oppositae, Radix), 9g
Fu Ling (Poriae Cocos, Sclerotium), 9g
Huang Lian (Coptidis Chinensis, Rhizoma), 7g
Han Lian Cao (Ecliptae Prostratae, Herba), 9g
Bai Shao (Paeoniae Lactiflorae, Radix Albus), 9g
Sheng Di Huang (Rehmanniae Glutinosae, uncooked Radix), 9g

MODIFICATION: If the bleeding does not stop, add *Xian He Cao* (Agrimoniae Pilosae, Herba).

COMMENTARY: In this pattern bleeding is the tip. The root consists of combinations of damp heat, blood heat, blood stasis, and blood vacuity. In most cases, one should treat the root first, then staunch bleeding. Blood-staunching medicinals may cause greater blood stasis. Blood stasis causes heat and blood vacuity leading to recurrent bleeding, thus defeating the strategy. However, if there is excessive bleeding, one must staunch bleeding first. Excessive bleeding will lead to severe blood vacuity and damage the true qi, hampering any further treatment.

ACUMOXIBUSTION: Choose from *Yin Bai* (Sp 1), *Xue Hai* (Sp 10), *Tai Xi* (Ki 3), *Gui Lai* (St 29), *Ge Shu* (Bl 17), *Pang Guang Shu* (Bl 28), *Shen Shu* (Bl 23), *Zhong Ji* (CV 3), and *Guan Yuan* (CV 4).

Case history from Dr. Wei Li's private practice: Lee, a 56 year-old female

Lee had overtaxed herself working night shifts seven days in a row. She felt feverish, very fatigued, and thirsty. She had urgent, painful, incomplete, and scanty urination, and there appeared to be fresh blood in her urine. Her tongue was red with yellow fur, and her pulse was slippery and fast. Dr. Li's diagnosis was blood strangury caused by damp heat in the lower burner. Her treatment strategy was to clear heat, cool blood, and staunch bleeding. She used *Xiao Ji Yin Zi* (Cephalanoplos Drink) plus *Huang Lian Jie Du Tang* (Coptis Toxin-resolving Decoction): *Xiao Ji* (Cephalanoplos, Herba), 9g, *Ou Jie* (Nelumbinis Nuciferae, Nodus Rhizomatis), 9g, stir-fried *Pu Huang* (Typhae, Pollen), 9g, *Sheng Di Huang* (Rehmanniae Glutinosae, uncooked Radix), 30g, *Mu Tong* (Akebiae, Caulis), 9g, *Dan Zhu Ye* (Lophatheri Graqcilis, Herba), 9g, *Zhi Zi* (Gardeniae Jasminoidis, Fructus), 9g, *Dang Gui* (Angelicae Sinensis, Radix), 9g, *Gan Cao Shao* (Glycyrrhizae Uralensis, Extremitas Radicis), 6g, *Huang Lian* (Coptidis Chinensis, Rhizoma), 9g, *Huang Qin* (Scutellariae Baicalensis, Radix), 9g, and *Huang Bai* (Phellodendri, Cortex), 9g.

Lee took this prescription for seven days and her symptoms disappeared. To consolidate the treatment by nourishing yin, Dr. Li prescribed *Liu Wei Di Huang Wan* (Six Flavors Rehmannia Pills). Lee finished her course of treatment by taking 10g of these pills two times a day for a month.

2. TRANSMISSION OF HEART FIRE TO THE SMALL INTESTINE

SIGNS & SYMPTOMS: Fresh red blood in the urine with a burning urination, vexation, thirst with desire to drink, and insomnia. The tongue is red with a red tip, and the pulse is fast.

TREATMENT PRINCIPLES: Clear and drain heart fire, cool the blood and staunch bleeding

REPRESENTATIVE FORMULAS: Modified *Dao Chi San* (Abduct the Red Powder)

Sheng Di Huang (Rehmanniae Glutinosae, uncooked Radix), 10g

Mu Tong (Akebiae, Caulis), 10g

Dan Zhu Ye (Lophatheri Gracilis, Herba), 10g

Gan Cao Shao (Glycyrrhizae Uralensis, Extremitas Radicis), 10g

Che Qian Zi (Plantaginis, Semen), 10g

Qu Mai (Dianthi, Herba), 10g

Bai Mao Gen (Imperatae Cylindricae, Rhizoma), 10g

Dang Gui (Angelicae Sinensis, Radix), 6g

Mu Dan Pi (Moutan, Cortex Radicis), 10g

Xiao Ji (Cephalanoplos, Herba), 10g

Fo Shou (Citri Sarcodactylis, Fructus), 10g

Dr. Li's empirical formula:

Lian Xin (Nelumbinis Nuciferae, Plumula), 6g

Mu Dan Pi (Moutan, Cortex Radicis), 9g

Sheng Di Huang (Rehmanniae Glutinosae, uncooked Radix), 9g

Huang Lian (Coptidis Chinensis, Rhizoma), 6g

Gan Cao Shao (Glycyrrhizae Uralensis, Extremitas Radicis), 3g

Dan Shen (Salviae Miltiorrhizae, Radix), 9g

Fu Ling (Poriae Cocos, Sclerotium), 9g

Zhi Mu (Anemarrhenae Asphodeloidis, Rhizoma), 9g

ACUMOXIBUSTION: Choose from *Zhong Ji* (CV 3), *Shui Dao* (St 28), *San Yin Jiao* (Sp 6), *Shao Fu* (Ht 8), *Yin Ling Quan* (Sp 9), *Lao Gong* (Per 8), *Zhao Hai* (Ki 6), *Nei Guan* (Per 6), and *Yin Tang* (M-HN-3).

3. YIN VACUITY-FIRE EFFULGENCE

SIGNS & SYMPTOMS: Difficult, painful, scanty urination with pale red blood, lower back and knee weakness, dizziness, and ear ringing. The tongue is red with little fur, and the pulse is thin and fast.

TREATMENT PRINCIPLES: Supplement the kidneys and nourish yin, clear vacuity heat

REPRESENTATIVE FORMULA: Augmented *Zhi Bai Di Huang Wan* (Anemarrhena & Phellodendron Rehmannia Pills)

Zhi Mu (Anemarrhenae Asphodeloidis, Rhizoma), 9g

Huang Bai (Phellodendri, Cortex), 9g

Shu Di Huang (Rehmanniae Glutinosae, cooked Radix), 12g

Shan Yao (Radix Dioscoreae Oppositae), 12g

Shan Zhu Yu (Corni Officinalis, Fructus), 12g

Ze Xie (Alismatis Orientalis, Rhizoma), 9g

Fu Ling (Poriae Cocos, Sclerotium), 9g

Mu Dan Pi (Moutan, Cortex Radicis), 9g

Pu Huang (Typhae, Pollen), 9g

Han Lian Cao (Ecliptae Prostratae, Herba), 12g

ACUMOXIBUSTION: Choose from *Ge Shu* (Bl 17), *Shen Shu* (Bl 23), *Pang Guang Shu* (Bl 28), *Zhong Ji* (CV 3), *Guan Yuan* (CV 4), *Zhao Hai* (Ki 6), *Tai Xi* (Ki 3), *Tai Chong* (Liv 3), *San Yin Jiao* (Sp 6), and *Xue Hai* (Sp 10).

4. KIDNEY YIN VACUITY

SIGNS & SYMPTOMS: Burning and painful urination with blood in the urine, night sweats, heat in the five hearts, dizziness, blurred vision, insomnia, tinnitus, low back pain, and seminal emission. The tongue is red with no fur. The pulse is thin and fast.

TREATMENT PRINCIPLES: Supplement the kidney and nourish yin, cool the blood and staunch bleeding

REPRESENTATIVE FORMULAS: Modified *Zhi Bai Di Huang Wan* (Anemarrhena & Phellodendron Rehmannia Pills) or modified *Da Bu Yin Wan* (Greatly Supplementing Yin Pills)

Zhi Bai Di Huang Wan (Anemarrhena & Phellodendron Rehmannia Pills):

Zhi Mu (Anemarrhenae Asphodeloidis, Rhizoma), 9g

Huang Bai (Phellodendri, Cortex), 9g

Shu Di Huang (Rehmanniae Glutinosae, cooked Radix), 12g

Shan Yao (Radix Dioscoreae Oppositae), 12g

Shan Zhu Yu (Corni Officinalis, Fructus), 12g

Ze Xie (Alismatis Orientalis, Rhizoma), 9g

Fu Ling (Poriae Cocos, Sclerotium), 9g

Mu Dan Pi (Moutan, Cortex Radicis), 9g

Da Bu Yin Wan (Greatly Supplementing Yin Pills)

Shu Di Huang (Rehmanniae Glutinosae, cooked Radix), 12g

deep-fried *Gui Ban* (Testudinis, Plastrum), 12g

stir-fried *Huang Bai* (Phellodendri, Cortex), 9g

wine stir-fried *Zhi Mu* (Anemarrhenae Asphodeloidis, Rhizoma), 9g

MODIFICATIONS: This formula was originally made in pill form combining the ground herbs with honey and pork marrow. These ingredients are more than binders. They are necessary to fully address concurrent essence insufficiency. Therefore, when one makes this formula as a decoction, one should cook the herbs with pork marrow and/or add honey (one tablespoon per dose). One may also add *Han Lian Cao* (Ecliptae Prostratae, Herba), *Nu Zhen Zi* (Ligustri Lucidi, Fructus), *Xiao Ji* (Cephalanoplos, Herba), *Ou Jie* (Nelumbinis Nuciferae, Nodus Rhizomatis), and *Xian He Cao* (Agrimoniae Pilosae, Herba).

Dr. Li's empirical formula:

Han Lian Cao (Ecliptae Prostratae, Herba), 10g

Nu Zhen Zi (Ligustri Lucidi, Fructus), 10g

Zhi Mu (Anemarrhenae Asphodeloidis, Rhizoma), 10g

Huang Bai (Phellodendri, Cortex), 10g

Sheng Di Huang (Rehmanniae Glutinosae, uncooked Radix), 15g

Shan Zhu Yu (Corni Officinalis, Fructus), 10g

Shan Yao (Radix Dioscoreae Oppositae), 10g

Qing Dai (Indigo Pulverata Levis), 5g

Huang Lian (Coptidis Chinensis, Rhizoma), 10g

Ban Xia (Pinelliae Ternatae, Rhizoma), 5g

Che Qian Zi (Plantaginis, Semen), 10g

Gui Ban (Testudinis, Plastrum), 15g

Mu Dan Pi (Moutan, Cortex Radicis), 10g

Chuan Xiong (Ligustici Wallichii, Radix), 10g

MODIFICATIONS: If there is nausea and gas, add *Huo Xiang* (Agastaches Seu Pogostemi, Herba) and *Pei Lan* (Eupatorii Fortunei, Herba). If there is diarrhea, add *Fu Ling* (Poriae Cocos, Sclerotium), *Bai Zhu* (Atractylodis Macrocephalae, Rhizoma), and *Chen Pi* (Citri Reticulatae, Pericarpium). If there is frequent diarrhea, add *Rou Dou Kou* (Myristicae Fragrantis, Semen). If there is low back pain, add *Niu Xi* (Achyranthis Bidentatae, Radix) and *Sang Ji*

Sheng (Ramulus Sangjisheng). For tinnitus, add *Huang Jing* (Polygonati, Rhizoma), *Shi Chang Pu* (Acori Graminei, Rhizoma), and *Ci Shi* (Magnititum). If there are night sweats, add *Di Gu Pi* (Lycii Chinensis, Cortex Radicis), *Fu Xiao Mai* (Tritici Aestivi, Semen Levis), *Wu Mei* (Pruni Mume, Fructus), *Wu Wei Zi* (Schizandrae Chinensis, Fructus), stir-fried *Suan Zao Ren* (Zizyphi Spinosae, Semen), and calcined *Mu Li* (Ostreae, Concha). One can also grind up *Wu Bei Zi* (Rhois Chinensis, Galla), mix it with vinegar, and put it on the patient's navel overnight. If there is dizziness, add *Gou Qi Zi* (Lycii Chinensis, Fructus), *Ju Hua* (Chrysanthemi Morifolii, Flos), *Mu Li* (Ostreae, Concha), and *Tian Ma* (Gastrodiae Elatae, Rhizoma). If there is insomnia, add *He Huan Pi* (Albizziae Julibrissinis, Cortex), *Ye Jiao Teng* (Polygoni Multiflori, Caulis), *Dan Shen* (Salviae Miltiorrhizae, Radix), and *Suan Zao Ren* (Zizyphi Spinosae, Semen).

ACUMOXIBUSTION: Choose from *Ge Shu* (Bl 17), *Shen Shu* (Bl 23), *Pang Guang Shu* (Bl 28), *Zhong Ji* (CV 3), *Guan Yuan* (CV 4), *Tai Xi* (Ki 3), *Zhao Hai* (Ki 6), *Yin Gu* (Ki 10), *San Yin Jiao* (Sp 6), *Xue Hai* (Sp 10), *Da Dun* (Liv 1), and *Yin Bai* (Sp 1).

5. SPLEEN-KIDNEY QI VACUITY

SIGNS & SYMPTOMS: Frequent urination, especially night urination, bloody urine with pink blood but without burning, dribbling urine, no appetite, loose stools, dizziness, shortness of breath, fatigue, seminal emission, low back and knee weakness. The tongue is pale, and the pulse is weak.

TREATMENT PRINCIPLES: Fortify the spleen and boost the qi, supplement the kidney and secure the essence

REPRESENTATIVE FORMULAS: *Wu Bi Shan Yao Wan* (Incomparable Dioscorea Pills)

Shan Yao (Dioscoreae Oppositae, Radix), 12g
Rou Cong Rong (Cistanchis Deserticolae, Herba), 9g
Shu Di Huang (Rehmanniae Glutinosae, cooked Radix), 12g

Shan Zhu Yu (Corni Officinalis, Fructus), 12g
Fu Ling (Poriae Cocos, Sclerotium), 12g
Tu Si Zi (Cuscutae Chinensis, Semen), 9g
Wu Wei Zi (Schisandrae Chinensis, Fructus), 9g
Chi Shi Zhi (Halloysitum, Rubrum), 9g
Ba Ji Tian (Morindae Officinalis, Radix), 9g
Ze Xie (Alismatis Orientalis, Rhizoma), 9g
Du Zhong (Eucommiae Ulmoidis, Cortex), 9g
Niu Xi (Achyranthis Bidentatae, Radix), 6g

MODIFICATIONS: One may add *Jing Ying Zi* (Rosae Laevigatae, Fructus), *Mu Li* (Ostreae, Concha), and *Long Gu* (Draconis, Os) and/or *Bu Zhong Yi Qi Tang* (Supplement the Center & Boost the Qi Decoction): *Huang Qi* (Astragali Membranacei, Radix), 12g, *Ren Shen* (Panacis Ginseng, Radix), 9g, *Bai Zhu* (Atractylodis Macrocephalae, Rhizoma), 12g, mix-fried *Gan Cao* (Glycyrrhizae Uralensis, Radix), 3g, *Dang Gui* (Angelicae Sinensis, Radix), 9g, *Chen Pi* (Citri Reticulatae, Pericarpium), 6g, *Sheng Ma* (Cimicifugae, Rhizoma), 9g, *Chai Hu* (Bupleuri, Radix), 6g.

Dr. Li's empirical formula:

Huang Jing (Polygonati, Rhizoma), 9g
Shan Zhu Yu (Corni Officinalis, Fructus), 9g
Fu Ling (Poriae Cocos, Sclerotium), 15g
Niu Xi (Achyranthis Bidentatae, Radix), 9g
Tu Si Zi (Cuscutae Chinensis, Semen), 9g
Wu Wei Zi (Schizandrae Chinensis, Fructus), 6g
Bu Gu Zhi (Psoraleae Corylifoliae, Fructus), 9g
Yin Yang Huo (Epimedii, Herba), 9g
Du Zhong (Eucommiae Ulmoidis, Cortex), 9g
Zhi Mu (Anemarrhenae Asphodeloidis, Rhizoma), 9g
Huang Bai (Phellodendri, Cortex), 9g
Chuan Xiong (Ligustici Wallichii, Radix), 9g
Rou Gui (Cinnamomi Cassiae, Cortex), 4.5-6g
Jin Ying Zi (Rosae Laevigatae, Fructus), 9g
Lian Zi (Nelumbinis Nuciferae, Semen), 9g

MODIFICATIONS: If there are loose stools, add *Bai Zhu* (Atractylodis Macrocephalae, Rhizoma), *Rou Dou Kou* (Myristicae Fragrantis, Semen), *Shan Yao* (Dioscoreae Oppositae, Radix), *Sha Ren* (Amomi, Fructus), and *Huo Xiang* (Agastaches Seu Pogostemi, Herba). If there is blood in the urine with a pale color, add *Huang Qi* (Astragali Membranacei, Radix), *Ren Shen* (Panacis Ginseng, Radix), *Dang Gui* (Angelicae Sinensis, Radix), and *San Qi* (Notoginseng, Radix). If there is dizziness, add *Huang Qi* (Astragali Membranacei, Radix), *Ren Shen* (Panacis Ginseng, Radix), and *Tian Ma* (Gastrodiae, Elatae, Rhizoma).

ACUMOXIBUSTION: Choose points to needle from *Yin Ling Quan* (Sp 9), *Tai Xi* (Ki 3), *Zu San Li* (St 36), *San Yin Jiao* (Sp 6), *Yin Bai* (Sp 1), *Zhong Ji* (CV 3), and *Qi Hai* (CV 6). Moxa *Qi Zhong* (CV 8) and *Bai Hui* (GV 20).

STONE STRANGURY

1. DAMP HEAT (WITH DAMPNESS MORE THAN HEAT)

SIGNS & SYMPTOMS: Frequent, painful urination with a dark color, commonly, cramping pain in the kidney area that may shoot down the interior of the leg or to the lower abdomen, sudden blockage of the urine and small stones in the urine. The tongue has thick or thin, yellow fur, and the pulse is bowstring, slippery, and fast.

TREATMENT PRINCIPLES: Clear heat, percolate dampness, and discharge stones

REPRESENTATIVE FORMULA: *Shi Wei San* (Pyrrosia Decoction)

Shi Wei (Pyrrosiae, Folium), 9g
Dong Kui Zi (Abutili Seu Malvae, Semen), 9g
Qu Mai (Dianthi, Herba), 9g
Hua Shi (Talcum), 6g
Che Qian Zi (Plantaginis, Semen), 9g

Dr. Li's empirical formula:

Bai Shao (Paeoniae Lactiflorae, Radix Albus), 12g
Gan Cao (Glycyrrhizae Uralensis, Radix), 6g
Niu Xi (Achyranthis Bidentatae, Radix), 9g
Jin Qian Cao (Lysimachiae, Herba), 12g
Hai Jin Sha (Lygodii Japonici, Spora), 9g
Ji Nei Jin (Gigeriae Galli, Endothelium Corneum), 9g
Che Qian Zi (Plantaginis, Semen), 9g
Qu Mai (Dianthi, Herba), 9g

Chuan Xiong (Ligustici Wallichii, Radix), 9g
Hua Shi (Talcum), 6g
Huang Bai (Phellodendri, Cortex), 9g
Zhi Mu (Anemarrhenae Asphodeloidis, Rhizoma), 9g

MODIFICATIONS: If there is severe cramping, add *Chuan Lian Zi* (Meliae Toosendan, Fructus) and *Yan Hu Suo* (Corydalis Yanhusuo, Rhizoma). If there is nausea, add *Zhu Ru* (Bambusae In Taeniis, Caulis) and *Huo Xiang* (Agastaches Seu Pogostemi, Herba).

ACUMOXIBUSTION: Use electroacupuncture on *Shen Shu* (Bl 23) (negative), *Pang Guang Shu* (Bl 28) (positive) for upper urethra stones and *Shen Shu* (Bl 23) (negative) and *Shui Dao* (St 28) (positive) for lower urethra stones. Use dense-disperse waves for 30 minutes, one time per day. Ten to 15 days constitute one course. The patient should rest 5-7 days between courses. Also, choose from the following points: *Wei Yang* (Bl 53), *San Yin Jiao* (Sp 6), *Yin Ling Quan* (Sp 9), *Chi Ze* (Liv 5), *Yun Men* (Liv 2), *Wai Guan* (TB 5), and *Yang Ling Quan* (GB 34).

One can use the following combination treatment once every two weeks if the patient's kidney function is not damaged. For upper urethra stones, employ the following schedule:

At 6:00 A.M., drink 500ml of green tea.
At 7:00 A.M., repeat.
At 8:00 A.M., repeat.
At 9:00 A.M., give an entire one-day dose of the patient's Chinese formula.
At 10:30 A.M., give the electro-acupuncture treatment mentioned above.
At 10:40 A.M., give local heat therapy with a heat lamp or heating pad.
At 11:30 A.M., the patient must get up and jump or dance.

For the lower urethra stones smaller than one centimeter, have the patient drink as much water or green tea as possible along with the patient's Chinese formula. Advise the patient to hold his or her urine as long as possible.

CAUTION: If the stones are bigger than 1cm, they must be broken up by ultrasound or some other method before using this combination therapy.

2. DAMP HEAT (WITH HEAT MORE THAN DAMPNESS)

SIGNS & SYMPTOMS: Fever, thirst, constipation, cramping in the kidney area or cramping that shoots to the lower abdomen, lower abdominal distention and pain, frequent, urgent, burning and sometimes bloody urination. The tongue has yellow, slimy fur and the pulse is bowstring, fast, slippery, and big.

TREATMENT PRINCIPLES: Clear heat, percolate dampness, and discharge stones

REPRESENTATIVE FORMULAS: *Jin Qian Cao San* (Lysimachia Powder)

Jin Qian Cao (Lysimachiae, Herba), 30g
Shi Wei (Pyrrosiae, Folium), 15g
Che Qian Zi (Plantaginis, Semen), 15g
Mu Tong (Akebiae, Caulis), 6g
Qu Mai (Dianthi, Herba), 12g
Bian Xu (Polygoni Avicularis, Herba), 15g
Zhi Zi (Gardeniae Jasminoidis, Fructus), 12g
Da Huang (Rhei, Radix Et Rhizoma), 9g
Hua Shi (Talcum), 9g
Gan Cao (Glycyrrhizae Uralensis, Radix), 9g

Dr. Li's empirical formula:

Bai Shao (Paeoniae Lactiflorae, Radix Albus), 12g
Gan Cao (Glycyrrhizae Uralensis, Radix), 6g
Niu Xi (Achyranthis Bidentatae, Radix), 9g
Jin Qian Cao (Lysimachiae, Herba), 12g
Hai Jin Sha (Lygodii Japonici, Spora), 9g
Ji Nei Jin (Gigeriae Galli, Endothelium Corneum), 9g
Che Qian Zi (Plantaginis, Semen), 9g
Qu Mai (Dianthi, Herba), 9g
Chuan Xiong (Ligustici Wallichii, Radix), 10g
Hua Shi (Talcum), 6g
Huang Bai (Phellodendri, Cortex), 10g
Zhi Mu (Anemarrhenae Asphodeloidis, Rhizoma), 10g
Huang Bai (Phellodendri, Cortex), 9g
Qing Dai (Indigo Pulverata Levis), 5g
Ban Xia (Pinelliae Ternatae, Rhizoma), 5g
Huang Lian (Coptidis Chinensis, Rhizoma), 9g

ACUMOXIBUSTION: Use electroacupuncture same as

above. Also choose other points from *Wei Zhong* (Bl 40), *Shao Fu* (Ht 8), *Yun Men* (Liv 2), *Chi Ze* (Liv 5), *Qu Chi* (LI 11), and *Wai Guan* (TB 5).

3. QI STAGNATION

SIGNS & SYMPTOMS: Distention and occasional pain in the low back, slight lower abdominal pain, or cramping in the kidney area. In some cases, the low back and knees are weak. The tongue is pale with thick, white fur, and the pulse is bowstring.

TREATMENT PRINCIPLES: Move the qi and percolate dampness, disinhibit urination and discharge stones

REPRESENTATIVE FORMULAS: *Niao Shi Yi Hao Fang* (Urine Stone Formula #1)

Jin Qian Cao (Lysimachiae, Herba), 9-15g
Hai Jin Sha (Lygodii Japonici, Spora), 9g
Shi Wei (Pyrrosiae, Folium), 9g
Che Qian Zi (Plantaginis, Semen), 9g
Mu Tong (Akebiae, Caulis), 9g

MODIFICATIONS: If there is serious pain, add *Yuan Hu Suo* (Corydalis Yanhusuo, Rhizoma) and *Chuan Lian Zi* (Meliae Toosendan, Fructus). If there is blood stasis, add *Pu Huang* (Typhae, Pollen) and *Wu Ling Zhi* (Trogopteri Seu Pteromi, Excrementum). If there is blood in the urine, add *Da Ji* (Cirsii Japonici, Herba Seu Radix), *Xiao Ji* (Cephalanoplos, Herba), and *Bai Mao Gen* (Imperatae Cylindricae, Rhizoma). If there is kidney yang vacuity, add *Rou Gui* (Cinnamomi Cassiae, Cortex), *Fu Zi* (Aconiti Carmichaeli, Radix Lateralis Praeparatus), and *Bu Gu Zhi* (Psoraleae Corylifoliae, Fructus). If there is kidney yin vacuity, add *Shu Di Huang* (Rehmanniae Glutinosae, cooked Radix), *Gou Qi Zi* (Lycii Chinensis, Fructus), and *Nu Zhen Zi* (Ligustri Lucidi, Fructus).

Dr. Li's empirical formula:

Bai Shao (Paeoniae Lactiflorae, Radix Albus), 9-15g
Gan Cao (Glycyrrhizae Uralensis, Radix), 3-6g
Bai Zhu (Atractylodis Macrocephalae, Rhizoma), 9-12g
Hua Shi (Talcum), 3-6g

Niu Xi (Achyranthis Bidentatae, Radix), 6-9g
Zhi Mu (Anemarrhenae Asphodeloidis, Rhizoma), 9g
Xiang Fu (Cyperi Rotundi, Rhizoma), 9g
Chuan Xiong (Ligustici Wallichii, Radix), 9g
Mu Dan Pi (Moutan, Cortex Radicis), 9g
Fo Shou (Citri Sarcodactylis, Fructus), 9g

ACUMOXIBUSTION: Use electroacupuncture same as above. Also, choose from the following points: *Tai Chong* (Liv 3), *Chi Ze* (Liv 5), *He Gu* (LI 4), and *Zu San Li* (St 36).

4. QI VACUITY WITH INHIBITED KIDNEY & BLADDER QI TRANSFORMATION

SIGNS & SYMPTOMS: Sudden stoppage of urine, urethral pain, lower abdomen distention and pain, difficult and painful urination with sand in the urine. The tongue is pale purple and the pulse is weak and bowstring.

TREATMENT PRINCIPLES: Supplement the qi and promote the bladder's qi transformation to transform dampness, warm yang and discharge stones

REPRESENTATIVE FORMULAS: Augmented *Wu Ling San* (Five [Ingredients] Poria Powder) and *Bao Yuan Tang* (Protect the Origin Decoction)

Wu Ling San (Five [Ingredients] Poria Powder)

Zhu Ling (Polypori Umbellati, Sclerotium), 9g
Fu Ling (Poriae Cocos, Sclerotium), 9g
Bai Zhu (Atractylodis Macrocephalae, Rhizoma), 9g
Ze Xie (Alismatis Orientalis, Rhizoma), 9g
Gui Zhi (Cinnamomi Cassiae, Ramulus), 9g
Hai Jin Sha (Lygodii Japonici, Spora), 15g
Jin Qian Cao (Lysimachiae, Herba), 20g
Ji Nei Jin (Gigeriae Galli, Endothelium Corneum), 9g
Bai Shao (Paeoniae Lactiflorae, Radix Albus), 9g
Hua Shi (Talcum), 9g
Niu Xi (Achyranthis Bidentatae, Radix), 9g
Che Qian Zi (Plantaginis, Semen), 9g
Bian Xu (Polygoni Avicularis, Herba), 9g

Bao Yuan Tang (Protect the Origin Decoction)

Huang Qi (Astragali Membranacei, Radix), 9-15g

Dang Shen (Codonopsis Pilosulae, Radix), 9-15g
Zhi Gan Cao (Glycyrrhizae Uralensis, Radix), 3-6g
Rou Gui (Cinnamonmi Cassiae, Cortex), 3-6g
Jin Qian Cao (Lysimachiae, Herba), 9-15g
Ji Nei Jin (Gigeriae Galli, Endothelium Corneum), 9g
Hu Tao Ren (Juglandis Regiae, Semen), 9g

MODIFICATIONS: If there is low back pain, add *Sang Ji Sheng* (Sangjisheng, Ramulus), *Du Zhong* (Eucommiae Ulmoidis, Cortex), *Yin Yang Huo* (Epimedii, Herba), and *Sheng Ma* (Cimicifugae, Rhizoma).

Dr. Li's empirical formula:

Huang Qi (Astragali Membranacei, Radix), 9-15g
Dang Shen (Codonopsis Pilosulae, Radix), 9-15g
Fu Ling (Poriae Cocos, Sclerotium), 15g
Bai Shao (Paeoniae Lactiflorae, Radix Albus), 9-15g
Zhi Gan Cao (Glycyrrhizae Uralensis, Radix), 3g
Jin Qian Cao (Lysimachiae, Herba), 15g
Hai Jin Sha (Lygodii Japonici, Spora), 9g
Niu Xi (Achyranthis Bidentatae, Radix), 9g
Hua Shi (Talcum), 3g
Chuan Xiong (Ligustici Wallichii, Radix), 9g
Che Qian Zi (Plantaginis, Semen), 9g
Qu Mai (Dianthi, Herba), 9g

ACUMOXIBUSTION: Use electroacupuncture same as above. Also choose from the following points: *Zhong Ji* (CV 3), *Guan Yuan* (CV 4), *Qi Hai* (CV 6), and *Zu San Li* (St 36).

Case history from Dr. Wei Li's private practice: Mike, a 53 year-old male

Mike had ultrasound to break up his kidney stones, but after one week, the stones still had not passed and were causing pain in his kidneys and low back. Dr. Li prescribed her empirical formula plus *Huang Bai* (Phellodendri, Cortex) and *Zhi Mu* (Anemarrhenae Asphodeloidis, Rhizoma). The stones started to pass within two days and completely passed out in five days.

Case history from Dr. Wei Li's private practice: Robert, a 47 year-old male

Robert experienced sudden, intense abdominal

cramps and proceeded to a hospital emergency room. Doctors discovered a 0.8cm stone stuck in the second level of his ureter. Dr. Li prescribed her empirical formula and also advised Robert to move more by walking, dancing, and even jumping. After taking this prescription for three days, Robert passed the stone.

5. KIDNEY YIN VACUITY

SIGNS & SYMPTOMS: Frequent, difficult, burning, painful urination with blood and sand, lower abdominal distention and pain, vexation, thirst, insomnia, dizziness, tinnitus or hearing loss, low back and knee soreness and weakness, blurred vision and dry eyes, dry mouth and thirst with desire to drink, heat in the five hearts, night sweats. The tongue is red with less than normal fur, and the pulse is thin and fast.

TREATMENT PRINCIPLES: Nourish yin, transform dampness, and discharge stones

REPRESENTATIVE FORMULAS: *Liu Wei Di Huang Wan* (Six Flavors Rehmannia Pills) plus *Zhu Ling Tang* (Polyporus Decoction)

Shu Di Huang (Rehmanniae Glutinosae, cooked Radix), 12g
Shan Zhu Yu (Corni Officinalis, Fructus), 12g
Shan Yao (Radix Dioscoreae Oppositae), 12g
Fu Ling (Poriae Cocos, Sclerotium), 12g
Ze Xie (Alismatis Orientalis, Rhizoma), 9g
Mu Dan Pi (Moutan, Cortex Radicis), 12g
Zhu Ling (Polypori Umbellati, Sclerotium), 9g
Hua Shi (Talcum), 12g
E Jiao (Corii Asini, Gelatinum), 9g
Ji Nei Jin (Gigeriae Galli, Endothelium Corneum), 9g
Che Qian Zi (Plantaginis, Semen), 12g
Hai Jin Sha (Lygodii Japonici, Spora), 12g
Bai Shao (Paeoniae Lactiflorae, Radix Albus), 12g
Niu Xi (Achyranthis Bidentatae, Radix), 9g

MODIFICATIONS: If there is dizziness and insomnia, add *Bai Zi Ren* (Biotae Orientalis, Semen) and *Ye Jiao Teng* (Polygoni Multiflori, Caulis). If there are night sweats, add *Wu Wei Zi* (Schizandrae Chinensis, Fructus) and *Huang Bai* (Phellodendri, Cortex).

Dr. Li's empirical formula:

Shan Zhu Yu (Corni Officinalis, Fructus), 9g
Shan Yao (Radix Dioscoreae Oppositae), 9g
Dan Shen (Salviae Miltiorrhizae, Radix), 9g
Mu Dan Pi (Moutan, Cortex Radicis), 9g
Niu Xi (Achyranthis Bidentatae, Radix), 6g
Tu Si Zi (Cuscutae Chinensis, Semen), 6g
Hai Jin Sha (Lygodii Japonici, Spora), 9g
Huang Bai (Phellodendri, Cortex), 15g
Zhi Mu (Anemarrhenae Asphodeloidis, Rhizoma), 15g
Di Gu Pi (Lycii Chinensis, Cortex Radicis), 9g
Hua Shi (Talcum), 3g
Ji Nei Jin (Gigeriae Galli, Endothelium Corneum), 9g
Shu Di Huang (Rehmanniae Glutinosae, cooked Radix), 9-15g

ACUMOXIBUSTION: Use electroacupuncture same as above. Also choose other points from *Zhao Hai* (Ki 6), *San Yin Jiao* (Sp 6), *Hou Xi* (SI 3), *Yin Xi* (Ht 6), and *Fu Liu* (Ki 7).

6. KIDNEY QI VACUITY

SIGNS & SYMPTOMS: Urinary difficulty and pain, pale yellow urine, low backache, weak knees. The pulse is deep and weak.

TREATMENT PRINCIPLES: Supplement the kidney qi and discharge stones

REPRESENTATIVE FORMULA: Modified *Jin Gui Shen Qi Wan* (*Golden Cabinet* Kidney Qi Pills)

Fu Zi (Aconiti Carmichaeli, Radix Lateralis Praeparatus), 9g
Rou Gui (Cinnamonmi Cassiae, Cortex), 5g
Shu Di Huang (Rehmanniae Glutinosae, cooked Radix), 12g
Shan Yao (Radix Dioscoreae Oppositae), 12g
Shan Zhu Yu (Corni Officinalis, Fructus), 12g
Ze Xie (Alismatis Orientalis, Rhizoma), 9g
Fu Ling (Poriae Cocos, Sclerotium), 12g
Mu Dan Pi (Moutan, Cortex Radicis), 9g
Hai Jin Sha (Lygodii Japonici, Spora), 9g
Ji Nei Jin (Gigeriae Galli, Endothelium Corneum), 9g
Jin Qian Cao (Lysimachiae, Herba), 9g
Bai Shao (Paeoniae Lactiflorae, Radix Albus), 12g

Hua Shi (Talcum), 9g

ACUMOXIBUSTION: Use electroacupuncture same as above. Choose other points from *Tai Xi* (Ki 3), *Zhong Ji* (CV 3), *Guan Yuan* (CV 4), *Qi Hai* (CV 6), and *Zu San Li* (St 36).

QI STRANGURY

1. LIVER DEPRESSION QI STAGNATION

SIGNS & SYMPTOMS: Lower abdominal distention and pain that is worse with pressure, painful, burning urination with an incomplete feeling and dribbling. The tongue has white fur, and the pulse is deep and bowstring. If depression transforms heat, then there will be burning urinary pain, a red tongue with possible dry fur, and a bowstring, rapid pulse.

TREATMENT PRINCIPLES: Course the liver and rectify the qi, percolate dampness and free the flow of strangury

REPRESENTATIVE FORMULAS: *Chen Xiang San* (Aquilaria Powder)

Chen Xiang (Aquilariae Agallochae, Lignum), 5g
Shi Wei (Pyrrosiae, Folium), 9g
Hua Shi (Talcum), 9g
Dang Gui (Angelicae Sinensis, Radix), 9g
Chen Pi (Citri Reticulatae, Pericarpium), 9g
Bai Shao (Paeoniae Lactiflorae, Radix Albus), 12g
Dong Kui Zi (Abutili Seu Malvae, Semen), 9g
Wang Bu Liu Xing (Vaccariae Segetalis, Semen), 9g
Gan Cao (Glycyrrhizae Uralensis, Radix), 6g
Mu Xiang (Aucklandiae Lappae, Radix), 9g
Qing Pi (Citri Reticulatae Viride, Pericarpium), 9g
Wu Yao (Linderae Strychnifoliae, Radix), 9g

MODIFICATIONS: If there is blood stasis, add *Hong Hua* (Carthami Tinctorii, Flos), *Chi Shao* (Paeoniae Lactiflorae, Radix Rubrus), and *Niu Xi* (Achyranthis Bidentatae, Radix). If there is burning urination, add *Hu Po* (Succinum).

Dr. Li's empirical formula:

Xiang Fu (Cyperi Rotundi, Rhizoma), 9g

Qing Pi (Citri Reticulatae Viride, Pericarpium), 9g
Chai Hu (Bupleuri, Radix), 3g
Bai Shao (Paeoniae Lactiflorae, Radix Albus), 9g
Huang Qin (Scutellariae Baicalensis, Radix), 9g
Mu Dan Pi (Moutan, Cortex Radicis), 9g
Zhi Zi (Gardeniae Jasminoidis, Fructus), 9g
Long Dan Cao (Gentiannae Longdancao, Radix), 9g
Che Qian Zi (Plantaginis, Semen), 9g
Sheng Di Huang (Rehmanniae Glutinosae, uncooked Radix), 3g
Chuan Xiong (Ligustici Wallichii, Radix), 9g

ACUMOXIBUSTION: Choose from *He Gu* (LI 4), *Tai Chong* (Liv 3), *Chi Ze* (Liv 5), *Nei Guan* (Per 6), *Gan Shu* (Bl 18), *San Jiao Shu* (Bl 22), *Pang Guang Shu* (Bl 28), *Shi Men* (CV 5), and *Qi Chong* (St 30).

2. CENTRAL QI FALLING DOWNWARD

SIGNS & SYMPTOMS: Lower abdominal distention with a feeling of heaviness and prolapse, urinary frequency and slight pain that is worse after urination and upon exertion, fatigue, reluctance to talk, dizziness. The tongue is pale with thin, white fur, and the pulse is slow and forceless.

NOTE: Water requires qi to move it. If there is qi vacuity, water and damp accumulate easily. Dampness is a "hot house." It can easily cause stagnation which engenders and envelops heat. One must be careful to treat any heat that is present or prevent its formation.

TREATMENT PRINCIPLES: Supplement the qi and lift the fallen

REPRESENTATIVE FORMULAS: *Bu Zhong Yi Qi Tang* (Supplement the Center & Boost the Qi Decoction)

Huang Qi (Astragali Membranacei, Radix), 12g
Ren Shen (Panacis Ginseng, Radix), 9g
Bai Zhu (Atractylodis Macrocephalae, Rhizoma), 12g
mix-fried *Gan Cao* (Glycyrrhizae Uralensis, Radix), 3g
Dang Gui (Angelicae Sinensis, Radix), 9g
Chen Pi (Citri Reticulatae, Pericarpium), 6g
Sheng Ma (Cimicifugae, Rhizoma), 9g
Chai Hu (Bupleuri, Radix), 6g

MODIFICATION: If there is frequent urination, add *Yi Zhi Ren* (Alpiniae Oxyphyllae, Fructus) and *Shan Zhu Yu* (Corni Officinalis, Fructus).

Dr. Li's empirical formula:

Ren Shen (Panacis Ginseng, Radix), 9g
Bai Zhu (Atractylodis Macrocephalae, Rhizoma), 9g
Chen Pi (Citri Reticulatae, Pericarpium), 9g
Fu Ling (Poriae Cocos, Sclerotium), 9g
Gui Zhi (Cinnamomi Cassiae, Ramulus), 6g
Zhu Ling (Polypori Umbellati, Sclerotium), 9g
Huang Bai (Phellodendri, Cortex), 12g
Huang Lian (Coptidis Chinensis, Rhizoma), 9g
Dan Zhu Ye (Lophatheri Gracilis, Herba), 9g
Shan Yao (Radix Dioscoreae Oppositae), 9g
Shan Zhu Yu (Corni Officinalis, Fructus), 9g

ACUMOXIBUSTION: Moxa *Zhong Ji* (CV 3) and *Bai Hui* (GV 20). Needle *Zu San Li* (St 36), *San Yin Jiao* (Sp 6), *Yin Ling Quan* (Sp 9), *Qi Hai* (CV 6), *Tai Chong* (Liv 3), *Tai Xi* (Ki 3), *Bai Hui* (GV 20), and *He Gu* (LI 4).

TAXATION STRANGURY

1. SPLEEN VACUITY

SIGNS & SYMPTOMS: No appetite, loose stool, fatigue, dizziness, short, or copious and difficult urination, urination difficulty upon exertion. The tongue is pale with thin, white fur, and the pulse is slow and forceless.

TREATMENT PRINCIPLES: Fortify the spleen and boost the qi, upbear yang and lift the fallen

REPRESENTATIVE FORMULAS: Augmented *Bu Zhong Yi Qi Tang* (Supplement the Center & Boost the Qi Decoction)

Huang Qi (Astragali Membranacei, Radix), 12g
Ren Shen (Panacis Ginseng, Radix), 9g
Bai Zhu (Atractylodis Macrocephalae, Rhizoma), 12g
Zhi Gan Cao (Glycyrrhizae Uralensis, Radix), 3g
Dang Gui (Angelicae Sinensis, Radix), 9g
Chen Pi (Citri Reticulatae, Pericarpium), 6g

Sheng Ma (Cimicifugae, Rhizoma), 9g
Chai Hu (Bupleuri, Radix), 6g
Yi Zhi Ren (Alpiniae Oxyphyllae, Fructus), 9g
Shan Zhu Yu (Corni Officinalis, Fructus), 12g

MODIFICATIONS: If there is no appetite, add *Sha Ren* (Amomi, Fructus) and *Mu Xiang* (Aucklandiae Lappae, Radix). If there is copious urination, add *Bu Gu Zhi* (Psoraleae Corylifoliae, Fructus) and *Wu Yao* (Linderae Strychnifoliae, Radix). If there are cold extremities, add *Fu Zi* (Aconiti Carmichaeli, Radix Lateralis Praeparatus) and *Rou Gui* (Cinnamonmi Cassiae, Cortex).

Dr. Li's empirical formula:

Ren Shen (Panacis Ginseng, Radix), 9g
Bai Zhu (Atractylodis Macrocephalae, Rhizoma), 9g
Chen Pi (Citri Reticulatae, Pericarpium), 9g
Fu Ling (Poriae Cocos, Sclerotium), 9g
Gui Zhi (Cinnamomi Cassiae, Ramulus), 6g
Zhu Ling (Polypori Umbellati, Sclerotium), 9g
Huang Bai (Phellodendri, Cortex), 12g
Huang Lian (Coptidis Chinensis, Rhizoma), 9g
Dan Zhu Ye (Lophatheri Gracilis, Herba), 9g
Shan Yao (Radix Dioscoreae Oppositae), 9g
Shan Zhu Yu (Corni Officinalis, Fructus), 9g

ACUMOXIBUSTION: Choose from *Guan Yuan* (CV 4), *Qi Hai* (CV 6), *Zu San Li* (St 36), *He Gu* (LI 4), *San Yin Jiao* (Sp 6), *Ci Liao* (Bl 32), *Bai Hui* (GV 20), *Lie Que* (Lu 7), and *Zhao Hai* (Ki 6).

Case history of Dr. Zhi Xiang-gong: Kan, a 36 year-old female[2]

Five years prior to Kan's first visit in July 1965, she was diagnosed with chronic pyelonephritis. A urine culture showed over 1million/ml bacteria. She had frequent, urgent, scanty, painful, and burning urination as well as fatigue, low back pain and weak legs. Her tongue had thin, white fur, and her pulse was bowstring, fast, thin, and forceless. Based on these symptoms, Dr. Zhi's pattern identification was qi and yin vacuity with damp heat in the lower burner. He prescribed modified *Qing Xin Lian Zi Yin* (Clear the Heart Lotus Seed Beverage): *Lian Zi* (Nelumbinis Nuciferae,

Semen), 15g, *Mai Men Dong* (Ophiopogonis Japonici, Tuber), 15g, *Huang Qi* (Astragali Membranacei, Radix), 30g, *Dang Shen* (Codonopsitis Pilosulae, Radix), 20g, *Huang Qin* (Scutellariae Baicalensis, Radix), 10g, *Chai Hu* (Bupleuri, Radix), 15g, *Di Gu Pi* (Lycii Chinensis, Cortex Radicis), 30g, *Fu Ling* (Poriae Cocos, Sclerotium), 12g, *Hua Shi* (Talcum), 20g, *Gan Cao* (Glycyrrhizae Uralensis, Radix), 6g, *Yin Hua Teng* (Lonicerae Japonicae, Caulis Et Folium), 30g, and *Che Qian Zi* (Plantaginis, Semen), 30g.

Kan took this prescription for 10 days and all her symptoms disappeared, but her urine culture was still positive. She took it another 15 days and her urine culture came back negative. Dr. Zhi then advised Kan to take *Bu Zhong Yi Qi Wan* (Supplement the Center & Boost the Qi Pills), 6g, in the morning and *Zhi Bai Di Huang Wan* (Anemarrhena & Phellodendron Rehmannia Pills), 6g, in the evening to consolidate the treatment. Kan took these pills for three months. A follow-up two years later found no recurrence.

2. KIDNEY YANG VACUITY

SIGNS & SYMPTOMS: Dizziness, tinnitus, low back and knee soreness and weakness, frequent, copious urination, impotence, seminal emission, frequent urination at night with dribbling after sexual intercourse. The tongue is pale with white fur, and the pulse is thin and forceless.

TREATMENT PRINCIPLES: Supplement the kidney and warm yang

REPRESENTATIVE FORMULA: *Shen Qi Wan* (Kidney Qi Pills)

Fu Zi (Aconiti Carmichaeli, Radix Lateralis Praeparatus), 3g
Rou Gui (Cinnamonmi Casiae, Cortex), 3g
Shu Di Huang (Rehmanniae Glutinosae, cooked Radix), 24g
Shan Yao (Radix Dioscoreae Oppositae), 12g
Shan Zhu Yu (Corni Officinalis, Fructus), 12g
Ze Xie (Alismatis Orientalis, Rhizoma), 9g
Fu Ling (Poriae Cocos, Sclerotium), 9g
Mu Dan Pi (Moutan, Cortex Radicis), 9g

MODIFICATIONS: If the qi vacuity is more severe, add *Huang Qi* (Astragali Membranacei, Radix) and *Dang Shen* (Codonopsitis Pilosulae, Radix). If the yang vacuity is more severe, add *Lu Jiao Jiao* (Cornu Cervi, Gelatinum) and *Yin Yang Huo* (Epimedii, Herba).

ACUMOXIBUSTION: Choose points to moxa from *Shen Shu* (Bl 23), *Ming Men* (GV 4), *Tai Xi* (Ki 3), *Guan Yuan* (CV 4), and *Qi Hai* (CV 6). Needle *Pang Guang Shu* (Bl 28) and *Zhong Ji* (CV 3).

Case history of Dr. Chang Qi: Gao, a 37 year-old female[3]

Gao's first visit was on Dec. 23, 1987. She suffered occasional recurrent strangury for over 10 years. Over the previous year, these recurrences became more frequent. Four months earlier, she had over-exerted herself and caught cold. At the time, she also had urgent, frequent, painful urination, low back pain, and lower abdominal pain. She took some antibiotics and these helped her recover. Then, just two weeks prior to the first visit, the symptoms returned. This time the antibiotics failed. At her first visit, Gao presented with lower back soreness, lower abdominal pain and distention, and frequent, urgent, painful urination. Her lower extremities were swollen. She was fatigued and always felt cold. Her tongue had white, glossy fur, and her pulse was deep and weak. Urinalysis showed protein 1+ and WBCs 0-2. A urine culture showed bacteria above 10,000/ml. The Western medical diagnosis was chronic pyelonephritis. Dr. Chang identified this disease as taxation strangury. The pattern identification was kidney yang vacuity and bladder damp heat.

Dr. Chang analyzed Gao's case as follows. Chronic damp heat had damaged kidney yin. Therefore, kidney yin failed to nourish kidney yang, and gradually kidney yang also became vacuous. The overuse of antibiotics exacerbated this kidney yang vacuity. (Antibiotics are bitter and very cold and tax yang.) Kidney yang vacuity resulted in failure of kidney and bladder qi transformation with symptoms of urinary frequency, lower abdominal pain, and water swelling. The painful, urgent urination indicated that the bladder damp heat was not completely eliminated. Dr. Chang's treatment strategy was to warm and invigorate kidney yang and clear damp heat. His formula consisted of: *Shu Di Huang* (Rehmanniae Glutinosae, cooked Radix), 20g, *Shan Zhu Yu* (Corni Officinalis, Fructus), 15g, *Rou Gui* (Cinnanmonmi Casiae, Cortex), 10g, *Fu Zi* (Aconiti Carmichaeli, Radix Lateralis Praeparatus), 10g, *Xiao Hui Xiang* (Foeniculi Vulgaris, Fructus), 10g, *Bu Gu Zhi* (Psoraleae Corylifoliae, Fructus), 10g, *Ze Xie* (Alismatis Orientalis, Rhizoma), 15g, *Huang Bai* (Phellodendri, Cortex), 15g, *Qu Mai* (Dianthi, Herba), 20g, *Bian Xu* (Polygoni Avicularis, Herba), 10g, *Pu Gong Yin* (Taraxaci Mongolici Cum Radice, Herba), 30g, *Bai Hua She She Cao* (Hedyotidis Diffusae, Herba), 30g, *Gan Cao* (Glycyrrhizae Uralensis, Radix), 10g.

Gao took this formula for 10 days and her urinary frequency, urgency, and pain disappeared. She still had lower back pain, lower abdominal pain, and edema in her lower extremities. Dr. Chang took out *Huang Bai* and *Bai Hua She She Cao* and added *Wu Yao* (Linderae Strychnifoliae, Radix), 15g, and *Du Zhong* (Eucommiae Ulmoidis, Cortex), 15g. Gao took this modified formula for 12 days, and her lower back and abdominal pain were lessened. The edema almost completely dissipated. Her tongue had thin, white fur, and her pulse was deep and slippery. By Jan. 22, all her symptoms had disappeared. Her urinalysis and urine culture were negative. Gao continued on this modified formula for 20 more days. A follow-up a half year later found no recurrence.

3. KIDNEY YIN VACUITY

SIGNS & SYMPTOMS: Dizziness, tinnitus, low back and knee soreness and weakness, frequent, copious urination, impotence, seminal emission, frequent urination at night with dribbling after sexual intercourse, a red facial complexion or malar flushing, vexation, heat in the five hearts, and a dry mouth. The tongue is red, and the pulse is fast and thin.

REPRESENTATIVE FORMULAS: Augmented *Liu Wei Di Huang Wan* (Six Flavors Rehmannia Pills)

Shu Di Huang (Rehmanniae Glutinosae, cooked Radix), 10-15g
Shan Zhu Yu (Corni Officinalis, Fructus), 12g

Shan Yao (Radix Dioscoreae Oppositae), 12g
Ze Xie (Alismatis Orientalis, Rhizoma), 9g
Fu Ling (Poriae Cocos, Sclerotium), 12g
Mu Dan Pi (Moutan, Cortex Radicis), 9g
Di Gu Pi (Lycii Chinensis, Cortex Radicis), 9g
Sang Piao Xiao (Mantidis, Ootheca), 9g
Fu Pen Zi (Rubi Chingii, Fructus), 9g

Dr. Li's empirical formula:

Shu Di Huang (Rehmanniae Glutinosae, cooked Radix), 9g
Shan Zhu Yu (Corni Officinalis, Fructus), 9g
Shan Yao (Radix Dioscoreae Oppositae), 9g
Yin Yang Huo (Epimedii, Herba), 9g
Bu Gu Zhi (Psoraleae Corylifoliae, Fructus), 9g
Sang Ji Sheng (Sangjisheng, Ramulus), 9g
Du Zhong (Eucommiae Ulmoidis, Cortex), 9g
Gou Qi Zi (Lycii Chinensis, Fructus), 9g
Huang Bai (Phellodendri, Cortex), 9g
Zhi Mu (Anemarrhenae Asphodeloidis, Rhizoma), 9g
Chuan Xiong (Ligustici Wallichii, Radix), 9g
Lian Zi (Nelumbinis Nuciferae, Semen), 12g

ACUMOXIBUSTION: Choose from *Shen Shu* (Bl 23), *Pang Guang Shu* (Bl 28), *Tai Xi* (Ki 3), *Zhao Hai* (Ki 6), *Tai Chong* (Liv 3), *Nei Guan* (Per 6), *Yin Xi* (Ht 6), *Zhong Ji* (CV 3), and *Guan Yuan* (CV 4).

UNCTUOUS STRANGURY

1. DAMP HEAT IN THE LOWER BURNER

SIGNS & SYMPTOMS: Urine like rice-washing water, painful, burning urination, a sticky, dry mouth. The tongue is red with yellow fur, and the pulse is bowstring and fast.

TREATMENT PRINCIPLES: Clear and eliminate dampness and heat, promote the separation of clear from turbid

REPRESENTATIVE FORMULAS: *Bei Xie Fen Qing Yin* (Dioscorea Hypolaguca Separate the Clear Beverage)

Bei Xie (Dioscoreae Hypolagucae, Rhizoma), 12g
Yi Zhi Ren (Alpiniae Oxyphyllae, Fructus), 9g

Wu Yao (Linderae Strychnifoliae, Radix), 9g
Shi Chang Pu (Acori Graminei, Rhizoma), 9g

MODIFICATIONS: If there is urination with burning pain, remove *Yi Zhi Ren* and add *Shi Wei* (Pyrrosiae, Folium), *Huang Bai* (Phellodendri, Cortex), *Che Qian Zi* (Plantaginis, Semen), and *Chuan Niu Xi* (Cyathulae, Radix). If there is a sticky mouth without thirst, add *Cang Zhu* (Atractylodis, Rhizoma), *Hou Po* (Magnoliae Officinalis, Cortex), and *Huang Bai* (Phellodendri, Cortex).

Dr. Li's empirical formula:

Bi Xie (Dioscoreae Hypoglaucae, Rhizoma), 9g
Yi Zhi Ren (Alpiniae Oxyphyllae, Fructus), 9g
Shi Wei (Pyrrosiae, Folium), 9g
Huang Bai (Phellodendri, Cortex), 9g
Zhi Mu (Anemarrhenae Asphodeloidis, Rhizoma), 9g
Shan Zhu Yu (Corni Officinalis, Fructus), 9g
Sheng Di Huang (Rehmanniae Glutinosae, uncooked Radix), 9g
Mu Dan Pi (Moutan, Cortex Radicis), 9g
Cang Zhu (Atractylodis, Rhizoma), 6g

ACUMOXIBUSTION: Choose from *San Jiao Shu* (Bl 22), *Pang Guang Shu* (Bl 28), *Zhong Ji* (CV 3), *Yin Ling Quan* (Sp 9), *San Yin Jiao* (Sp 6), *Shui Dao* (St 28), *Yang Ling Quan* (GB 34), *Feng Long* (St 40), and *Fu Liu* (Ki 7).

2. KIDNEY QI VACUITY

SIGNS & SYMPTOMS: Urine like rice-washing water, constitutional weakness, dizziness, fatigue, low back and knee soreness and weakness, impotence, seminal emission. No pain upon urination, but when protein, fat, and carbohydrates are eaten, the urine becomes more turbid. The tongue is pale with less than normal fur, and the pulse is weak.

TREATMENT PRINCIPLES: Supplement and secure the kidney

REPRESENTATIVE FORMULAS: Modified *Tu Si Zi Wan* (Cuscuta Pills)

Tu Si Zi (Cuscutae Chinensis, Semen), 9g

Lu Rong (Cervi, Cornu Parvum), 6g
Rou Cong Rong (Cistanchis Deserticolae, Herba), 9g
Shan Yao (Dioscoreae Oppositae, Radix), 12g
Fu Zi (Aconiti Carmichaeli, Radix Lateralis Praeparatus), 3g
Wu Yao (Linderae Strychnifoliae, Radix), 9g
Wu Wei Zi (Schizandrae Chinensis, Fructus), 12g
Yi Zhi Ren (Alpiniae Oxyphyllae, Fructus), 9g
calcined *Mu Li* (Ostreae, Concha), 9g
Ji Nei Jin (Gigeriae Galli, Endoethelium Corneum), 9g

MODIFICATIONS: If there is low back and knee soreness and limpness, add *Shu Di Huang* (Rehmanniae Glutinosae, cooked Radix), *Chuan Niu Xi* (Cyathulae, Radix), Ramulus Sangjisheng (*Sang Ji Sheng*), and *Yin Yang Huo* (Epimedii, Herba). If there is dizziness and shortness of breath, add *Huang Qi* (Astragali Membranacei, Radix) and *Dang Shen* (Codonopsitis Pilosulae, Radix). If the urination is frequent and profuse, add *Shan Zhu Yu* (Corni Officinalis, Fructus) and *Bu Gu Zhi* (Psoraleae Corylifoliae, Fructus).

Dr. Li's empirical formula:

Tu Si Zi (Cuscutae Chinensis, Semen), 9g
Shan Yao (Dioscoreae Oppositae, Radix), 9g
Lian Zi (Nelumbinis Nuciferae, Semen), 9g
Fu Ling (Poriae Cocos, Sclerotium), 9g
Gou Qi Zi (Lycii Chinensis, Fructus), 9g
Huang Jing (Polygonati, Rhizoma), 9g
He Shou Wu (Polygoni Multiflori, Radix), 6g
Dang Gui (Angelicae Sinensis, Radix), 6g
Huai Niu Xi (Achyranthis Bidentatae, Radix), 9g
Sang Ji Sheng (Sangjisheng, Ramulus), 9g
Yin Yang Huo (Epimedii, Herba), 9g
Huang Bai (Phellodendri, Cortex), 9g
Zhi Mu (Anemarrhenae Asphodeloidis, Rhizoma), 9g
Shan Zhu Yu (Corni Officinalis, Fructus), 9g

ACUMOXIBUSTION: Choose from *Pang Guang Shu* (Bl 28), *Zhong Ji* (CV 3), *Guan Yuan* (CV 4), *Yin Ling Quan* (Sp 9), *Tai Xi* (Ki 3), *Qi Hai* (CV 6), *Bai Hui* (GV 20), *Si Feng* (M-UE-9), and *Feng Long* (St 40).

Case history of Dr. Zhi Xiang-gong: Dai, a 36 year-old female[4]

Dai was diagnosed with chronic pyelonephritis 10 years previous to visiting Dr. Zhi. She caught cold easily. She had frequent pyelonephritis recurrences with symptoms of copious, frequent, but incomplete urine, edema in the lower extremities, a cold feeling in the lower half of her body, low back pain, dizziness and tinnitus, dry throat, and no thirst. Her urine was turbid with a white hue. Collected urine had much oil and many bubbles floating on the surface. At Dai's first visit, her face was pale, and she had a pale tongue with white, slimy fur. Her pulse was thin and slow, with the cubit position especially deep and weak. The Western medical diagnosis was chronic pyelonephritis with lowered kidney function. Dr. Zhi's pattern identification was kidney yin and yang vacuity. His treatment strategy was to warm and boost kidney yang, nourish kidney yin, supplement the qi, and quicken the blood. He used a version of *Shen Qi Wan* (Kidney Qi Pills) with modifications: *Shu Di Huang* (Rehmanniae Glutinosae, cooked Radix), 15g, *Mu Dan Pi* (Moutan, Cortex Radicis), 10g, *Shan Zhu Yu* (Corni Officinalis, Fructus), 15g, *Shan Yao* (Radix Dioscoreae Oppositae), 30g, *Fu Ling* (Poriae Cocos, Sclerotium), 15g, *Gou Qi Zi* (Lycii Chinensis, Fructus), 15g, *Rou Gui* (Cinnamonmi Cassiae, Cortex), 6g, *Fu Zi* (Aconiti Carmichaeli, Radix Lateralis Praeparatus), 18g (cooked two hours longer), *Huang Qi* (Astragali Membranacei, Radix), 30g, *Dang Gui* (Angelicae Sinensis, Radix), 10g, and *He Shou Wu* (Polygoni Multiflori, Radix), 30g. Dr. Zhi would add *Sha Ren* (Amomi, Fructus), 6g, whenever Dai's appetite was not good and *Suan Sao Ren* (Zizyphi Spinosae, Semen), 15g, when she had insomnia. Dai took this formula for three months. Even though all her symptoms were better, she sometimes had recurrences. Dr. Zhi felt his treatment was less than excellent. Dai decided to stop taking the formula and died two years later.

CLINICAL TIPS

1. Patients with acute strangury usually present a pattern of repletion marked by symptoms of fever, night sweats, low back pain, burning urine, etc., and pathologically large amounts of WBCs or RBCs in their urine. Some patients may even have pus in their urine. Indeed, this may be the only symptom. Patients with chronic strangury may present with patterns of repletion but often have underlying vacuity patterns marked by symptoms of low back pain, weak knees, ear ringing, fatigue, etc. In most cases the acute stage is more replete while the chronic stage is more vacuous. When treating acute strangury, one should 1) flush out the kidney/bladder by having the patient drink more water and by prescribing water-disinhibiting, dampness-percolating medicinals, and 2) clear heat (including damp heat and toxins) by prescribing heat-clearing, toxin-resolving medicinals. One should control the symptoms in three days but continue the treatment for 1-2 weeks.

When treating chronic strangury, one should 1) boost the right qi by prescribing the appropriate supplements, 2) clear heat and resolve toxins, 3) flush out the kidney-bladder,[5] and 4) rectify qi and blood. One may need to treat chronic strangury for 3-6 months. (Please see Chart 1.2.) Thus for chronic strangury one must employ a treatment strategy that combines supplementing as well as clearing and draining. For example, in chronic strangury cases one often finds that damp heat has burnt the yin resulting in yin vacuity. Yin vacuity causes dryness and irritation and exacerbates heat. Since yin is part of the right qi, yin vacuity also weakens the right qi. A weakened right qi is less able to oppose evils, thus making recurrences more likely. To put this in Western medical terms, chronic urinary tract infections can easily recur because the patient's resistance, immunity, or strength is low. Using antibiotics is equivalent to attacking the evil without supporting the correct; this will not strengthen the patient. When using Chinese medicinals one can clear damp heat while supplementing yin. This is equivalent to fighting the infection and boosting the immunity at the same time.

2. The overuse of antibiotics for recurrent UTIs may cause bacteria to become resistant to them. However, Chinese medicinals may succeed even when antibiotics become ineffective. Chinese medicinals have complex constituents, and bacteria do not become resistant to them as readily. For instance, the *Zhong Yao Da Zi Dian* (*The Great Dictionary of Chinese Medicinals*) reports that repeated use of *Huang Lian* (Rhizoma Coptidis Chinensis) and green tea did not result in bacterial resistance.[6] Many Chinese medicinals have secondary functions that are also important. For instance, *Mu Dan Pi* (Moutan, Cortex Radicis) clears heat but also quickens the blood and dispels stasis. There are also Chinese medicinals that treat both the root and tip at one and the same time. For instance, *Zhi Mu* (Anemarrhenae Asphodeloidis, Rhizoma) and *Sheng Di* (Rehmanniae Glutinosae, uncooked Radix) clear heat as well as nourish yin fluids.

3. A long-term urinary tract infection scars the renal pelvis. (This can often be seen in an x-ray.) Bacteria may populate the area around the scar tissue where it is difficult for antibiotics to penetrate. Once the antibiotics are withdrawn, the remaining bacteria may become active leading to a recurrence. Scarring is equivalent to qi stagnation and blood stasis, and, in this case, one may need to rectify the qi, quicken blood, and dispel stasis as well as clear and eliminate dampness and heat and supplement any underlying vacuity.

Type of Strangury	Treatment Strategy	Medicinal Categories
Acute strangury (Usually replete) Control symptoms in three days; continue to treat for 1-2 weeks	**1.** Disinhibit water & percolate dampness	Water-disinhibiting dampness-percolating
	2. Clear heat & resolve toxins	Heat-clearing, fire-draining Heat-clearing, dampness-eliminating Heat-clearing, blood-cooling Heat-clearing, toxin-resolving
Chronic strangury (Usually vacuity) Treat from 3-6 months	**1.** Boost the right qi	Qi-supplementing Blood-supplementing Yin-supplementing Yang-supplementing
	2. Clear heat & resolve toxins	Heat-clearing, fire-draining Heat-clearing, dampness-eliminating Heat-clearing, blood-cooling Heat-clearing, toxin-resolving Vacuity heat-clearing
	3. Disinhibit water & percolate dampness	Water-disinhibiting, dampness-percolating
	4. Rectify the qi & blood	Qi-rectifying, stasis-dispelling, blood-quickening

Chart 1.2. Common treatment strategies for acute & chronic strangury

Endnotes

[1] *Chang Qi Ling Chuan Jing Yan Ji Yao* (*The Clinical Experience of Chang Qi*), China Medical Science Publishing Company, Beijing, 1998, p. 87
[2] Yu Guan-shi & Shui Jian-shen, *Dong Dai Ming Yi Ling Zheng Jing Hua* (*Collection of Clinical Case Histories of Modern Famous Doctors*), Ancient Chinese Medicine Book Publishing Company, Beijing, 1998, p. 386
[3] Chang Qi, *op. cit.*, p. 88
[4] Yu Guan-shi and Shui Jian-shen, *op. cit.*, p. 389
[5] Patients with chronic strangury often have patterns of blood stasis. (This includes scarring of the renal pelvis.) In these cases, flushing out the kidney/bladder may be ineffective, and the prolonged use of water-disinhibiting dampness-percolating medicinals may damage yin.
[6] *Zhong Yao Da Zi Dian* (*The Great Dictionary of Chinese Medicinals*), Shanghai Science Technology Publishing Co., 1991, p. 2022

CHAPTER 2
INTERSTITIAL CYSTITIS (IC)

Interstitial cystitis (IC), also called painful bladder syndrome and frequency-urgency-dysuria syndrome, is a complex, chronic disorder of unknown etiology characterized by inflammation and irritation of the bladder wall which can lead to scarring and stiffening of the bladder, decreased bladder capacity, pinpoint bleeding, and, in rare cases, ulceration of the bladder lining.

NOSOLOGY

Interstitial cystitis is divided into two types. The first in non-ulcerative IC. It primarily affects young and middle-aged women. Ulcerative IC affects middle-aged to older women.

EPIDEMIOLOGY

Ninety percent of patients are women, and, although it may strike at any age, two-thirds of sufferers are between 20-40 years old. It is estimated that there may be a half million sufferers in the U.S.

ETIOLOGY & PATHOPHYSIOLOGY

Although the etiology of this condition is currently officially listed as unknown, it may be an autoimmune condition as a reaction to a leaky bladder lining. Seventy percent of IC patients do have a leaky bladder.

RISK FACTORS

Foods which may aggravate this condition include alcohol, tomatoes, spices, chocolate, caffeinated and citrus beverages, and high acid foods.

SYMPTOMATOLOGY

In general, the symptoms of IC are decreased bladder capacity, an urgent need to urinate, urinary frequency both day and night, pressure, pain, and tenderness around the bladder and perineum, painful intercourse, and worsening of pain around menstruation.

DIAGNOSIS

There is no definitive Western medical test for interstitial cystitis, and its diagnosis depends mostly on ruling out other diseases. Uroscopy or cystoscopy confirms the diagnosis by visualization of small hemorrhages in the bladder wall. Small bladder capacity (less than 400mm) is an additional confirmation.

DIFFERENTIAL DIAGNOSIS

Endometriosis
Kidney stones
Sexually transmitted disease
Chronic bacterial and nonbacterial prostatitis
Urinary tract infections
Vaginal tract infections

STANDARD WESTERN MEDICAL TREATMENT & MANAGEMENT

Intravesical DMSO and bladder distention with water provide symptomatic relief but are rarely curative. Physicians typically prescribe antiallergenic, immunosuppressive, and anti-inflammatory drugs, but may also prescribe antibiotics. Transcutaneous electrical stimulation (TENS) may also be used as well as surgery.

PROGNOSIS & COMPLICATIONS

Overall, Western medical treatment has limited success with this condition. Common complications include depression and anxiety, and bladder ulcers may develop over time.

CHINESE MEDICAL DISEASE CATEGORIZATION

Interstitial cystitis corresponds to the following diseases in Chinese medicine: heat strangury, blood strangury, stone strangury, qi strangury, and taxation strangury.

TREATMENT BASED ON PATTERN IDENTIFICATION

NOTE: For more information on pattern identification, treatment principles, and representative formulas for interstitial cystitis see the Chinese medical disease identifications in the previous chapter on urinary tract infections.

1. DAMP HEAT POURING DOWNWARD

SIGNS & SYMPTOMS: Frequent, urgent, painful urination with a burning hot feeling in the urethra, short, dark-colored, turbid urination, a sticky, dry mouth, thirst without desire to drink, lower abdominal distention and fullness, constipation, a red tongue with slimy, yellow fur, and a slippery, rapid pulse

TREATMENT PRINCIPLES: Clear heat and disinhibit dampness

REPRESENTATIVE FORMULA: *Ba Zheng San* (Eight [Ingredients] Rectification Powder)

Hua Shi (Talcum), 18g
Che Qian Zi (Plantaginis, Semen), 12g
Qu Mai (Dianthi, Herba), 9g
Da Huang (Rhei, cooked Radix Et Rhizoma), 9g
Zhi Zi (Gardeniae Jasminoidis, Fructus), 9g
Bian Xu (Polygoni Avicularis, Herba), 9g
Gan Cao Shao (Glycyrrhizae Uralensis, Radix Tenuis), 6g
Mu Tong (Akebiae, Caulis), 6g

MODIFICATIONS: For nausea from taking this formula, subtract *Mu Tong* and *Da Huang* and add *Sheng Jiang* (Zingiberis, uncooked Rhizoma) and ginger-processed *Ban Xia* (Pinelliae Ternatae, Rhizoma). For concomitant qi vacuity with fatigue, abdominal distention after meals, and loose stools, subtract *Mu Tong* and *Da Huang*, and add *Huang Qi* (Astragali Membranacei, Radix), *Dang Shen* (Codonopsitis Pilosulae, Radix), and *Fu Ling* (Poriae Cocos, Sclerotium). For concomitant liver depression, add *Chai Hu* (Bupleuri, Radix), *Bai Shao* (Paeoniae Lactiflorae, Radix Albus), and *Chuan Lian Zi* (Meliae Toosendan, Fructus). For concomitant kidney vacuity, add *Tu Si Zi* (Cuscutae Chinensis, Semen) and *Rou Gui* (Cinnamomi Cassiae, Cortex). For constipation, add *Zhi Shi* (Citri Aurantii, Fructus Immaturus) and replace cooked *Da Huang* with uncooked *Da Huang*. For hematuria, add *Xiao Ji* (Cephalanoplos Segeti, Herba), *Da Ji* (Cirsii Japonici, Herba Seu Radix), and *Bai Mao Gen* (Imperatae Cylindricae, Radix). For damp heat damaging yin with thirst and a desire to drink, and a dry mouth and throat, subtract *Da Huang* and add *Zhi Mu* (Anemarrhenae Aspheloidis, Rhizoma), *Sheng Di Huang* (Rehmanniae Glutinosae, uncooked Radix), and *Bai Mao Gen* (Imperatae Cylindricae, Radix). If this formula is too bitter and heat-clearing as written above, one can subtract *Mu Tong* and *Da Huang*, increase the dosage of *Hua Shi* up to 25g, and add *Fu Ling* (Poriae Cocos, Sclerotium) and *Da Zao* (Zizyphi Jujubae, Fructus).

For alternating fever and chills, a bitter taste in the mouth, dry throat, and nausea, add *Xiao Chai Hu Tang* (Minor Bupleurum Decoction): *Chai Hu* (Bupleuri, Radix), *Huang Qin* (Scutellariae Baicalensis, Radix), and *Ban Xia* (Pinelliae Ternatae, Rhizoma), 9g each, *Dang Shen* (Codonopsitis Pilosulae, Radix) and *Sheng Jiang* (Zingiberis Officinalis, uncooked Rhizoma), 6g each, and *Da Zao* (Zizyphi Jujubae, Fructus), 4 pieces.

ACUMOXIBUSTION: Needle *Zhong Ji* (CV 3), *Zhi Bian* (Bl 54), *San Yin Jiao* (Sp 6), and *Qu Quan* (Liv 8).

MODIFICATIONS: For fever, a bitter taste in the mouth, nausea, and vomiting, add *San Jiao Shu* (Bl 22) and *Ye Men* (TB 3). For constipation, add *Zhao Hai* (Ki 6) and *Zhi Gou* (TB 6). For fever, add *Qu Chi* (LI 11). For colicky pain in the abdomen and low back, add *Xiao Chang Shu* (Bl 27). For severely painful and/or burning urination, add *Shui Quan* (Ki 5). For concomitant qi vacuity, add *Tai Bai* (Sp 3) and *Zu San Li* (St 36). For concomitant liver depression, add *Xing Jian* (Liv 2) and *Jian Shi* (Per 5). For concomitant kidney vacuity, add *Tai Xi* (Ki 3). For hematuria, add *Xue Hai* (Sp 10). For nausea, add *Shang Wan* (CV 13) or *Nei Guan* (Per 6).

Case history from Dr. Wei Li's private practice: Sarah, a 27 year-old female

Sarah had burning, painful, frequent, and incomplete urination off and on since high school. She was usually warm or hot and had night sweats and kidney-bladder area pain. Western doctors could find no bacteria or other causes of the symptoms. Nevertheless, they prescribed several courses of antibiotics which were ineffective. They finally diagnosed the patient with interstitial cystitis. When Sarah came to see Dr. Li, she had the symptoms listed above plus digestive problems, including nausea and constipation. She had a red tongue with yellow fur and a slippery, fast pulse. Dr. Li's pattern identification was damp heat pouring downward with yin vacuity. She employed the three major principles for clearing heat described in the wind heat kidney wind section: clearing four aspect heat, draining fire, and discharging fire. Her formula was modified *Huang Lian Jie Du Tang* (Coptis Toxin-resolving Decoction) plus *Zhi Bai Di Huang Wan* (Anemarrhena & Phellodendron Rehmannia Pills): *Huang Lian* (Coptidis Chinensis, Rhizoma), 6g, *Xuan Shen* (Scrophulariae Ningpoensis, Radix), 5g, *Huang Qin* (Scutellariae Baicalensis, Radix), 9g, *Huang Bai* (Phellodendri, Cortex), 9g, *Zhi Mu* (Anemarrhenae Aspheloidis, Rhizoma), 9g, *Sheng Di Huang* (Rehmanniae Glutinosae, uncooked Radix), 15g, *Shan Zhu Yu* (Corni Officinalis, Fructus), 5g, *Shan Yao* (Dioscoreae Oppositae, Radix), 10g, *Fu Ling* (Poriae Cocos, Sclerotium), 5g, *Mu Dan Pi* (Moutan, Cortex Radicis), 5g, *Dan Zhu Ye* (Lophatheri Gracilis, Herba), 9g, *Che Qian Zi* (Plantaginis, Semen), 9g, *Mai Men Dong* (Ophiopogonis Japonici, Tuber), 9g, and *Feng Mi* (Mel), 1 tablespoon with each dose to protect the middle burner.

For this type of case, Dr. Li usually uses *Shi Gao* (Gypsum Fibrosum) and *Qing Dai* (Indigonis, Pulvis). But because Sarah had digestive problems, Dr. Li left these out. After taking the above medicinals, the patient's constipation improved. If it had not, Dr. Li would have added *Da Huang* (Rhei, Radix Et Rhizoma). As she continued with these herbs, Sarah's other symptoms began to decline. In the beginning, if she discontinued the formula, the symptoms would recur. After two months of taking these medicinals, Sarah's symptoms were practically gone. However, Dr. Li felt she must continue on this formula for another three months to consolidate the results, making the course of treatment five months. In such cases, the practitioner should expect a course of treatment to last from 3-6 months.

2. LIVER DEPRESSION & DAMP ACCUMULATION

SIGNS & SYMPTOMS: Frequent urination, an unfinished feeling after voiding, rib-side discomfort, lower abdominal distention and fullness, irritability, possible premenstrual or menstrual breast distention and pain, menstrual lower abdominal distention and pain, a normal or possibly dark, somewhat swollen tongue with slimy, white fur, and a bowstring pulse

TREATMENT PRINCIPLES: Course the liver and rectify the qi, eliminate dampness and disinhibit urination

REPRESENTATIVE FORMULA: Augmented *Chai Hu Shu Gan San Jia Wei* (Bupleurum Course the Liver Powder)

Hua Shi (Talcum), 18g
Che Qian Zi (Plantaginis, Semen), 12g
Chai Hu (Bupleuri, Radix), 9g
Bai Shao (Paeoniae Lactiflorae, Radix Albus), 9g
Zhi Ke (Citri Aurantii, Fructus), 9g
Xiang Fu (Cyperi Rotundi, Rhizoma), 9g
Chuan Lian Zi (Meliae Toosendan, Fructus), 9g
Ze Xie (Alismatis, Rhizoma), 9g
Yu Jin (Curcumae, Tuber), 9g
Chen Pi (Citri Reticulatae, Pericarpium), 6g
Chuan Xiong (Ligustici Wallichii, Radix), 6g
Gan Cao (Glycyrrhizae Uralensis, Radix), 6g

MODIFICATIONS: For blood stasis signs and symptoms such as a dark purple tongue or static macules on the tip and edges of the tongue, add *Chi Shao* (Paeoniae Lactiflorae, Radix Rubrus), *Dan Shen* (Salviae Miltiorrhizae, Radix), and *Hong Hua* (Carthami Tinctorii, Flos). For acid regurgitation, dry throat, and a red tongue, add *Zhi Zi* (Gardeniae Jasminoidis, Fructus) and *Mu Dan Pi* (Moutan, Cortex Radicis). For depressive heat in the liver and stomach, add *Huang Qin* (Scutellariae Baicalensis, Radix). For painful menstruation, add *Yi Mu Cao* (Leonuri Heterophylli, Herba) and *Dang Gui* (Angelicae Sinensis, Radix). For chest oppression, add *Jie Geng* (Platycodi Grandiflori, Radix). For frequent belching, add *Chen Xiang* (Aquilariae Agallochae, Lignum) and *Xuan Fu Hua* (Inulae Racemosae, Flos). For severe liver depression, add *Qing Pi* (Citri Reticulatae Viride, Pericarpium) and *Fo Shou* (Citri Sacrodactylis, Fructus). For concomitant spleen qi vacuity, add *Bai Zhu* (Atractylodis Macrocephalae, Rhizoma), *Fu Ling* (Poriae Cocos,

Sclerotium), and *Dang Shen* (Codonopsitis Pilosulae, Radix). For severe lower abdominal distention and pain, add *Yan Hu Suo* (Corydalis Yanhusuo, Rhizoma). If the condition gets worse with emotional disturbances, such as anger, frustration, and depression, add *Suan Zao Ren* (Zizyphi Spinosae, Semen), *He Huan Pi* (Albizziae Julibrissinis, Cortex), and *Ye Jiao Teng* (Polygoni Multiflori, Caulis).

ACUMOXIBUSTION: Needle *Xing Jian* (Liv 2), *Zhong Feng* (Liv 4), *Qu Quan* (Liv 8), *Qu Gu* (CV 2), and *Zhi Bian* (Bl 54).

MODIFICATIONS: For concomitant blood stasis, add *Xue Hai* (Sp 10) and *San Yin Jiao* (Sp 6). For depressive heat in the liver and stomach, add *Nei Ting* (St 44). For painful menstruation, add *Gui Lai* (St 29). For chest oppression, add *Nei Guan* (Per 6). For frequent belching, add *Jiu Wei* (CV 15). For severe liver depression, add *Jian Shi* (Per 5). For concomitant spleen qi vacuity, add *Zu San Li* (St 36). For severely painful and/or burning urination, add *Shui Quan* (Ki 5). For lower abdominal distention and pain, add *Yin Bao* (Liv 9). For frequent sighing, add *Yang Ling Quan* (GB 34). For rib-side pain, add *Qi Men* (Liv 14). For a bitter taste in the mouth due to depressive heat, add *Xia Xi* (GB 43).

3. SPLEEN QI VACUITY

SIGNS & SYMPTOMS: Frequent, long, clear urination, possible urinary incontinence or enuresis, pale lips, a pale facial complexion, fatigue, lassitude of the spirit, lack of strength, dizziness, shortage of qi, lack of warmth in the four limbs, possible facial edema, reduced food intake, and loose stools. There is a pale, fat tongue with white fur and a vacuous, weak pulse.

TREATMENT PRINCIPLES: Fortify the spleen and boost the qi

REPRESENTATIVE FORMULA: Augmented *Bu Zhong Yi Qi Tang* (Supplement the Center & Boost the Qi Decoction)

Huang Qi (Astragali Membranacei, Radix), 15g
Dang Shen (Codonopsitis Pilosulae, Radix), 9g

Bai Zhu (Atractylodis Macrocephalae, Rhizoma), 9g
Wu Wei Zi (Schisandrae Chinensis, Fructus), 9g
Fu Ling (Poriae Cocos, Sclerotium), 9g
Dang Gui (Angelicae Sinensis, Radix), 6g
Chen Pi (Citri Reticulatae, Pericarpium), 6g
mix-fried *Gan Cao* (Glyrrhizae Uralensis, Radix), 6g
Sheng Ma (Cimicifugae, Rhizoma), 4.5g
Chai Hu (Bupleuri, Radix), 3g

MODIFICATIONS: For severe frequent urination due to spleen disease reaching the kidneys, add *Qian Shi* (Euryalis Ferocis, Semen), *Jin Ying Zi* (Rosae Laevigatae, Fructus), and *Tu Si Zi* (Cuscutae Chinensis, Semen). For susceptibility to common cold, add *Fang Feng* (Ledebouriellae Divaricatae, Radix). For phlegm dampness obstructing the lungs manifesting as cough with white phlegm, add *Ban Xia* (Pinelliae Ternatae, Rhizoma) and *Jie Geng* (Platycodi Grandiflori, Radix). For food stagnation with loss of appetite, abdominal distention, and loss of taste, add *Mai Ya* (Hordei Vulgaris, Fructus Germinatus), *Lai Fu Zi* (Raphani Sativi, Semen), and stir-fried *Shan Zha* (Crataegi, Fructus).

For heart-spleen dual vacuity, replace *Bu Zhong Yi Qi Tang* with modified *Gui Pi Tang* (Return the Spleen Decoction): *Huang Qi* (Astragali Membranacei, Radix), 15g, *Bai Zhu* (Atractylodis Macrocephalae, Rhizoma), 12g, *Dang Gui* (Angelicae Sinensis, Radix), *Long Yan Rou* (Euphoriae Longanae, Arillus), *Dang Shen* (Codonopsitis Pilosulae, Radix), and *Yi Zhi Ren* (Alpiniae Oxyphyllae, Fructus), 9g each, *Mu Xiang* (Auklandiae Lappae, Radix), *Suan Zao Ren* (Zizyphi Spinosae, Semen), *Yuan Zhi* (Polygalae Tenuifoliae, Radix), and *Fu Ling* (Poriae Cocos, Sclerotium), 6g each, and mix-fried *Gan Cao* (Glycyrrhizae Uralensis, Radix), 3g.

For both qi and blood vacuity, replace *Bu Zhong Yi Qi Tang* with modified *Ba Zhen Tang* (Eight Pearls Decoction): *Shu Di Huang* (Rehmanniae Glutinosae, cooked Radix), 18g, *Bai Zhu* (Atractylodis Macrocephalae, Rhizoma) and *Huang Qi* (Astragali Membranacei, Radix), 15g each, *Bai Shao* (Paeoniae Lactiflorae, Radix Albus), *Dang Gui* (Angelicae Sinensis, Radix), and *Dang Shen* (Codonopsitis Pilosulae, Radix), 9g each, and *Fu Ling* (Poriae Cocos, Sclerotium), *Gui Zhi* (Cinnamomi Cassiae,

Ramulus), *Chuan Xiong* (Ligustici Wallichii, Radix), and mix-fried *Gan Cao* (Glycyrrhizae Uralensis, Radix), 6g each.

ACUMOXIBUSTION: Needle and/or moxibustion *Guan Yuan* (CV 4), *Qi Hai* (CV 6), *Bai Hui* (GV 20), *Zu San Li* (St 36), and *San Yin Jiao* (Sp 6).

MODIFICATIONS: For severe frequent urination, add *Zhong Ji* (CV 3) with supplementing method. For susceptibility to common cold, add *He Gu* (LI 4) and *Da Zhui* (GV 14). For phlegm dampness obstructing the lungs manifesting as cough with profuse white phlegm, add *Feng Men* (Bl 12) and *Fei Shu* (Bl 13). For food stagnation, add *Liang Men* (St 21). For concomitant kidney qi vacuity, add *Tai Xi* (Ki 3). For heart-spleen dual vacuity, add *Shen Men* (Ht 7).

4. STRAITENED SPLEEN

SIGNS & SYMPTOMS: Frequent, possibly dark-colored urination, a tendency to dry, hard stools, rapid hungering and large appetite, possible abdominal fullness, possible fatigue, a fat, enlarged tongue with yellow, possibly dry tongue fur, and a slippery, bowstring pulse which is often also floating in the right bar

NOTE: Straitened spleen refers to a replete stomach with a vacuous spleen. It is said that the kidneys are the sluicegate of the stomach. Therefore, there is a close reciprocal relationship between the stomach and kidneys. If the stomach is hot, it hyperfunctions. Since one of its functions are to downbear turbidity, a hyperfunctioning stomach disperses food too quickly on the one hand, while downbearing fluids too quickly to the bladder on the other. This gives rise to rapid hungering and frequent urination accompanied by a tendency to constipation. This is a common pattern in Western clinical practice. In real life, it is typically complicated by liver depression/depressive heat.

TREATMENT PRINCIPLES: Clear the stomach and moisten the intestines, fortify the spleen and supplement the qi, move the qi and free the flow of the stools

REPRESENTATIVE FORMULA: Modified *Xiao Chai Hu*

Tang (Minor Bupleurum Decoction) plus *Ma Zi Ren Wan* (Cannabis Seed Pills)

Huang Qin (Scutellariae Baicalensis, Radix), 12g
Chai Hu (Bupleuri, Radix), 9g
Dang Shen (Codonopsitis Pilosulae, Radix), 9g
Ban Xia (Pinelliae Ternatae, Rhizoma), 9g
Huo Ma Ren (Cannabis Sativae, Semen), 9g
Hou Po (Magnoliae Officinalis, Cortex), 9g
Bai Shao (Paeoniae Lactiflorae, Radix Albus), 9g
Zhi Shi (Citri Aurantii, Fructus Immaturus), 6g
Xing Ren (Pruni Armeniacae, Semen), 6g
mix-fried *Gan Cao* (Glycyrrhizae Uralensis, Radix), 6g
Da Zao (Zizyphi Jujubae, Fructus), 3 pieces

MODIFICATIONS: If constipation is severe, add *Da Huang* (Rhei, Radix Et Rhizoma). If there are no dry stools, delete *Huo Ma Ren* and *Xing Ren*. If spleen vacuity with dampness is marked, add *Bai Zhu* (Atractylodis Macrocephalae, Rhizoma) and *Fu Ling* (Poriae Cocos, Sclerotium). If *Huo Ma Ren* is difficult to find, replace with *Tao Ren* (Pruni Persicae, Semen).

ACUMOXIBUSTION: Needle *Wei Shu* (Bl 21), *Zhao Hai* (Ki 6), *San Yin Jiao* (Sp 6), *Nei Ting* (St 44), and *Zhi Gou* (TB 6).

MODIFICATIONS: For concomitant difficult, painful urination and constipation, add *Zhi Bian* (Bl 54). For concomitant liver depression, add *Zhong Feng* (Liv 4) and *Qu Quan* (Liv 8). For abdominal pain, add *Da Heng* (Sp 15). For bad breath, add *Jie Xi* (St 41). For heart vexation, add *Shen Men* (Ht 7). If constipation is severe, add *Shang Ju Xu* (St 37). If there are no dry stools, subtract *Zhao Hai*. If spleen vacuity with dampness is marked, add *Yin Ling Quan* (Sp 9) and *Tai Bai* (Sp 3). For severely painful and/or burning urination, add *Shui Quan* (Ki 5). For lower abdominal distention and pain, add *Yin Bao* (Liv 9). For rib-side pain, add *Qi Men* (Liv 14). For a bitter taste in the mouth due to depressive heat, add *Xia Xi* (GB 43).

5. BLOOD STASIS OBSTRUCTING INTERNALLY

SIGNS & SYMPTOMS: Frequent, painful urination with dark-colored, turbid urine and possible purple clots in the urine, dribbling urination, lower abdominal distention and pain which refuses pressure, a dark tongue with static macules or spots, and a bowstring and/or choppy pulse

NOTE: This pattern mainly complicates other patterns associated with frequent urination.

TREATMENT PRINCIPLES: Quicken the blood and transform stasis, free the flow of and disinhibit urination

REPRESENTATIVE FORMULA: Augmented *Shao Fu Zhu Yu Tang Jia Wei* (Lower Abdomen Dispel Stasis Decoction)

Che Qian Zi (Plantaginis, Semen), 12g
Dang Gui (Angelicae Sinensis, Radix), 9g
Chuan Xiong (Ligustici Wallichii, Radix), 9g
Chi Shao (Paeoniae Lactiflorae, Radix Rubrus), 9g
Pu Huang (Typhae, Pollen), 9g
Wu Ling Zhi (Trogopteri Seu Pteromi, Feces), 9g
Yan Hu Suo (Corydalis Yanhusuo, Rhizoma), 9g
Mo Yao (Myrrhae, Resina), 9g
Ze Xie (Alismatis, Rhizoma), 9g
Zhu Ling (Polypori Umbellati, Sclerotium), 9g
Xiao Hui Xiang (Feoniculi Vulgaris, Fructus), 6g
Rou Gui (Cinnamomi Cassiae, Cortex), 3g

MODIFICATIONS: For hematuria, subtract *Rou Gui* and add *San Qi* (Notoginseng, Radix) and *Hu Po* (Succinum), powdered and taken with the strained decoction. For painful urination, add *Dan Zhu Ye* (Lophatheri Gracilis, Herba), *Gan Cao Shao* (Glycyrrhizae Uralensis, Radix Tenuis), and *Hua Shi* (Talcum). For absence of cold and the presence of heat, subtract *Xiao Hui Xiang* and *Rou Gui* and add *Mu Dan Pi* (Moutan, Cortex Radicis) and *Dan Shen* (Salviae Miltiorhizzae, Radix). For severe pain, add *Bai Shao* (Paeoniae Lactiflorae, Radix Albus), *Jin Qian Cao* (Lysimachiae, Herba), and *Gan Cao* (Glycyrrhizae Uralensis, Radix).

ACUMOXIBUSTION: Needle *Zhong Ji* (CV 3), *Zhi Bian* (Bl 54), *San Yin Jiao* (Sp 6), and *Shui Quan* (Ki 5).

MODIFICATIONS: For concomitant urethral distention and pain, add *Zhong Fu* (Liv 4). For lower abdominal or umbilical region distention and pain, add *Qi Hai* (CV 6). For stone strangury, add *Wei Yang* (Bl 39) and *Ran Gu* (Ki 2).

6. KIDNEY YIN VACUITY

SIGNS & SYMPTOMS: Frequent, short, dark-colored urination, tinnitus, dizziness, a dry throat and mouth, red cheeks and lips, vacuity vexation and insomnia, low back and knee soreness and limpness, steaming bones and taxation fever, vexatious heat in the five hearts, night sweats, and dry stools. There is a red tongue with scanty fur and a fine, fast pulse.

TREATMENT PRINCIPLES: Enrich yin and downbear fire

REPRESENTATIVE FORMULA: Augmented *Zhi Bai Di Huang Wan* (Anemarrhena & Phellodendron Rehmannia Pills)

Shu Di Huang (Rehmanniae Glutinosae, cooked Radix), 12g
Shan Zhu Yu (Corni Officinalis, Fructus), 9g
Shan Yao (Dioscoreae Oppositae, Radix), 9g
Fu Ling (Poriae Cocos, Sclerotium), 9g
Mu Dan Pi (Moutan, Cortex Radicis), 9g
Ze Xie (Alismatis, Rhizoma), 9g
Zhi Mu (Anemarrhenae Aspheloidis, Rhizoma), 9g
Huang Bai (Phellodendri, Cortex), 9g
Niu Xi (Achyranthis Bidentatae, Radix), 9g

MODIFICATIONS: For tidal heat and steaming bones, add *Di Gu Pi* (Lycii Chinensis, Cortex Radicis), *Qing Hao* (Artemisiae Annuae, Herba), and *Yin Chai Hu* (Stellariae Dichotomae, Radix). For night sweats, add *Wu Wei Zi* (Schisandrae Chinensis, Fructus) and *Suan Zao Ren* (Zizyphi Spinosae, Semen). For thirst and a dry mouth and throat at night, add *Xuan Shen* (Scrophulariae Ningpoensis, Radix) and *Mai Men Dong* (Ophiopogonis Japonici, Tuber). For severe kidney yin vacuity, add *Er Zhi Wan* (Two Ultimate Pills), *i.e.*, *Nu Zhen Zi* (Ligustri Lucidi) and *Han Lian Cao* (Ecliptae Prostratae, Herba). For vexatious heat in the chest, add *Zhi Zi* (Gardeniae Jasminoidis, Fructus). For insomnia, add *Suan Zao Ren* (Zizyphi Spinosae, Semen). For concomitant spleen qi vacuity, add *Huang Qi* (Astragali Membranacei, Radix),

Dang Shen (Codonopsitis Pilosulae, Radix) and *Bai Zhu* (Atractylodis Macrocephalae, Rhizoma). If there is concomitant liver depression, add *Chuan Lian Zi* (Meliae Toosendan, Fructus). For concomitant kidney yang vacuity with cold limbs, aversion to cold, and decreased sexual desire, add *Fu Zi* (Aconiti Carmichaeli, Radix Lateralis Praeparatus), *Rou Gui* (Cinnamomi Cassiae, Cortex), and *Ba Ji Tian* (Morindae Officinalis, Radix).

ACUMOXIBUSTION: Needle *Fu Liu* (Ki 7), *Zhao Hai* (Ki 6), *Ran Gu* (Ki 2), *San Yin Jiao* (Sp 6), and *Guan Yuan* (CV 4).

MODIFICATIONS: For heart palpitations and insomnia, add *Xin Shu* (Bl 15). For just insomnia, add *Shen Men* (Ht 7). For vexatious heat of the five hearts and night sweats, add *Yin Xi* (Ht 6). For seminal emission, add *Zhi Shi* (Bl 52). For scanty menstruation or blocked menstruation, *i.e.*, amenorrhea, add *Xue Hai* (Sp 10) and *Gui Lai* (St 29). For constipation, add *Zhao Hai* (Ki 6). For severe kidney yin vacuity with effulgent fire, add *Yin Gu* (Ki 10), *Zhao Hai* (Ki 6), and *Jiao Xing* (Ki 8) to enrich yin, downbear fire, and free the flow of urination. For hematuria, add *Xue Hai* (Sp 10).

Case history from Dr. Wei Li's private practice: Nancy, a 45 year-old female

Nancy first visited Dr. Li in 1993. She had urinary frequency, burning, pain, and discomfort for over 10 years. She had to urinate 20-30 times a day, and she dribbled so constantly she had to wear a diaper. Western urinalysis revealed no bacteria. Nevertheless, Western doctors tried many types of antibiotics, even antituberculosis medications. Some of these drugs relieved her symptoms temporarily but did not resolve her condition. Nancy's tongue was devoid of fur, and her pulse was bowstring and forceful. Dr. Li's pattern identification was kidney yin vacuity with internal heat and blood stasis. The representative formula for kidney yin vacuity with internal heat is *Zhi Bai Di Huang Wan* (Anemarrhena & Phellodendron Rehmannia Pills). However, since blood stasis was an important part of the patient's overall pattern, Dr. Li chose to use variations of *Si Wu Tang* (Four Materials Decoction):

Shu Di Huang (Rehmanniae Glutinosae, cooked Radix), 6g, *Sheng Di Huang* (Rehmanniae Glutinosae, uncooked Radix), 6g, *Dang Gui Wei* (Angelicae Sinensis, Extremitas Radicis), 9g, *Chi Shao* (Paeoniae Lactiflorae, Radix Rubrus), 9g, *Chuan Xiong* (Ligustici Wallichii, Radix), 9g, *Mu Dan Pi* (Moutan, Cortex Radicis), 9g, and *Shan Zhu Yu* (Corni Officinalis, Fructus), 9g. After taking this prescription for one week, Nancy felt she was 50% better. After taking variations of this formula for one year, she had nearly normal urination. She did not require a diaper, the burning was gone, and the frequency was nearly normal. The patient still had some urgency and dribbling when her bladder was full. Dr. Li felt that the chronic inflammation had caused some structural damage to the bladder, perhaps some local scar tissue. Thus, while the bladder function was almost normal, the structural damage could only be improved to 90-95%.

7. KIDNEY YANG VACUITY

SIGNS & SYMPTOMS: Frequent, long, clear urination, possible urinary incontinence or enuresis, a bright white facial complexion, dizziness, tinnitus, shortage of qi, lack of strength in the low back and knees, and lack of warmth in the limbs. There is a pale, fat tongue with thin, white fur and a deep, fine, weak pulse.

TREATMENT PRINCIPLES: Supplement the kidneys and invigorate yang

REPRESENTATIVE FORMULA: Augmented *You Gui Wan Jia Wei* (Restore the Right [Kidney] Pills)

Shu Di Huang (Rehmanniae Glutinosae, cooked Radix), 12g
Tu Si Zi (Cuscutae Chinensis, Semen), 12g
Shan Yao (Dioscoreae Oppositae, Radix), 9g
Shan Zhu Yu (Corni Officinalis, Fructus), 9g
Gou Qi Zi (Lycii Chinensis, Fructus), 9g
Du Zhong (Eucommiae Ulmoidis, Cortex), 9g
Yi Zhi Ren (Alpiniae Oxyphyllae, Fructus), 9g
Sang Piao Xiao (Mantidis, Ootheca), 9g
Dang Gui (Angelicae Sinensis, Radix), 6g
Lu Jiao Jiao (Cervi, Gelatinum Cornu), 6g
Fu Zi (Aconiti Carmichaeli, Radix Lateralis Praeparatus), 3g

Rou Gui (Cinnamomi Cassiae, Cortex), 3g

MODIFICATIONS: For severe frequent, long, clear urination, enuresis, urinary incontinence, or nocturia, add *Jin Ying Zi* (Rosae Laevigatae, Fructus) and *Fu Pen Zi* (Rubi Chingii, Fructus). For heart palpitations and a bound or regularly intermittent pulse, add mix-fried *Gan Cao* (Glycyrrhizae Uralensis, Radix) and *Dan Shen* (Salviae Miltiorrhizae, Radix). For hasty panting and spontaneous perspiration, add *Ren Shen* (Panacis Ginseng, Radix) and *Wu Wei Zi* (Schisandrae Chinensis, Fructus). For seminal emission, vaginal discharge, or diarrhea, add *Bu Gu Zhi* (Psoraleae Corylifoliae, Fructus). For lower limb edema, subtract *Yi Zhi Ren, Tu Si Zi,* and *Sang Piao Xiao* and add *Wu Jia Pi* (Acanthopanacis Gracilistylis, Cortex Radicis), *Ze Xie* (Alismatis, Rhizoma), and *Fu Ling* (Poriae Cocos, Sclerotium). For decreased sexual desire or impotence, add *Xian Mao* (Curculiginis Orchioidis, Rhizoma) and *Yin Yang Huo* (Epimedii, Herba). For liver depression qi stagnation, increase *Chai Hu* to nine grams. For spleen vacuity, add *Huang Qi* (Astragali Membranacei, Radix), *Dang Shen* (Codonopsitis Pilosulae, Radix), and *Bai Zhu* (Atractylodis Macrocephalae, Rhizoma).

ACUMOXIBUSTION: Needle *Tai Xi* (Ki 3) and *San Ying Jiao* (Sp 6) and moxibustion *Guan Yuan* (CV 4), *Shen Shu* (Bl 23), and *Zhi Shi* (Bl 52).

MODIFICATIONS: For panting counterflow, add *Ran Gu* (Ki 2). For dribbling urination, add *Pang Guang Shu* (Bl 28). For frequent night-time urination, add *Zhao Hai* (Ki 6). For clear, thin vaginal discharge, add *Dai Mai* (GB 26).

CLINICAL TIPS

1. Practitioners should take care not to allow the word "cystitis" in interstitial cystitis to seduce them into immediately thinking of damp heat strangury. Most patients with interstitial cystitis do not exhibit the signs and symptoms of an acute damp heat pattern, such as burning hot urinary pain.

2. Interstitial cystitis is particularly recalcitrant and treatment may require more than the rote application of a representative formula for the appropriate pattern identification. One must carefully analyze and treat both the tip and root. Interstitial cystitis can be seen as a struggle between evils and the righteous qi. In this case, the evils or tip are typically some combination of heat, dampness, qi stagnation, and blood stasis, while the root is a righteous qi vacuity. Yin is often vacuous, either constitutionally or due to damage by enduring heat. During the course of this disease, if the pattern is more replete, one must focus on attacking evils. If the pattern is more vacuous, one must focus on supporting the righteous. In other words, one must pay special attention to the relative strength of evils and the righteous qi in the pattern identification. Tongue and pulse diagnosis are extremely important in making this assessment. One's treatment principles and formula must combine attacking evils and supporting the righteous in direct relation to the relative strength of each through the vicissitudes of the disease. This means that one will typically have to modify these principles and formulas as the patient progresses over time.

3. Patients with interstitial cystitis have often been given one or more courses of antibiotics or immunosuppressive and anti-inflammatory drugs. These drugs tend to injure the central and true qi. Therefore, one may need to start treatment by focusing on harmonizing the center and supporting the true qi before aggressively attacking evils. On the other hand, if there is prominent blood stasis or heat, one must not be reluctant to use the appropriate blood-quickening, stasis-dispelling or heat-clearing medicinals.

CHAPTER 3
NEPHROTIC SYNDROME (NS)

Nephrotic syndrome (NS) refers to a predictable complex of signs and symptoms characterized by increased glomerular permeability to proteins resulting in massive loss of proteins in the urine, edema, hypoalbuminemia, hyperlipidemia, and hypercoagulability. This syndrome can be caused by several different types of glomerular injury resulting from a broad array of diseases, such as diabetes mellitus, amyloidosis, vasculitis, systemic lupus erythmatosus, and toxic injury to the kidneys by drugs.

NOSOLOGY

Nephrotic syndrome is categorized by whether it is due to primary glomerular disease or is secondary to some other, nonrenal disease. Primary glomerular diseases include minimal change disease (MCD), focal segmental glomerulosclerosis (FSGS), membranous glomerulonephritis (MGN), membranoproliferative glomerulonephritis (MPGN), mesangial proliferative glomerulonephritis (GN), IgA nephropathy, rapidly progressive glomerulonephritis, and fibrillary glomerulonephritis. Secondary renal diseases resulting in NS may be divided into metabolic (such as diabetes mellitus), immunogenic (such as SLE, RA, and Sjögren's syndrome), neoplastic (such as leukemia), nephrotoxic, allergenic, infectious (including bacterial, viral, protozoal, and helminthic), heredofamilial (such as sickle-cell anemia), and miscellaneous (such as due to toxemia of pregnancy, malignant hypertension, and transplant rejection).

EPIMIOLOGY

Children between the ages of one and eight are most frequently affected, boys slightly more than girls. Therefore, nephrotic syndrome is also commonly called childhood nephrotic syndrome. Minimal change disease is the most common form of the syndrome in children. It is characterized by normal or nearly normal biopsies of the kidneys.

ETIOLOGY & PATHOPHYSIOLOGY

Minimal change disease (MCD) in children typically follows an upper respiratory infection. Periorbital edema and swelling of the ankles or testicles may be noted. In most cases, however, the cause of nephrotic syndrome in children is idiopathic or unknown. Slow moving infections, such as hepatitis, and allergic or adverse drug reactions may be implicated.

In adults there are a host of diseases that are known to be risk factors for nephrotic syndrome. These include poorly controlled diabetes mellitus, certain cancers such as leukemia and lymphoma, and some snakebite poisonings. Amyloidosis, which is characterized by fibrous protein deposition, may result in nephrotic syndrome due to its hardening of the kidneys. Pre-eclampsia of pregnancy is also marked by heavy proteinuria but is rarely associated with true nephrotic syndrome. The most significant risk factor for nephrotic syndrome is chronic kidney disease, especially glomerulonephritis. Those disorders, which directly damage the filtration system, are most likely to result in nephrosis.

SYMPTOMATOLOGY

An early sign of NS is frothy urine due to protein. Other symptoms include anorexia, malaise, pugy eyelids, retinal sheen, abdominal pain, and wasting of the muscles. Anasarca with ascites and pleural effusions may occur. Focal edema may present as difficulty breathing, substernal chest pain, scrotal swelling, and swollen abdomen. Most often, edema is mobile. For instance, it is detected in the eyelids in the morning and in the ankles after walking. This edema may also mask muscle wasting. Parallel white lines in the fingernail beds may be due to subungual edema. Oliguria or acute renal failure may develop, and children may present with orthostatic hypotension and even shock. The hyperlipidemia that often accompanies this syndrome may lead to symptoms caused by atherosclerosis. Adults may be hypotensive, normotensive, or hypertensive depending on the degree of angiotensin II production.

DIAGNOSIS

The diagnosis of NS is suggested by the clinical features and laboratory findings and confirmed by renal biopsy. Nephrotic syndrome is typically first suspected in-office due to a urine dip-stick analysis. Elevated marks on this test necessitate the use of a 24 hour urine collection. Additionally, blood tests are usually done in order to look for decreased albumin and increased cholesterol or triglycerides. Eventually, a biopsy may be performed in order to understand the extent of the kidney damage.

DIFFERENTIAL DIAGNOSIS

Many conditions are characterized by mild elevations in protein in the urine. These include pyelonephritis, tubular necrosis, analgesic nephropathy and hypokalemia. These should be included in the differential diagnosis of nephrotic syndrome.

WESTERN MEDICAL TREATMENT

Western medical treatment of NS is directed at the underlying pathogenic process and is dependent on the renal pathology. Minimal change disease is the most common form of nephrosis. Children with this disorder are commonly prescribed corticosteroids, typically prednisone. The mechanism of action of steroids is to decrease the loss of proteins from the blood into the urine. Angiotensin-converting enzyme (ACE) inhibitors, a common class of antihypertensive medications, have also been used to slow the loss of protein. Initially, along with steroids, intravenous albumin is often administered to replenish the lost protein. Diuretics are then prescribed to eliminate the excess fluid. Adults are treated in a similar manner to children. Treatment is chiefly geared to managing the fluid levels and electrolyte balance.

PROGNOSIS & COMPLICATIONS

The prognosis for nephrotic syndrome is dependent on that of the underlying disorder. Both acute and chronic renal failures are associated with nephrosis and, for this reason, it must be considered a life-threatening complication. Some patients are also at an increased risk for developing blood clots. Increased permeability of the glomerular filtration system can result in hypercoagulability states.

CHINESE MEDICAL DISEASE CATEGORIZATION

Because the clinical manifestations of NS are relatively various, this disease corresponds to a diverse and indeterminate group of traditional Chinese disease categories: kidney wind, block and repulsion, dribbling urinary block, water swelling, kidney taxation or vacuity taxation and taxation wind, phlegm rheum, lumbar pain, turbid condition, abdominal distention, dizziness.

TREATMENT BASED ON PATTERN IDENTIFICATION

Nephrotic syndrome always presents a pattern of cold dampness. However, this may be complicated with either a qi vacuity pattern or a qi and yang vacuity pattern. Cold dampness may also stagnate, causing heat, or may be complicated by a contraction of damp heat. (Please see Figure 3.1.)

1. COLD DAMPNESS WITH QI VACUITY

SIGNS AND SYMPTOMS: Edema, a pale facial complexion, fatigue, no appetite, loose stools, abdominal distention, heart palpitations, dizziness, insomnia, difficult urination. The tongue is big and swollen with thin, white fur, and the pulse is thin and forceless.

TREATMENT PRINCIPLES: Fortify the spleen and supplement the kidney, eliminate dampness and dispel cold

REPRESENTATIVE FORMULA: *Bu Zhong Yi Qi Tang* (Supplement the Center & Boost the Qi Decoction) plus *Ju Yuan Jian* (Origin-lifting Brew) with modifications

Huang Qi (Astragali Membranacei, Radix), 12g
Ren Shen (Panacis Ginseng, Radix), 9g
Bai Zhu (Atractylodis Macrocephalae, Rhizoma), 12g
mix-fried *Gan Cao* (Glycyrrhizae Uralensis, Radix), 3g
Dang Gui (Angelicae Sinensis, Radix), 9g

Chen Pi (Citri Reticulatae, Pericarpium), 6g
Sheng Ma (Cimicifugae, Rhizoma), 9g
Chai Hu (Bupleuri, Radix), 6g

MODIFICATIONS: For prominent edema, combine with *Shi Pi Yin* (Bolster the Spleen Beverage), *Wu Ling San* (Five [Ingredients] Poria Powder), or *Wu Pi Yin* (Five Peels Beverage). If the patient is cold, add *Gui Zhi* (Cinnamomi Cassiae, Ramulus) and *Fu Zi* (Aconiti Carmichaeli, Radix Lateralis Praeparatus). For low appetite, add *Shan Zha* (Crataegi, Fructus), *Lai Fu Zi* (Raphani Sativi, Semen), and *Shen Qu* (Massa Medica Fermentata). For qi stagnation with abdominal distention and gas, add *Fo Shou* (Citri Sacrodactylis, Fructus), *Xiang Fu* (Cyperi Rotundi, Rhizoma), *Lai Fu Zi* (Raphani Sativi, Semen), and *Gan Jiang* (Zingiberis Officinalis, dry Rhizoma). For loose stools, add *Yi Yi Ren* (Coicis Lachryma-jobi, Semen), *Huo Xiang* (Agastachis Seu Pogostemi, Herba), and *Pei Lan* (Eupatorii Fortunei, Herba). For nausea, add *Ban Xia* (Pinelliae Ternatae, Rhizoma), *Hou Po* (Magnoliae Officinalis, Cortex), and *Huo Xiang* (Agastachis Seu Pogostemi, Herba).

ACUMOXIBUSTION: Choose from *Pi Shu* (Bl 20), *Shen Shu* (Bl 23), *Da Chang Shu* (Bl 25), *Ming Men* (GV 4), *Tai Bai* (Sp 3), *Tai Xi* (Ki 3), *San Yin Jiao* (Sp 6), *Zu San Li* (St 36), *Guan Yuan* (CV 4), *Qi Hai* (CV 6), *Zhong Wan* (CV 12), *Tian Shu* (St 25), *Yin Ling Quan* (Sp 9), *Fu Liu* (Ki 7), *Zhong Ji* (CV 3), and *Pang Guang Shu* (Bl 28).

Case history of Dr. Pei Ran-chu: A seven year-old boy[1]

This child was diagnosed with nephrotic syndrome and chronic renal failure (CRF). He was treated with

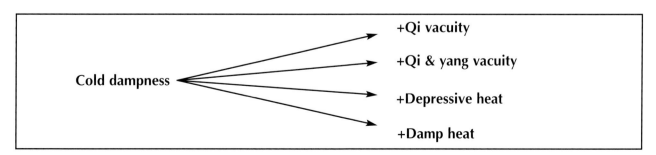

Figure 3.1. Nephrotic syndrome pattern identifications

Western medicine in the hospital, including hormones and other drugs, for over two months without any improvement. The doctors gave notice to his family that he might die at any time. Therefore, the family decided to consult Dr. Pei. At the time of examination, Dr. Pei found the boy very fatigued and in a lethargic state. He had a very pale face, his whole body was edematous, he had drum-like abdominal distention, his chest was full and round, his testicles were big and swollen, and he had great difficulty urinating and would only dribble. His tongue was puffy, big, swollen, and pale with very wet, slimy fur. His pulse was fine and faint, being only barely perceptible. Based on the above signs and symptoms, Dr. Pei concluded that the boy was suffering from qi exhaustion. Long-term illness had severely damaged the boy's body and spirit. His qi was so vacuous that qi transformation was severely inhibited and water could not be transformed. Instead, it accumulated to form water swelling. He felt this boy's prognosis was not good. Dr. Pei decided to try the following formula: *Sheng Di Huang* (Rehmanniae Glutinosae, uncooked Radix), 50g, *Tu Fu Ling* (Smilacis Glabrae, Rhizoma), 30g, *Hei Da Dou* (Glycines, Semen Atrum), 30g, *Da Zao* (Zizyphi Jujubae, Fructus), 7 pieces, and *Mu Li* (Ostreae, Concha), 30g.

After three days, the boy's urination began to become disinhibited. His edema reduced, he had more energy, and his pulse was stronger. Dr. Pei decided to augment the prescription with the following: *Ba Ji Tian* (Morindae Officinalis, Radix), 15g, *Huang Bai* (Phellodendri, Cortex), 15g, *Ze Xie* (Alismatis Orientalis, Rhizoma), 18g. After one week on the augmented formula, the boy's 24 hour urine output reached 1500ml. His water swelling dissipated greatly, his testicle size reduced to almost normal, he regained some appetite, and he became more active. His tongue returned to normal with thin, white fur. His pulse was still fine but stronger. Therefore, Dr. Pei prescribed this same formula with modifications for three months. All the boy's symptoms disappeared and he recovered completely. On follow-up after two years, there had been no recurrence.

Case history of Dr. Ke Wan-chen: Yong, a 45 year-old male[2]

Yong had chronic nephritis for 10 years. He was treated for half a year without a change in the abnormal level of his urine protein. He had edema in both legs and his kidney function was compromised. Dr. Ke prescribed *Huang Qi Chi Xiao Dou Tang* (Astragalus & Red Bean Decoction): *Huang Qi* (Astragali Membranacei, Radix), 100g, and *Chi Xiao Dou* (Phaseoli Calcarati, Semen), 30g, cooked at a low temperature until completely soft. This formula was divided into two servings and taken twice a day.

Yong took this formula every day for approximately one and a half months. His edema completely dissipated and his proteinuria disappeared. He continued on it for another month and a half to consolidate the results. Yong recovered completely. In fact, he passed his entrance exam for graduate school and became a college teacher. Yearly follow-ups found no recurrence.

2. COLD DAMPNESS WITH QI & YANG VACUITY

SIGNS & SYMPTOMS: Edema, a pale facial complexion, fatigue, no appetite, loose stools, abdominal distention, feeling cold with a cold back and a sensation like sitting in water, difficult but profuse urination. The tongue is pale and swollen, and the pulse is deep and slow.

TREATMENT PRINCIPLES: Fortify the spleen and boost the qi, supplement the kidney and invigorate yang, eliminate dampness

REPRESENTATIVE FORMULA: Modified *Zhen Wu Tang* (True Warrior Decoction), *Shi Pi Yin* (Bolster the Spleen Beverage) & *Wu Ling San* (Five [Ingredients] Poria Powder)

Shu Fu Zi (Aconiti Carmichaeli, Radix Lateralis Praeparatus), 3-6g
Gan Jiang (Zingiberis Officinalis, dry Rhizoma), 3g
Gui Zhi (Cinnamomi Cassiae, Ramulus), 3g
Bai Zhu (Atractylodis Macrocephalae, Rhizoma), 9g
Fu Ling (Poriae Cocos, Sclerotium), 9g
Sheng Jiang (Zingiberis Officinalis, uncooked Rhizoma), 6g
Bai Shao (Paeoniae Lactiflorae, Radix Albus), 6g
Mu Gua (Chaenomelis Lagenariae, Fructus), 6g

Hou Po (Magnoliae Officinalis, Cortex), 6g
Mu Xiang (Auklandiae Lappae, Radix), 3g
Da Fu Pi (Arecae Catechu, Pericarpium), 6g
Cao Guo (Amomi Tsao-ko, Fructus), 6g
mix-fried *Gan Cao* (Glycyrrhizae Uralensis, Radix), 3g
Ze Xie (Alismatis Orientalis, Rhizoma), 6g
Zhu Ling (Polypori Umbellati, Sclerotium), 6g

MODIFICATIONS: If the patient is severely fatigued, add *Huang Qi* (Astragali Membranacei, Radix) and *Ren Shen* (Panacis Ginseng, Radix). For low appetite, add *Shan Zha* (Crataegi, Fructus), *Lai Fu Zi* (Raphani Sativi, Semen), and *Shen Qu* (Massa Medica Fermentata). If the patient is bleeding, add *San Qi* (Notoginseng, Radix), *Fu Ling Gan* (Terra Flava Usta), and *E Jiao* (Asini, Gelatinum Corii). If the patient is losing protein, add *Huang Qi* (Astragali Membranacei, Radix), *Dang Shen* (Codonopsitis Pilosulae, Radix), and *Chi Xiao Dou* (Phaseoli Calcarati, Semen).

ACUMOXIBUSTION: Choose points to needle from *Yin Ling Quan* (Sp 9), *Fu Liu* (Ki 7), *Zhong Ji* (CV 3), and *Pang Guang Shu* (Bl 28). Choose points to moxa from *Pi Shu* (Bl 20), *Shen Shu* (Bl 23), *Da Chang Shu* (Bl 25), *Ming Men* (GV 4), *Tai Bai* (Sp 3), *Tai Xi* (Ki 3), *San Yin Jiao* (Sp 6), *Zu San Li* (St 36), *Guan Yuan* (CV 4), *Qi Hai* (CV 6), *Zhong Wan* (CV 12), and *Tian Shu* (St 25).

Case history of Dr. Pei Zhang: Wang, a 35 year-old female worker[3]

Wang had repeatedly recurring edema for four years for which she had been admitted to the hospital twice. Two months prior to her first visit, her face became edematous. She also had abdominal distention, lack of appetite, and loose stool. Her urinalysis showed her urine protein at 3+, with a few RBCs, a few granular casts, BUN at 56mg%, Cr at 3mg%. Her tongue was covered with thick, white, slimy fur, and her pulse was slow and deep. Based on these signs and symptoms: Dr. Pei's pattern identification was spleen yang vacuity with water accumulation. His treatment strategy was to warm yang and transform damp. His formula was modified *Shi Pi Yin* (Bolster the Spleen Beverage) and *Si Ling San* (Four

[Ingredients] Poria Powder): *Shu Fu Zi* (Aconiti Carmichaeli, Radix Lateralis Praeparatus), 10g, *Bai Zhu* (Atractylodis Macrocephalae, Rhizoma), 10g, *Da Fu Pi* (Arecae Catechu, Pericarpium), 15g, *Rou Dou Kou* (Myristicae Fragrantis, Semen), 10g, *Fu Ling Pi* (Poriae Cocos, Cortex Sclerotii), 30g, *Zhu Ling* (Polypori Umbellati, Sclerotium), 10g, *Ze Xie* (Alismatis Orientalis, Rhizoma), 10g, *Yi Mu Cao* (Leonuri Heterophylli, Herba), 30g, *Tu Si Zi* (Cuscutae Chinensis, Semen), 10g, and *Fu Pen Zi* (Rubi Chingii, Fructus), 30g. Dr. Pei also recommended a low salt diet.

After Wang took this formula, her edema and abdominal distention decreased. Therefore, she continued taking the formula for 50 days and all her blood analyses returned to normal. Then Dr. Pei prescribed modified *Shen Ling Bai Zhu San* (Ginseng, Poria & Atractylodes Powder) to be taken for a half a year to consolidate the results. Wang took this formula and completely recovered.

Case history of Dr. Sun Mo-zheng: Zheng, a 12 year-old female[4]

Zheng's first visit was in May 1984. She had been diagnosed with nephrotic syndrome a year and a half earlier. She had been hospitalized for a few months and was given hormone therapy. The hormones made her very fat but did not improve her condition. A week after she stopped hormone therapy, she had a urinalysis that showed her protein at 2+, with a few RBCs. When she came to see Dr. Sun, Zheng's face and whole body were edematous. She had lack of appetite and thirst, nausea, abdominal distention, wheezing that was worse upon exertion, scanty urination, and loose stools a few times a day. Dr. Sun's pattern identification was spleen qi vacuity and qi stagnation, kidney qi vacuity, and kidney nonabsorption of qi. His first treatment strategy was to open the lung, descend the qi, and harmonize the water passageways. His formula consisted of: *Zi Su Ye* (Perillae Frutescentis, Folium), 6g, *Mu Dan Pi* (Moutan, Cortex Radicis), 8g, *Chan Tui* (Cicadae, Periostracum), 3g, *Huang Qi* (Astragali Membranacei, Radix), 18g, *Shan Yao* (Radix Dioscoreae Oppositae), 15g, *Fu Ling* (Poriae Cocos, Sclerotium), 10g, *Yi Mu Cao* (Leonuri Heterophylli,

Herba), 12g, *Che Qian Cao* (Plantaginis, Herba), 2 pieces, *Ze Xie* (Alismatis Orientalis, Rhizoma), 10g, and *Fu Ping* (Lemnae Seu Spirodelae, Herba), 10g.

By May 18, Zheng's second visit, she had taken the formula for three days. Her facial edema had dissipated but her abdomen was still quite edematous. Her appetite was better, but she still had stomach bloating and nausea. She also had blurred vision and asthma. Dr. Sun decided to modify the formula by adding *Dang Gui Wei* (Angelicae Sinensis, Extremitas Radicis), 6g, in order to quicken the blood and transform stasis. Zheng took this new formula for three more days, but, on May 31, her third visit, her appetite was still not good and her urination became profuse. Urinalysis showed a little protein and a few RBCs. Dr. Sun decided to change the treatment strategy to open the lung and supplement the kidney. His formula consisted of: *Huang Qi* (Astragali Membranacei, Radix), 12g, *Shu Di Huang* (Rehmanniae Glutinosae, cooked Radix), 18g, *Niu Xi* (Achyranthis Bidentatae, Radix), 10g, *Chen Pi* (Citri Reticulatae, Pericarpium), 3g, *Yi Mu Cao* (Leonuri Heterophylli, Herba), 12g, *Zi Su Ye* (Perillae Frutescentis, Folium), 5g, *Shan Yao* (Radix Dioscoreae Oppositae), 18g, *Tu Si Zi* (Cuscutae Chinensis, Semen), 9g, and *Fu Ling* (Poriae Cocos, Sclerotium), 10g. Zheng took this new formula and started using food therapy to supplement her qi and yang. She drank a soup made of 250g of lamb cooked together with 30g of *Huang Qi* (Astragali Membranacei, Radix) twice a week. After five days, she noticed an improvement in her condition. She continued on this regimen and, in three months, staged a complete recovery. A follow-up visit three years later found no recurrence.

3. COLD DAMPNESS WITH DEPRESSIVE HEAT

SIGNS & SYMPTOMS: Edema, fatigue, a pale facial complexion, dry mouth, thirst, dry stool, feels warm instead of cold, possible red eyes. The tongue is red with thick, yellow fur, and the pulse is fast and slippery.

NOTE: In the beginning, the tongue may have been pale and swollen, but it then becomes slightly red with yellow fur. This is because damp accumulation

has caused depression that produces heat. This depressive heat then combines with the dampness to form damp heat. It is also possible that some of these patients have been given medicinals to warm the interior and transform dampness. These medicinals may have caused excess dryness and heat that have combined with dampness to also create damp heat.

TREATMENT PRINCIPLES: Clear heat and eliminate dampness

REPRESENTATIVE FORMULA: *Ba Zheng San* (Eight [Ingredients] Rectification Powder)

Mu Tong (Akebiae Mutong, Caulis), 9g
Qu Mai (Dianthi, Herba), 9g
Bian Xu (Polygoni Avicularis, Herba), 9g
Hua Shi (Talcum), 6g
Deng Xin Cao (Junci Effusi, Medulla), 9g
Che Qian Zi (Plantaginis, Semen), 9g
Zhi Zi (Gardeniae Jasminoidis, Fructus), 9g
Da Huang (Rhei, Radix Et Rhizoma), 9g
Gan Cao (Glycyrrhizae Uralensis, Radix), 9g
Huang Bai (Phellodendri, Cortex), 9g
Zhi Mu (Anemarrhenae Asphodeloidis, Rhizoma), 9g

ACUMOXIBUSTION: Choose from *He Gu* (LI 4), *Qu Chi* (LI 11), *Pi Shu* (Bl 20), *Shen Shu* (Bl 23), *Pang Guang Shu* (Bl 28), *Wei Zhong* (Bl 40), *Yin Ling Quan* (Sp 9), *Yang Ling Quan* (GB 34), and *Tai Xi* (Ki 3).

Case history of Dr. Zhen Shen-shi: Ling, a 20 year-old female[5]

Ling's face and lower extremities had been edematous for six months. She was admitted to the hospital where Chinese doctors prescribed spleen yang invigorating, damp-transforming formulas such as *Shi Pi Yin* (Bolster the Spleen Beverage), *Wei Ling Tang* (Stomach Poria Decoction), and *Chuan Ze Tang* (Spring Pond Decoction). *Wei Ling Tang* consists of: *Zhu Ling* (Polypori Umbellati, Sclerotium), 9g, *Ze Xie* (Alismatis Orientalis, Rhizoma), 9g, *Bai Zhu* (Atractylodis Macrocephalae, Rhizoma), 9g, *Fu Ling* (Poriae Cocos, Sclerotium), 9g, *Rou Gui* (Cinnamonmi Casiae, Cortex), 6g, *Cang Zhu* (Atractylodis, Rhizoma), 9g, *Hou Po* (Magnoliae

Officinalis, Cortex), 9g, *Chen Pi* (Citri Reticulatae, Pericarpium), 6g, *Gan Cao* (Glycyrrhizae Uralensis, Radix), 3g, *Sheng Jiang* (Zingiberis Officinalis, uncooked Rhizoma), 3g, and *Da Zao* (Zizyphi Jujubae, Fructus), 5 pieces. *Chuan Ze Tang* consists of: *Zhu Ling* (Polypori Umbellati, Sclerotium), 9g, *Ze Xie* (Alismatis Orientalis, Rhizoma), 9g, *Bai Zhu* (Atractylodis Macrocephalae, Rhizoma), 9g, *Fu Ling* (Poriae Cocos, Sclerotium), 9g, *Gui Zhi* (Cinnamomi Cassiae, Ramulus), 9g, *Ren Shen* (Panacis Ginseng, Radix), 4.5g, *Chai Hu* (Bupleuri, Radix), 3g, and *Mai Men Dong* (Ophiopogonis Japonici, Tuber), 4.5g. After using these, Ling's urine output started to increase, going from 500-600ml to 1000-1500ml. After a while, however, her urine output started to decline and her water swelling worsened. Dr. Zhen decided that damp accumulation and stagnation had created damp heat. Accordingly, he changed the formula to a heat-clearing, dampness-percolating formula based on *Ba Zheng San* (Eight [Medicinals] Rectification Powder). After taking this new formula, Ling's urine increased to 1500ml per day and her edema completely dissipated.

COMMENTARY: Dampness is a "hot house." It causes stagnation that engenders and then envelopes heat. In this pattern, cold damp with stagnant heat, cold is the root and heat is the tip. One may treat this pattern in two ways. One may first clear heat, then supplement qi and yang; or one may invigorate yang and clear heat at the same time. For the latter, one may combine formulas such as *Shi Pi Yin* (Bolster the Spleen Beverage) with *Ba Zheng San* (Eight [Medicinals] Rectification Powder). However, if one uses this sort of combination, one must be especially careful with the warming medicinals and adjust the formula according to changes in the pattern.

4. COLD DAMPNESS WITH DAMP HEAT

SIGNS & SYMPTOMS: Edema of the face and lower extremities, a sore or red throat, feeling cold, low back pain, fatigue, low appetite, normal or loose stools, lots of bubbles in the urine. The tongue is pale red with thick, yellow fur, and the pulse is fast.

NOTE: In this pattern, kidney vacuity is often the root. The tip is an external attack on the lung.

Because the true qi is debilitated, it cannot contain the evils in the upper burner and the heat moves down to the kidney.[6] In this case, one must open the lung to drain dampness, "opening a hole in the teapot's lid."[7] The lung governs the qi and is the upper source of the water passageways. When evils inhibit the lung's diffusion and downbearing, this compromises qi transformation in other organs and inhibits urination. When dealing with inhibited urination, it is often not enough to simply disinhibit the urination with bland, dampness-percolating medicinals. One must also diffuse the lung to open the water passageways. Besides opening the lung, one must pay special attention to clearing heat.

TREATMENT PRINCIPLES: Diffuse the lung and resolve exterior wind heat or damp heat, supplement the kidney and transform water

REPRESENTATIVE FORMULA: *Yin Qiao San* (Lonicera & Forsythia Powder) plus *Huang Lian Jie Du Tang* (Coptis Toxin-resolving Decoction) plus *Shen Qi Wan* (Kidney Qi Pills)

Jin Yin Hua (Lonicerae Japonicae, Flos), 9-15g
Lian Qiao (Forsythiae Suspensae, Fructus), 9-15g
Jie Geng (Platycodi Grandiflori, Radix), 3-6g
Niu Bang Zi (Arctii Lappae, Fructus), 9-12g
Bo He (Menthae Haplocalycis, Herba), 3-6g
Dan Dou Chi (Sojae Praeparatus, Semen), 3-6g
Jing Jie (Schizonepetae Tenuifoliae, Herba Seu Flos), 6-9g
Dan Zhu Ye (Lophatheri Gracilis, Herba), 3-6g
fresh *Lu Gen* (Phragmitis Communis, Rhizoma), 15-30g
Gan Cao (Glycyrrhizae Uralensis, Radix), 3-6g
Huang Lian (Coptidis Chinensis, Rhizoma), 6-9g
Huang Qin (Scutellariae Baicalensis, Radix), 6-9g
Huang Bai (Phellodendri, Cortex), 6-9g
Zhi Zi (Gardeniae Jasminoidis, Fructus), 6-9g
Shu Fu Zi (Aconiti Carmichaeli, Radix Lateralis Praeparatus), 3-6g
Rou Gui (Cinnamonmi Casiae, Cortex), 3-6g
Shu Di Huang (Rehmanniae Glutinosae, cooked Radix), 9-12g
Shan Yao (Radix Dioscoreae Oppositae), 9-12g
Shan Zhu Yu (Corni Officinalis, Fructus), 9g
Ze Xie (Alismatis Orientalis, Rhizoma), 9g

Fu Ling (Poriae Cocos, Sclerotium), 9-12g
Mu Dan Pi (Moutan, Cortex Radicis), 9-12g

ACUMOXIBUSTION: Choose from *He Gu* (LI 4), *Qu Chi* (LI 11), *Pi Shu* (Bl 20), *Shen Shu* (Bl 23), *Pang Guang Shu* (Bl 28), *Wei Zhong* (Bl 40), *Zhong Ji* (CV 3), *Yin Ling Quan* (Sp 9), *Yang Ling Quan* (GB 34), and *Tai Xi* (Ki 3).

Case history of Dr. Jing Hua-ye: Chen, a 35 year-old female[8]

Chen was often edematous and urinalysis showed protein in her urine at 1-2+, but there were no RBCs and she did not have hypertension. Chen had a pale facial complexion, low back and knee soreness and limpness, shortness of breath, fatigue, dizziness, and constipation. She had a sore throat once a week. Her tongue was pale red, and her pulse was soggy. Based on these signs and symptoms, Dr. Jing's treatment principles were to supplement the spleen and kidney qi, secure and astringe the kidney essence, clear heat and free the flow of the throat. To this end, he prescribed modified *Liu Wei Di Huang Wan* (Six Flavors Rehmannia Pills): *Huang Qi* (Astragali Membranacei, Radix), 30g, *Cang Zhu* (Atractylodis, Rhizoma), 15g, *Fu Ling* (Poriae Cocos, Sclerotium), 15g, *Hei Da Dou* (Glycines, Semen Atrum), 15g, *Du Zhong* (Eucommiae Ulmoidis, Cortex), 15g, *Jue Chuang* (Rostellulariae Procumbentis, Herba), 15g, *Shan Yao* (Radix Dioscoreae Oppositae), 15g, *Shan Zhu Yu* (Corni Officinalis, Fructus), 10g, *Mu Dan Pi* (Moutan, Cortex Radicis), 10g, *Zhi Mu* (Anemarrhenae Asphodeloidis, Rhizoma), 10g, and *Huang Bai* (Phellodendri, Cortex), 15g.

After taking this formula for 14 days, Chen returned for her second visit. Her appetite was better, she had less fatigue, she no longer had sore throats, but she still had low back and knee soreness. Dr. Jing decided to add *Dang Shen* (Codonopsitis Pilosulae, Radix), 15g, and *Gou Ji* (Cibotii Barometsis, Rhizoma), 15g, to her formula. Chen took this new prescription for 14 days, and, at her third visit, all her symptoms were reduced. Urinalysis showed her urine protein was 1+. Thus, Dr. Jing decided to add *Bu Gu Zhi* (Psoraleae Corylifoliae, Fructus), 9g, and *Tu Si Zi* (Cuscutae Chinensis, Semen), 9g, to her formula. Chen took

this formula for 14 days and returned to see Dr. Jing. Dr. Jinge continued to modify Chen's formula every two weeks for the next six months. Chen's urinalysis returned to normal, but she still had slight edema and low back soreness. Dr. Jinge decided to add *Ze Xie* (Alismatis Orientalis, Rhizoma), 10g, to more strongly percolate dampness. After another six months, all Chen's Western medical tests were normal. She had completely recovered.

CLINICAL TIPS

1. From a Chinese medical perspective, nephrotic syndrome always presents a pattern of cold damp at the tip. However, the root is usually yang and qi vacuity. The kidney is vacuous and loses its securing of the essence. Some patients may also contract damp heat because of yang qi vacuity. In this case, the defensive qi is weak and cannot resist external evils. Nevertheless, this disease may also start with a damp heat contraction that damages the kidney resulting in yang and qi vacuity and loss of essence.

To relate it to Western thought, loss of large amounts of protein through the urine equates to loss of kidney essence. Loss of protein leads to weakened immunity and increased likelihood of bacterial or viral infections exacerbating the nephrotic syndrome. (Note that a microbial infection may lead to nephrotic syndrome in the first place.) This leads to a vicious cycle as described by the Figure 3.2 on the next page.

2. The Chinese medical treatment strategy of NS depends on the patient's personal pattern identification. If the patient shows more vacuity, one should primarily supplement. In cases of repletion, meaning mostly damp heat and toxins, one should begin treatment by clearing the external evils. After dispelling these evils, one may supplement, secure, and astringe. According to Chinese medical thinking, one should never retain or "lock in" evils by employing securing and astringing medicinals before evils have been eliminated. One must be certain the evils have been eliminated, and then cautiously and gradually supplement, secure, and astringe. However, if the patient is extremely vacuous, one may clear and supplement at the same time. The following case history illustrates these points.

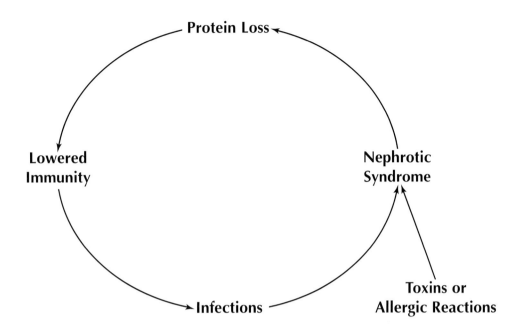

Figure 3.2. Nephrotic syndrome's vicious cycle

Case history from Dr. Wei Li's private practice: Donald, a 52 year-old man

Donald's first visit was on Nov. 11, 2000. He had large amounts of protein in his urine, up to 4+. He was always tired and had chronic urinary tract infections. He also had chronic throat infections. His throat was dry and he was almost always hoarse, even losing his voice at times. Western medical doctors had diagnosed his condition as IgA nephritis with nephrotic syndrome. They gave him Western drugs to improve his kidney function. These seemed to work, and his proteinuria came down to 2+. But the proteinuria leveled off at 2+ and could not be further reduced. His doctors told Donald that his kidneys were going to fail and he needed to start dialysis and contemplate a kidney transplant.

Donald presented with a red tongue with teeth-marks on its edges, and a soggy pulse, with the inch position pulse especially deep. Dr. Li's pattern identification was wind heat and toxins with spleen and kidney qi vacuity. She analyzed the case as follows: There are only two places where IgA exists, in the digestive tract and the respiratory tract. Donald's major symptoms were in the respiratory tract.

Therefore, this must be the place to start. (One theory is that the IgA that the body produces to fight lung infections also attacks the kidney.) She had to completely eliminate the heat and toxins to address the root of the problem. The Western medical therapy had only treated the tip, the kidney function, but did not address the root, the infection. Dr. Li used modified *Yin Qiao San* (Lonicera & Forsythia Powder): *Jin Yin Hua* (Lonicerae Japonicae, Flos), 15g, *Ban Lan Gen* (Isatidis Seu Baphicacanthi, Radix), 10g, *Lian Qiao* (Forsythiae Suspensae, Fructus), 10g, *Huang Lian* (Coptidis Chinensis, Rhizoma), 6g, *Mai Men Dong* (Ophiopogonis Japonici, Tuber), 10g, *Xuan Shen* (Scrophulariae Ningpoensis, Radix), 6g, and *Sheng Di Huang* (Rehmanniae Glutinosae, uncooked Radix), 9g. In this formula, *Jin Yin Hua* and *Lian Qiao* clear defensive aspect heat. With *Ban Lan Gen*, they resolve toxins. *Huang Lian* clears qi aspect heat. *Sheng Di Huang* and *Xuan Shen* clear constructive and blood aspect heat. With *Mai Men Dong*, they preserve the yin. Dr. Li also employed acupuncture to boost the qi as well as to assist clearing heat and resolving toxins. She chose the following points: *He Gu* (LI 4), *Lie Que* (Lu 7), *Qu Chi* (LI 11), *San Yin Jiao* (Sp 6), *Zu San Li* (St 36), and *Tai Xi* (Ki 3).

After four weeks, Donald's protein urinalyses were usually negative, with just an occasional trace. His tongue and pulse were basically normal. In other words, his tongue was pink with thin, white fur, and his pulse was bowstring but not too forceful, perhaps a little weak at times. Donald felt good, had more energy, and no longer had a hoarse voice. Dr. Li considered this a clinical cure. A Western biopsy would be needed to declare Donald totally cured, but the patient did not feel a need to do this. Since the evils had been cleared, Dr. Li started supplementing with *Zhi Bai Di Huang Wan* (Anemarrhena & Phellodendron Rehmannia Pills): *Huang Bai* (Phellodendri, Cortex), 9g, *Zhi Mu* (Anemarrhenae Asphodeloidis, Rhizoma), 9g, *Sheng Di Huang* (Rehmanniae Glutinosae, uncooked Radix), 12g, *Shan Zhu Yu* (Corni Officinalis, Fructus), 12g, *Shan Yao* (Radix Dioscoreae Oppositae), 12g, *Fu Ling* (Poriae Cocos, Sclerotium), 9g, *Ze Xie* (Alismatis Orientalis, Rhizoma), 9g, and *Mu Dan Pi* (Moutan, Cortex Radicis), 9g. After Donald took this formula for three months, Dr. Li reviewed the formula and added qi and yang supplements as needed.

3. The root pattern of nephrotic syndrome is qi and yang vacuity and thus supplementing qi and yang must be part of any treatment strategy. The best single medicinal for supplementing qi in nephrotic syndrome is *Huang Qi* (Astragali Membranacei, Radix). For yang vacuity, the best single medicinal is *Zi He Che* (Hominis, Placenta). This may be added to the formulas that are typically used: *You Gui Wan* (Restore the Right [Kidney] Pills) or *You Gui Yin* (Restore the Right [Kidney] Beverage).

4. Profuse urination can be a species of loss of essence. In this case, one must use the treatment principles of securing and astringing. In order to accomplish this, one may use the following:

A. Apply nine grams of powdered *Wu Bei Zi* (Rhois Chinensis, Galla) mixed with vinegar, or saliva mixed with water, to (Ki 1) or *Qi Zhong* (CV 8).

B. Ingest two grams of calcined *Wu Mei* (Pruni Mume, Fructus) powder per day.

C. Ingest nine grams each of *Fu Pen Zi* (Rubi

Chingii, Fructus), *Sang Shen* (Mori Albi, Fructus), *Mu Li* (Ostreae, Concha), etc. per day.

5. The kidney is the source of former heaven qi, while the spleen is the source of latter heaven qi, and former and latter heavens are mutually engendering and bolstering. Therefore, when supplementing the qi, it is necessary for the middle burner to function properly to absorb the finest essence of the grain qi, and harmonizing the middle burner insures that this finest essence can be absorbed, transformed, and moved. The major medicinals for supplementing and harmonizing the middle burner are *Ren Shen* (Panascis Ginseng, Radix), *Dang Shen* (Codonopsitis Pilosulae, Radix), *Bai Zhu* (Atractylodis Macrocephalae, Rhizoma), *Sheng Jiang* (Zingiberis Officinalis, uncooked Rhizoma), *Shan Yao* (Radix Dioscoreae Oppositae), *Da Zao* (Zizyphi Jujubae, Fructus), and *Gan Cao* (Glycyrrhizae Uralensis, Radix). The most common formulas are *Shen Ling Bai Zhu San* (Ginseng, Poria & Atractylodes Powder) and *Si Jun Zi Tang* (Four Gentlemen Decoction). *Shen Ling Bai Zhu San* (Ginseng, Poria & Atractylodes Powder) consists of:

Ren Shen (Panacis Ginseng, Radix), 9g, *Bai Zhu* (Atractylodis Macrocephalae, Rhizoma), 9g, *Fu Ling* (Poriae Cocos, Sclerotium), 9g, mix-fried *Gan Cao* (Glycyrrhizae Uralensis, Radix), 3g, *Shan Yao* (Radix Dioscoreae Oppositae), 9g, *Bai Bian Dou* (Dolichoris Lablab, Semen), 9g, *Lian Zi* (Nelumbinis Nuciferae, Semen), 9g, *Yi Yi Ren* (Coicis Lachryma-jobi, Semen), 9g, *Sha Ren* (Amomi, Fructus), 3g, and *Jie Geng* (Platycodi Grandiflori, Radix), 6g. *Si Jun Zi Tang* consists of: *Ren Shen* (Panacis Ginseng, Radix), 9g, *Bai Zhu* (Atractylodis Macrocephalae, Rhizoma), 9g, *Fu Ling* (Poriae Cocos, Sclerotium), 9g, and mix-fried *Gan Cao* (Glycyrrhizae Uralensis, Radix), 3g.

6. In nephrotic syndrome, replenishing the essence is generally achieved through food therapy, especially by eating more animal protein, such as meat and eggs. Seafood should be avoided. (Seafood is *fa wu*, *i.e.*, emitting substances which are thought to make diseases recur.) The patient can follow a high animal protein diet unless renal failure develops.

7. In NS, one should use yin-supplementing medicinals with caution. These enriching, cool medicinals can exacerbate dampness and cold, leading to more qi and yang vacuity.

8. Use water-disinhibiting, dampness-percolating medicinals, water-expelling medicinals, dampness-dispelling formulas, and water-expelling formulas appropriately. These formulas are usually divided into three levels. The drastic water-expelling formulas are the strongest. One should not use the strongest ones when initially treating nephrotic syndrome. One must always supplement qi and yang as well as disinhibit water. (This strategy is significantly different than the Western approach.) For nephrotic syndrome, one usually starts with a mildly draining formula such as *Wu Ling San* (Five [Ingredients] Poria Powder). If this does not work well, one may try the second level, moderate to strongly draining formulas, such as *Zhen Wu Tang* (True Warrior Decoction) and *Shi Pi Yin* (Bolster the Spleen Beverage). If these are not strong enough, one may add one of the drastic formulas, *Shi Zao Tang* (Ten Dates Decoction), *Kong Xian Dan* (Drool-controlling Elixir), or *Zhou Che Wan* (Vessel & Vehicle Pills) to the moderate formulas. These formulas, which should be appropriately modified, are as follows:

Wu Ling San: *Ze Xie* (Alismatis Orientalis, Rhizoma), 9g, *Fu Ling* (Poriae Cocos, Sclerotium), 9g, *Zhu Ling* (Polypori Umbellati, Sclerotium), 9g, *Bai Zhu* (Atractylodis Macrocephalae, Rhizoma), 9g, and *Gui Zhi* (Cinnamomi Cassiae, Ramulus), 6g

Zhen Wu Tang: *Shu Fu Zi* (Aconiti Carmichaeli, Radix Lateralis Praeparatus), 9g, *Bai Zhu* (Atractylodis Macrocephalae, Rhizoma), 6g, *Fu Ling* (Poriae Cocos, Sclerotium), 9g, *Bai Shao* (Paeoniae Lactiflorae, Radix Albus), 9g, and *Sheng Jiang* (Zingiberis Officinalis, uncooked Rhizoma), 9g

Shi Pi Yin: *Shu Fu Zi* (Aconiti Carmichaeli, Radix Lateralis Praeparatus), 3g, *Gan Jiang* (Zingiberis Officinalis, dry Rhizoma), 3g, *Fu Ling* (Poriae Cocos, Sclerotium), 6g, *Bai Zhu* (Atractylodis Macrocephalae, Rhizoma), 9g, *Mu Gua* (Chaenomelis Lagenariae, Fructus), 6g, *Hou Po* (Magnoliae Officinalis, Cortex), 6g, *Mu Xiang* (Aucklandiae Lappae, Radix), 3g, *Da Fu Pi* (Arecae Catechu, Pericarpium), 9g, *Cao Guo* (Amomi Tsao-ko, Fructus), 3g, mix-fried *Gan Cao* (Glycyrrhizae Uralensis, Radix), 3g, *Sheng Jiang* (Zingiberis Officinalis, uncooked Rhizoma), 3g, *Da Zao* (Zizyphi Jujubae, Fructus), 5 piece

Shi Zao Tang: *Gan Sui* (Euphorbiae Kansui, Radix), 0.2-0.3g, *Jing Da Ji* (Euphorbiae Seu Knoxiae, Radix), 0.2-0.3g, *Yuan Hua* (Daphnis Genkwae, Flos), 0.2-0.3g, and *Da Zao* (Zizyphi Jujubae, Fructus), 10 pieces. Grind the first three ingredients into powder and take with a decoction made from the last ingredient

Kong Xian Dan: *Gan Sui* (Euphorbiae Kansui, Radix), 9g, *Da Ji* (Cirsii Japonici, Herba Seu Radix), 9g, *Bai Jie Zi* (Sinapis Albae, Semen), 9g. These three medicinals are ground to a powder and made into small pills. The pills are taken at 0.2g twice a day after meals

Zhou Che Wan: *Gan Sui* (Euphorbiae Kansui, Radix), 30g, *Yuan Hua* (Daphnis Genkwae, Flos), 30g, *Jing Da Ji* (Euphorbiae Seu Knoxiae, Radix), 30g, *Qian Niu Zi* (Pharbitidis, Semen), 120g, *Da Huang* (Rhei, Radix Et Rhizoma), 60g, *Qing Pi* (Citri Reticulatae Viride, Pericarpium), 15g, *Chen Pi* (Citri Reticulatae, Pericarpium), 15g, *Bin Lan* (Arecae Catechu, Semen), 15g, *Mu Xiang* (Aucklandiae Lappae, Radix), 15g, and *Qing Fen* (Calomelas), 3g. Grind into a powder and take a 3-6 gram dose. This should only be done once the patient has regained their strength or remains strong

CAUTION: When using the drastic formulas one must be very cautious and observe the following:

A. One should not use these formulas alone. These drastic formulas are extremely draining and one must be sure to support the righteous at the same time. One should combine a drastic formula with a formula that strengthens the spleen and kidney, such as *Zhen Wu Tang* (True Warrior Decoction), *Shi Pi Yin* (Bolster the Spleen Beverage), etc.

B. One must start with a small dosage of these formulas and be careful with the toxic medicinals.

C. What has been described in the ancient literature as "stone water" is probably not a kidney disease. It most likely equates to liver cirrhosis or the effects of an abdominal tumor. In kidney diseases, edema starts on the extremities and the face. Stone water starts in the abdomen or just affects the abdomen because it is due to portal vein obstruction caused by cirrhosis or a tumor. When treating stone water, *i.e.*, ascites, one must be careful using the moderate to strongly draining formulas, and one should not use the drastic formulas unless one has had vast experience with them. The danger lies in draining the abdominal water too quickly. This may reduce blood pressure suddenly, leading to heart failure and death. Even if it does not lead to heart failure, the patient's health may still be at risk from drastic draining. To reiterate, one must be especially careful using the draining method with stone water.

D. Edema may also be due to heart failure. For patients with heart disease who are edematous, one should use only the mildly draining formulas. The second level formulas contain *Fu Zi* (Aconiti Carmichaeli, Radix Lateralis Praeparatus). *Fu Zi* can increase the strength of the heartbeat and may conflict with Western heart-strengthening drugs. *Fu Zi* may also cause toxic reactions or make it difficult to control other drug dosages. Mildly draining formulas do not cause these problems. Drastic formulas are absolutely forbidden.

E. Even when edema is due to a kidney disease, one must be especially careful if there is renal failure. All the formulas listed above are popularly used for kidney diseases, but, in renal failure, the kidney function is especially low. Normally, there are two ways in which medicinals and drugs are metabolized and excreted—either via the liver through the stool or via the kidney through the urine. In renal failure, the kidney metabolizes medicinals only very slowly. If certain medicinals are metabolized in the liver, they can still exit normally by the stool. But if they have to be metabolized and excreted via the kidney and urine, they will build up quickly when the kidney function is low. Therefore, what may otherwise be normal dosages of medicinals may become toxic because they are not metabolized and excreted.

F. Even when the patient has recovered and the edema has completely dissipated, one should still use dampness-dispelling formulas. One can use a formula that is milder than the initial one and have the patient continue on it for 1-2 weeks. Then one should follow up with a formula like *Shen Qi Wan* (Kidney Qi Pills) for 2-3 months to build up yin and yang. This will consolidate the results and prevent recurrences.

9. Blood is the mother of the qi, and qi is the commander of blood. Therefore, it follows that qi vacuity may cause blood stasis. Hence, when one supplements the qi, one should add some stasis-dispelling, blood-quickening medicinals, such as *Chi Shao* (Paeoniae Lactiflorae, Radix Rubrus), *Hong Hua* (Carthami Tinctorii, Flos), *Dang Gui* (Angelicae Sinensis, Radix), *Chuan Xiong* (Ligustici Wallichii, Radix), and *Dan Shen* (Salvia Miltiorrhizae, Radix). These medicinals should be added only in small dosages because dispelling stasis is an attacking therapy and dispelling stasis too strongly can further weaken the qi. One can start with one-third the normal dosage. Stasis-dispelling, blood-quickening medicinals are contraindicated when first treating patients with severe qi vacuity to prevent dangerously depleting the qi.

10. There are four types of primary nephrotic syndrome patients who come to Chinese medicine. 1) Patients whose symptoms include severe edema, low appetite, poor digestion, low energy, and insomnia and are not being treated with Western medicine. These patients use Chinese medicine to improve their general health, including improving their appetite, digestion, and sleep, before employing Western hormone therapy. 2) Patients who have tried Western hormone therapy but whose conditions have not improved. 3) Patients who have responded to Western hormone therapy but whose symptoms start to recur when they start to withdraw from the therapy or after they stop the therapy. 4) Patients who have undesirable side effects from Western hormone therapy. (Please see Chart 3.1.) Chinese medical practitioners usually treat type 2, 3, and 4 patients.

Type 1	Not on Western therapy
Type 2	Have tried Western hormone therapy but have not improved
Type 3	Have responded to Western therapy but have symptoms recur during or after withdrawl
Type 4	Have undesirable side effects from Western hormone therapy

Chart 3.1. Four types of NS patients who come to Chinese medicine

Usually, NS patients see a Western physician before coming to a Chinese medical practitioner and, in that case, Chinese medicine is used as an adjunctive therapy. It is important that such patients have a clear Western medical diagnosis. A Western medical diagnosis based on Western medical tests can help the Chinese practitioner judge patients' progress. In addition, some Western medical treatment is efficacious. Nephrotic syndrome is a serious disease, and it is incumbent upon the Chinese practitioner to make patients feel confident they have not overlooked anything; that they have the best diagnosis, lab work, treatment, and medicine. The Chinese practitioner must be pragmatic and remain open to all treatment options.

11. Chinese medical treatment for nephrotic syndrome takes a significant amount of time to effect a cure. A reasonable estimate is from a minimum of three months to over a year. Although the course is long, the results of Chinese medical treatment are very stable.

ENDNOTES

[1] *Shui Zhong Guan Ge Jun* (*Water Swelling and Block & Repulsion*, Volume 2), Chinese Medicine Publishing Company, Beijing, 1998, p. 46
[2] *Ibid.*, p. 176
[3] *Ibid.*, p. 128
[4] *Ibid.*, p. 192
[5] *Ibid.*, p. 71
[6] In classical literature, when cold is the exogenous attacking evil, this is called "lung cold moves to the kidney" (*fei yi han yu shen*). However, there is no reason that this mechanism must be limited to cold, and in our experience, lung heat may also move to the kidney.
[7] This metaphor refers to boring a hole in a teapot's lid in order to allow tea to pour out of a teapot unobstructed. "Opening a hole in a teapot's lid" is also called "raising the pot and removing the lid" (*ti hu jie gai fa*).
[8] *Shui Zhong Guan Ge Jun* (*Water Swelling and Block & Repulsion*, Volume 2), *op. cit.*, p. 41

Nephritis means inflammation of the kidney. Such inflammation may be caused by bacteria or their toxins, autoimmune disorders, or toxic chemicals. Acute nephritis is also known as acute glomerulonephritis (AGN) and is one of the diseases which may result in nephrotic syndrome. It refers to a specific set of renal diseases in which an immunologic mechanism triggers inflammation and proliferation of glomerular tissue. This condition is characterized by an abrupt onset of hematuria and proteinuria. The patient classically experiences pruritis, edema, nausea, constipation, hypertension, and oliguria.

NOSOLOGY

Acute glomerulonephritis may be subcategorized as degenerative, diffuse, suppurative, hemorrhagic, interstitial, or parenchymal depending on the portion of the kidney involved.

EPIDEMIOLOGY

Glomerulonephritis represents 10-15% of glomerular diseases. Variable incidence has been reported due, in part, to the subclinical nature of the disease in more than one-half the affected population. Despite sporadic outbreaks, with the widespread use of antibiotics, the incidence of post-streptococcal glomerulonephritis (PSGN) has fallen over the last few decades. Other factors responsible for this decline may include better health care delivery and improved socioeconomic conditions. However, AGN remains a common disorder in regions of Africa, the Caribbean, India, and South America. This disease is more common in children over the age of three, with most sufferers being between 5-15 years of age. Only 10% of AGN sufferers are over 40 years old. It is also more common in males than females at a ratio of 2:1.

ETIOLOGY & PATHOPHYSIOLOGY

Causes of acute glomerulonephritis include postinfectious, renal, and systemic etiologies. The most common cause is postinfectious *Streptococcus* species (*i.e.*, group A, beta-hemolytic). Post-streptococcal nephritis due to an upper respiratory infection occurs primarily in the winter months, and post-streptococcal nephritis due to a skin infection is usually observed in the summer and fall and is more prevalent in southern regions of the U.S. Other bacterial causes include diplococcal, staphylococcal, or mycobacterial. *Salmonella typhosa*, *Brucella suis*, *Treponema pallidum*, *Corynebacterium bovis*, and *actinobacilli* also have been identified. Other specific agents include viruses and parasites, visceral abscesses, endocarditis, infected grafts or shunts, and pneumonia. However, cytomegalovirus, coxsackievirus, Epstein-Barr virus, hepatitis B, rubella, rickettsial scrub typhus, and mumps are accepted as viral causes only if it can be documented that a recent group A beta-hemolytic streptococcal infection did not occur. Similarly, attributing glomerulonephritis to a parasitic or fungal etiology requires the exclusion of a streptococcal infection. Identified organisms include *Coccidioides immitis* and the following parasites: *Plasmodium malariae*, *Plasmodium falciparum*, *Schistosoma mansoni*, *Toxoplasma gondii*, filariasis, trichinosis, and trypanosomes.

As for systemic causes, Wegener granulomatosis causes glomerulonephritis that combines upper and lower granulomatous nephritises. Hypersensitivity vasculitis encompasses a heterogeneous group of disorders featuring small vessel and skin disease, while cryoglobulinemia causes abnormal quantities of cryoglobulin in plasma that result in repeated episodes of widespread purpura and cutaneous ulcerations upon crystallization. Systemic lupus erythematous causes glomerulonephritis through renal deposition of immune complexes, and polyarteritis nodosa causes nephritis from a vasculitis involving the renal arteries. Henoch-Schönlein purpura causes a generalized vasculitis resulting in glomerulonephritis. Goodpasture syndrome causes circulating antibodies to type IV collagen and often results in a rapidly progressive oliguric renal failure (weeks to months). Recent studies also indicate the possibility of AGN due to reactions to vaccines.

There are also several renal diseases which may result in AGN. For instance, membranoproliferative glomerulonephritis is due to the expansion and proliferation of mesangial cells as a consequence of the deposition of complements. Berger disease (IgG-immunoglobulin A [IgA] nephropathy) glomerulonephritis results from a diffuse mesangial deposition of IgA and IgG, while idiopathic rapidly progressive glomerulonephritis is a form of glomerulonephritis characterized by the presence of glomeru-

lar crescents. Three types have been distinguished. Type I is an antiglomerular basement membrane disease, type II is mediated by immune complexes, and type III is identified by antineutrophil cytoplasmic antibody. It is believed that poor diet and food sensitivities play a role in the mechanism and onset of these diseases.

RISK FACTORS

Post-streptococcal glomerulonephritis is more likely to develop in environments of overcrowding and poor hygiene. It may also develop secondarily to untreated skin conditions such as scabies.

SYMPTOMATOLOGY

The onset of symptoms in AGN is typically abrupt. Initial signs may include puffiness of the eyelids and facial edema. The urine is usually dark and scanty, and blood pressure is elevated. There is usually a latent period of 1-3 weeks from infection to the development of acute nephritis. If AGN occurs within four days of infection, this indicates a prior renal disease. Other symptoms include fever, malaise, headache and nausea. With children, gross hematuria may be seen. Shortness of breath and dyspnea on exertion may be seen in adults, but are less common in children. Patients with worsening hypertension may present with marked confusion. Costovertebral tenderness is common on palpation.

DIAGNOSIS

The Western medical diagnosis of AGN is based on the patient's history, signs and symptoms, and urine analysis. It is essential in making a diagnosis of AGN to determine any recent history of streptococcal infection. Questions should also be asked regarding any recent history of fatigue, headache, anorexia, and fever. Hypertensive retinopathy revealed by opthalmoscopy may also be present. However, urine analysis (UA), both macro- and microscopic examination, provides the best indications of AGN. Gross hematuria may be present. Although RBC casts are the "classic" finding for AGN, they are actually only rarely seen. It is more common to spot large numbers of hyaline and granular casts and WBCs. Increased protein may be excreted. Blood testing may reveal elevated BUN and creatinine and mild, normochromic anemia. Antistreptolysin O (ASO) titer may be elevated. It usually rises in weeks one and two following infection. Ultrasound may be useful in distinguishing enlarged (acute) from shrunken (chronic) kidney disease.

DIFFERENTIAL DIAGNOSIS

As previously mentioned, PSGN should develop at least 1-3 weeks following an infection. If it develops at the same time as a sore throat, pharyngitis, or skin rash, there is greater likelihood of a pre-existing renal condition. Diagnosis should focus on underlying conditions, whether infectious, autoimmune, or renal.

Angioedema
Guillain-Barré syndrome
Hypertensive emergencies
Impetigo
Necrotizing fasciitis
Pediatrics, fever
Pediatrics, pharyngitis
Pharyngitis
Renal failure, acute
Rheumatic fever
Scarlet fever
Serum sickness
Systemic lupus erythematosus
Thrombocytopenic purpura
Transplants, renal

WESTERN MEDICAL TREATMENT

Modern Western medicine has no specific treatment for AGN. Infection is treated with antibiotics, although this does not serve to halt the process of glomerular damage. If there is fluid retention, diuretics or thiazides are used. If there is hypertension, beta-blockers and vasodilators are typically prescribed. Dialysis is indicated in cases of severe renal failure. Body weight is checked daily, and there is careful monitoring of complications such as hypertensive encephalopathy and heart failure. Although Western medicine routinely treats inflammation with corticosteroids, in the case of AGN, such treat-

ment is contraindicated since it may seriously compromise the integrity of the nephrons.

PROGNOSIS & COMPLICATIONS

Acute glomerulonephritis is generally considered a self-limiting illness. Most cases of AGN go unnoticed, and up to 95% will heal completely. Oliguria and heart involvement as well as proteinuria longer than three weeks typically indicate worse outcomes. Children with AGN fare far better than adults. Ultimately, 5-20% of sufferers may develop a progressive disease.

CHINESE MEDICAL DISEASE CATEGORIZATION

In Chinese medicine, the clinical manifestations of acute nephritis correspond to the traditional disease categories of kidney wind, block and repulsion, dribbling urinary block, bloody urine, water swelling, kidney taxation or vacuity taxation and taxation wind, lumbar pain, abdominal distention, and dizziness.

TREATMENT BASED ON PATTERN IDENTIFICATION

In Chinese medicine, acute nephritis is usually caused by a contraction of external evils, *i.e.*, some combination of wind, cold, heat, and/or dampness. Wind is "the spearhead of a thousand diseases," and it often leads other evils into the body. When a contraction of wind is accompanied by edema, it is called "wind water." For this reason, all AGN patterns have "wind water" in their names, *e.g.*, wind water wind heat, wind water wind cold, etc. (Please see Chart 4.1.)

1. WIND WATER WIND HEAT

SIGNS & SYMPTOMS: Chills and fever, sinus congestion with yellow nasal mucus, sore throat, cough, facial and generalized edema, dark, scanty urination, and sore joints. The tongue is red with yellow fur, and the pulse is floating and fast.

	EVILS AND UNDERLYING VACUITY	PATTERN IDENTIFICATIONS
WIND WATER	Wind cold	1. Wind water wind cold
	Wind heat	2. Wind water wind cold
	Wind cold + yang vacuity	3. Wind water wind cold with yang vacuity
	Damp heat	4. Wind water damp heat
	Damp heat + yin vacuity	5. Wind water damp heat with yin vacuity

Chart 4.1. Acute nephritis pattern identification

TREATMENT PRINCIPLES: Course wind, clear heat, and drain water

REPRESENTATIVE FORMULAS: Modified *Yin Qiao San* (Lonicera & Forsythia Powder)

Jin Yin Hua (Lonicerae Japonicae, Flos), 20g
Lian Qiao (Forsythiae Suspensae, Fructus), 15g
Jing Jie (Schizonepetae Tenuifoliae, Herba Seu Flos), 15g
Fu Ping (Lemnae Seu Spirodelae, Herba), 9g
Ban Lan Gen (Isatidis Seu Baphicacanthi, Radix), 15g
Da Qing Ye (Daqingye, Folium), 15g
Shi Gao (Gypsum Fibrosum), 6g
Huang Qin (Scutellariae Baicalensis, Radix), 9g
Che Qian Zi (Plantaginis, Semen), 15g
Bai Mao Gen (Imperatae Cylindricae, Rhizoma), 15g

Modified *Ma Huang Lian Qiao Chi Xiao Dou Tang* (Ephedra, Forsythia & Red Bean Decoction)

Ma Huang (Ephedrae, Herba), 9g
Lian Qiao (Forsythiae Suspensae, Fructus), 15g
Chi Xiao Dou (Phaseoli Calcarati, Semen), 15g
Da Fu Pi (Arecae Catechu, Pericarpium), 9g
Che Qian Cao (Plantaginis, Herba), 15g
Han Fang Ji (Stephaniae Tetrandrae, Radix), 9g
Fu Ling (Poriae Cocos, Sclerotium), 15g
Huang Lian (Coptidis Chinensis, Rhizoma), 9g
Jin Yin Hua (Lonicerae Japonicae, Flos), 15g
Lian Qiao (Forsythiae Suspensae, Fructus), 15g
Ban Lan Gen (Isatidis Seu Baphicacanthi, Radix), 15g
Da Qing Ye (Daqingye, Folium), 15g
Bai Mao Gen (Imperatae Cylindricae, Rhizoma), 15g

Modified *Yue Bi Tang* (Maidservant from Yue Decoction)

Ma Huang (Ephedrae, Herba), 9g
Shi Gao (Gypsum Fibrosum), 48g
Sheng Jiang (Zingiberis Officinalis, uncooked Rhizoma), 9g
Gan Cao (Glycyrrhizae Uralensis, Radix), 6g
Da Zao (Zizyphi Jujubae, Fructus), 10 pieces

ACUMOXIBUSTION: Choose from the following for all types of wind water: *Shui Fen* (Ren 9), *Qi Hai* (Ren 6), *Zhong Ji* (CV 3), *San Jiao Shu* (Bl 22), *Zu San Li* (St 36), *Feng Men* (Bl 12), *Fei Shu* (Bl 13), *Da Zhu* (Bl 11), *Shen Shu* (Bl 23), *Pang Guang Shu* (Bl 28), *Feng Chi* (GB 20), *Wai Guan* (TB 5), *Hu Gu* (LI 4), *Qu Chi* (LI 11), *Chi Ze* (Lu 5), *Lie Que* (Lu 7), *San Yin Jiao* (Sp 6), and *Yin Ling Quan* (Sp 9). For wind heat with high fever, add *Du Zhui* (GV 14) and prick *Shi Xuan* (M-UE-1) to bleed.

Case history 1: Huang, a 12 year-old boy[1]

Huang was diagnosed with acute nephritis. His whole body became edematous after he caught cold and had chills, fever, and sore throat for a week. Urinalysis showed protein 2+ and RBCs 2+. Granular cast was 0-1. Huang was referred to a Chinese medical clinic for treatment, and his first visit was in April 1980. His presenting symptoms were fever without sweating, sore throat, generalized edema, yellow, scanty urination, and constipation. His tongue was covered with thin, yellow, slimy fur, and his pulse was floating and fast. The Chinese medical diagnosis was wind heat kidney wind. The treatment strategy was to clear and diffuse the lung, transform water and drain dampness. The prescription was *Ma Huang Lian Qiao Chi Xiao Dou Tang* (Ephedra, Forsythia & Red Bean Decoction) plus *Huang Lian Jie Du Tang* (Coptis Toxin-Resolving Decoction) with modifications: *Ma Huang*

(Ephedrae, Herba), 10g, *Lian Qiao* (Forsythiae Suspensae, Fructus), 20g, *Sang Bai Pi* (Mori Albi, Cortex Radicis), 20g, *Xing Ren* (Pruni Armeniacae, Semen), 8g, *Huang Qin* (Scutellariae Baicalensis, Radix), 10g, *Zhi Zi* (Gardeniae Jasminoidis, Fructus), 10g, *Da Huang* (Rhei, Radix Et Rhizoma), 5g, *Jie Geng* (Platycodi Grandiflori, Radix), 15g, *Bo He* (Menthae Haplocalycis, Herba), 10g, *Sheng Gan Cao* (Glycyrrhizae Uralensis, Radix), 8g, and *Chi Xiao Dou* (Phaseoli Calcarati, Semen), 20g.

After two days, Huang experienced a proper sweat[2] and his fever broke. He was able to pass more urine, the edema greatly decreased, and his constipation abated. His doctor then removed *Da Huang* from Huang's prescription, and, after taking this new prescription for two more days, the edema completely dissipated. His doctor then gave him a different prescription to harmonize the middle burner and clear heat. Huang took this for another three weeks and had a complete recovery.

Case history 2: Sun, a 10 year-old boy[3]

Prior to Sun's first visit in May 1977, he contracted mumps and had a sore throat for eight days. When the facial swelling had almost disappeared, his face suddenly became edematous and pitting edema spread throughout his entire body. Urinalysis showed protein 3+, RBCs 4+. Sun presented with fever, thirst, headache, and low back pain. His urine was scanty and colored like red tea. His tongue was red with yellow, slimy fur, and his pulse was slippery and fast. The Chinese medical diagnosis was wind, heat, and dampness kidney wind. The treatment principles were to clear heat and resolve toxins, cool the blood and eliminate dampness. The prescription was modified *Qing Shen Xiao Du Yin* (Kidney-clearing, Toxin-dispersing Beverage). A one-day dose consisted of: *Lian Qiao* (Forsythiae Suspensae, Fructus), 20g, *Zhi Zi* (Gardeniae Jasminoidis, Fructus), 10g, *Huang Bai* (Phellodendri, Cortex), 10g, *Da Qing Ye* (Daqingye, Folium), 15g, *Jin Yin Hua* (Lonicerae Japonicae, Flos), 20g, *Sheng Di Huang* (Rehmanniae Glutinosae, uncooked Radix), 15g, *Mu Dan Pi* (Moutan, Cortex Radicis), 10g, and *Xiao Ji* (Cephalanoplos Segeti, Herba), 15g. Sun took this

prescription for three days and had a slight, proper sweat. After this, his urination and defecation returned to normal and his edema greatly dissipated. After six days of this formula, his edema had completely disappeared. He was given a new prescription to clear heat and eliminate dampness. He took this formula for three weeks and completely recovered. Subsequent urinalyses were normal.

COMMENTARY: Zhu Dan-xi, in his *Dan Xi Xin Fa (Dan-xi's Heart Methods)*, stated that symptoms of whole body water swelling, heat effusion, and aversion to cold, sore throat, cough, thirst, vexation, dark, scanty urination, and constipation indicate yang water. In yang water, external wind and internal damp heat damage both the lung and kidney. Wind attacks and constrains the lung, obstructing the lung's functions of diffusing and depurative downbearing and impairing its regulation of the water passageways. Water accumulates, becomes water swelling, and inhibits kidney qi transformation. Wind and damp heat block the triple burner causing additional water accumulation.

When there is wind, heat, and dampness, one must deal with three evils. In this case, water or dampness is the result of wind heat and is the tip. The root is wind heat. When wind and heat combine, one must focus on heat. Heat is the first concern, wind second, and dampness third. Heat can stir wind, but wind can also stir or fan heat (as when wind fans up a forest fire). Wind can fan heat even if there is only slight heat or depressed heat. Therefore, while one must focus on heat, one must also address wind to prevent it from fanning heat.

One must also "stay ahead" of the penetration of heat into the four aspects. Heat can move into deeper aspects quickly, causing toxins. When using medicinals that clear heat, one must prescribe them according to the aspect the heat has entered and then also add some medicinals for the next deepest aspect. For the defensive aspect, one should employ acrid, cool, exterior-resolving medicinals plus certain heat-clearing medicinals such as *Jin Yin Hua* (Lonicerae Japonicae, Flos), *Lian Qiao* (Forsythiae Suspensae, Fructus), *Ban Lan Gen* (Isatidis Seu Baphicacanthi, Radix), *Da Qing Ye* (Daqingye,

Folium), and *Niu Bang Zi* (Arctii Lappae, Fructus). For the qi aspect with symptoms and signs such as a big pulse, high fever, profuse sweating, and great thirst, one should use medicinals such as *Huang Lian* (Coptidis Chinensis, Rhizoma), *Huang Qin* (Scutellariae Baicalensis, Radix), and *Huang Bai* (Phellodendri, Cortex). For the yin or blood aspect, when there is blood in the urine, one should add medicinals such as *Mu Dan Pi* (Moutan, Cortex Radicis), *Sheng Di Huang* (Rehmanniae Glutinosae, uncooked Radix), *Chi Shao* (Paeoniae Lactiflorae, Radix Rubrus), and *Dan Shen* (Salvia Miltiorrhizae, Radix).

If one is using blood-stanching medicinals, one must remember to also quicken the blood to prevent stasis. One must also choose those medicinals with the proper temperature. Here one is treating heat. So one should use cool blood-stanching medicinals. According to Chinese medical theory, this is called straight or correct treatment. In other words, a heat pattern is treated with cold medicinals and vice versa.

When coursing wind in wind water with edema, one often uses acrid, warm, exterior-resolving medicinals. This has to do with the nature of dampness and water. These are both yin evils associated with cold. Therefore, one must use warm medicinals to overcome their cold nature. Cold medicinals tend to reinforce water's cold and congealing nature. If one must use many cold medicinals to clear heat, one must add some warm medicinals to overcome this tendency.

It may seem that the medicinals needed to clear wind heat and those needed to eliminate dampness will interfere with each other. Properly used, however, warm medicinals need not compromise cold medicinals' effects. In fact, they may balance each other as in *Ma Huang Lian Qiao Chi Xiao Dou Tang* (Ephedra, Forsythia & Red Bean Decoction). In this ancient formula, *Ma Huang* (Ephedrae, Herba) is warm and balances the effects of cold *Lian Qiao* (Forsythiae Suspensae, Fructus).

After the symptoms have subsided and one is sure the wind, heat, and dampness have been eliminated, one must harmonize the lung, spleen, and kidney.

This includes supplementing the lung, spleen, and kidney to strengthen their ability to govern and transform water, supplementing the kidney to secure former heaven qi, and supplementing the spleen and stomach to produce latter heaven qi.

2. WIND WATER WIND COLD

SIGNS & SYMPTOMS: Chills and fever, generalized heaviness, heavy, achy joints and muscles, edema starting on the face and possibly spreading to the whole body, difficult urination. The tongue is covered with thin, white fur, and the pulse is floating and tight.

TREATMENT PRINCIPLES: Warm and resolve the exterior, open the lung and transform water

REPRESENTATIVE FORMULA: Modified *Ma Huang Jia Zhu Tang* (Ephedra Plus Atractylodes Decoction) plus *Wu Pi Yin* (Five Peels Beverage)

Ma Huang (Ephedrae, Herba), 9g
Gui Zhi (Cinnamomi Cassiae, Ramulus), 9g
Xing Ren (Pruni Armeniacae, Semen), 9g
mix-fried *Gan Cao* (Glycyrrhizae Uralensis, Radix), 3g
Cang Zhu (Atractylodis, Rhizoma), 9g
Chen Pi (Citri Reticulatae, Pericarpium), 9g
Fu Ling Pi (Poriae Cocos, Cortex Sclerotii), 15g
Da Fu Pi (Arecae Catechu, Pericarpium), 15g
Sang Bai Pi (Mori Albi, Cortex Radicis), 15g
Sheng Jiang Pi (Zingiberis Officinalis, uncooked Cortex), 6g

MODIFICATIONS: For asthma and wheezing, add *Xi Xin* (Asari, Herba Cum Radice) and *Wu Wei Zi* (Schisandrae Chinensis, Fructus). For cough, add *Qian Hu* (Peucedani, Radix), *Jie Geng* (Platycodi Grandiflori, Radix), and *Zhi Ke* (Citri Aurantii, Fructus). For phlegm, add *Ban Xia* (Pinelliae Ternatae, Rhizoma). For low appetite, add *Shan Zha* (Crataegi, Fructus) and *Mai Ya* (Hordei Vulgaris, Fructus Germinatus). If there is dribbling urine, please refer to Part 2, Chapter 3 on dribbling urinary block.

ACUMOXIBUSTION: Choose from the acupoints

given above for all types of wind water. Use moxibustion on *Da Zhui* (GV 14), *Feng Men* (Bl 12), and *Fei Shu* (Bl 13).

Case history of Dr. Yi Ma: Xu, a 54 year-old male[4]

Xu's first visit was in November 1978. Xu had been traveling when he caught cold with fever and chills, a heavy feeling in his joints, and discomfort throughout his entire body. Three days later, edema first appeared on his eyelids. It spread to his face and then to his entire body. The Western medical diagnosis was acute nephritis. When he came to see Dr. Yi, Xu's tongue had thin, white fur, and his pulse was floating and tight. Dr. Yi's pattern identification was wind cold kidney wind. His treatment strategy was to diffuse the lung and release the exterior, transform dampness and drain water. His herbal prescription was *Ma Huang Jia Zhu Tang* (Ephedra Plus Atractylodes Decoction) plus *Wu Pi Yin* (Five Peel Beverage) with modifications: *Ma Huang* (Ephedrae, Herba), 15g, *Gui Zhi* (Cinnamomi Cassiae, Ramulus), 15g, *Xing Ren* (Pruni Armeniacae, Semen), 10g, *Cang Zhu* (Atractylodis, Rhizoma), 15g, *Chen Pi* (Citri Reticulatae, Pericarpium), 20g, *Fu Ling Pi* (Poriae Cocos, Cortex Sclerotii), 25g, *Da Fu Pi* (Arecae Catechu, Pericarpium), 20g, *Sang Bai Pi* (Mori Albi, Cortex Radicis), 20g, *Sheng Jiang Pi* (Zingiberis Officinalis, Cortex Rhizomatis), 15g, *Di Fu Zi* (Kochiae Scopariae, Fructus), 20g, and *Fu Ping* (Lemnae Seu Spirodelae, Herba), 20g.

Xu took this prescription for three days and had a mild proper sweat. His urination began to flow easily and his edema dissipated, but he was still fatigued. His tongue fur was slimy and his pulse was slow. Therefore, Dr. Yi decided to change the prescription to one that eliminates dampness: *Fu Ling Pi* (Poriae Cocos, Cortex Sclerotii), 15g, *Sang Bai Pi* (Mori Albi, Cortex Radicis), 20g, *Che Qian Zi* (Plantaginis, Semen), 20g, *Shi Wei* (Pyrrosiae, Folium), 10g, *Bai Mao Gen* (Imperatae Cylindricae, Rhizoma), 25g, *Chen Pi* (Citri Reticulatae, Pericarpium), 15g, and *Dan Zhu Ye* (Lophatheri Gracilis, Herba), 10g.

Xu took this prescription for three days and the slimy fur on his tongue disappeared, but he was still fatigued. Dr. Yi changed the prescription to one that

harmonizes the middle burner and transforms dampness. He directed Xu to take it for one week. By the time Xu finished this last formula, he had completely recovered. A follow-up on May 15, 1981 found no recurrence.

3. WIND WATER WIND COLD WITH YANG VACUITY

SIGNS & SYMPTOMS: Fever and chills, headache, body aches, a pale facial complexion, cold extremities, edema of the lower extremities, urinary difficulty. The tongue is pale with white, slimy fur, and the pulse is deep and slow.

TREATMENT PRINCIPLES: Warm and resolve the exterior and open the lung, warm the interior and transform dampness

REPRESENTATIVE FORMULA: Modified *Ma Huang Fu Zi Xi Xin Tang* (Ephedra, Aconite & Asarum Decoction) plus *Wu Ling San* (Five [Ingredients] Poria Powder)

Ma Huang (Ephedrae, Herba), 9g
Shu Fu Zi (Aconiti Carmichaeli, Radix Lateralis Praeparatus), 9g
Xi Xin (Asari, Herba Cum Radice), 3g
Zhu Ling (Polypori Umbellati, Sclerotium), 9g
Ze Xie (Alismatis Orientalis, Rhizoma), 9g
Bai Zhu (Atractylodis Macrocephalae, Rhizoma), 9g
Fu Ling (Poriae Cocos, Sclerotium), 9g
Gui Zhi (Cinnamomi Cassiae, Ramulus), 9g

MODIFICATIONS: For wheezing due to the kidney's inability to grasp or absorb the qi, add *Jing Gui Shen Qi Wan* (*Golden Cabinet* Kidney Qi Pills). For seminal emission, add *You Gui Wan* (Restore the Right [Kidney] Pills). For constipation, add *Rou Cong Rong* (Cistanchis Deserticolae, Herba). For chronic low back pain and knee pain, add *Du Zhong* (Eucommiae Ulmoidis, Cortex), *Gou Ji* (Cibotii Barometsis, Rhizoma), and *Niu Xi* (Achyranthis Bidentatae, Radix). If the patient's tongue and face are always puffy, add *Ba Ji Tian* (Morindae Officinalis, Radix) to supplement yang and drain water.

ACUMOXIBUSTION: Choose from the acupoints given above for all types of wind water. Use moxibustion on *Shen Shu* (Bl 23), *Ming Men* (GV), and *Tai Xi* (Ki 3).

Case history: Lee, a 56 year-old male[5]

Lee's first visit was in February 1973. Lee caught cold and then, one morning when he got up, he found that his eyelids were swollen. Gradually, his whole body became edematous. His lower extremities were especially swollen. He had fever, chills, difficult urination, fatigue, and his trunk and extremities felt heavy. His tongue was pale and had teeth-marks on its edges with thin, white fur, and his pulse was fine and forceless. Lee always felt cold and had to wear a lot of clothes. His doctor believed this indicated Lee had habitual or constitutional yang vacuity. His diagnosis was cold damp kidney wind. His treatment strategy was to diffuse the lung and drain water, warm the interior and expel cold. He prescribed *Ma Huang Fu Zi Xi Xin Tang* (Ephedra, Aconite & Asarum Decoction) plus *Wu Ling San* (Five [Ingredients] Poria Powder) with modifications: *Ma Huang* (Ephedrae, Herba), 10g, *Shu Fu Zi* (Aconiti Carmichaeli, Radix Lateralis Praeparatus), 10g, *Xi Xin* (Asari, Herba Cum Radice), 3g, *Zhu Ling* (Polypori Umbellati, Sclerotium), 15g, *Ze Xie* (Alismatis Orientalis, Rhizoma), 15g, *Cang Zhu* (Atractylodis, Rhizoma), 15g, *Fu Ling* (Poriae Cocos, Sclerotium), 20g, *Gui Zhi* (Cinnamomi Cassiae, Ramulus), 15g, *Ren Shen* (Panacis Ginseng, Radix), 10g, and *Sheng Jiang* (Zingiberis Officinalis, uncooked Rhizoma), 5g. Lee took this formula for four days and the edema began to dissipate. After two weeks, it had completely disappeared. The doctor modified his formula somewhat. Lee took this new formula for a month and completely recovered.

4. WIND WATER DAMP HEAT

SIGNS & SYMPTOMS: Generalized edema, difficult urination, dark, scanty urination or bloody urination, constipation, lower back distention and pain, fever, vexation and agitation, thirst, sore throat. The tongue is red with yellow, dry or yellow, slimy fur, and the pulse is slippery and fast.

TREATMENT PRINCIPLES: Clear kidney heat and toxins, eliminate dampness and disperse swelling

REPRESENTATIVE FORMULA: *Qing Shen Xiao Du Yin* (Kidney-clearing, Toxin-dispersing Beverage)

Lian Qiao (Forsythiae Suspensae, Fructus), 20g
Jin Yin Hua (Lonicerae Japonicae, Flos), 30g
Da Qing Ye (Daqingye, Folium), 30g
Pu Gong Ying (Taraxaci Mongolici, Herba Cum Radice), 25g
Hua Shi (Talcum), 30g
Dong Kui Zi (Abutili Seu Malvae, Semen), 25g
Di Fu Zi (Kochiae Scopariae, Fructus), 25g
Mu Dan Pi (Moutan, Cortex Radicis), 15g
Zhi Zi (Gardeniae Jasminoidis, Fructus), 15g
Dan Zhu Ye (Lophatheri Gracilis, Herba), 9g

MODIFICATIONS: If there is constipation, add *Da Huang* (Rhei, Radix Et Rhizoma). If there is bloody urine, add *Sheng Di Huang* (Rehmanniae Glutinosae, uncooked Radix), *Xiao Ji* (Cephalanoplos Segeti, Herba), and *Bai Mao Gen* (Imperatae Cylindricae, Rhizoma).

ACUMOXIBUSTION: Choose from the acupoints given above for all types of wind water and add *Yang Ling Quan* (GB 34) and *Yin Ling Quan* (Sp 9).

Case history 1: Chang, a 17 year-old female student[6]

On Oct. 12, 1976, Chang ran a high fever. Four days later, she had facial edema. On October 24, she was admitted to the hospital, at which time, she had fatigue, no appetite, a dry, sore throat, and low back soreness. Her urine protein was 3+ and there were RBCs and casts in her urine. Her blood pressure was120/70mmHg, her heartbeat was 100bpm, and her WBCs were 22,400/cubic ml. Her tongue had thick, slimy fur, and her pulse was fine and fast. Based on these signs and symptoms, the Chinese medical diagnosis was damp heat water swelling. The treatment strategy was to clear heat and drain dampness. Chang's prescription consisted of: *Chen Pi* (Citri Reticulatae, Pericarpium), 12g, *Ban Xia* (Pinelliae Ternatae, Rhizoma), 12g, *Fu Ling* (Poriae Cocos, Sclerotium), 18g, *Zhu Ru* (Bambusae In Taeniis, Caulis), 6g, *Zhu Ye* (Lophatheri Gracilis, Herba), 6g, *Hua Shi* (Talcum), 18g, *Gan Cao* (Glycyrrhizae Uralensis, Radix), 6g, *Che Qian Cao* (Plantaginis, Herba), 12g, *Bai Mao Gen* (Imperatae

Cylindricae, Rhizoma), 18g, and *Shen Qu* (Massa Medica Fermentata), 10g. By October 29, Chang's urine had increased, her edema had dissipated, and her appetite was better. Her tongue had white, slimy fur, and her pulse was fine. Her urine protein was 2+, WBCs were 1-2, and RBCs were 5-10. Her blood WBC count was 9800. Treatment continued using the same formula.

Case history of Dr. Yu Xiong-zao: Yu, a 12 year-old male[7]

Yu's first visit was on Apr. 12, 1973. Yu had scarlet fever in March. By April, he started to have edema on his face and in his extremities. He had a high fever and his throat was red, with swollen tonsils (two degrees) and swollen lymph glands that were painful upon palpation. Urinalysis showed urine casts at 2+, pus at 2+, and some RBCs. The Western medical diagnosis was acute nephritis and, for this, his doctors prescribed penicillin. However, this produced no change in Yu's condition. He still had a fever. Therefore, on April 12, Yu came to see Dr. Yu. Yu presented with fever without sweating, a sore throat, dry lips, dry skin, and a rash. His tongue was red and swollen with gray-black fur. Dr. Yu's diagnosis was wind water kidney heat. His treatment strategy was to expel wind, clear and resolve heat toxins, and transform phlegm dampness. His prescription consisted of: *Lian Qiao* (Forsythiae Suspensae, Fructus), 12g, *Niu Bang Zi* (Arctii, Fructus), 9g, *Qian Hu* (Peucedani, Radix), 9g, *Jin Yin Hua* (Lonicerae Japonicae, Flos), 30g, *Jiang Can* (Bombyx Batryticatus), 15g, *Xuan Shen* (Scrophulariae Ningpoensis, Radix), 15g, *Lu Dou Yi* (Glycines Seu Sojae, Testa), 24g, *Bai Xian Pi* (Dictamni Dasycarpi, Cortex Radicis), 12g, *Jie Geng* (Platycodi Grandiflori, Radix), 6g, *Sheng Di Huang* (Rehmanniae Glutinosae, uncooked Radix), 12g, *Nan Sha Shen* (Adenophorae Strictae, Radix), 15g, and stir-fried *Huang Qin* (Scutellariae Baicalensis, Radix), 1.8g.

By April 14, Yu's second visit to Dr. Yu, he still had a fever but his body temperature was down to 38.5° C. The sides of his tongue were red and peeled, his left tonsil was swollen, his lips were dry and cracked, and he had a little nose-bleeding. His BUN was

60.1mg%. His tongue fur was still gray-black. Dr. Yu decided Yu had lung and stomach toxic heat and that phlegm heat was still steaming the interior. Therefore, he prescribed the following medicinals to clear heat and resolve toxins: *Bo He* (Menthae Haplocalycis, Herba), 2.4g, *Ma Bo* (Lasiosphaerae Seu Calvatiae, Fructificatio), 1.2g, *Jie Geng* (Platycodi Grandiflori, Radix), 6g, *Jiang Can* (Bombyx Batryticatus), 12g, *Jin Yin Hua* (Lonicerae Japonicae, Flos), 45g, *Lian Qiao* (Forsythiae Suspensae, Fructus), 12g, *Xuan Shen* (Scrophulariae Ningpoensis, Radix), 24g, *Mai Men Dong* (Ophiopogonis Japonici, Tuber), 12g, *Shi Hu* (Dendrobii, Herba), 24g, *Shi Chang Pu* (Acori Graminei, Rhizoma), 24g, *Zhi Zi* (Gardeniae Jasminoidis, Fructus), 3g, *Yuan Zhi* (Polygalae Tenuifoliae, Radix), 6g, *Chuan Bei Mu* (Fritillariae Cirrhosae, Bulbus), 4.5g, *Lu Dou Yi* (Glycines Seu Sojae, Testa), 24g, *Lu Gen* (Phragmitis Communis, Rhizoma), 120g (used as an infusion instead of water to cook the other medicinals), plus *Xi Lei San* (Tin-like Powder),[8] 600mg (to be blown into the throat).

By April 16, Yu's third visit, he felt better and his sore throat was gone, but, in the evening, his body temperature would still go up to 38° C. His tongue fur was gray but not black, and his nose-bleeding had stopped. His pulse was fine and he looked anemic. Therefore, Dr. Yu changed the treatment strategy to clearing heat and nourishing yin. His prescription consisted of: *Bo He* (Menthae Haplocalycis, Herba), 1.5g, *Jin Yin Hua* (Lonicerae Japonicae, Flos), 30g, *Xuan Shen* (Scrophulariae Ningpoensis, Radix), 24g, *Gou Qi Zi* (Lycii Chinensis, Fructus), 12g, *Mai Men Dong* (Ophiopogonis Japonici, Tuber), 9g, *Jie Geng* (Platycodi Grandiflori, Radix), 3g, *Jiang Can* (Bombyx Batryticatus), 12g, *Shi Hu* (Dendrobii, Herba), 18g, *Lian Qiao* (Forsythiae Suspensae, Fructus), 30g, *Lu Dou Yi* (Glycines Seu Sojae, Testa), 24g, powdered *Chuan Bei Mu* (Fritillariae Cirrhosae, Bulbus), 3g, *Lu Gen* (Phragmitis Communis, Rhizoma), 60g, and *Bai Mao Gen* (Imperatae Cylindricae, Rhizoma), 60g.

Yu took this prescription until the end of April. His tonsils were no longer swollen, but he still had fever in the evenings and blood in his urine. His rash was completely gone, but his face was still slightly swollen and he had dry, peeling skin. His BUN would go up to 70.7mg%, and his creatinine was 4.2mg%. He had a low appetite and lots of sweating. His tongue had a white, slimy coat, and his pulse was fine and bowstring. Dr. Yu thought that the toxins had not been completely cleared but that there was underlying kidney qi vacuity. Hence, he decided to add qi-supplementing and securing and astringing medicinals. His new prescription consisted of: *Huang Qi* (Astragali Membranacei, Radix), 18g, *Jin Yin Hua* (Lonicerae Japonicae, Flos), 30g, *Lian Qiao* (Forsythiae Suspensae, Fructus), 12g, *Xuan Shen* (Scrophulariae Ningpoensis, Radix), 12g, *Lu Dou Yi* (Glycines Seu Sojae, Testa), 18g, *Bai Mao Gen* (Imperatae Cylindricae, Rhizoma), 60g, *Lu Gen* (Phragmitis Communis, Rhizoma), 60g, *Mu Dan Pi* (Moutan, Cortex Radicis), 9g, *Chi Shao* (Paeoniae Lactiflorae, Radix Rubrus), 9g, *Yi Yi Ren* (Coicis Lachryma-jobi, Semen), 18g, *Fu Ling* (Poriae Cocos, Sclerotium), 12g, and *Nuo Dao Gen Xu* (Oryzae Glutinosae, Radix Et Rhizoma), 12g.

After Yu took this prescription, his body temperature, BUN, and creatinine came down. Dr. Yu decided to increase the dose of *Huang Qi* up to 30 grams and to add 12 grams of *Ci Shi* (Magnititum) to supplement the kidney and nourish the blood. Yu continued to improve and, by May 2, his BUN was 53mg%, his creatinine was 2.2mg%, and his blood pressure was 118/70mmHg. However, he still had a low-grade fever in the afternoon and continued to look anemic. His tongue had thin, white fur, and his pulse was fine and bowstring. Dr. Yu now added some kidney-supplementing and spleen-fortifying medicinals. His prescription consisted of: *Huang Qi* (Astragali Membranacei, Radix), 30g, *Jin Yin Hua* (Lonicerae Japonicae, Flos), 12g, *Lu Dou Yi* (Glycines Seu Sojae, Testa), 12g, *Mu Dan Pi* (Moutan, Cortex Radicis), 9g, *Chi Shao* (Paeoniae Lactiflorae, Radix Rubrus), 9g, *Er Zhi Wan* (Two Ultimates Pills),[9] 12g, *Shan Yao* (Radix Dioscoreae Oppositae), 12g, *Ci Shi* (Magnititum), 12g, *Fu Ling* (Poriae Cocos, Sclerotium), 9g, *Gou Qi Zi* (Lycii Chinensis, Fructus), 12g, *Fo Shou* (Citri Sarcodactylis, Fructus), 12g, *Bai Mao Gen* (Imperatae Cylindricae, Rhizoma), 60g, *Lu Gen* (Phragmitis Communis, Rhizoma), 60g, and *Nuo Dao Gen Xu* (Oryzae Glutinosae, Radix Et Rhizoma), 90g.

Yu took this prescription until June 8. He felt better, but he still had a low-grade fever in the afternoon and he occasionally got a sore throat. Urinalysis showed a mild protein content with some RBCs. His tongue had yellow fur, and his pulse was fine. Dr. Yu thought that Yu had both qi and yin vacuity. He decided to focus on supplementing qi and yin but also to clear the lung and drain fire. His prescription consisted of: *Huang Qi* (Astragali Membranacei, Radix), 30g, *Di Gu Pi* (Lycii Chinensis, Cortex Radicis), 9g, *Bai Wei* (Cynanchi Baiwei, Radix), 9g, *Fu Ling* (Poriae Cocos, Sclerotium), 12g, *Yi Yi Ren* (Coicis Lachryma-jobi, Semen), 12g, *Dong Chong Xia Cao* (Cordyceps Sinensis), 9g, *Gu Sui Bu* (Gusuibu, Rhizoma), 9g, *Ci Shi* (Magnititum), 15g, *Xuan Shen* (Scrophulariae Ningpoensis, Radix), 12g, *Fo Shou* (Citri Sarcodactylis, Fructus), 9g, *E Jiao* (Corii Asini, Gelatinum), 3g, *Nan Sha Shen* (Adenophorae Structae, Radix), 9g, *Bei Sha Shen* (Glenhniae Littoralis, Radix), 9g, *Lu Gen* (Phragmitis Communis, Rhizoma), 60g, and *Bai Mao Gen* (Imperatae Cylindricae, Rhizoma), 60g.

Yu took this formula until July 2 and felt much better. Although his urinalysis was normal, his face was not anemic looking, and he felt strong, he still had low back soreness. Dr. Yu decided to give him medicinals to supplement the kidney and spleen as well as medicinals to clear and eliminate damp heat: *Huang Qi* (Astragali Membranacei, Radix), 15g, *Gou Qi Zi* (Lycii Chinensis, Fructus), 12g, *Tu Si Zi* (Cuscutae Chinensis, Semen), 12g, *Qian Shi* (Euryales Ferocis, Semen), 9g, *Xuan Shen* (Scrophulariae Ningpoensis, Radix), 9g, *Dong Chong Xia Cao* (Cordyceps Sinensis), 9g, *Lu Dou Yi* (Glycines Seu Sojae, Testa), 12g, *Nan Sha Shen* (Adenophorae Strictae, Radix), 9g, fresh *Lu Gen* (Phragmitis Communis, Rhizoma), 60g, *Liu Yi San* (Six-to-One Powder),[10] 9g, and fresh *He Ye* (Nelumbinis Nuciferae, Folium), 1 piece. At this point, Yu was considered cured.

5. WIND WATER DAMP HEAT WITH YIN VACUITY

SIGNS & SYMPTOMS: Edema, fever, sore throat, thirst, night sweats, constipation, low back and knee soreness and limpness, dark urine with hematuria, and fatigue. The tongue is red with lack of fur or thin, yellow fur. The pulse is fine, bowstring, forceful, and fast.

TREATMENT PRINCIPLES: Clear heat and resolve toxins in the upper burner, supplement kidney yin and quell vacuity fire, cool the blood and drain water

REPRESENTATIVE FORMULA: Modified *Zhi Bai Di Huang Wan* (Anemarrhena & Phellodendron Rehmannia Pills)

Zhi Mu (Anemarrhenae Asphodeloidis, Rhizoma), 9g
Huang Bai (Phellodendri, Cortex), 9g
Sheng Di Huang (Rehmanniae Glutinosae, uncooked Radix), 12-15g
Shan Yao (Radix Dioscoreae Oppositae), 12g
Shan Zhu Yu (Corni Officinalis, Fructus), 12g
Fu Ling (Poriae Cocos, Sclerotium), 9g
Ze Xie (Alismatis Orientalis, Rhizoma), 9g
Mu Dan Pi (Moutan, Cortex Radicis), 12g
Xuan Shen (Scrophulariae Ningpoensis, Radix), 6-9g
Han Lian Cao (Ecliptae Prostratae, Herba), 6-9g
Nu Zhen Zi (Ligustri Lucidi, Fructus), 6-9g
Di Gu Pi (Lycii Chinensis, Cortex Radicis), 9g
Chi Shao (Paeoniae Lactiflorae, Radix Rubrus), 3-6g

ACUMOXIBUSTION: Choose from the acupoints given above for all types of wind water. Add *Yang Ling Quan* (GB 34), *Yin Ling Quan* (Sp 9), and *Zhao Hai* (Ki 6).

Case history of Dr. Dan Zhu-li: Xu, a 13 year-old girl[11]

In August 1981, Xu started to experience edema and scanty urination. She was admitted to the hospital and treated with cortisone and anti-immune drugs, but she did not improve. At the same time, she was diagnosed with a diabetic complication. She also had an infection on her left eyelid and in her left ear. Urinalysis showed protein at 2+, urine sugar at 2+, WBCs at 2-5/HP, RBCs at 8-10/HP, granular casts at 2-4/HP, ESR at 45 mm/hour, and cholesterol at 345mg/dL. Her blood total was 48.8g/L, her albumin was 25g/L, and her blood sugar was 255mg/dL. Xu presented with edema over her entire body, low back pain, weak legs, scanty urination, and loose stools. Her tongue was pale with teeth-marks on its edges and white fur. Her pulse was deep, fine, and forceless. Dr. Dan's pattern identification was spleen and kidney vacuity with water swelling. His formula was modified *Liu Wei Di Huang Wan* (Six Flavors Rehmannia Pills): *Sheng Di Huang* (Rehmanniae Glutinosae, uncooked Radix), 20g, *Shan Yao* (Radix Dioscoreae Oppositae), 20g, *Shan Zhu Yu* (Corni Officinalis, Fructus), 15g, *Ze Xie* (Alismatis Orientalis, Rhizoma), 12g, *Mu Dan Pi* (Moutan, Cortex Radicis), 12g, *Huang Qi* (Astragali Membranacei, Radix), 15g, *He Shou Wu* (Polygoni Multiflori, Radix), 15g, *Tu Si Zi* (Cuscutae Chinensis, Semen), 15g, *Ba Ji Tian* (Morindae Officinalis, Radix), 12g, *Fu Ling Pi* (Poriae Cocos, Cortex Sclerotii), 15g, *Gou Qi Zi* (Lycii Chinensis, Fructus), 20g, *Di Gu Pi* (Lycii Chinensis, Cortex Radicis), 20g, *Di Yu* (Sanguisorbae Officinalis, Radix), 15g, and *Shi Hu* (Dendrobii, Herba), 15g.

Meanwhile, Dr. Dan started to reduce the amount of cortisone Xu was given. By June, the cortisone treatments were stopped altogether. Then Xu caught cold with a sore throat, low back pain, and difficult urination. Her tongue was red with thin, yellow fur and her pulse was fine and fast. Dr. Dan gave Xu a formula to clear heat and resolve toxins for one week. Xu recovered from the cold and then continued on Dr. Dan's previous formula. In October, Xu began having symptoms of genital redness, swelling, and itchiness. Her urine was burning hot and she became edematous over her whole body. Dr. Dan gave her another formula to clear and resolve heat toxins. Xu took this formula for 10 days and the symptoms disappeared. He then prescribed the following as a base formula: *Sang Shen Zi* (Mori Albi, Fructus), 15g, *He Shou Wu* (Polygoni Multiflori, Radix), 15g, *Huang Qi* (Astragali Membranacei, Radix), 15g, *Gou Qi Zi* (Lycii Chinensis, Fructus), 12g, *Nu Zhen Zi* (Ligustri Lucidi, Fructus), 12g, *Bai Zhu* (Atractylodis Macrocephalae, Rhizoma), 12g, *Bai Shao* (Paeoniae Lactiflorae, Radix Albus), 12g, *Dang Shen* (Codonopsitis Pilosulae, Radix), 12g, *Shu Di Huang* (Rehmanniae Glutinosae, cooked Radix), 15g, *Huang Jing* (Polygonati, Rhizoma), 12g, and *Mu Dan Pi* (Moutan, Cortex Radicis), 12g. Xu took variations of this formula for two years and she completely recovered. All her tests returned to normal, and a follow-up seven years later showed no recurrence.

CLINICAL TIPS

1. Warning: Acute nephritis is a serious and potentially life threatening disease. Chinese medical practitioners are not equipped to diagnose acute nephritis. When they suspect their patient has AGN, they should have the patient consult a Western physician. The Chinese medical practitioner should also consult with a Western physician to review urinalyses and blood tests. These tests indicate the disease progression as well as the effectiveness of Chinese medical therapy. Chinese medical practitioners must appreciate that some AGN patients need dialysis immediately. They should not attempt to dissuade the patient from employing dialysis while beginning Chinese medical therapy.

2. There are two types of AGN patients that come to Chinese medicine: 1) those who do not adequately respond to Western medical diuretic therapy and/or do not adequately respond to antibiotics, or 2) those who respond to Western medical therapy and whose symptoms disappear but who still have abnormal urinalysis. Patients may not adequately respond to Western diuretic therapy because of a weak constitution or a lingering pathogen. Edema indicates that kidney function is damaged. If the edema is allowed to remain for a protracted period, acute nephritis can become chronic and may even lead to renal failure. Patients use dialysis to rid the body of the edema, but dialysis cannot eliminate lingering pathogens, nor does it support the patient's constitution. Thus the edema may easily return.

Patients may not adequately respond to antibiotics because various pathogens, such as streptococcus or staphylococcus, viruses, or parasites (such as malaria), have become resistant to them. The cause of primary acute nephritis is often bacterial. Antibiotic therapy is an extremely important aspect of Western medical therapy. If the antibiotics are not completely successful in controlling the infection, the patient has little chance for cure with Western medicine. However, a combination of Western and Chinese medicine has proven to be an effective treatment approach for many primary acute nephritis patients as well as some drug-induced secondary acute nephritis patients. Ongoing Chinese medical therapy after cessation of Western therapy addresses and resolves underlying disharmonies as revealed in improved urinalysis results.

3. Chinese medicine does not distinguish between primary and secondary glomerular diseases. Pattern identification is used for all types of acute nephritis. On the other hand, Chinese medicine makes a distinction between the root and the tip of the disease. Analyzing primary glomerular diseases, one usually finds the root is spleen and kidney vacuity. This leads to a vacuity of defensive and righteous qi. When defensive and righteous qi are vacuous, it is easy for an external evil to invade and to penetrate deeply into the interior. In secondary (multisystem disease-associated) glomerular diseases, the causal agent may be an environmental toxin (such as heavy metal contamination) or a toxic drug reaction. While this represents the tip, one must focus on it. At the same time, one must identify the root pattern and begin treating it.

ENDNOTES

[1] Yu Wong-shi, *Dong Dai Ming Yi Ling Zhen Jing Hua* (*Modern Famous Doctors Clinic Collection*), Chinese Ancient Book Publishing Co., Beijing, 1991, p. 8

[2] In this book we use the term "proper sweat" (*zhen han*) to indicate correctly releasing the surface. A proper sweat is a light sweat over the entire body with, perhaps, a little heavier sweat on the nose.

[3] Yu Guan-shi and Shui Jian-shen, *Dong Dai Ming Yi Lin Zheng Jing Hua* (*Collection of Clinical Case Histories of Modern Famous Doctors*), Ancient Chinese Medicine Book Publishing Company, Beijing, 1998, pg. 9

[4] Yu Wong-shi, *op. cit.*, p. 6

[5] *Ibid.*, p. 9

[6] *Ibid.*, p. 72

[7] *Ibid.*, p. 25

[8] *Xi Lie San* (Tin-like Powder) consists of *Xiang Ya Xue* (Elephas Maximus), *Zhen Zhu* (Margarita), *Qing Dai* (Indigonis, Pulvis), *Bing Pian* (Borneol), *Niu Huang* (Bovis, Calculus), and *Bi Qian* (Uroctea Compactilis)

[9] *Er Zhi Wan* (Two Ultimates Pills) consists of *Nu Zhen Zi* (Ligustri Lucidi, Fructus) and *Han Lian Cao* (Ecliptae Prostratae, Herba)

[10] *Liu Yi San* (Six-to-One Powder) consists of six parts of *Hua Shi* (Talcum) to one part of *Gan Cao* (Glycyrrhizae Uralensis, Radix)

[11] *Shui Zhong Guan Ge Jun* (*Water Swelling and Block & Repulsion*), Vol. 2, Chinese Medicine Publishing Company, Beijing, 1998, p. 56

Chronic nephritis is also known as chronic nephritic-proteinuric syndrome and chronic glomerulonephritis (CGN). Chronic glomerulonephritis is more aptly named slowly progressive glomerular disease. It is marked by chronic inflammation and gradual destruction of the glomeruli. Lesions are focused on the glomerular region but may spread to other structures.

EPIDEMIOLOGY

The incidence of CGN is rare. Approximately only four per 100,000 people will be affected. One-quarter of those diagnosed with CGN have no prior history of kidney illness. Investigations into the cause of a patient's hypertension or routine physical examination and urine analysis may reveal CGN.

ETIOLOGY & PATHOPHYSIOLOGY

The precise etiology of CGN is currently unknown. Histological evidence of antibody formation in the glomeruli suggests a possible immune etiology. Infection, toxicity, metabolic disorders, and intrarenal coagulation are all theoretical etiologies for CGN. Direct links have not been found. Mercury

toxicity, organic solvents, and NSAIDs may play a role in causation. As for pathophysiology, early and extensive damage to the interstitium typically occurs. Tubule atrophy and vascular lesions are diffuse, and cell adhesions may fill up to 50% of the glomerular cavity.

SYMPTOMATOLOGY

Most patients with CGN remain asymptomatic for years. Eventually, symptoms of blood in the urine or dark and foamy urine may appear. This may be combined with nonspecific symptoms of weight loss, malaise, general malaise, headaches, itching, oliguria, easy bruising, nosebleeds, and decreased mental clarity. Hypertension is a common finding.

DIAGNOSIS

Often patients present with seemingly normal renal function, but urinalysis reveals proteinuria and hematuria. Diagnosis often occurs during routine medical screening. An appreciable rise in BUN and creatinine levels only occurs after more than 50% of the functioning nephrons have been destroyed. Urinalysis and blood work, therefore, may or may not offer direct indications of CGN. During the early stages, renal biopsy may prove useful to distinguish CGN from similar disorders. Kidneys that have been reduced in size (due to chronicity) are not suited for biopsy.

DIFFERENTIAL DIAGNOSIS

Chronic glomerulonephritis may be confused with the following disorders: idiopathic recurrent hematuria, nonglomerular disease, such as tubulointerstitial disease, focal segmental glomerulosclerosis, membranous glomerulonephritis, and IgA nephropathy.

WESTERN MEDICAL TREATMENT

The primary goal of Western medical treatment for this condition is to control and address symptoms. Hypertension, commonly associated with CGN, is often the most important and difficult issue. Unlike AGN, the use of corticosteroids and other immunosuppressant medications may be warranted. Dietary protein, salt, and fluid intake is regulated. Dialysis becomes necessary with progression of the disease.

PROGNOSIS & COMPLICATIONS

The prognosis and progression of this disease vary widely depending on the extent of glomerular damage, and spontaneous remission is possible. Uncontrolled nephrotic syndrome is likely to develop into end-stage renal disease. Complications include nephrotic syndrome, acute glomerulonephritis, chronic renal failure, hypertension and malignant hypertension, edema, fluid overload, congestive heart failure, urinary tract infections, chronic, recurrent, and increased susceptibility to infection.

CHINESE MEDICAL DISEASE CATEGORIZATION

In Chinese medicine, the clinical signs and symptoms of chronic nephritis correspond to the following traditional disease categories: kidney wind, dribbling urinary block, bloody urine, water swelling, kidney taxation or vacuity taxation and taxation wind, phlegm rheum, lumbar pain, abdominal distention, and dizziness.

TREATMENT BASED ON PATTERN IDENTIFICATION

PROTEIN ONLY IN THE URINE

1. SPLEEN-KIDNEY QI VACUITY

SIGNS & SYMPTOMS: Fatigue, heart palpitations, shortness of breath, no appetite, loose stools, a pale facial complexion, low back and knee soreness and limpness. The tongue is pale with thin, white fur and the pulse is weak and slow or fine and weak.

TREATMENT PRINCIPLES: Supplement the center and boost the qi

REPRESENTATIVE FORMULAS: *Fang Ji Huang Qi Tang* (Stephania & Astragalus Decoction)

Huang Qi (Astragali Membranacei, Radix), 12g
Han Fang Ji (Stephaniae Tetrandrae, Radix), 9g
Bai Zhu (Atractylodis Macrocephalae, Rhizoma), 9g
mix-fried *Gan Cao* (Glycyrrhizae Uralensis, Radix), 3g
Sheng Jiang (Zingiberis Officinalis, uncooked Rhizoma), 4 pieces
Da Zao (Zizyphi Jujubae, Fructus), 3 pieces

Bu Zhong Yi Qi Tang (Supplement the Center & Boost the Qi Decoction)

Huang Qi (Astragali Membranacei, Radix), 12g
Ren Shen (Panacis Ginseng, Radix), 9g
Bai Zhu (Atractylodis Macrocephalae, Rhizoma), 12g
mix-fried *Gan Cao* (Glycyrrhizae Uralensis, Radix), 3g
Dang Gui (Angelicae Sinensis, Radix), 9g
Chen Pi (Citri Reticulatae, Pericarpium), 6g
Sheng Ma (Cimicifugae, Rhizoma), 9g
Chai Hu (Bupleuri, Radix), 6g

MODIFICATIONS: If the patient has insomnia, add *Da Zao* (Zizyphi Jujubae, Fructus), *Long Yan Rou* (Euphoriae Longanae, Arillus), *Suan Zao Ren*

(Zizyphi Spinosae, Semen), and *Ci Wu Jia* (Eleuthrococci Senticosi, Radix). For profuse menstruation, add steamed *San Qi* (Notoginseng, Radix) after the first day. If the patient has profuse abnormal vaginal discharge, one may add *Bai Zhu* (Atractylodis Macrocephalae, Rhizoma), *Fu Ling* (Poriae Cocos, Sclerotium), *Shan Yao* (Dioscoreae Oppositae, Radix), *Lian Zi* (Nelumbinis Nuciferae, Semen), and *Ban Xia* (Pinelliae Ternatae, Rhizoma). One may also add astringents such as *Wu Mei* (Pruni Mume, Fructus), *Wu Wei Zi* (Schisandrae Chinensis, Fructus), and *Jin Ying Zi* (Rosae Laevigatae, Fructus). For visceral prolapse, add a larger dose of *Huang Qi*, up to 50 grams per day for three months. If the patient has high blood pressure, add *Niu Xi* (Achyranthis Bidentae, Radix) and *Du Zhong* (Eucommiae Ulmoidis, Cortex) or switch to *Tian Ma Gou Teng Yin* (Gastrodia & Uncaria Beverage) plus medicinals to supplement the qi. If there is blood in the urine, one should focus on boosting the spleen and kidney qi to treat the root. If one wants to add medicinals that stanch bleeding, one must add medicinals which quicken the blood and stop bleeding, such as *San Qi*, or which supplement the qi and stanch bleeding, such as *Xian He Cao* (Agrioniae Pilosae, Herba). One can also use *Huang Qi* combined with *Shui Zhi* (Hirudo Seu Whitmania).

If there is stasis, one may need to employ blood-quickening, stasis-dispelling medicinals, such as *Tao Ren* (Persicae, Semen), *Hong Hua* (Carthami Tinctorii, Flos), *Dan Shen* (Salvia Miltiorrhizae, Radix), *Chi Shao* (Paeoniae Lactiflorae, Radix Rubrus), *Niu Xi* (Achyranthis Bidentatae, Radix), *Shui Zhi* (Hirudo Seu Whitmania), *Chuan Xiong* (Ligustici Wallichii, Radix), *Dang Gui* (Angelicae Sinensis, Radix), and *Mu Dan Pi* (Moutan, Cortex Radicis). However, when using such attacking medicinals, one should always consider the strength of the patient. Overuse of blood-quickening, stasis-dispelling medicinals can lead to greater vacuity.

Caution: Patients must maintain a healthy diet with a high protein content to make up for the protein loss through proteinuria. Patients should also avoid cold and damp weather conditions and heavy exertion.

Acumoxibustion: Choose from *Pi Shu* (Bl 20),

Shen Shu (Bl 23), *Qi Hai* (CV 6), *Zhong Wan* (CV 12), *Guan Yuan* (CV 4), *Zu San Li* (St 36), *Tai Bai* (Sp 3), *Gong Sun* (Sp 4), *San Yin Jiao* (Sp 6), *Yin Ling Quan* (Sp 9), *Tai Xi* (Ki 3), and *Zhao Hai* (Ki 6).

Case history of Dr. Ke Wan-chen: Yong, a 45 year-old male[1]

Yong suffered with chronic nephritis for 10 years. He was treated for half a year without any change in his proteinuria. His kidney function was damaged and he had edema in both legs. Dr. Ke prescribed *Huang Qi Chi Xiao Dou Tang* (Astragalus & Red Bean Decoction): *Huang Qi* (Astragali Membranacei, Radix), 100g, *Chi Xiao Dou* (Phaseoli Calcarati, Semen), 30g (cooked at a low temperature until completely soft).

This formula was divided into two servings. Yong ate one serving two times a day for a month and a half. His edema completely dissipated and his urinalysis returned to normal. He continued on this regimen for another month and a half to consolidate the results. Yong completely recovered. Later, he passed his entrance examination for graduate school and became a college teacher. Follow-ups once a year found no recurrence.

2. Spleen-kidney yang vacuity

Signs & symptoms: Feeling cold, cold hands and feet, fatigue, no appetite, water swelling (ascites). The tongue is pale and puffy with thin, white fur, and the pulse is deep, fine, and forceless.

Treatment principles: Fortify the spleen, warm the kidney, and transform water

Representative formulas: *Zhen Wu Tang* (True Warrior Decoction)

Shu Fu Zi (Aconiti Carmichaeli, Radix Lateralis Praeparatus), 9g
Bai Zhu (Atractylodis Macrocephalae, Rhizoma), 6g
Fu Ling (Poriae Cocos, Sclerotium), 9g
Bai Shao (Paeoniae Lactiflorae, Radix Albus), 9g
Sheng Jiang (Zingiberis Officinalis, uncooked Rhizoma), 9g

Shi Pi Yin (Bolster the Spleen Beverage)

Shu Fu Zi (Aconiti Carmichaeli, Radix Lateralis Praeparatus), 3g
Gan Jiang (Zingiberis Officinalis, dry Rhizoma), 3g
Fu Ling (Poriae Cocos, Sclerotium), 9g
Bai Zhu (Atractylodis Macrocephalae, Rhizoma), 9g
Mu Gua (Chaenomelis Lagenariae, Fructus), 9g
Hou Po (Magnoliae Officinalis, Cortex), 9g
Mu Xiang (Aucklandiae Lappae, Radix), 3g
Da Fu Pi (Arecae Catechu, Pericarpium), 9g
Cao Guo (Amomi Tsao-ko, Fructus), 3g
mix-fried *Gan Cao* (Glycyrrhizae Uralensis, Radix), 3g

MODIFICATIONS: If there is scanty urination, add *Zhu Ling* (Polypori Umbellati, Sclerotium), *Ze Xie* (Alismatis Orientalis, Rhizoma), and *Gui Zhi* (Cinnamomi Cassiae, Ramulus). If the face and head are swollen, add *Ma Huang* (Ephedrae, Herba). *Ma Huang* helps open the exterior and upper orifices ("making a hole in the teapot's lid").

Shen Qi Wan (Kidney Qi Pills)

Shu Fu Zi (Aconiti Carmichaeli, Radix Lateralis Praeparatus), 3g
Rou Gui (Cinnamonmi Casiae, Cortex), 3g
Shu Di Huang (Rehmanniae Glutinosae, cooked Radix), 12-15g
Shan Yao (Radix Dioscoreae Oppositae), 12g
Shan Zhu Yu (Corni Officinalis, Fructus), 12g
Ze Xie (Alismatis Orientalis, Rhizoma), 9g
Fu Ling (Poriae Cocos, Sclerotium), 9g
Mu Dan Pi (Moutan, Cortex Radicis), 9g

MODIFICATIONS: *Che Qian Zi* (Plantaginis, Semen) and *Niu Xi* (Achyranthis Bidentatae, Radix) may be added to enhance this formula's effect. *Che Qian Zi* drains dampness, while *Niu Xi* guides the other medicinals to the kidney. It also harmonizes the water passageways.

One should continue to prescribe *Shen Qi Wan* after the edema has dissipated. Ongoing supplementation of kidney yin and yang consolidates the results and stops recurrences.

CAUTION: Patients must maintain a healthy diet with a high protein content to make up for the protein loss through proteinuria. Patients should also avoid cold and damp weather conditions and heavy exertion.

ACUMOXIBUSTION: Choose points to moxa from *Pi Shu* (Bl 20), *Shen Shu* (Bl 23), *Ming Men* (GV 4), *Guan Yuan* (CV 4), *Qi Hai* (CV 6), *Zhong Wan* (CV 12), *Zu San Li* (St 36), *Tai Bai* (Sp 3), *Gong Sun* (Sp 4), *San Yin Jiao* (Sp 6), *Yin Ling Quan* (Sp 9), *Tai Xi* (Ki 3), and *Zhao Hai* (Ki 6).

Case history of Dr. He Ho-ling: Yin, a six year-old boy[2]

Nine months prior to Yin's first visit on Sept. 18, 1985, he suddenly developed acute nephritis. After Western medical treatment, the edema dissipated, but every time the young boy caught a cold, it would return. Two months prior to his first visit, his face and whole body became edematous (pitting edema). He had a pale facial complexion, spontaneous perspiration, loose stools, and scanty urination. His tongue had thin, white fur, and his pulse was deep and fine. The Western medical diagnosis was chronic nephritis. The Chinese medical department tried interior-warming and water-disinhibiting, dampness-percolating medicinals for over a month without success. Yin's urinalysis still showed protein at 2+-3+ and casts at 0-3. Therefore, Dr. He's treatment strategy was to warm the kidney and fortify the spleen, resolve toxins and eliminate dampness, for which he prescribed the following: *Huang Qi* (Astragali Membranacei, Radix), 9g, *Fu Ling* (Poriae Cocos, Sclerotium), 9g, *Zao Pi* (Zizyphi Jujubae, Cortex), 9g, *Dang Shen* (Codonopsitis Pilosulae, Radix), 9g, *Yi Mu Cao* (Leonuri Heterophylli, Herba), 9g, *Chi Xiao Dou* (Phaseoli Calcarati, Semen), 10g, *Ban Bian Lian* (Lobeliae Chinensis, Herba Cum Radice), 10g, *Rou Gui* (Cinnamonmi Casiae, Cortex), 7g, *Bai Hua She Cao* (Oldenlandiae Diffusae, Herba), 12g, *Yu Mi Xu* (Zeae Maydis, Stylus), 15g, and *Da Zao* (Zizyphi Jujubae, Fructus), 5 pieces. Yin took this formula for 15 days and his edema dissipated, his appetite improved, and his urinalysis returned to normal. He took it for another three months and had a complete recovery. A follow-up after one year showed no recurrence.

Case history of Dr. Huo Ren-chen: Nie, a male child of unstated age[3]

Nie first came in to see Dr. Huo on Feb. 9, 1961. He had edema for two and one half years and was treated by both Chinese and Western medical practitioners. While he was being treated, the edema would dissipate, but it always returned after the treatments ended. When seen by Dr. Huo, the boy had pitting edema over his entire body but especially in his face and upper extremities. His abdomen was very bloated and he had loose stools, low appetite, and scanty urination. His tongue was pale, and his pulse was soggy and forceless. Based on these signs and symptoms, Dr. Huo's pattern identification was spleen-kidney yang vacuity with vacuity cold yin water. Therefore, he prescribed modified *Shi Pi Yin* (Bolster the Spleen Beverage).

Dr. Huo analysis was as follows: Children's organs are fragile. External cold and dampness had taken advantage of Nie's spleen-kidney yang vacuity. Therefore, Nie's kidney qi transformation had become severely inhibited and this further compromised spleen yang, resulting in abdominal bloating. Nie's former doctors principal treatment strategy had been to disinhibit water. They relied on water-disinhibiting, dampness-percolating medicinals, but these medicinals had damaged Nie's true qi. Because the true qi was vacuous, edema would always return. Dr. Huo believed the treatment strategy should focus on warming the kidney and fortifying the spleen in order to transform water and move the qi. His prescription consisted of: *Fu Ling* (Poriae Cocos, Sclerotium), 6g, *Bai Zhu* (Atractylodis Macrocephalae, Rhizoma), 6g, *Mu Gua* (Chaenomelis Lagenariae, Fructus), 6g, *Hou Po* (Magnoliae Officinalis, Cortex), 6g, *Zhu Ling* (Polypori Umbellati, Sclerotium), 6g, *Xiang Fu* (Cyperi Rotundi, Rhizoma), 6g, *Che Qian Zi* (Plantaginis, Semen), 6g, *Da Fu Pi* (Arecae Catechu, Pericarpium), 6g, *Zi Su Zi* (Perillae Frutescentis, Fructus), 6g, *Cao Dou Kou* (Alpiniae Katsumadai, Semen), 6g, mix-fried *Fu Zi* (Aconiti Carmichaeli, Radix Lateralis Praeparatus), 6g, *Qu Mai* (Dianthi, Herba), 6g, *Mu Xiang* (Aucklandiae Lappae, Radix), 3g, *Gan Cao* (Glycyrrhizae Uralensis, Radix), 3g,

and *Dong Gua Pi* (Benincasae Hispidae, Semen), 24g. This is a one day dose.

Nie took this formula and returned on Feb. 13. His urination had increased and the edema had disappeared from his face and upper extremities, but his lower extremities and genitals were still swollen. Dr. Huo thought the prescription needed more medicinals to warm kidney yang and fortify the spleen in order to fully transform water. Thus, he added *Qian Niu Zi* (Pharbitidis, Semen), nine grams, and increased *Fu Zi* to nine grams. He also added one pill of *Shen Qi Wan* (Kidney Qi Pills) twice a day to Nie's regimen. When Nie returned on Feb. 27, he had a healthy appetite, all his edema dissipated, and his stool and urination had returned to normal. Dr. Huo decided to reduce the medicinals to one bolus of *Shen Qi Wan* twice a day plus one bolus of *Gui Pi Wan* (Restore the Spleen Pills) once a day. A follow-up after three years showed no recurrence.

COMMENTARY: As mentioned above, when kidney and spleen yang vacuity cause edema, one cannot rely only on water-disinhibiting, dampness-percolating medicinals. These can easily damage the true qi. If the true qi is damaged, the patient can never fully recover and edema will recur. Of course, one must percolate dampness, but one must also supplement any constitutional yang and qi vacuity. Even if the edema is completely gone, one must continue to supplement the spleen and kidney for 3-6 months, using formulas such as *Shen Qi Wan* (Kidney Qi Pills).

3. KIDNEY YIN & YANG VACUITY

SIGNS & SYMPTOMS: Feeling cold during the day, cold hands and feet, pale face, fatigue, low appetite; feeling hot during the night with night sweats. The tongue is pale red and puffy, and the pulse is bowstring but fine and forceless.

TREATMENT PRINCIPLES: Supplement yin and yang and secure the essence

REPRESENTATIVE FORMULA: Modified *Liu Wei Di Huang Wan* (Six Flavors Rehmannia Pills)

Shu Di Huang (Rehmanniae Glutinosae, cooked Radix), 12g

Shan Zhu Yu (Corni Officinalis, Fructus), 12g

Shan Yao (Radix Dioscoreae Oppositae), 12g

Fu Ling (Poriae Cocos, Sclerotium), 12g

Ze Xie (Alismatis Orientalis, Rhizoma), 9g

Mu Dan Pi (Moutan, Cortex Radicis), 12g

Zhu Ling (Polypori Umbellati, Sclerotium), 9g

MODIFICATIONS: One can also add powdered *Huang Qi* (Astragali Membranacei, Radix) to reduce the blood protein level. This must be used cautiously, however, because *Huang Qi* is warming and can increase night sweats.[4]

NOTE: One might think that one should prescribe *Jin Gui Shen Qi Wan* (*Golden Cabinet* Kidney Qi Pills) for this condition, but this depends whether yin or yang vacuity is greater. If a patient has severe night sweats, one should start with a yin-supplementing formula, such as *Liu Wei Di Huang Wan* (Six Flavors Rehmannia Pills) or even *Zhi Bai Di Huang Wan* (Anemarrhena & Phellodendron Rehmannia Pills). When the night sweats have resolved, one can switch to *Jin Gui Shen Qi Wan*.

When using *Liu Wei Di Huang Wan* or *Zhi Bai Di Huang Wan*, one may add securing and astringing medicinals to help reduce protein loss. (See the list of securing and astringing medicinals in the discussion of the spleen-kidney qi vacuity pattern above.) Adding these tends to cause stagnation, however, and there is already a tendency for protein loss to cause stagnation. In order to counter such possible stagnation, one may add blood-quickening medicinals, such as *Tao Ren* (Pruni Persicae, Semen), *Hong Hua* (Carthami Tinctorii, Flos), *Dan Shen* (Salviae Miltiorrhizae, Radix), *Chi Shao* (Paeoniae Lactiflorae, Radix Rubrus), *Niu Xi* (Achyranthis Bidentatae, Radix), *Shui Zhi* (Hirudo Seu Whitmania), *Chuan Xiong* (Ligustici Wallichii, Radix), *Dang Gui* (Angelicae Sinensis, Radix), and *Mu Dan Pi* (Moutan, Cortex Radicis).

CAUTION: Patients must maintain a healthy diet with a high protein content to make up for the protein loss through proteinuria. Patients should also avoid cold and damp weather conditions and heavy exertion.

ACUMOXIBUSTION: Choose from *Pi Shu* (Bl 20), *Shen Shu* (Bl 23), *Zhi Shi* (Bl 52), *Ming Men* (GV 4), *Qi Hai* (CV 6), *Qi Zhong* (CV 8), *Guan Yuan* (CV 4), *Zhong Wan* (CV 12), *Yong Quan* (Ki 1), *Tai Xi* (Ki 3), *Zhao Hai* (Ki 6), *He Gu* (LI 4), and *Fu Liu* (Ki 7).

Case history from Dr. Wei Li's private practice: Shen, a 14 year-old boy

Shen's first visit was in October 1989. His symptoms included low appetite and sore throat. Urinalysis showed protein at 3+. During the day, Shen's hands and feet felt cold. In the evening, however, he always felt hot. Even in the dead of winter, he could only have a thin blanket covering him at night. He would still sweat and have to change his bedclothes a few times. Shen's tongue was pale and puffy with a red tip and thin, white fur, and his pulse was bowstring. Dr. Li's pattern identification was kidney yin and yang vacuity with spleen qi vacuity. She prescribed modified *Zhi Bai Di Huang Wan* (Anemarrhena & Phellodendron Rehmannia Pills): *Fu Pen Zi* (Rubi Chingii, Fructus), 10g, *Sang Shen* (Mori Albi, Fructus), 10g, *Wu Mei* (Pruni Mume, Fructus), 10g, calcined, powdered *Mu Li* (Ostreae, Concha), 6g, *Hu Zhang* (Polygoni Cuspidati, Radix Et Rhizoma), 10g, *Dan Shen* (Salviae Miltiorrhizae, Radix), 5g, *Jin Yin Hua* (Lonicerae Japonicae, Flos), 15g, *Lian Qiao* (Forsythiae Suspensae, Fructus), 15g, *Zhi Mu* (Anemarrhenae Asphodeloidis, Rhizoma), 7g, *Huang Bai* (Phellodendri, Cortex), 7g, *Sheng Di Huang* (Rehmanniae Glutinosae, uncooked Radix), 15g, *Shan Zhu Yu* (Corni Officinalis, Fructus), 7g, *Fu Ling* (Poriae Cocos, Sclerotium), 7g, *Shan Yao* (Radix Dioscoreae Oppositae), 7g, *Mu Dan Pi* (Moutan, Cortex Radicis), 5g, and *Ze Xie* (Alismatis Orientalis, Rhizoma), 5g. Dr. Li also used moxibustion on *Shen Shu* (Bl 23), *Zhi Shi* (Bl 52), *Qi Zhong* (CV 8), and *Yong Quan* (Ki 1) for a half hour once a day.

Shen took Dr. Li's prescription for three days and his night sweats almost completely disappeared. His urine protein reduced to 1-2+. He took the prescription for seven days and his urine protein became negative, he stopped having night sweats, he slept very soundly, and his appetite and energy returned. However, in the following month, his symptoms reoccurred. Dr. Li changed Shen's prescription to:

uncooked, powdered *Huang Lian* (Coptidis Chinensis, Rhizoma), 1g, *Feng Mi* (Mel, honey), 1 teaspoon, and *Xi Gua Zhi* (Citrulli, Succus Fructi, watermelon juice), 2-3 cups. Shen was to take this prescription two times per day for one month. After this regimen, Shen's symptoms completely disappeared and his urinalysis returned to normal. A follow-up three months later found no recurrence.

Case history of Dr. Sun Lian-xu: Yao, a 35 year-old male[5]

Yao's first visit was on Feb. 21, 1980. He had been suffering with nephritis since 1973. His urine protein was 3+. His face and feet had slight edema, and he experienced fatigue and low back soreness. His tongue was red with thin, white fur, and his pulse was fine. Dr. Sun's pattern identification was kidney yin and yang vacuity. He used a formula called *Gu Shen Feng* (Secure the Kidney Decoction).[6] To this he added *Jin Ying Zi* (Rosae Laevigatae, Fructus), 30g, and *Sang Shen* (Mori Albi, Fructus), 30g. Yao took this formula for eight months. By the end of this course of treatment, his urinalysis was normal and he was symptom free. A follow-up six months later found that he had had a complete recovery.

COMMENTARY: The three patterns discussed above are always accompanied by some degree of dampness. Sometimes they even have damp heat. When damp heat is involved, the patient will have fever, thirst, constipation, sore throat, and dark, scanty, and/or painful urination. The tongue will be red with yellow fur, and the pulse will be slippery and fast. When damp heat is involved, one must determine what level the heat is in. If it is in the defensive aspect, one may use *Jin Yin Hua* (Lonicerae Japonicae, Flos), *Lian Qiao* (Forsythiae Suspensae, Fructus), *Ban Lan Gen* (Isatidis Seu Baphicacanthi, Radix), *Da Qing Ye* (Daqingye, Folium), etc. If the heat is in the qi aspect, one may use *Huang Lian* (Coptidis Chinensis, Rhizoma), *Huang Qin* (Scutellariae Baicalensis, Radix), *Huang Bai* (Phellodendri, Cortex), *Zhi Zi* (Gardeniae Jasminoidis, Fructus), *Zhi Mu* (Anemarrhenae Asphodeloidis, Rhizoma), etc. If the heat is in the constructive/blood aspect, one may use blood-cooling, stasis-dispelling medicinals such as *Mu Dan Pi* (Moutan, Cortex Radicis) and *Chi*

Shao (Paeoniae Lactiflorae, Radix Rubrus) plus medicinals that clear defensive and qi aspect heat.

PROTEIN, BLOOD & CASTS IN THE URINE

1. SPLEEN-KIDNEY QI & YANG VACUITY WITH DAMP HEAT

SIGNS & SYMPTOMS: Fever, dry mouth with a bitter taste, desire for cold drinks. These are in addition to fatigue, heart palpitations, shortness of breath, no appetite, loose stools, a pale facial complexion, low back and knee soreness and limpness, feeling cold, cold hands and feet, and edema. The tongue is red and the pulse is floating and fast.

TREATMENT PRINCIPLES: First, clear and eliminate dampness and heat and quicken the blood; secondly, supplement yang and qi

REPRESENTATIVE FORMULAS: *Yin Qiao San* (Lonicera & Forsythia Powder)

Jin Yin Hua (Lonicerae Japonicae, Flos), 9-15g
Lian Qiao (Forsythiae Suspensae, Fructus), 9-15g
Jie Geng (Platycodi Grandiflori, Radix), 3-6g
Niu Bang Zi (Arctii Lappae, Fructus), 9-12g
Bo He (Menthae Haplocalycis, Herba), 3-6g
Dan Dou Chi (Sojae, Semen Praeparatum), 3-6g
Jing Jie (Schizonepetae Tenuifoliae, Herba Seu Flos), 6-9g
Dan Zhu Ye (Lophatheri Gracilis, Herba), 3-6g
fresh *Lu Gen* (Phragmitis Communis, Rhizoma), 15-30g
Gan Cao (Glycyrrhizae Uralensis, Radix), 3-6g

Sang Ju Yin (Morus & Chrysanthemum Beverage)

Sang Ye (Mori Albi, Folium), 9-12g
Ju Hua (Chrysanthemi Morifolii, Flos), 9-12g
Lian Qiao (Forsythiae Suspensae, Fructus), 9-12g
Bo He (Menthae Haplocalycis, Herba), 6g
Jie Geng (Platycodi Grandiflori, Radix), 9g
Xing Ren (Pruni Armeniacae, Semen), 9g
Lu Gen (Phragmitis Communis, Rhizoma), 9-12g
Gan Cao (Glycyrrhizae Uralensis, Radix), 3g

These two formulas clear defensive aspect heat.

Huang Lian Jie Du Tang (Coptis Toxin-resolving Decoction)

Huang Lian (Coptidis Chinensis, Rhizoma), 9g
Huang Qin (Scutellariae Baicalensis, Radix), 9g
Huang Bai (Phellodendri, Cortex), 9g
Zhi Zi (Gardeniae Jasminoidis, Fructus), 9g

This formula clears qi aspect heat, including damp heat.

MODIFICATIONS: One may also need to clear deeper constructive and blood aspect heat, especially if the patient has swollen glands and/or tonsillitis. (Red and swollen glands indicate there is blood heat stasis and stagnation, for which one must cool and quicken the blood.) In this case, one can choose from medicinals such as *Xuan Shen* (Scrophulariae Ningpoensis, Radix), *Sheng Di Huang* (Rehmanniae Glutinosae, uncooked Radix), and *Chi Shao* (Paeoniae Lactiflorae, Radix Rubrus) to cool the blood aspect. Clearing heat is key; nephritis cannot be cured if heat is not eliminated.

COMMENTARY: According to Western medical theory, this type of nephritis is caused by an antibody/antigen reaction from an upper respiratory infection. Therefore, one must resolve the upper respiratory infection to resolve the nephritis. In terms of the five phases, metal (lung) generates water (kidney). Thus metal is the mother of water. If the mother is sick, the child suffers, and, to cure the child, one must treat the mother. After the evils have been cleared, one must supplement. To supplement yang qi one must follow the principles discussed under spleen-kidney yang vacuity above. In this pattern, there are blood and casts in the urine (in addition to protein). Besides clearing heat, one must also cool and quicken the blood even if there are no swollen glands. Gentle blood-quickening medicinals are not strong enough. One must use strong stasis-dispelling medicinals, such as *Dan Shen* (Salviae Miltiorrhizae, Radix), *Shui Zhi* (Hirudo Seu Whitmania), *San Leng* (Sparganii Stoloniferi, Rhizoma), or *Yi Mu Cao* (Leonuri Heterophylli, Herba). Dispelling stasis is extremely important in this pattern. One can hardly succeed without it.

ACUMOXIBUSTION: Choose points to needle from

Zhi Gou (TB 6), *Wei Yang* (Bl 53), *He Gu* (LI 4), *Yang Ling Quan* (GB 34). Choose points to moxa from *Pi Shu* (Bl 20), *Shen Shu* (Bl 23), *Ming Men* (GV 4), *Qi Hai* (CV 6), *Guan Yuan* (CV 4), *Zhong Wan* (CV 12), *Qi Hai* (CV 6), *Qi Zhong* (CV 8), *Zu San Li* (St 36), *Tai Bai* (Sp 3), *Gong Sun* (Sp 4), *San Yin Jiao* (Sp 6), *Yin Ling Quan* (Sp 9), *Yong Quan* (Ki 1), *Tai Xi* (Ki 3), and *Zhao Hai* (Ki 6).

2. SPLEEN-KIDNEY QI & YANG VACUITY WITH DAMPNESS

SIGNS & SYMPTOMS: Feeling cold, cold hands and feet, fatigue, no appetite, water swelling (ascites). The tongue is pale and puffy with thin, white fur, and the pulse is deep, thin, and forceless.

TREATMENT PRINCIPLES: Fortify the spleen, warm the kidney, and transform water

REPRESENTATIVE FORMULAS: Modified *Zhen Wu Tang* (True Warrior Decoction), *Shi Pi Yin* (Bolster the Spleen Beverage), and *Shen Qi Wan* (Kidney Qi Pills); see pattern 2 above.

NOTE: The difference between this pattern and pattern 2, spleen-kidney qi vacuity, is egregious blood stasis[7] resulting in microcirculation problems. Therefore, one must add strong stasis-dispelling medicinals, such as *Dan Shen* (Salviae Miltiorrhizae, Radix), *Shui Zhi* (Hirudo Seu Whitmania), *Yi Mu Cao* (Leonuri Heterophylli, Herba), *Tao Ren* (Pruni Persicae, Semen), *Chi Shao* (Paeoniae Lactiflorae, Radix Rubrus), *Mu Dan Pi* (Moutan, Cortex Radicis), etc. to the formulas found in pattern 2 above.

ACUMOXIBUSTION: Choose points to moxa from *Pi Shu* (Bl 20), *Shen Shu* (Bl 23), *Ming Men* (GV 4), *Qi Hai* (CV 6), *Zhong Wan* (CV 12), *Guan Yuan* (CV 4), *Zu San Li* (St 36), *Tai Bai* (Sp 3), *Gong Sun* (Sp 4), *San Yin Jiao* (Sp 6), *Yin Ling Quan* (Sp 9), *Tai Xi* (Ki 3), *Zhao Hai* (Ki 6); needle *Xue Hai* (Sp 10) and *Ge Shu* (Bl 17).

Case history of Dr. Sun Lian-xu: Wang, a 46 year-old male[8]

Wang first came to see Dr. Sun on Feb. 4, 1980. He

became ill two years earlier, in April 1978. Urinalysis showed protein at 2+ and RBCs at 1-2+. His kidney function was mildly damaged. Wang felt weak and dizzy and had a pale yellow facial complexion. His low back and knees were weak and sore and his lower extremities were edematous. His tongue was pale with thin, white fur, and his pulse was fine, soft, and soggy. Dr. Sun's pattern identification was qi and yang vacuity with blood stasis. His treatment strategy was to fortify the spleen, supplement the qi, and quicken the blood. His prescription consisted of: *Dang Shen* (Codonopsitis Pilosulae, Radix), 15g, *Bai Zhu* (Atractylodis Macrocephalae, Rhizoma), 15g, *Fu Ling* (Poriae Cocos, Sclerotium), 15g, mix-fried *Gan Cao* (Glycyrrhizae Uralensis, Radix), 6g, *Sang Shen* (Mori Albi, Fructus), 30g, *Huang Qi* (Astragali Membranacei, Radix), 30g, *Dan Shen* (Salviae Miltiorrhizae, Radix), 30g, uncooked *Di Yu* (Sanguisorbae Officinalis, Radix), 30g, *Ma Bian Cao* (Verbena Officinalis, Herba), 30g, *Huang Lian* (Coptidis Chinensis, Rhizoma), 3g, *Pao Jiang* (Zingiberis Officinalis, blast-fried Rhizoma), 3g, and *Da Zao* (Zizyphi Jujubae, Fructus), 5 pieces. Wang took this prescription for five months. All his symptoms disappeared and his laboratory tests returned to normal.

Later, Wang caught a cold and his symptoms returned. His urine protein went up to 1+ and RBCs to 1+. Dr. Sun prescribed a formula to clear and resolve heat toxins and drain dampness, adding *Sheng Ma* (Cimicifugae, Rhizoma), 9g, and *Dang Shen* (Codonopsitis Pilosulae, Radix), 15g. Wang took this new prescription for a month. After finishing this regimen, he no longer had symptoms of an exterior pattern, but he still had red blood cells in his urine. Dr. Sun decided to change the prescription back to one that supplemented the qi and quickened the blood. After Wang finished this last formula, his laboratory tests returned to normal. A follow-up eight months later showed no recurrence.

3. KIDNEY YIN VACUITY WITH DAMPNESS

SIGNS & SYMPTOMS: Dizziness, headache, dry eyes, tinnitus, edema in the lower extremities or whole body, low back and knee soreness and limpness, irascibility and insomnia, hot palms and soles. The tongue is red and without fur, and the pulse is fine, fast, and forceful.

TREATMENT PRINCIPLES: Nourish kidney yin, subdue yang, and drain water

REPRESENTATIVE FORMULA: *Liu Wei Di Huang Wan* (Six Flavors Rehmannia Pills)

Shu Di Huang (Rehmanniae Glutinosae, cooked Radix), 12g
Shan Yao (Dioscoreae Oppositae, Radix), 12g
Shan Zhu Yu (Corni Officinalis, Fructus), 12g
Ze Xie (Alismatis Orientalis, Rhizoma), 9g
Fu Ling (Poriae Cocos, Sclerotium), 9g
Mu Dan Pi (Moutan, Cortex Radicis), 9g

MODIFICATIONS: For night sweats, add *Huang Bai* (Phellodendri, Cortex), *Zhi Mu* (Anemarrhenae Aspheloidis, Rhizoma), *Sang Ye* (Mori Albi, Folium), *Xuan Shen* (Scrophulariae Ningpoensis, Radix), and *Han Lian Cao* (Ecliptae Prostratae, Herba). Fro dry throat and mouth, add *Jin Yin Hua* (Lonicerae Japonicae, Flos), *Xuan Shen* (Scrophulariae Ningpoensis, Radix), *Mu Hu Die* (Oroxyli Indici, Semen), and *Fang Huang Yi* (chicken egg membrane). If the patient has bloody urine, add *Da Ji* (Cirsii Japonici, Herba Seu Radix), *Xiao Ji* (Cephalanoplos Segeti, Herba), *Dan Shen* (Salviae Miltiorrhizae, Radix), and *Han Lian Cao* (Ecliptae Prostratae, Herba). If the patient has high blood pressure, add *Niu Xi* (Achyranthis Bidentatae, Radix), *Sheng Di Huang* (Rehmanniae Glutinosae, uncooked Radix), *Bai Shao* (Paeoniae Lactiflorae, Radix Albus), *Gou Qi Zi* (Lycii Chinensis, Fructus), and *Ju Hua* (Chrysanthemi Morifolii, Flos). For insomnia, add *Tian Wang Bu Xi Dan* (Heavenly Emperor Supplement the Heart Elixir). For constipation, add *Zeng Ye Cheng Qi Tang* (Increase Humors Order the Qi Decoction).

ACUMOXIBUSTION: Choose from *Shen Shu* (Bl 23), *Tai Xi* (Ki 3), *Zhao Hai* (Ki 6), *Tai Chong* (Liv 3), *Nei Guan* (Per 6), *Yin Ling Quan* (Sp 9), and *Zu San Li* (St 36).

Case history of Dr. Xi Shuan-chang: Huo, a 20 year-old female[9]

Huo had yin vacuity water swelling. Her face and body were edematous with pitting, and she had tidal fever and heat in the five hearts. She could urinate only one time per day, and her urine was red and her urination was rough. Her left pulse was bowstring and fine, while her right pulse was bowstring, forceful, and fast. Based on these signs and symptoms, Dr. Xi thought there were three causes of Huo's difficult urine: vacuity heat damaging the kidney, liver disharmony, and stomach heat descending. The liver disharmony was indicated by Huo's bowstring and fine left pulse. The liver channel transverses the genital area and, if the liver's coursing function is weak, it can cause urinary difficulty. Stomach heat descending was indicated by Huo's bowstring, forceful right pulse. Therefore, Dr. Xi prescribed the following: *Shan Yao* (Radix Dioscoreae Oppositae), 50g, *Sheng Di Huang* (Rehmanniae Glutinosae, uncooked Radix), 18g, *Bai Shao* (Paeoniae Lactiflorae, Radix Albus), 18g, *Xuan Shen* (Scrophulariae Ningpoensis, Radix), 15g, *Gou Qi Zi* (Lycii Chinensis, Fructus), 15g, *Sha Shen* (Glenhniae Littoralis, Radix), 12g, and *Hua Shi* (Talcum), 9g.

Huo took this formula for four days, and her urine became easy, her edema dissipated by half, and her tidal fever disappeared. However, she still had heat in the five hearts and a fast pulse. Dr. Xi changed the formula, prescribing the following: *Shu Di Huang* (Rehmanniae Glutinosae, cooked Radix), 50g, *Bai Shao* (Paeoniae Lactiflorae, Radix Albus), 18g, *Shan Yao* (Radix Dioscoreae Oppositae), 15g, *Gou Qi Zi* (Lycii Chinensis, Fructus), 15g, *Bai Zi Ren* (Biotae Orientalis, Semen), 12g, *Xuan Shen* (Scrophulariae Ningpoensis, Radix), 12g, *Sha Shen* (Glenhniae Littoralis, Radix), 9g, *Che Qian Zi* (Plantaginis, Semen), 9g, *Fu Ling* (Poriae Cocos, Sclerotium), 6g, and *Bai Mao Gen* (Imperatae Cylindricae, Rhizoma), 15g. After six days of the new formula, Huo's edema completely dissipated and her pulse returned to normal. Dr. Xi discontinued the formula and advised Huo to take 50 grams of *Shan Yao* (Radix Dioscoreae Oppositae) powder mixed with fresh pear juice every day to consolidate the results.

4. KIDNEY YIN VACUITY WITH DAMP HEAT

SIGNS & SYMPTOMS: Low back and knee soreness and limpness, fatigue, thirst, dizziness, tinnitus, tidal fever, night sweats, irascibility, and insomnia. The tongue is red with yellow fur, and the pulse is fine, bowstring, forceful, and fast.

TREATMENT PRINCIPLES: Supplement the kidney and enrich yin, clear heat and eliminate dampness

REPRESENTATIVE FORMULA: *Zhi Bai Di Huang Wan* (Anemarrhena & Phellodendron Rehmannia Pills)

Zhi Mu (Anemarrhenae Asphodeloidis, Rhizoma), 9g
Huang Bai (Phellodendri, Cortex), 9g
Shu Di Huang (Rehmanniae Glutinosae, cooked Radix), 12g
Shan Yao (Radix Dioscoreae Oppositae), 12g
Shan Zhu Yu (Corni Officinalis, Fructus), 12g
Ze Xie (Alismatis Orientalis, Rhizoma), 9g
Fu Ling (Poriae Cocos, Sclerotium), 9g
Mu Dan Pi (Moutan, Cortex Radicis), 9g

MODIFICATIONS: If heat is more pronounced, one may add *Huang Lian* (Coptidis Chinensis, Rhizoma), *Huang Qin* (Scutellariae Baicalensis, Radix), and *Zhi Zi* (Gardeniae Jasminoidis, Fructus).

ACUMOXIBUSTION: Choose from *Shen Shu* (Bl 23), *Yin Ling Quan* (Sp 9), *Tai Xi* (Ki 3), *Zhao Hai* (Ki 6), *Yang Ling Quan* (GB 34), *Zhi Gou* (TB 6), *Wei Yang* (Bl 53), *He Gu* (LI 4), and *San Yin Jiao* (Sp 6).

Case history of Dr. Zhi Xian-gong: Li, a 28 year-old female[10]

Li was having an acute episode of her chronic pyelonephritis when she came to see Dr. Zhi. Urinalysis showed her urine protein at 1+, pus cells at 3+, and RBCs at 3+. Her urine bacterial culture was more than one million. The patient presented with urinary urgency, frequency, burning, and scanty, dark yellow urine. She also had low back pain, lower abdominal cramping, shortness of breath, fatigue, dry throat without thirst, night sweats, dizziness, and tinnitus. Her tongue was red without fur, and her pulse was fine and fast. Based on these signs and symptoms, Dr. Zhi's pattern identification was kidney qi and yin vacuity with damp heat. Therefore, he prescribed modified *Zhi Bai Di Huang Wan* (Anemarrhena &

Phellodendron Rehmannia Pills): *Sheng Di Huang* (Rehmanniae Glutinosae, uncooked Radix), 20g, *Mu Dan Pi* (Moutan, Cortex Radicis), 10g, *Nu Zhen Zi* (Ligustri Lucidi, Fructus), 30g, *Han Lian Cao* (Ecliptae Prostratae, Herba), 30g, *Shan Yao* (Radix Dioscoreae Oppositae), 20g, *Fu Ling* (Poriae Cocos, Sclerotium), 12g, *Ze Xie* (Alismatis Orientalis, Rhizoma), 12g, *Huang Qi* (Astragali Membranacei, Radix), 30g, *Tai Zi Shen* (Pseudostellariae Heterophyllae, Radix), 20g, *Zhi Mu* (Anemarrhenae Asphodeloidis, Rhizoma), 12g, *Huang Bai* (Phellodendri, Cortex), 12g, *Jin Yin Hua* (Lonicerae Japonicae, Flos), 30g, and *Che Qian Zi* (Plantaginis, Semen), 30g.

Li took this formula for five days and all her symptoms were better except for her urination. Dr. Zhi decided to add 20 grams of *Liu Yi San* (Six-to-One Powder).[11] Li took this new formula for 10 days. All her symptoms disappeared except for low back soreness. Accordingly, Dr. Zhi prescribed the following formula: *Shu Di Huang* (Rehmanniae Glutinosae, cooked Radix), 15g, *Mu Dan Pi* (Moutan, Cortex Radicis), 10g, *Shan Zhu Yu* (Corni Officinalis, Fructus), 15g, *Shan Yao* (Radix Dioscoreae Oppositae), 20g, *Fu Ling* (Poriae Cocos, Sclerotium), 12g, *Zhi Mu* (Anemarrhenae Asphodeloidis, Rhizoma), 12g, *Huang Bai* (Phellodendri, Cortex), 12g, *Huang Qi* (Astragali Membranacei, Radix), 30g, *Dang Shen* (Codonopsitis Pilosulae, Radix), 15g, *Gou Qi Zi* (Lycii Chinensis, Fructus), 15g, *Jin Yin Teng* (Lonicerae Japonicae, Caulis), 30g, and *Che Qian Zi* (Plantaginis, Semen), 30g. Li took this formula for 15 days and her low back pain improved. A urine culture was negative. Dr. Zhi advised her to take six grams of *Zhi Bai Di Huang Wan* twice a day for three months to consolidate the results. A follow-up one year later showed no recurrence.

5. KIDNEY YIN VACUITY WITH BLOOD STASIS

SIGNS & SYMPTOMS: Low back and knee soreness and limpness, fatigue, thirst, dizziness, tinnitus, tidal fever, night sweats, irascibility, insomnia, dry mouth, thirst without a desire to drink, low-grade fever, and purple patches (purpura). The tongue is red with dark, purple, stasis speckles. The pulse is fine and choppy.

TREATMENT PRINCIPLES: Supplement the kidney and nourish yin, quicken the blood and transform stasis

REPRESENTATIVE FORMULA: Modified *Zhi Bai Di Huang Wan* (Anemarrhena & Phellodendron Rehmannia Pills) plus *Xue Fu Zhu Yu Tang* (Blood Mansion Dispel Stasis Decoction)

Zhi Mu (Anemarrhenae Asphodeloidis, Rhizoma), 9g
Huang Bai (Phellodendri, Cortex), 9g
Shu Di Huang (Rehmanniae Glutinosae, cooked Radix), 12g
Shan Yao (Radix Dioscoreae Oppositae), 12g
Shan Zhu Yu (Corni Officinalis, Fructus), 12g
Ze Xie (Alismatis Orientalis, Rhizoma), 9g
Fu Ling (Poriae Cocos, Sclerotium), 9g
Mu Dan Pi (Moutan, Cortex Radicis), 9g
Tao Ren (Pruni Persicae, Semen), 9g
Hong Hua (Carthami Tinctorii, Flos), 6g
Chuan Xiong (Ligustici Wallichii, Radix), 9g
Dang Gui (Angelicae Sinensis, Radix), 9g
Chi Shao (Paeoniae Lactiflorae, Radix Rubrus), 9g
Niu Xi (Achyranthis Bidentatae, Radix), 9g
Chai Hu (Bupleuri, Radix), 3g
Sheng Di Huang (Rehmanniae Glutinosae, uncooked Radix), 9g
Jie Geng (Platycodi Grandiflori, Radix), 9g
Zhi Ke (Citri Aurantii, Fructus), 6g
Gan Cao (Glycyrrhizae Uralensis, Radix), 3g
Shui Zhi (Hirudo Seu Whitmania), 1.5-3g

NOTE: The most effective blood-quickening medicinal for this condition is *Shui Zhi* (Hirudo Seu Whitmania).

MODIFICATIONS: For edema, add *Yi Mu Cao* (Leonuri Heterophylli, Herba) and *Ze Lan* (Lycopi Lucidi, Herba). If the patient has high blood pressure, one must use medicinals which move the blood and subdue yang, such as *Niu Xi, Chi Shao,* and *Dan Shen* (Salviae Miltiorrhizae, Radix). For constipation, add *Da Huang* (Rhei, Radix Et Rhizoma). One must be careful when precipitating, however, as this can damage yin. To avoid this, one can add yin-supplementing medicinals. If there is bleeding, be sure to use medicinals which both stanch bleeding and quicken the blood as mentioned above.

ACUMOXIBUSTION: Choose from *Ge Shu* (Bl 17), *Shen Shu* (Bl 23), *Kun Lun* (Bl 60), *Tai Xi* (Ki 3), *Zhao Hai* (Ki 6), *Xue Hai* (Sp 10), *Yun Men* (Liv 2), and *Tai Chong* (Liv 3).

Case history of Dr. Hou Rian-chen: Qu, a 25 year-old female[12]

Qu had chronic nephritis for five years. While she frequently had blood and protein in her urine, typically she had only blood. She had tried Western medications with no success. Therefore, she turned to Chinese medicine and tried *Lui Wei Di Huang Wan* (Six Flavors Rehmannia Pills) and *Xiao Ji Yin Zi* (Cephalanoplos Beverage) to nourish yin and cool the blood. This combination improved her condition for a while, but then there was a recurrence. She tried the same combination again, but it did not work the second time. On the contrary, it seemed to cause difficult urination.

Qu was skinny with a dark face. She had dizziness and low back soreness. Her mouth was dry, and she was thirsty without the desire to drink. She also had purple spots on her body. Her tongue was dark red with purple speckles, and her pulse was bowstring, fine, and choppy. Urinalysis showed RBCs at 3+ and protein at 1+. Dr. Hou's pattern identification was yin vacuity heat with obstruction in the kidney channel. He thought that the use of *Liu Wei Di Huang Wan* and *Xiao Ji Yin Zi* had relied too heavily on supplementing yin and stanching bleeding without attending to blood stasis. Thus, his treatment strategy was to supplement the kidney and nourish yin, clear heat and dispel stasis. His formula consisted of: *Sheng Di Huang* (Rehmanniae Glutinosae, uncooked Radix), 12g, *Shu Di Huang* (Rehmanniae Glutinosae, cooked Radix), 12g, *Han Lian Cao* (Ecliptae Prostratae, Herba), 15g, *He Shou Wu* (Polygoni Multiflori, Radix), 9g, *Huang Bai* (Phellodendri, Cortex), 9g, *Da Ji* (Cirsii Japonici, Herba Seu Radix), 15g, *Xiao Ji* (Cephalanoplos Segeti, Herba), 15g, *Chi Shao* (Paeoniae Lactiflorae, Radix Rubrus), 9g, *Mu Dan Pi* (Moutan, Cortex Radicis), 6g, *Tao Ren* (Pruni Persicae, Semen), 9g, *Dang Gui* (Angelicae Sinensis, Radix), 9g, *Hong Hua* (Carthami Tinctorii, Flos), 4.5g, *Bie Jia* (Amydae Sinensis, Carapax), 15g, *Niu Xi* (Achyranthis Bidentatae, Radix), 15g, uncooked

Gan Cao (Glycyrrhizae Uralensis, Radix), 6g, and *Yi Mu Cao* (Leonuri Heterophylli, Herba), 12g. Qu took this prescription for seven days and her urine became disinhibited. Her urinalysis showed RBCs at 1+ with negative protein. Dr. Hou removed *Mu Dan Pi* and Qu continued on the modified formula for 14 more days. By that time, her urine returned to normal.

COMMENTARY: Quickening the blood and dispelling stasis is an extremely important strategy for chronic nephritis. Dr. Hou's formula is called *Tong Yu Tang* (Free the Flow of Stasis Decoction). It supplements yin as well as quickens the blood and dispels stasis. *Mu Dan Pi, Chi Shao, Niu Xi,* and *Yi Mu Cao* free the flow of the channels in the lower burner to remove stasis. These also clear the extravasated blood and help generate new blood. (When one removes old blood, one should also generate new blood.) The additions *Han Lian Cao, He Shou Wu, Shu Di Huang,* and *Bie Jia* supplement the kidney and enrich yin. *Huang Bai, Da Ji, Sheng Di Huang,* and *Xiao Ji* clear heat and drain fire, cool the blood and stanch bleeding.

When treating yin vacuity with blood stasis, the treatment strategy should include nourishing yin, clearing heat, dispelling stasis, and stopping bleeding. (When there is stasis heat, the symptoms often include thirst without a desire to drink, a low-grade fever, purpura, and a red tongue with dark, purple stasis speckles.) If one uses only kidney yin-supplementing medicinals, one may cause more stagnation. If one employs only heat-clearing and blood-stanching medicinals, one may make urinary difficulties worse. Therefore, one must combine medicinals to fulfill all the elements of the treatment strategy at the same time.

CLINICAL TIPS

1. There are two categories of Clinical Nephrology patients who come to Chinese medical practitioners. The first, Category A, includes patients who have had Western drug therapy but have not achieved completely satisfactory results. There are three reasons for this. First, the patient may not have responded to Western drug therapy. Second, the patient may have responded favorably to Western drug therapy but has recurrences when the drug ther-

apy is discontinued. Third, the patient may have had favorable results to the Western drug therapy, but symptoms start to recur when beginning withdrawal. Category B includes patients who have abnormal urinalyses but are not ill and have no symptoms.

Furthermore, all Clinical Nephrology patients may be divided into two types according to the results of their urinalysis. Type 1 are those patients who have protein only in the urine. Type 2 are patients who have protein, abnormal amounts of red blood cells, and casts in the urine. Category B, type 1 patients, asymptomatic patients with protein only in their urine, have either "posture protein" or mesangiopathic nephritis. Posture protein is usually found in children. Proteinuria only occurs when the child is in a certain posture. This is because bones impinge on the child's kidney vein when the child stands up and causes proteinuria. When lying down, these bones do not impinge on the kidney vein and the proteinuria disappears. Mesangiopathic nephritis is often caused by mild damage to the kidney membrane and is usually self-limiting. Western physicians do not treat posture protein and mesangiopathic nephritis. However, some of these patients do develop more serious conditions and they should be carefully monitored.

Category B, type 2 patients, asymptomatic patients with protein, abnormal amounts of red blood cells, and casts in the urine, are usually given Western medical treatment even though they have no symptoms. These patients often have a positive response to Chinese medicine.

2. Pattern identification of Clinical Nephrology in the modern Chinese medical clinic is based on the results of urinalysis.

A. Patients with protein only in their urine usually have one of the following patterns: spleen and kidney qi vacuity, spleen and kidney yang vacuity, or kidney yin and yang vacuity. Any of these may be complicated with patterns of dampness or damp heat.

B. Patients with protein, casts, and blood cells in their urine usually have either spleen and kidney qi and yang vacuity or yin vacuity. Both these patterns may be complicated with patterns of dampness or damp heat. Yin vacuity may also be complicated with patterns of blood stasis.

3. There is an alternative Chinese medicinal therapy for Category A patients, those who have tried Western drug therapy but who do not respond or have started to have recurrences during or after withdrawing from these drugs. This consists of a few standard formulas not based on pattern identification but used to replace Western hormone therapy.

Figure 5.1 summarizes the above, *i.e.*: while standard hormone replacement formulas are useful in some instances, the following pattern identifications are useful for all Clinical Nephrology patients.

In the modern TCM clinic determining treatment by patterns identified (*bian zheng lun zhi*) is used to analyze the functional effects of chronic nephritis as

Category A: Clinical Nephrology patients who have tried Western medicine.		Chinese formulas to replace Western hormone therapy
Category B: Clinical Nephrology patients without symptoms.		
	Pattern identification:	**May combine with:**
Type 1: Patients with protein only in their urine	1. Spleen-kidney qi vacuity 2. Spleen-kidney yang vacuity 3. Kidney yin & yang vacuity	Dampness or damp heat Dampness or damp heat Dampness or damp heat
Type 2: Patients with protein, casts, and blood in their urine	4. Spleen-kidney qi & yang vacuity 5. Yin vacuity	Dampness or damp heat Dampness, damp heat, or blood stasis

Figure 5.1. Chinese medical therapy for Clinical Nephrology patients

determined by urinalysis. Pattern identification is used for both Category A and Category B patients. The patterns fall under rubrics with the same defining characteristics as type 1 and type 2 clinical nephrology patients, that is patients with protein only in the urine or patients with protein, casts, and blood in the urine. (See Figure 5.1.) In addition, there are a few standard formulas that are used for Category A patients. These are found under item 5 below. These standard formulas are not based on pattern identification, but are used in a broad way to replace Western hormone therapy.

4. Important considerations for all patterns of chronic nephritis:

A. Chronic nephritis patients usually have underlying vacuity patterns and, therefore, supplementation is often the treatment strategy of choice. However, one must identify which aspect or humor is vacuous and supplement accordingly. For yin vacuity one must supplement yin, for qi vacuity one must supplement qi, and so on. While *Huang Qi* (Astragali Membranacei, Radix) is good for all clinical nephrology patterns with protein in the urine, if a patient has yin vacuity, one should supplement yin first with formulas like *Liu Wei Di Huang Wan* (Six Flavors Rehmannia Pills). However, while *Liu Wei Di Huang Wan* is very good for improving the kidney function,[13] it is too cold for qi and yang vacuity patterns. In that case, one must add qi and yang supplementing medicinals, such as *Huang Qi* (Astragali Membranacei, Radix), *Dang Shen* (Codonopsitis Pilosulae, Radix), *Dong Chong Xia Cao* (Cordyceps Sinensis), *Yin Yang Huo* (Epimedii, Herba), *Du Zhong* (Eucommiae Ulmoidis, Cortex), *Fu Zi* (Aconiti Carmichaeli, Radix Lateralis Praeparatus), *Rou Gui* (Cinnamonmi Casiae, Cortex), *Gan Jiang* (Zingiberis Officinalis, dry Rhizoma), *Wu Zhu Yu* (Evodiae Rutaecarpae, Fructus), etc.

B. When one supplements edematous clinical nephrology patients, one must open and drain at the same time. To percolate dampness, one may choose medicinals such as *Ze Xie* (Alismatis Orientalis, Rhizoma), *Che Qian Zi* (Plantaginis, Semen), *Bai Mao Gen* (Imperatae Cylindricae, Rhizoma), *Yi Mu Cao* (Leonuri Heterophylli, Herba), *Shi Wei* (Pyrrosiae, Folium), and *Chi Xiao Dou* (Phaseoli Calcarati, Semen).

One can see this dual strategy at work in a formula such as *Liu Wei Di Huang Wan* from the *Xiao Er Yao Zheng Shi Jue* (*The Craft of Medicinal Treatment for Childhood Disease Patterns*) mentioned above. In this formula, *Shu Di Huang* strongly supplements the kidney, while *Ze Xie* and *Fu Ling* percolate dampness, thereby combining the strategies of supplementation and draining.[14] *Liu Wei Di Huang Wan* also uses *Shan Zhu Yu* (Fructus Corni Officinalis) to secure the essence. An important principle in Chinese medicine is to avoid retaining (or "locking in") evils when securing or supplementing. In *Liu Wei Di Huang Wan*, the draining medicinals counterbalance the securing medicinals to avoid this pitfall.

Another important formula used for chronic nephritis that supplements and drains is *Li Yu Huang Qi Tang* (Carp & Astragalus Decoction): *Li Yu* (Cyprinus Carpio), 1 piece, and *Huang Qi* (Astragali Membranacei, Radix), 50-100g. These are cooked together and one eats both the soup and the carp.

C. One often has to continue to eliminate external evils. Lingering evils are the primary reason acute nephritis becomes chronic. One can eliminate evils and supplement vacuities simultaneously.

5. Formulas to replace hormone therapy for Category A patients:

As stated above, Category A patients are those who have tried Western drug therapy but have not had complete success. One may always treat them with the standard Chinese medical approach, *i.e.*, by identifying patterns and basing treatment on these patterns. However, one may also prescribe one of a few standard formulas that replace hormone therapy.

Hormonal therapy is the Western therapy of choice for treating chronic nephritis. Patients given hormonal therapy have an increased amount of exogenous hormones in their blood. These exogenous hormones cause the endocrine glands to reduce the secretion of natural hormones. This is especially true of the hypothalamus, pituitary, and adrenal glands. When the patient withdraws from hormonal drug therapy, the endocrine glands usually resume their normal functioning. In other words, they begin to secrete hormones at a normal rate. However, in some cases, these glands begin to atrophy and become unable to resume their normal functioning. In these cases, symptoms of nephritis may reappear during withdrawal or after withdrawal.

The Chinese formulas that replace Western hormonal therapy have a different therapeutic mechanism and do not cause the endocrine glands to atrophy. These formulas have a positive effect on the endocrine glands, harmonizing their functions so that they can naturally produce the correct amount of hormones.

GENERAL COMMENTS ON SUBSTITUTING CHINESE MEDICINALS FOR HORMONE THERAPY

A. Acute nephritis is often caused by external evils: wind, heat, dampness, or toxins. Even if the patient's symptoms start to improve and most of the evils are eliminated, there is usually lingering heat as well as damage to yin from the heat toxins. In view of this, one should not use yang-invigorating medicinals even if there is yang vacuity. In this case, one may add only *Huang Qi* (Astragali Membranacei, Radix) to heat-clearing and toxin-resolving medicinals.

B. Patients who have been given large amounts of hormones or immunosuppressant drugs often contract infection diseases, especially urinary tract infections and upper respiratory infections. (These infections may not show very severe symptoms because the patient's immunity is compromised.) In treating these patients, one should first clear damp-heat toxins and then harmonize the spleen and stomach. Only after one is sure that the evils have been eliminated and the spleen and stomach are strong can one start to supplement kidney yin and yang.

C. Kidney patients usually have yin and yang vacuity since these are interdependent. They may also have hypertension. In a hypertensive patient, invigorating yang may damage yin, resulting in further yin-yang disharmony. In that case, one must nourish yin and subdue rising yang. However, if there is egregious yang vacuity, one may cautiously invigorate yang at the same time. One should also avoid the use

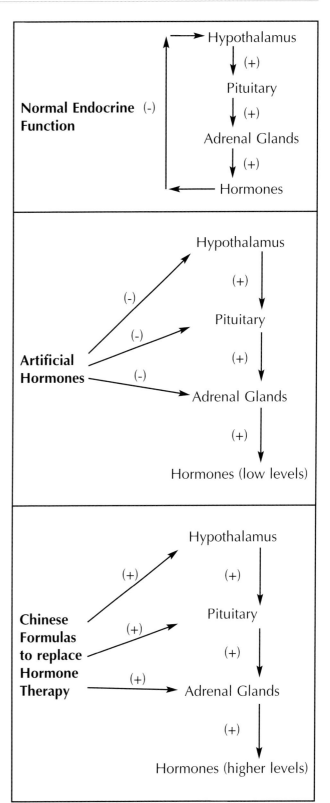

Figure 5.2. Comparison of normal endocrine function with hormone therapy and Chinese medicinal therapy

of medicinals that may raise blood pressure, such as *Ren Shen* (Panacis Ginseng, Radix) and *Huang Qi* (Astragali Membranacei, Radix).

The following are typical formulas to replace Western hormone therapy:

REPLACE HORMONE FORMULA #1

He Shou Wu (Polygoni Multiflori, Radix), 30g
Shan Yao (Radix Discoreae Opposiate), 30g
Huang Qi (Astragali Membranacei, Radix), 30g
Tai Zi Shen (Pseudostellariae Heterophyllae, Radix), 18g
Gan Cao (Glycyrrhizae Uralensis, Radix), 9g
Zi He Che (Hominis, Placenta), 3g

Case history of Dr. De Qian-yan: Li, a nine year-old boy[15]

Li was diagnosed with nephritis. Doctors gave him cortisone for 30 days without success. He had severe edema, fatigue, a pale facial complexion, low blood protein, high cholesterol, and urine protein at 4+. Dr. De prescribed Replace Hormone Formula #1. Li took this formula for a half year and all his symptoms disappeared and all Western medical tests returned to normal. Li was followed for 20 years and there was no recurrence. At his last visit, he was healthy, married, and had one six year-old child.

COMMENTARY: For cases such as this with severe edema, high urine protein, high cholesterol, and low blood protein, one must warm and invigorate kidney yang and fortify the spleen. The most important medicinal here is *Zi He Che* (Hominis, Placenta). Processed, dried *Zi He Che* from China is very effective.

Case history from Dr. Wei Li's private practice: Wu, a 14 month-old baby boy

Dr. Li saw Wu in 1983. Wu had been diagnosed a year previously with nephritis syndrome. He was treated with cortisone and all his symptoms disappeared, but, later, he suffered a recurrence. Wu was given cortisone again, but his parents insisted on concurrent Chinese medical therapy. Therefore, Dr. Li prescribed fresh *Zi He Che* (Hominis, Placenta).

In this case, the tendrils of aborted fetuses were used. Tendrils from a single aborted fetus were divided into seven daily doses. Wu took a dose a day for eight weeks and completely recovered. Follow-up 19 years later showed no recurrence.

Case history of Dr. Xin Jun-hang: Chao, a 13 year-old boy[16]

Chao's first visit was on Nov. 2, 1995. He had been having recurrent bouts of protein in his urine for 12 years. He had taken cortisone for 10 years but had five major recurrences. When Chao came to see Dr. Xin, he was on 20ml of cortisone per day. He had a moon face, lots of hair on an undersized body, and easily caught colds. He had thin tongue fur and a fine pulse. Dr. Xin gave Chao the formula below plus 40ml of cortisone every other day. Then he started reducing the dose of cortisone by 5ml every two weeks, meanwhile increasing the dosage of *Yin Yang Huo* (Epimedii, Herba) to 15g per day. By June 1996, the artificial hormones were completely eliminated. Chao continued on this formula for six months and completely recovered. A follow-up one year later found no recurrences. His moon face had disappeared and he had grown to a normal size.

Modified *Liu Wei Di Huang Wan* (Six Flavors Rehmannia Pills) plus *Yu Ping Feng San* (Jade Windscreen Powder):

Huang Qi (Astragali Membranacei, Radix), 30g
Sheng Di Huang (Rehmanniae Glutinosae, uncooked Radix), 15g
Shan Zhu Yu (Corni Officinalis, Fructus), 10g
Shan Yao (Radix Dioscoreae Oppositae), 10g
Mu Dan Pi (Moutan, Cortex Radicis), 10g
Bai Zhu (Atractylodis Macrocephalae, Rhizoma), 10g
Fang Feng (Ledebouriellae Divaricatae, Radix), 6g
Fu Ling (Poriae Cocos, Sclerotium), 10g
Gan Cao (Glycyrrhizae Uralensis, Radix), 4g
Yi Mu Cao (Leonuri Heterophylli, Herba), 40g
Mu Li (Ostreae, Concha), 30g
Yin Yang Huo (Epimedii, Herba), 10-15g

REPLACE HORMONE FORMULA #2[17]

Dang Shen (Codonopsitis Pilosulae, Radix), 12g

Huang Qi (Astragali Membranacei, Radix), 15g

Fu Ling (Poriae Cocos, Sclerotium), 15g

Bai Zhu (Atractylodis Macrocephalae, Rhizoma), 12g

Sheng Di Huang (Rehmanniae Glutinosae, uncooked Radix), 15g

Yin Yang Huo (Epimedii, Herba), 9g

Jing Ying Zi (Rosae Laevigatae, Fructus), 12g

Qian Shi (Euryalis Ferocis, Semen), 15g

Yu Mi Xu (Zeae Maydis, Stylus), 15g

Hong Hua (Carthami Tinctorii, Flos), 6g

E Zhu (Curcumae Zedoariae, Rhizoma), 12g

Yi Mu Cao (Leonuri Heterophylli, Herba), 12g

Xiang Fu (Cyperi Rotundi, Rhizoma), 12g

This is Dr. Jian's formula. He believes the best medicinals to supplement the kidney are *Yin Yang Huo* and *Rou Cong Rong* (Cistanches Deserticolae, Herba). These two medicinals warm yang without drying and invigorate yang without damaging yin. While both *Yin Yang Huo* and *Rou Cong Rong* invigorate yang, *Rou Cong Rong* moistens the intestines and is appropriate if the patient has constipation. If the patient has loose stool, one should use *Yin Yang Huo*. If the patient's stool is normal, one may use either or both. For most cases, the effective dosage is nine grams of *Yin Yang Huo* and 12 grams of *Rou Cong Rong* per day. Dr. Jian combines these with *Qian Shi* and *Jin Ying Zi* to supplement and secure the kidney. He uses *Hong Hua*, *E Zhu*, and *Yi Mu Cao* to quicken blood. This is based on the saying, "If blood moves, water moves." Dr. Jian combines 30-40 grams of *Sheng Di Huang* with either *Yin Yang Huo* or *Rou Cong Rong* to increase the immune function. This combination supplements both yin and yang and seems to work like a hormone.

Case history of Dr. Yu Ping-gong: Gu, a 23 year-old female[18]

Gu first came to see Dr. Yu on Dec. 22, 1991. One half year previously, she began to develop edema on her face and eyes. Urinalysis revealed a high protein level. The Western medical diagnosis was chronic nephritis. Therefore, doctors prescribed large dosages of cortisone and she improved for a while. Then, two months before her visit to Dr. Yu, she worsened. She began to have symptoms of dizziness, fatigue, low back soreness and weakness, stomachache after eat-

ing (her stomach was inflamed), and painful menstruation. When Gu came in, her tongue tip was red with thin, white fur, and her pulse was fine. Her blood pressure, BUN, and creatinine were normal. Urinalysis showed protein at 4+. Dr. Yu's pattern identification was spleen-kidney vacuity, damp stagnation, blood stasis, and stomach disharmony. He prescribed Replace Hormone Formula #2. After taking this formula for 14 days, all Gu's symptoms disappeared and her urinalysis returned to normal. She continued on it for three months, at which time she was stable and her urinalyses remained normal. A follow-up one year later showed no recurrences even after catching colds.

6. According to *The Great Dictionary of Chinese Medicinals*,[19] the use of powdered, uncooked *Huang Qi* (Astragali Membranacei, Radix) at dosages up to 30 grams per day can remarkably reduce protein in the urine. In addition, animal tests have shown that if powdered, uncooked *Huang Qi* is given two days before researchers artificially induce nephritis in animals, symptoms are milder and the animals recover faster. However, one must use the uncooked powder. Water decoctions of *Huang Qi* do not achieve the same effect. *Huang Qi* also percolates dampness.

7. A good combination of medicinals for spleen-kidney qi vacuity pattern of clinical nephrology is powdered *Huang Qi* with decocted *Dang Shen* (Codonopsitis Pilosulae, Radix) and *Hu Zhang* (Polygoni Cuspidati, Radix Et Rhizoma). The two formulas mentioned above under this pattern already have *Huang Qi* and *Dang Shen* in them. Thus only *Hu Zhang* needs to be added. *Hu Zhang* is neutral, nontoxic, and has been shown to be an effective antimicrobial. Chronic nephritis patients with qi vacuity are especially susceptible to contraction of external evils that may further damage the true qi. An external attack may also force one to discontinue the use of supplementing medicinals while concentrating on such an attack. Using *Hu Zhang* or other medicinals with antimicrobial functions hinder such attacks.

8. One should also add securing and astringing medicinals to the above formulas for the long-term loss of protein through proteinuria. This protein loss is equivalent to the loss of kidney essence. If kidney essence is lost, the kidney (water) will not be strong enough to nourish the heart (fire). If heart fire becomes vacuous, it will not be able to generate spleen (earth) yang. Vacuous spleen (earth) yang cannot send fluids to the lungs (metal). Vacuous lungs will then lose governance of the triple burner water passageways, and, ultimately, this pathological process results in edema. Securing and astringing medicinals that help reduce the loss of kidney essence include *Jin Ying Zi* (Rosae Laevigatae, Fructus), *Bai Guo* (Ginkgo Bilobae, Semen), *Fu Pen Zi* (Rubi Chingii, Fructus), *Sang Shen Zi* (Mori Albi, Fructus), *Wu Mei* (Pruni Mume, Fructus), *Wu Wei Zi* (Schisandrae Chinensis, Fructus), *Shan Zhu Yu* (Corni Officinalis, Fructus), *Wu Bei Zi* (Rhois Chinensis, Galla), *Fu Xiao Mai* (Tritici Aestivi, Semen Levis), calcined *Mu Li* (Ostreae, Concha), and calcined *Long Gu* (Draconis, Os).

To help determine if there is a large loss of protein in the urine, one can examine clinical nephrology patients' fingernails. A large loss of protein through the urine can cause the blood protein level to drop and lead to high blood cholesterol. High cholesterol causes patients' fingernails to have white streaks in them. High blood cholesterol can also lead to blood stasis. This is analogous to sediment in a river that precipitates out. The sediment will eventually clog the river, reducing its free flow (one definition of stasis).

ENDNOTES

1 *Shui Zhong Guan Ge Jun* (*Water Swelling and Block and Repulsion*, Volume 2), Chinese Medicine Publishing Company, Beijing, 1998, p. 176

2 Yu Wong-shi, *Dong Dai Ming Yi Lin Zhen Jing Hua* (*Modern Famous Doctors Clinic Collection*), Chinese Ancient Book Publishing Co., Beijing, 1991, p. 182

3 Qing He-chen, *Dong Dai Ming Lao Zhong Yi Lin Zheng Hui Cui* (*Modern Famous Old Doctors Clinical Collection*), Guandong Science & Technology Publishing Company, Guanzhou, 1991, p. 347

4 Some sources suggest that *Huang Qi* (Astragali Membranacei, Radix) reduces night sweats because it consolidates the surface, but in Wei Li's experience it often exacerbates them.

5 *Dong Dai Ming Lao Zhong Yi Ling Zheng Hui Cui* (*A Collection of Modern Famous Chinese Doctors' Clinical Experiences*) Guandong Science and Technology Publishing Company, Guanzhou, 1987, p. 376

6 *Gu Shen Feng* (Secure the Kidney Decoction) is a common name for formulas that supplement kidney yin and yang, but the exact formula was not given.

7 As mentioned above, blood and casts in the urine indicate blood stasis.

8 *Dong Dai Ming Long Zhong Yi Ling Zheng Hui Cui* (*Modern Famous Old Chinese Doctors Clinical Case Collection*), *op. cit.*, p. 381

9 *Shui Zhong Guan Ge Jun* (*Water Swelling and Block & Repulsion*), Volume 1, Chinese Medicine Publishing Company, Beijing, 1998, p. 170

10 *Ibid.*, p. 387

11 *I.e.*, *Hua Shi* (Talcum), 6 parts, and *Gan Cao* (Glycyrrhizae Uralensis, Radix), 1 part

12 Qing He-chen, *op. cit.*, p. 363

13 *Zhong Yao Da Zi Dian* (*The Great Dictionary of Chinese Medicinals*), Shanghai Science & Technology Publishing Co., 1991

14 In Western terms, one could say that Clinical Nephrology patients' kidneys are swollen and that one must relieve the swelling as well as strengthening kidney function.

15 *Ibid.*, p. 207

16 *Ibid.*, p. 589

17 Yu Ping-gong, "The Experience of Jian Hua-hu Using *Yin Yang Huo* (Epimedii, Herba) and *Rou Cong Rong* (Cistanches Deserticolae, Herba)" *Zhong Yi Za Zhi* (Journal of Chinese Medicine), #6, 1998, p. 334

18 *Ibid.*, p. 334

19 *Zhong Yao Da Zi Dian* (*The Great Dictionary of Chinese Medicinals*), *op. cit.*

Acute renal failure (ARF) is defined as an abrupt reduction in the glomerular filtration rate (GFR). This decrease in GFR leads to a sudden retention of endogenous and exogenous metabolites. These include urea, potassium, phosphate, sulfate, creatinine and administered drugs. The increase of nitrogenous waste is referred to as uremia or azotemia. Urine output volume decreases in 70% of the cases of ARF. Scanty urination is called oliguria. It is defined as less than 400ml/day in adults or less than 24ml/kg of body weight in children. Anuria refers to output of less than 100ml/day. Acute renal failure is a critical, medical emergency and is associated with significant morbidity and mortality. Mortality from ARF is approximately 30-50%. Mortality rates are generally lower for nonoliguric ARF patients than for oliguric ARF patients. (There are 35,000 deaths annually due to kidney disease.) A wide range of other disturbances may accompany ARF. These will depend on the duration and severity of the kidney dysfunction and may include metabolic acidosis, hyperkalemia and disturbances of body fluid balance.

NOSOLOGY

There are three types of acute renal failure. Each type is defined by the anatomical location of the inciting cause. These are prerenal, renal (also described as intrarenal, intrinsic, or parenchymal), and postrenal. Intrarenal ARF is subdivided into four categories: glomerular, tubular, vascular and interstitial diseases.

EPIDEMIOLOGY

Acute renal failure is commonly encountered in intensive care units and emergency rooms and is less commonly seen in general practice. Emergency department physicians play a critical role in recognizing early ARF, preventing iatrogenic injury, and reversing its course. Acute renal failure affects approximately 1% of patients on admission to the hospital, 2-5% during the hospital stay, and 4-15% after cardiopulmonary bypass surgery. This disorder is more common in adults than children.

ETIOLOGY & PATHOPHYSIOLOGY

Abrupt renal decline and failure is the end result of a number of disease processes. The most common cause of acute prerenal failure is dehydration. Other causes include hemorrhage, congestive heart failure, heatstroke, renal artery atherosclerosis, malignant hypertension, ACE inhibitors, NSAIDss, aristolochic acid,[1] cyclosporine, shock and vascular collapse, for example from sepsis, burns or trauma. The pathophysiology of prerenal ARF results from a decrease in the renal blood flow. The GFR is reduced and the kidney retains water and salt. This causes oliguria, production of concentrated urine and a progressive inability to excrete nitrogenous wastes. The most common cause of intrarenal ARF is acute or rapidly progressive glomerulonephritis. Other causes include pyelonephritis, acute and chronic tubular necrosis, interstitial nephritis, disseminated intravascular coagulation, nephrolithiasis, myeloma, nephritic syndrome, pre-eclampsia and adverse drug reactions. In intrarenal ARF the renal parenchyma is injured causing impaired sodium reabsorption. Glomerulonephritis is characterized by proteinuria, hematuria and hypertension. Most of the types of glomerulonephritis (discussed in a following section) are associated with chronic renal disease. Rapidly progressive glomerulonephritis (RPGN) and acute glomerulonephritis (AGN), however, may cause ARF. Acute glomerulonephritis may occur in patients with postinfectious conditions and bacterial endo-carditis. Acute tubular necrosis is the most common cause of intrarenal ARF in hospitalized patients. Ischemia or toxins usually induce this condition. Macro- and microvascular diseases can cause glomerular capillary thrombosis and occlusion. This may be accompanied by thrombocytopenia. A classic example of this is the HELLP syndrome (hemolysis, elevated liver enzymes and low platelets).

Acute interstitial nephritis leading to ARF is usually the result of an allergic drug reaction. It may also be caused by an autoimmune disease, infection or infiltrative disease. An inflammatory process is initiated in the renal interstitium. This is in response to a wide variety of stimuli (toxic, metabolic, infectious, immune or infiltrative). Acute postrenal failure is usually due to urine outflow obstruction. This may be due to benign prostatic hyperplasia, bilateral urethral obstruction, kidney and bladder stones (especially seen in patients with one kidney), bladder tumors, cervical cancer, retroperitoneal disorders and renal vein stenosis. A functional or mechanical obstruction to the free flow of urine precludes its excretion.

SYMPTOMATOLOGY

Though the symptoms will vary depending on the type of ARF, the following signs and symptoms may be indicative of any of the three types of ARF: weakness, cardiac dysrhythmia, apathy, decreased appetite, lethargy, fatigue, nausea, vomiting, itching, changes in mental status, shortness of breath, seizures, peripheral and pulmonary edema, elevated right atrial pressure, deep and frequent respiration, ascites, increasing metabolic acidosis, coma. Oliguria or anuria is present 70% of the time. Voiding of dark-colored urine (preceding oliguria) may occur. Prerenal ARF may manifest in the following ways: dehydration, thirst, dizziness (especially when standing), history of fluid loss during the preceding hours or day, poor skin turgor, dry mucous membranes, orthostatic hypotension, and collapsed neck veins. Intrarenal ARF may manifest with a recent history of sore throat, upper respiratory infection, diarrhea, antibiotic and/or IV drug use, severe back pain, and gross hematuria. Postrenal ARF may be marked by kidney tenderness and pain (at times exquisite), incontinence (especially postoperative), and abdominal distention.

DIAGNOSIS

Acute renal failure is diagnosed using urine, blood, and imaging examinations. A rise in serum creatinine and an increase in the BUN/creatinine ratio are indicative of ARF. Examination of the urine by dipstick often reveals proteinuria. A marked, positive finding should be followed up by a 24 hour urine analysis. Red blood cells are usually not present in prerenal ARF but may be noted in intrarenal and postrenal ARF. Urinalysis is often not possible in postrenal ARF. Catheterization may be used to release urinary retention.

Microscopic urine examination may show RBCs, WBCs, and cellular and granular casts for postrenal ARF. Tubular, brown granular and red cell casts may be seen in intrarenal ARF. Casts are usually not present in prerenal ARF. Blood serum analysis is critical for monitoring BUN (blood urea nitrogen) and creatinine levels. Serum tests also are used to monitor possible states of metabolic acidosis, hyperkalemia, hyponatremia, and anemia. The most important imaging examination for ARF is by ultrasonography. It is a sensitive test for obstruction and kidney size. Computed tomography (CT) is useful in visualizing ureteral obstruction. The chest x-ray is used to monitor possible fluid overload. Renal biopsy may be indicated in rapidly progressing disease. Chest ECG monitoring is indicated if there is a possibility of hyperkalemia and/or atrial fibrillation.

DIFFERENTIAL DIAGNOSIS

A host of disorders and diseases may mimic and lead to ARF. The following is a partial list of disorders to consider during a workup for acute renal failure:

Abdominal aneurysm
Acute glomerulonephritis
Adverse drug reaction
Alcohol toxicity
Cirrhosis
Congestive heart failure
Dehydration
Dialysis complications
Diarrhea
Endocarditis
Hemolytic uremic syndrome
Hemorrhage
Henoch-Schönlein purpura
Hyperkalemia
Hypermagnesemia
Hypernatremia
Hypertension
Ketoacidosis (alcoholic or diabetic)
Kidney stones
Nephrotic syndrome
Neurogenic bladder
Over-diuresis
Post-streptococcal and pneumococcal infections
Pyelonephritis
Sepsis
Sickle-cell anemia
Urinary obstruction
Urinary tract infection
Vomiting

WESTERN MEDICAL TREATMENT

Western medical treatment of acute renal failure is guided by precision of diagnosis. Understanding that acute renal failure is often the final result of numerous conditions, treatment includes both support for the kidneys and identifying and treating the underlying cause. Hospitalization is required for treatment and monitoring. If available, initial treatment is dialysis. Dialysis should be administered urgently in cases of hyperkalemia with cardiac dysrhythmia, anuria, and obstinate metabolic acidosis. Fluid and salt intake are severely restricted. Dietary intakes of substances, which are excreted by the kidneys, are minimized. Diet plans high in carbohydrates and low in protein, sodium and potassium are encouraged. Nephrotoxic medications and all drugs requiring renal excretion are closely monitored or discontinued. Antibiotics may be used to prevent infection. One of the priorities in treatment is to control episodes of hyperkalemia (excess blood potassium). Intravenous calcium is one method to control potassium overload. Vasopressor drugs, such as dopamine (Intropin), may be prescribed in order to elevate the blood pressure and maintain adequate renal blood flow. Diuretics may worsen renal failure but may be necessary to prevent pulmonary edema. In general, potassium-sparing diuretics should be avoided because of the high-risk of hyperkalemia. A common diuretic is furosemide (Lasix). Kidney patients, especially those undergoing habitual dialysis, are encouraged to attend support groups.

PROGNOSIS & COMPLICATIONS

Acute renal failure is a life-threatening, medical emergency. Uremic syndrome defines the condition. Fluid overload is an inevitable consequence. Serum potassium may rise, seriously compromising the stable rhythm of the heart. Metabolic acidosis may develop. Mild hyperphosphatemia and gastrointestinal bleeding frequently occur. Anemia is quick to develop in ARF. Infection and cardiorespiratory complications account for the majority of deaths in acute renal failure. The survival rate for ARF has remained at 60% for the past 40 years. This is due in part to the severity of the co-morbid conditions, *e.g.*, sepsis, burns, pulmonary failure, and the older age of the affected patients. Survival rates are not likely to improve with Western medicine.

CHINESE MEDICAL DISEASE CATEGORIZATION

The clinical manifestations of acute renal failure correspond to the following traditional Chinese medical disease categories: kidney wind, block and repulsion, dribbling urinary block, bloody urine, and water swelling.

TREATMENT BASED ON PATTERN IDENTIFICATION

In the modern Chinese medical clinic, the patterns of ARF are listed under the rubrics of scanty urination and profuse urination. Scanty urination patterns include: 1) wind cold, 2) wind heat, 3) toxic poisoning, 4) blood stasis, and 5) fluid exhaustion. Profuse urination patterns include: 1) lingering damp heat and 2) qi and yin vacuity.

SCANTY URINATION[2]

1. WIND COLD

SIGNS & SYMPTOMS: Chills, no sweating, coughing, nasal congestion and dripping, low back pain, aching joints, edema, and scanty urination. The tongue is pale red with thin, white fur, and the pulse is floating and tight.

NOTE: This pattern usually occurs because of true qi vacuity often due to kidney vacuity. This, in turn, causes defensive qi vacuity. External evils can then attack and penetrate deeply inside the body. The righteous qi and these evils engage in an acute struggle resulting in disharmony of yin and yang of the organs and channels. Wind cold is a combination of wind and cold. Wind, a yang pathogen described as "light and floating," tends to attack the upper part of the body first. Cold, a yin pathogen associated with pain, tends to descend. Here, wind first attacks the (upper) lung, while cold moves down to the (lower) kidney. This is called "lung cold moves to the kidney" and results in kidney wind.

TREATMENT PRINCIPLES: Expel wind and open the lung, warm the interior and disinhibit water

REPRESENTATIVE FORMULA: Modified *Ma Huang Zhu Ling Tang* (Ephedra & Polyporus Decoction)[3]

Ma Huang (Ephedrae, Herba), 9g
Xing Ren (Pruni Armeniacae, Semen), 9g
Gui Zhi (Cinnamomi Cassiae, Ramulus), 9g
Fu Ling (Poriae Cocos, Sclerotium), 9g
Tu Fu Ling (Smilacis Glabrae, Rhizoma), 50g
Bai Mao Gen (Imperatae Cylindricae, Rhizoma), 25g
Huo Xiang (Agastachis Seu Pogostemi, Herba), 9g
Gan Jiang (Zingiberis Officinalis, dry Rhizoma), 3g
Zhu Ling (Polypori Umbellati, Sclerotium), 9g
Yi Mu Cao (Leonuri Heterophylli, Herba), 9g

MODIFICATIONS: If the patient has severe fatigue, supplement the qi and yang with such medicinals as *Huang Qi* (Astragali Membranacei, Radix), *Ren Shen* (Panacis Ginseng, Radix), *Yin Yang Huo* (Epimedii, Herba), and *Du Zhong* (Eucommiae Ulmoidis, Cortex). If the patient has a purple tongue and a choppy pulse, add *Ze Lan* (Lycopi Lucidi, Herba), *Yi Mu Cao* (Leonuri Heterophylli, Herba), *Hong Hua* (Carthami Tinctorii, Flos), *Dan Shen* (Salviae Miltiorrhizae, Radix), and *Shui Zhi* (Hirudo Seu Whitmania). If the patient has serious edema, drain water through the stool using *Da Cheng Qi Tang* (Major Order the Qi Decoction) or *Shi Zao Tang* (Ten Dates Decoction) along with the methods used above to strongly promote sweating and free urination.[4] If the patient has abdominal distention, add *Hou Po* (Magnoliae Officinalis, Cortex), *Da Fu Pi* (Arecae Catechu, Pericarpium), *Chen Pi* (Citri Reticulatae, Pericarpium), *Zhi Ke* (Citri Aurantii, Fructus), and *Mu Xiang* (Auklandiae Lappae, Radix).

CAUTION: If the patient has hypertension, be careful with the dosage of *Ma Huang* (Ephedrae, Herba).

ACUMOXIBUSTION: Choose points to needle from *Tai Xi* (Ki 3), *Yin Ling Quan* (Sp 9), *Lie Que* (Lu 7), *He Gu* (LI 4), *Da Zhui* (GV 14), *Fei Shu* (Bl 13), *Gan Shu* (Bl 18), *Pi Shu* (Bl 20), and *Shen Shu* (Bl 23) and moxibustion *Qi Zhong* (CV 8), *Yong Quan* (Ki 1), *Shen Shu* (Bl 23), and/or *Hua Tuo Jia Ji* on the lumbar vertebrae. Choose six points each treatment.

Case history from Dr. Wei Li's private practice:
Xu, an 18 year-old male soldier

Xu had been playing basketball and had become hot and sweaty. He undressed, was caught in a draft, and caught cold. A week later, he could not urinate and his whole body became edematous. The Western medical diagnosis was ARF. Dr. Li's disease identification was kidney wind. She identified the pattern as wind cold, evil wind, and evil water. She prescribed a variation of *Ma Huang Zhu Shi Tang* (Ephedra Expel Dampness Decoction). The patient also received dialysis. In six weeks, the patient staged a complete recovery.

2. WIND HEAT

SIGNS & SYMPTOMS: Fever, sweating, a red facial complexion, distending headache, sore throat, cough, nasal congestion with yellow discharge, edema, red, difficult, scanty urination, and low back pain. The tongue is red with thin, yellow fur, and the pulse is deep or floating and fast.

TREATMENT PRINCIPLES: Clear the lung and resolve toxins, harmonize and open the water passageways

REPRESENTATIVE FORMULA: Modified *Qing Wen Bai Du Yin* (Scourge-clearing, Toxin-vanquishing Beverage)

Shi Gao (Gypsum Fibrosum), 20g
Sheng Di Huang (Rehmanniae Glutinosae, uncooked Radix), 20g
Huang Lian (Coptidis Chinensis, Rhizoma), 9g
Huang Qi (Astragali Membranacei, Radix), 12g
Zhi Zi (Gardeniae Jasminoidis, Fructus), 9g
Zhi Mu (Anemarrhenae Asphodeloidis, Rhizoma), 9g
Xuan Shen (Scrophulariae Ningpoensis, Radix), 9g
Lian Qiao (Forsythiae Suspensae, Fructus), 15g
Chi Shao (Paeoniae Lactiflorae, Radix Rubrus), 9g
Mu Dan Pi (Moutan, Cortex Radicis), 9g
Tu Fu Ling (Smilacis Glabrae, Rhizoma), 40g
Bai Mao Gen (Imperatae Cylindricae, Rhizoma), 30g
Ma Huang (Ephedrae, Herba), 10g

Huo Xiang (Agastachis Seu Pogostemi, Herba), 15g
Gui Zhi (Cinnamomi Cassiae, Ramulus), 9g

MODIFICATIONS: If the patient has high fever and irritability, add *Jian Can* (Bombyx Batryticatus), *Sheng Ma* (Cimicifugae, Rhizoma), *Qing Dai* (Indigonis, Pulvis), *Ban Lan Gen* (Isatidis Seu Baphicacanthi, Radix), and *Tian Ma* (Gastrodia Elatae, Rhizoma). If the patient has lung heat, add *Di Gu Pi* (Lycii Chinensis, Cortex Radicis), *Sang Bai Pi* (Mori Albi, Cortex Radicis), and *Gan Cao* (Glycyrrhizae Uralensis, Radix). If the patient cannot pass urine, use *Da Huang* (Rhei, Radix Et Rhizoma), 20g, and *Mang Xiao* (Mirabilitum), 20g, as an enema.

NOTE: In China, there are many incidences of epidemic hemorrhagic fever causing ARF. A number of famous hospitals, including the Anhui Medical University Hospital, the Nanjing Chinese Medical Hospital, and the Zhong Ying Zou Hospital, report treating this condition successfully using formulas similar to the one described above. The following case history is an example.

Case history from Dr. Wei Li's private practice:
Hua, a 34 year-old farmer's wife

Hua was three months pregnant. She suddenly had chills and a high fever and thought she had caught cold. The condition soon became much more serious and she started bleeding. She had occult blood in her urine and stool and there were streaks of blood like scratches in her armpits. When her eyelids were lifted, there were spots of blood inside. Her urination was normal and she was not edematous. (As mentioned above, while most patients have edema and scanty urination, there are some that do not display these symptoms.) The Western medical diagnosis was acute renal failure and epidemic hemorrhagic fever. Dr. Li's disease identification was dribbling urinary block and bloody urination. Her pattern identification was wind heat penetrating the qi and blood aspects. Therefore, she prescribed *Qing Wen Bai Du Yin* (Scourge-clearing, Toxin-vanquishing Beverage) with modifications. The patient took this formula for two months and completely recovered.
ACUMOXIBUSTION: Choose from *Qu Chi* (LI 11), *He*

Gu (LI 4), *Yin Ling Quan* (Sp 9), *San Yin Jiao* (Sp 6), *Tai Xi* (Ki 3), *Tai Chong* (Liv 3), *Wai Guan* (TB 5), *Shui Dao* (St 28), *Zhong Ji* (CV 3), *Pang Guang Shu* (Bl 28), *Shen Shu* (Bl 23), *Da Zhui* (GV 14), and *Wei Zhong* (Bl 40).

3. TOXIC POISONING

SIGNS & SYMPTOMS: Sudden scanty urination or anuria, coma or a sleepy, lethargic state, nausea and vomiting. The tongue has thick, slimy fur, and the pulse is soggy or thin and slippery.

EMERGENCY TREATMENT: It is of utmost importance to get the patient to an emergency room as soon as possible. If this is impossible, in the case of a snake bite, one may apply a tourniquet and eliminate as much poison as possible. In the case of mushroom poisoning, one should try inducing vomiting and purging the bowels.

TREATMENT PRINCIPLES: Guide out toxins and open the orifices, downbear the turbid and disperse stagnation

REPRESENTATIVE FORMULA: *San Huang Xia Du Tang* (Three Yellows Precipitate Toxins Decoction)

Huang Lian (Coptidis Chinensis, Rhizoma), 9g
Huang Qi (Astragali Membranacei, Radix), 9g
Huang Bai (Phellodendri, Cortex), 9g
Zhi Zi (Gardeniae Jasminoidis, Fructus), 9g
Lu Dou (Phaseoli Radiati, Semen), 100g
Gan Cao (Glycyrrhizae Uralensis, Radix), 9g

MODIFICATIONS: If the patient has toxic neurological symptoms, such as numbness, dizziness, and loss of balance, add *Ban Bian Lian* (Lobeliae Chinensis, Herba Cum Radice), *Ye Ju Hua* (Chrysanthemi Indici, Flos), *Bei Mu* (Fritillariae Thumbergii, Bulbus or Fritillariae Cirrhosae, Bulbus), *Long Dan Cao* (Gentiannae Longdancao, Radix), *Jian Can* (Bombyx Batryticatus), *Quan Xie* (Buthus Martensis), *Wu Gong* (Scolopendra Subspinipes), and *Chan Tui* (Cicadae, Periostracum). If the patient has toxins in the blood aspect, add *Ban Bian Lian* (Lobeliae Chinensis, Herba Cum Radice), *Sheng Di Huang* (Rehmanniae Glutinosae, uncooked Radix), *Mu Dan*

Pi (Moutan, Cortex Radicis), *Chi Shao* (Paeoniae Lactiflorae, Radix Rubrus), and *She Gan* (Belmancandae Chinensis, Rhizoma).

ACUMOXIBUSTION: Bleed the well points, needle *Qu Chi* (LI 11), *Zu San Li* (St 36), *Ren Zhong* (GV 26), *San Yin Jiao* (Sp 6), *Zhong Ji* (CV 3), and *Lin Qi* (GB 41), and moxibustion *Bai Hui* (GV 20) and *Yong Quan* (Ki 1).

4. BLOOD STASIS

SIGNS & SYMPTOMS: Large areas of bruising, generalized pain, bloody urination, scanty urine, or anuria, nausea and vomiting. The tongue is purple with thin, slimy fur, and the pulse is choppy.

TREATMENT PRINCIPLES: Move the qi and quicken the blood, downbear the turbid and expel toxins

REPRESENTATIVE FORMULA: Modified *Xue Fu Zhu Yu Tang* (Blood Mansion Stasis-dispelling Decoction) plus *Cheng Qi Tang* (Order the Qi Decoction)[5]

Tao Ren (Pruni Persicae, Semen), 9g
Hong Hua (Carthami Tinctorii, Flos), 6g
Chuan Xiong (Ligustici Wallichii, Radix), 15g
Dang Gui (Angelicae Sinensis, Radix), 9g
Chi Shao (Paeoniae Lactiflorae, Radix Rubrus), 9g
Mu Dan Pi (Moutan, Cortex Radicis), 9g
Chai Hu (Bupleuri, Radix), 3g
Niu Xi (Achyranthis Bidentatae, Radix), 9g
Sheng Di Huang (Rehmanniae Glutinosae, uncooked Radix), 9g
Da Huang (Rhei, Radix Et Rhizoma), 9g
Shui Zhi (Hirudo Seu Whitmania), 9g
Mang Xiao (Mirabilitum), 9g

MODIFICATIONS: If the patient has anxiety and insomnia, add *Tian Ma* (Gastrodia Elatae, Rhizoma), *Ju Hua* (Chrysanthemi Morifolii, Flos), *Zhen Zhu Mu* (Margaritaferae, Concha), *He Huan Pi* (Albizziae Julibrissinis, Cortex), *Ye Jiao Teng* (Polygoni Multiflori, Caulis), *Dan Shen* (Salviae Miltiorrhizae, Radix), *Suan Sao Ren* (Zizyphi Spinosae, Semen), and *Hu Po* (Succinum). If the patient has tidal fever or night sweats,[6] add *Zhi Mu* (Anemarrhenae Asphodeloidis,

Rhizoma), *Huang Bai* (Phellodendri, Cortex), *Bie Jia* (Amydae Sinensis, Carapax), and *Di Gu Pi* (Lycii Chinensis, Cortex Radicis). If the patient is bleeding, especially internally, one must be very careful prescribing stasis-dispelling, blood-quickening medicinals, especially in the first 24 hours. However, one can administer a retention enema consisting of *Da Huang* (Rhei, Radix Et Rhizoma), *Mang Xiao* (Mirabilitum), *Gui Zhi* (Cinnamomi Cassiae, Ramulus), *Huai Hua Mi* (Sophorae Japonicae, Flos Immaturus), *Fu Ling* (Poriae Cocos, Sclerotium), *Chi Shao* (Paeoniae Lactiflorae, Radix Rubrus), and *Zhu Ling* (Polypori Umbellati, Sclerotium). This enema should be administered twice a day and held in as long as possible.

ACUMOXIBUSTION: Choose from *Ge Shu* (Bl 17), *Shen Shu* (Bl 23), *Pang Guang Shu* (Bl 28), *He Gu* (LI 4), *Tai Chong* (Liv 3), *Yin Ling Quan* (Sp 9), *Xue Hai* (Sp 10), *Tai Xi* (Ki 3), and *Zhong Ji* (CV 3).

5. FLUID EXHAUSTION

SIGNS & SYMPTOMS: Scanty urination, low blood pressure (below 80/60mmHg), sweating, cold extremities. The tongue is pale, and the pulse is fine and forceless.

TREATMENT PRINCIPLES: Rescue yang and supplement the qi and blood

REPRESENTATIVE FORMULAS: Modified *Si Ni Tang* (Four Counterflows Decoction) plus *Ba Zhen Tang* (Eight Pearls Decoction)[7]

Ren Shen (Panacis Ginseng, Radix), 9g
Fu Zi (Aconiti Carmichaeli, Radix Lateralis Praeparatus), 9g
Gan Jiang (Zingiberis Officinalis, dry Rhizoma), 9g
Mai Men Dong (Ophiopogonis Japonici, Tuber), 9g
Wu Wei Zi (Schisandrae Chinensis, Fructus), 6g
Shu Di Huang (Rehmanniae Glutinosae, cooked Radix), 9g
Dang Gui (Angelicae Sinensis, Radix), 9g
Bai Shao (Paeoniae Lactiflorae, Radix Albus), 9g
Chuan Xiong (Ligustici Wallichii, Radix), 9g
Fu Ling (Poriae Cocos, Sclerotium), 9g
Bai Zhu (Atractylodis Macrocephalae, Rhizoma), 9g
mix-fried *Gan Cao* (Glycyrrhizae Uralensis, Radix), 3g

Modified *Shen Fu Tang* (Ginseng & Aconite Decoction) plus *Dang Gui Bu Xue Tang* (Dang Gui Supplement the Blood Decoction)

Ren Shen (Panacis Ginseng, Radix; must use Korean white Ginseng), 9g
Fu Zi (Aconiti Carmichaeli, Radix Lateralis Praeparatus), 9g
Shu Di Huang (Rehmanniae Glutinosae, cooked Radix), 9g
Dang Gui (Angelicae Sinensis, Radix), 9g
Bai Shao (Paeoniae Lactiflorae, Radix Albus), 9g
Chuan Xiong (Ligustici Wallichii, Radix), 9g
Huang Qi (Astragali Membranacei, Radix), 15g

MODIFICATIONS: If the patient has heart palpitations, add mix-fried *Gan Cao* (Glycyrrhizae Uralensis, Radix), *Sheng Di Huang* (Rehmanniae Glutinosae, uncooked Radix), *Gui Zhi* (Cinnamomi Cassiae, Ramulus), and *E Jiao* (Asini, Gelatinum Corii). If the patient has a low appetite, add *Shan Zha* (Crataegi, Fructus), *Shen Qu* (Massa Medica Fermentata), and *Ji Nei Jin* (Gigeriae Galli, Endothelium Corneum).

If the patient has insomnia, add *He Huan Pi* (Albizziae Julibrissinis, Cortex), *Ye Jiao Teng* (Polygoni Multiflori, Caulis), and *Suan Sao Ren* (Zizyphi Spinosae, Semen). If the patient is depressed, add *Huang Jing* (Polygonati, Rhizoma), *Xiang Fu* (Cyperi Rotundi, Rhizoma), and *He Huan Pi* (Albizziae Julibrissinis, Cortex). If the patient is anxious, add *Bai He* (Lilii, Bulbus), *Tian Ma* (Gastrodia Elatae, Rhizoma), and *He Huan Pi* (Albizziae Julibrissinis, Cortex).

ACUMOXIBUSTION: Choose from *Hui Yin* (CV 1), *Chang Qiang* (GV 1), *Tai Xi* (Ki 3), *San Yin Jiao* (Sp 6) and moxibustion *Ming Men* (GV 4), *Qi Zhong* (CV 8), and *Bai Hui* (GV 20).

PROFUSE URINATION[8]

1. LINGERING DAMP HEAT

SIGNS & SYMPTOMS: Dizziness, irritability, loss of appetite, nausea, vomiting, profuse urination. The tongue has slimy, yellow fur, and the pulse is forceful.

NOTE: When a lack of treatment or incorrect treatment has not entirely cleared and drained damp heat, it lingers or endures. This smoldering heat has the potential to flare up and should be cleared completely.

TREATMENT PRINCIPLES: Clear heat and eliminate dampness

REPRESENTATIVE FORMULA: Modified *San Ren Tang* (Three Nut Decoction)

Xing Ren (Pruni Armeniacae, Semen), 9g
Yi Yi Ren (Coicis Lachryma-jobi, Semen), 30g
Bai Dou Kou (Cardamomi, Fructus), 9g
Ban Xia (Pinelliae Ternatae, Rhizoma), 9g
Hou Po (Magnoliae Officinalis, Cortex), 9g
Hua Shi (Talcum), 6g
Dan Zhu Ye (Lophatheri Gracilis, Herba), 9g
Huang Lian (Coptidis Chinensis, Rhizoma), 9g
Huang Qi (Astragali Membranacei, Radix), 9g
Zhu Ru (Bambusae In Taeniis, Caulis), 9g
Fu Ling (Poriae Cocos, Sclerotium), 9g
Zhu Ling (Polypori Umbellati, Sclerotium), 9g

MODIFICATIONS: If the patient has dark urine and constipation, add *Che Qian Zi* (Plantaginis, Semen), *Yin Chen Hao* (Artemisiae Yinchenhao, Herba), *Huang Bai* (Phellodendri, Cortex), *Zhi Mu* (Anemarrhenae Asphodeloidis, Rhizoma), *Da Huang* (Rhei, Radix Et Rhizoma), *Tao Ren* (Pruni Persicae, Semen), and *Mang Xiao* (Mirabilitum). If the patient has thick, white, slimy tongue fur and a soggy, slow pulse, add *Huo Xiang* (Agastachis Seu Pogostemi, Herba) *Pei Lan* (Eupatorii Fortunei, Herba), and *Hou Po* (Magnoliae Officinalis, Cortex). If the patient has tidal fever, this is often caused by yang ming heat burning and consuming yin. In that case, add *Zhi Mu* (Anemarrhenae Asphodeloidis, Rhizoma), *Huang Bai* (Phellodendri, Cortex), *Sheng Di Huang* (Rehmanniae Glutinosae, uncooked Radix), and *Chi Shao* (Paeoniae Lactiflorae, Radix Rubrus). If the patient's pulse becomes big and vacuous, this is caused by great heat damaging and depleting true qi. In that case, add *Ren Shen* (Panacis Ginseng, Radix) or *Dang Shen* (Codonopsitis Pilosulae, Radix).

ACUMOXIBUSTION: Choose from *Qu Chi* (LI 11), *Wei Zhong* (Bl 40), *Yin Ling Quan* (Sp 9), *Yang Ling Quan* (GB 34), *Zu San Li* (St 36), *Nei Guan* (Per 6), *Shen Shu* (Bl 23), *Pang Guang Shu* (Bl 28), *Zhong Ji* (CV 3), and *Tai Xi* (Ki 3).

2. QI & YIN VACUITY

SIGNS & SYMPTOMS: Profuse urination, fatigue, dry throat with thirst for warm drinks, possible low backache. The tongue is dry with a pale red body and little or no fur. The pulse is fine and forceless.

TREATMENT PRINCIPLES: Fortify the spleen and boost the qi, supplement the kidney and enrich yin

REPRESENTATIVE FORMULA: Modified *Bu Zhong Yi Qi Tang* (Supplement the Center & Boost the Qi Decoction) plus *Sheng Mai San* (Generate the Pulse Powder)

Ren Shen (Panacis Ginseng, Radix), 9g
Huang Qi (Astragali Membranacei, Radix), 9g
Dang Gui (Angelicae Sinensis, Radix), 9g
Mai Men Dong (Ophiopogonis Japonici, Tuber), 9g
Wu Wei Zi (Schisandrae Chinensis, Fructus), 6g
Bai Zhu (Atractylodis Macrocephalae, Rhizoma), 9g
mix-fried *Gan Cao* (Glycyrrhizae Uralensis, Radix), 3g
Xuan Shen (Scrophulariae Ningpoensis, Radix), 6g
Sha Shen (Glehniae Litoralis, Radix), 9g
Shi Hu (Dendrobii, Herba), 9g
Tian Hua Fen (Trichosanthis Kirilowii, Radix), 15g
Ge Gen (Puerariae, Radix), 10g

MODIFICATIONS: If the patient has concurrent liver yin vacuity (with vision problems, anxiety, and mood swings), add *Gou Qi Zi* (Lycii Chinensis, Fructus), *Ju Hua* (Chrysanthemi Morifolii, Flos), *Nu Zhen Zi* (Ligustri Lucidi, Fructus), *Han Lian Cao* (Ecliptae Prostratae, Herba), *Bie Jia* (Amydae Sinensis, Carapax), and *Gui Ban* (Testudinis, Plastrum). If the patient has concurrent heart yin vacuity (with heart palpitations, impaired memory, and insomnia), add *Wu Wei Zi* (Schisandrae Chinensis, Fructus), *Xuan Shen* (Scrophulariae Ningpoensis, Radix), *Sheng Di Huang* (Rehmanniae Glutinosae, uncooked Radix), *E Jiao* (Asini,

Gelatinum Corii), mix-fried *Gan Cao* (Glycyrrhizae Uralensis, Radix), and *Ren Shen* (Panacis Ginseng, Radix). If the patient has concurrent lung yin vacuity (with dry cough, dry throat, and thirst), add *Bei Sha Shen* (Glenhniae Littoralis, Radix), *Shi Hu* (Dendrobii, Herba), *Tian Hua Fen* (Trichosanthis Kirlowii, Radix), and *Lu Gen* (Phragmitis Communis, Rhizoma).

ACUMOXIBUSTION: Choose from *Zu San Li* (St 36), *San Yin Jiao* (Sp 6), *Zhong Ji* (CV 3), *Guan Yuan* (CV 4), *Qi Hai* (CV 6), *Lie Que* (Lu 7), *Bai Hui* (GV 20), *Tai Xi* (Ki 3) or *Zhao Hai* (Ki 6), *Shen Shu* (Bl 23), *Wai Guan* (TB 5), and the following ear points: Kidney, Urinary Bladder, Triple Burner, and Endocrine. Choose four to six points each time.

CLINICAL TIPS

1. COMMON PROTOCOLS FOR ALL TYPES OF ARF

A. Moxibustion

Moxibustion is an important treatment method for acute renal failure. Moxa *Guan Yuan* (CV 4), *Qi Hai* (CV 6), *Shen Shu* (Bl 23), *Yong Quan* (Ki 1), and *Qi Zhong* (CV 8). One may also burn direct moxa on salt or ginger in the umbilicus, *Qi Zhong* (CV 8), or one may use the TDP lamp on *Yong Quan* (Ki 1) or *Shen Shu* (Bl 23).

B. External medicinals

One may apply the ingredients in *Xue Fu Zhu Yu Tang* (Blood Mansion Stasis-dispelling Decoction) as a poultice over the kidney area. One may also use an infusion of *Gan Jiang* (Zingiberis Officinalis, dry Rhizoma) as a poultice or smash up fresh garlic, *Da Suan* (Alli Sativi, Bulbus), and apply it over the kidneys. Any of these medicinals will increase blood circulation and disperse kidney blood stasis for every pattern of ARF.

C. Western dietary recommendations

It is extremely important that the patient limit salt, protein, and water intake. The intake of water should equal the output of fluids (urine, stool, vomitus, oozing of fluids from wounds, etc.) plus 500ml per day. The extra 500ml equals the amount of water lost by the skin and lungs. The patient should eat 1500 calories a day. Patients with ARF cannot excrete protein properly. This often leads to azotemia. The patient must limit protein to 0.38 gm/kg of body weight. Sugar intake should be around 150gm per day. The patient should have very little fat in the diet. The patient should consult with a Western dietitian.

D. Chinese dietary recommendations

i. *Yu Mi Xu* (Zeae Maydis, Stylus): For wind heat type edema, decoct 50 grams of the medicinal in 600ml of water for 20-30 minutes. Then boil it down to 300-400ml of decoction. Remove the dregs and divide the resulting medicinal liquid into two doses per day.

ii. *Bai Mao Gen* (Imperatae Cylindricae, Rhizoma): This is one of the best water-disinhibiting, dampness-percolating medicinals for edema and bloody urination. Decoct a one day dose of 60 grams fresh or 30 grams dried *Bai Mao Gen* in water and have the patient drink it frequently over the course of a day.

iii. *Dong Gua* (Benincasae Hispidae, Fructus): For wind heat type ARF with edema, make a soup with 500 grams of *Dong Gua*. Have the patient drink one-third of the soup per day over three days.

iv. *Li Yu* (Cyprinus Carpio, carp), and *Chi Xiao Dou* (Phaseoli Calcarati, Semen): For distinct edema with dark or difficult urination, stew these two medicinals together to make a soup. (Salt should be avoided.) Have the patient eat the fish and beans and drink the liquid at one meal.

v. *Ji Dan* (Ovum Galli, chicken egg) and *Hu Jiao* (Piperis Nigri, Fructus, black pepper): For each egg, add seven grams of pepper. Make a hole in the shell of the raw egg and put in the pepper. Use flour to close the hole. Wet some paper, wrap up the egg, and then steam the egg for one-half hour. Remove the shell and eat the egg. The dosage is two eggs per day for adults and one egg per day for children. This is a general supplement for kidney essence vacuity and spleen qi vacuity.

vi. *Hei Dou* (Phaseoli Vulgaris, Semen, black beans): To supplement the kidney and drain dampness causing edema, cook with water or use in soup.

CAUTION: Fish, eggs, and beans contain protein and one must be careful to stay within the allowable protein limits per day.

2. Acute renal failure generally corresponds to kidney wind, and Chapter 14 of the *Nei Jing Su Wen*, "*Tang Ye Lao Li Lun* (On Rice Soup, Turbid Wine & Sweet Wine)" describes how to treat kidney wind.

> In treating this condition, one should eliminate water by dispelling static blood[9] and make the patient exercise his extremities gently to cause the yang energy to spread gradually . . . Then strongly promote sweating[10] and free the urination.[11]

The contraction of external evils and the resultant edema constitute the tip of this disease. The root is usually a spleen-kidney qi and yang vacuity. The treatment strategy for the tip is resolving the exterior and disinhibiting water. Resolving the exterior includes opening the lung as well as opening the pores. Resolving the exterior not only expels the evils but also helps disinhibit water.

The most important method of resolving the exterior is to strongly promote sweating. "Strongly promote sweating" does not mean to promote strong sweating. The induction of sweating must conform to proper sweating. Proper sweating indicates a mild, whole body sweat with a little extra sweating on the nose. One must avoid inducing excessive sweating. If there is excessive sweating and the pores are open for a long time, the righteous qi effuses with the sweat and evils can re-enter the body. The more vacuous the righteous qi, the more easily and deeply evils can penetrate.

If a patient has ARF as a result of wind cold contraction, one must choose the appropriate warm, acrid,

exterior-resolving medicinals from such medicinals as *Ma Huang* (Ephedrae, Herba), *Jing Jie* (Schizonepetae Tenuifoliae, Herba Seu Flos), *Fang Feng* (Ledebouriellae Divaricatae, Radix), *Fu Ping* (Lemnae Seu Spirodelae, Herba), *Da Fu Pi* (Arecae Catechu, Pericarpium), *Zi Su Ye* (Perillae Frutescentis, Folium), and *Qiang Huo* (Notopterygii, Rhizoma Et Radix). The strength of the medicinals needed to strongly promote sweating varies from case to case. Some cases may need a strong medicinal, such as *Ma Huang*; some only the relatively milder *Qiang Huo*. *Ma Huang* is indicated when one observes the following: The patient has strong chills. (The patient cannot stop shivering even after bundling up.) The patient is wheezing. (This indicates severe impediment and stagnation of lung qi by wind cold.) *Shen Jiang* (Zingiberis Officinalis, uncooked Rhizoma) tea has failed to release the exterior.

In severe cases, one must use larger dosages of a warm, acrid, exterior-resolving medicinal than in mild cases. One must also take note of the season, climate, and geography. For example, one must use a smaller dosage of the warm and strong diaphoretic *Ma Huang* in the south than in the north. Because the weather is hotter, a dosage that might be correct in the north will cause too much sweating in the south. In summer, one often substitutes *Xiang Ru* (Elsholtziae Seu Moslae, Herba) for *Ma Huang*.

Medicinals used to resolve the exterior open the pores and lung to expel wind cold. This is an important strategy to drain water. The lung governs the water passageways. Therefore, it must be open for the triple burner to function properly. Disinhibiting water or keeping urination unobstructed by opening the lung is described metaphorically as "making a hole in the teapot's lid."[12] (In order to facilitate the pouring of tea a teapot's lid is made with a hole in it. The hole allows a release of pressure that allows the tea to flow out of the spout unobstructed.)

Freeing the flow of urination to resolve edema is second in importance in ARF. This strategy requires water-disinhibiting, dampness-percolating medicinals. The most important ones are *Fu Ling* (Poriae Cocos, Sclerotium), *Zhu Ling* (Polypori Umbellati,

Sclerotium), *Ze Xie* (Alismatis Orientalis, Rhizoma), *Che Qian Zi* (Plantaginis, Semen), *Qu Mai* (Dianthi, Herba), *Dong Gua Pi* (Benincasae Hispidae, Semen), *Sheng Jiang Pi* (Zingiberis Officinalis, Cortex Rhizomatis), *Fu Ling Pi* (Poriae Cocos, Cortex Sclerotii), *Da Fu Pi* (Arecae Catechu, Pericarpium), *Yi Yi Ren* (Coicis Lachryma-jobi, Semen), *Chi Xiao Dou* (Phaseoli Calcarati, Semen), *Yu Mi Xu* (Zeae Maydis, Stylus), and *Fang Ji* (Stephaniae Tetrandrae, Radix).

To treat the root, one must use the warming method. Water is yin (associated with cold) and requires warmth to transform and resolve it. When the kidney yang is strong, the kidney's qi transformation (or steaming function) is strong and water can be eliminated. Interior-warming medicinals, *Fu Zi* (Aconiti Carmichaeli, Radix Lateralis Praeparatus), *Rou Gui* (Cinnamomi Cassiae, Cortex), *Gan Jiang* (Zingiberis Officinalis, dry Rhizoma), etc., are often prescribed for kidney wind to strengthen kidney yang's steaming function. However, one must not confuse the interior-warming method with the supplementation method. The later is used to supplement the qi. Some scholars believe that qi supplementation should not be used in ARF. Qi supplementing medicinals can secure and astringe or close the pores. (Note that patients with qi vacuity often have spontaneous sweating because the qi is not strong enough to close the pores.) Closing the pores is counterproductive when trying to drain water. This school of thought contends that supplementing medicinals, such as *Ren Shen* (Panacis Ginseng, Radix) and *Huang Qi* (Astragali Membranacei, Radix), are contraindicated. Other scholars support the opposite contention that it is proper to use supplementing medicinals for ARF. They argue that, since qi and yang depend on each other, one should supplement while warming. Even though there is disagreement about the supplementation method, all authorities agree that the interior-warming method must be used.

Since this is a problem of tip and root, one must pay attention to both. The question of the relative importance of relieving the exterior or warming the interior must be decided on a case by case basis. Because the rule is to treat the tip in acute situations

and to treat the root in chronic situations, one usually weighs treating the tip by putting greater emphasis on relieving the surface in ARF.

3. *Su Wen*, Chapter 3, "*Sheng Qi Tong Tian Lun* (On the Union Heaven & Living Beings)" states:

> When dampness invades the body, one's head will feel heavy and distended as if being tightly bandaged. Prolonged dampness will turn to heat. If this is not eliminated in time, the heat will damage the yin blood, causing malnourishment of the sinews. The large sinews will become rigid with cramping and spasms, the small ones will become flaccid and atrophy. When wind invades, swelling will occur. First one, then another of the extremities will swell. This indicates exhaustion of yang qi.

In treating the pattern of wind heat as in treating wind cold, one must address both the tip and root. With wind heat, the tip consists of both edema and toxins (that cannot be eliminated through urination). The root is spleen-kidney qi vacuity. If one just treats the tip without the root, one may not be able to completely rid the body of water. If one just treats the root and not the tip, one may cause more stagnation. In this case, the best strategy is to first focus on the tip. After the exterior pattern, water, and toxins have been resolved, one can focus on the root using supplementation. Focusing on supplementation in the acute phase may exacerbate the problem by causing more stagnation resulting in greater toxicity.

One must carefully monitor the dosage of all the medicinals. Using too many cooling medicinals can further damage spleen and kidney qi. Using too many water-disinhibiting, dampness-percolating medicinals may also harm the qi by draining water too quickly. To successfully treat this condition, one must skillfully weigh the medicinals to combine three treatment strategies: 1) clearing wind heat, 2) draining water, and 3) supplementing (usually after the evils have been eliminated).

ENDNOTES

1 Aristolochic acid is a constituent of some Chinese medicinals. Overdoses of it have been implicated in renal failure.

[2] In scanty urination the urine volume is less than 400ml/day (oliguric) or less than 100ml/day (anuric).

[3] This is Dr. Wei Li's formula.

[4] See footnotes 5 and 6

[5] The practitioner should choose the appropriate *Cheng Qi Tang* (Order the Qi Decoction).

[6] Blood stasis causes a reduced blood flow. Blood belongs to yin, and a reduction in blood flow is similar to a loss of yin. This causes heat similar to yin vacuity heat.

[7] *Zhong Yi Lin Chuang Shen Zang Bing Xue* (*Clinical Nephrology in Chinese Medicine*), Shanghai Science and Technology Publishing Co., 1998, p. 292 reports that the Beijing Guan An Men Hospital used *Ba Zhen Tang* (Eight Pearls Decoction) and *Dang Gui Bu Xue Tang* (Dang Gui Supplement the Blood Decoction) to treat ARF caused by blood loss from trauma with good results.

[8] In profuse urination the urine volume is increased to over 1500ml per 24 hours (postoliguric). Sometimes a patient first has scanty urination, followed by copious urination. The prognosis is better if the patient only has copious urination. It is essential to monitor the electrolyte balance when the patient has copious urination. The electrolytes pass out with the urine causing imbalances. In Chinese medicine, one must boost qi and nourish yin.

[9] Wiseman translates *qu wan chen cuo* as "eliminate stale water." However, *wan* is "purple" and refers to static blood. *Chen cuo* is old abnormal or harmful body fluids. This is close to one meaning of *shui* or "water." Thus we translate *qu wan chen cuo* as "eliminate water by dispelling static blood."

[10] *Kai gui men* literally means "open the ghost gate." The "ghost gate" is a sweat pore. Since this statement refers to the necessity of strongly overcoming blockage to cause sweating when a replete evil blocks the pores, we have translated *kai gui men* as "strongly promote sweating."

[11] Wiseman translates *jie jing fu* as "cleansing the clean bowel [the bladder]," a literal translation. We have chosen "free the urination" or "freeing urination," to distinguish *jie jing fu* from *li shui shen shi*, "disinhibiting water and percolating dampness," a similar concept.

[12] This is also called "raising the pot and removing the lid" (*ti hu jie gai fa*).

Chronic renal failure (CRF)is defined as the significant insufficiency in renal regulatory and excretory functions regardless of the cause. A diagnosis of implies that nephron destruction and resultant GFR decline have occurred for at least 3-6 months. Unlike ARF with its sudden and reversible kidney function, CRF is slowly progressive and is considered irreversible, in terms of healthy kidney function. Chronic renal failure typically involves widespread metabolic problems and multiple systems. Chronic renal failure is also called chronic renal insufficiency or uremia and may progress to end-stage renal disease (ESRD). Chronicity of renal disease is marked by associated laboratory findings of anemia, hyperphosphatemia, or hypocalcemia.

NOSOLOGY

There are five stages used to describe the progression to end-stage renal failure. The first stage, which is not pathological and has no metabolic consequences, relates with a creatinine clearance greater than 90ml/mn/1.73m^2. The second stage is called early renal insufficiency and is correlated with a creatinine clearance between 60-89. The metabolic consequence is an increase in serum parathyroid hormone. The third stage is described as chronic renal failure and is marked by a creatinine clearance between 30-59. Another way to describe this is to say that CRF equates with a glomerular filtration rate of less than 60ml/min. Metabolically, the body reacts with an increase in calcium absorption and anemia. The fourth stage is pre-end stage failure. Creatinine clearance is between 15-29, and the body enters a state of acidosis. The fifth and final stage is ESRD. Creatinine clearance is less than 15. The metabolic consequence is uremia.

EPIDEMIOLOGY

In the United States, chronic renal failure occurs in about two per 10,000 people annually. Precise statistics are difficult to gauge because symptoms of CRF may not be detected until 90% destruction of the nephrons has occurred. Annual statistics are made by tracking the number of patients using dialysis and by the number of deaths yearly due to ESRD. Annual prevalence of ESRD in the United States in 1997 was 361,031. Of those cases, 62% were Caucasian, 31% were African American, 3% were Asian, 2% were Native American, 1.5% were other, and the ethnicity of 0.5% was unknown. In terms of ages, 41% of those cases were 60-79 years old, 35% were 40-59. Fifteen percent were 20-39, 7% were 80 and above, and only 2% were 0-19 years of age.

ETIOLOGY & PATHOPHYSIOLOGY

Diabetes and hypertension account for two-thirds of all CRF cases. Glomerulonephritis, acute or chronic, is another major cause. Less common causes include kidney stones, kidney infection, obstructive uropathies, polycystic kidney disease, Alport syndrome, reflux neuropathy, and analgesic nephropathy. Like acute renal failure, CRF leads to an accumulation of fluid and waste. This is termed azotemia and uremia. Uremia is defined as the condition of illness as a result of renal failure. Azotemia is the build-up of waste compounds.

The etiology of CRF is noted by the location of the offending, original lesion. Metabolic and autoimmune diseases tend to lodge in the glomerulus. Toxins and infections lodge in either the tubules or the interstitium. Thromboses and atherosclerosis affect the blood vessels. Ultimately the basement membrane of the glomerulus thickens and becomes diffusely sclerotic. Surrounding cells proliferate and eventually become fibrotic. ESRD is accompanied by renal papillary necrosis.

To summarize the pathophysiology, filtration is reduced. Secondary hyperparathyroidism compensates for the nephron loss. Mineral and fluid balance becomes significantly disrupted and results in edema and hypertension. Two critical endocrine functions of the kidney, vitamin D activation and erythropoietin production (EPO), become impaired. Without adequate vitamin D, osteodystrophy results and without erythropoietin chronic anemia is inevitable. The gastrointestinal tract is affected and micronutrients are less readily absorbed.

SYMPTOMATOLOGY

Initially symptoms may be nonspecific. These can include pruritus, weight loss, nausea and vomiting, fatigue, and headaches. As CRF progresses, urine output may decrease or increase. There may be increased urinary frequency and urgency at night.

Bleeding and bruising may become common, and there may be blood in the stools or vomitus. Mental focus becomes impaired. This may extend from drowsiness to coma. There may be muscle spasms, twitches, and cramps. Peripheral neuropathy is common, especially in patients with diabetes. The term "uremic frost" is used for the white, crystal deposition in and on the skin. Additional symptoms may include excessive thirst, change in skin color, light or dark abnormalities of the nails, ammonia breath, and increased agitation. Abnormally high cholesterol may be the first indicator of CRF and calls for further testing.

DIAGNOSIS

A variety of tests are useful for diagnosing CRF. Physical examination, urine and blood testing, imaging, and biopsy may be indicated. Classically, urinalysis reveals broad waxy casts in the sediment, though this is not always seen. Urinary osmolality usually closely matches that of plasma, 300-320 Osm/kg. Ultrasound or intravenous pyelography may show bilateral reduction of kidney size. Biopsy gives definitive diagnosis. Progressive increases in creatinine and urea are useful indicators for CRF. A serum concentration of creatinine is greater than 1.5 to 2 mg/dL is a likely indicator of CRF. It is also noted that a 50% reduction in the glomerular filtration rate correlates with a doubling of the creatinine value. If the creatinine value lies within the reference range but is seen to double (e.g., 0.6-1.2 mg/dL) in a patient, this indicates a loss of 50% of the functioning nephron mass. Concentrations of plasma sodium may be normal or low. Serum potassium may be normal or slightly elevated, usually less than 6 mmol/L. (Potassium levels will vary depending on the concurrent use of potassium-sparing diuretics, ACE inhibitors, or other heart/blood pressure medications.) Hypocalcemia and hyperphosphatemia are common as are moderate acidosis and anemia. Plasma content of CO_2 is between 15-20 mmol/L. The anemia in chronic renal failure is normochromic and normocytic. The hematocrit typically reads between 20-30%. (If a patient has polycystic kidney disease, this may increase to between 35-50%.)

Once a diagnosis has been made, it is important to do

a physical exam at least once yearly and laboratory testing at least twice yearly. Physical examination should pay special attention to mental status. Lab tests monitor for microalbuminuria, WBCs, and broad waxy casts. Chemistry screens check protein/albumin, liver function, electrolytes and BUN/creatinine.

DIFFERENTIAL DIAGNOSIS

Several conditions must be considered in addition to CRF during the diagnosis. These include:

> Rhabdomyolysis
> Nephrotic syndrome
> Carcinoma

Non-proteinuric conditions such as:

> Tubular disorders
> Chronic pyelonephritis
> Polycystic kidneys

WESTERN MEDICAL TREATMENT

Initially, Western medical treatment focuses on diet with close monitoring of dietary protein intake as well as phosphorous, potassium, and sodium. The patient's weight is checked daily. In cases of acidosis, bicarbonate is used to buffer. Recombinant erythropoietin may be supplemented in cases of anemia. Erythropoietin injections remain important therapy for patients on dialysis. With the development of secondary hyperparathyroidism and uremic osteodystrophy, close attention is paid to the calcium and phosphorous balance. Vitamin D supplementation is typical, but it raises the possibility of metastatic calcifications. Angiotensin-converting enzyme (ACE) inhibitors are also often used with CRF patients to control hypertension.

As electrolyte balance becomes increasingly disordered, for example hyperkalemia exceeding 7mmol/L on a consistent basis, patients need to be dialyzed. Peritoneal dialysis is used in patients for whom there are insufficient vascular access. More commonly, hemodialysis is used. Grafting and catheterization is performed in order to allow repetitive entrance into the vascular system. Patients usually undergo thrice

weekly treatments, lasting 3-5 hours. Dialysis machines serve as a membrane filter in place of and in addition to the nephrons. Hemodialysis may be done in clinical settings or at home.

Renal transplantation is a viable option for patients who are less than 70 years old and who have a life expectancy greater than five years. Renal transplantation allows patients a normalized body chemistry and physiology and frees them from the exhausting routine of dialysis. Transplants are considered in the context of the following factors: cardiac status, disease malignancy, infection status, systemic and metabolic disease, gastrointestinal disease, genitourinary tract anomalies, and distal urinary obstruction.

SIDE EFFECTS & DRAWBACKS OF WESTERN MEDICAL THERAPY

Dialysis patients are susceptible to infections, fever, sepsis, bone abnormalities, and persistent anemia. Technical (human) errors are common, especially given the frequency of treatment. Hypotension and arrhythmias can occur. Atherosclerosis is common in dialysis patients given the high rates of hyperhomocysteinemia and hyperlipidemia. Dementia from dialysis is a possible side effect due to toxic aluminum overload from the filtration system. Psychological problems are also frequently associated with long-term dialysis treatments.

PROGNOSIS & COMPLICATIONS

Before the advent of dialysis, chronic renal failure was a terminal illness. Today, the most common complication associated with chronic renal failure is atherosclerosis. This may lead to a myocardial infarction and/or stroke. Patients with CRF more commonly die from the primary etiological factor of CRF rather than renal failure itself.

CHINESE MEDICAL DISEASE CATEGORIZATION

In Chinese medicine, the clinical manifestations of CRF correspond to the traditional disease categories of: block and repulsion, dribbling urinary block, water swelling, kidney taxation or vacuity taxation and taxation wind, phlegm rheum, lumbar pain, abdominal distention, and dizziness.

TREATMENT BASED ON PATTERN IDENTIFICATION

1. SPLEEN-KIDNEY QI & YANG VACUITY

SIGNS & SYMPTOMS: Fatigue, shortness of breath, frequent colds, abdominal distention, lack of appetite, loose stools, profuse urination, feeling cold, thirst without desire to drink, a pale facial complexion, low back and knee soreness and limpness, possible edema depending on the stage. The tongue is pale and puffy with teeth-marks on its edges and white, slimy fur. The pulse is weak.

TREATMENT PRINCIPLES: Supplement the spleen and kidney qi, warm spleen and kidney yang, transform dampness

REPRESENTATIVE FORMULAS: *Xiao Jian Zhong Tang* (Minor Fortify the Center Decoction)

Yi Tang (Saccharum Granorum), 18-30g
Gui Zhi (Cinnamomi Cassiae, Ramulus), 9g
Bai Shao (Paeoniae Lactiflorae, Radix Albus), 18g
mix-fried *Gan Cao* (Glycyrrhizae Uralensis, Radix), 6g
Da Zao (Zizyphi Jujubae, Fructus), 12 pieces

Wen Shen San (Warm the Kidney Powder)

Rou Cong Rong (Cistanchis Deserticolae, Herba), 400g
Mai Men Dong (Ophiopogonis Japonici, Tuber), 400g
Niu Xi (Achyranthis Bidentatae, Radix), 400g
Wu Wei Zi (Schisandrae Chinensis, Fructus), 400g
Ba Ji Tian (Morindae Officinalis, Radix), 400g
Gan Cao (Glycyrrhizae Uralensis, Radix), 400g
Fu Shen (Poriae Cocos, Sclerotium Pararadicis), 250g
Gan Jiang (Zingiberis Officinalis, dry Rhizoma), 250g
Du Zhong (Eucommiae Ulmoidis, Cortex), 150g

Grind all the above ingredients into a fine powder and take six grams with wine 2-3 times per day.

Da Tu Si Zi Wan (Major Cuscuta Pills)

Lu Rong (Cervi, Cornu Parvum), 100g
Ze Xie (Alismatis Orientalis, Rhizoma), 400g
Fu Zi (Aconiti Carmichaeli, Radix Lateralis Praeparatus), 200g
Rou Gui (Cinnamonmi Casiae, Cortex), 200g
Shu Di Huang (Rehmanniae Glutinosae, cooked Radix), 400g
Niu Xi (Achyranthis Bidentatae, Radix), 400g
Fu Ling (Poriae Cocos, Sclerotium), 400g
Shan Zhu Yu (Corni Officinalis, Fructus), 400g
Xu Duan (Dipsaci Asperi, Radix), 400g
Fang Feng (Ledebouriellae Divaricatae, Radix), 400g
Du Zhong (Eucommiae Ulmoidis, Cortex), 400g
Ba Ji Tian (Morindae Officinalis, Radix), 400g
Chen Xiang (Aquilariae Agallochae, Lignum), 200g
Xiao Hui Xiang (Foeniculi Vulgaris, Fructus), 200g
Wu Wei Zi (Schisandrae Chinensis, Fructus), 400g
Chuan Xiong (Ligustici Wallichii, Radix), 400g
Rou Cong Rong (Cistanchis Deserticolae, Herba), 400g
Tu Si Zi (Cuscutae Chinensis, Semen), 400g
Bu Gu Zhi (Psoraleae Corylifoliae, Fructus), 400g
Bi Ba (Piperis Longi, Fructus), 200g
Sang Piao Xiao (Mantidis, Ootheca), 400g
Fu Pen Zi (Rubi Chingii, Fructus), 400g
Shi Long Rui (Ranunculi Sclerati, Semen), 400g

Grind all the above ingredients into a fine powder and take six grams with wine 2-3 times per day.

Bu Tian Da Zao Wan (Supplement Heaven Great Creation Pills)

Ren Shen (Panacis Ginseng, Radix), 100g
Huang Qi (Astragali Membranacei, Radix), 150g
Bai Zhu (Atractylodis Macrocephalae, Rhizoma), 150g
Dang Gui (Angelicae Sinensis, Radix), 75g
Suan Zao Ren (Zizyphi Spinosae, Semen), 75g
Yuan Zhi (Polygalae Tenuifoliae, Radix), 75g
Gan Cao (Glycyrrhizae Uralensis, Radix), 75g
Bai Shao (Paeoniae Lactiflorae, Radix Albus), 75g
Shan Yao (Dioscoreae Oppositae, Radix), 75g
Fu Ling (Poriae Cocos, Sclerotium), 75g
Gou Qi Zi (Lycii Chinensis, Fructus), 200g
Shu Di Huang (Rehmanniae Glutinosae, cooked Radix), 200g
Zi He Che (Hominis, Placenta), 1 whole piece
Gan Cao (Glycyrrhizae Uralensis, Radix), 1 scoop
Lu Jiao (Cervi, Cornu), 1 scoop

Gui Ban (Testudinis, Plastrum), 400g

Cook the last three ingredients together to make *Gui Ban Jiao* (Turtle Plastron Gelatin). Then mix the resulting gelatin with all the rest of the powdered medicinals to make pills and take 12 grams one time per day.

Shi Pi Yin (Bolster the Spleen Beverage)

Shu Fu Zi (Aconiti Carmichaeli, Radix Lateralis Praeparatus), 3g
Gan Jiang (Zingiberis Officinalis, dry Rhizoma), 3g
Fu Ling (Poriae Cocos, Sclerotium), 9g
Bai Zhu (Atractylodis Macrocephalae, Rhizoma), 9g
Mu Gua (Chaenomelis Lagenariae, Fructus), 9g
Hou Po (Magnoliae Officinalis, Cortex), 6g
Mu Xiang (Aucklandiae Lappae, Radix), 3g
Da Fu Pi (Arecae Catechu, Pericarpium), 9g
Cao Guo (Amomi Tsao-ko, Fructus), 6g
mix-fried *Gan Cao* (Glycyrrhizae Uralensis, Radix), 3g
Sheng Jiang (Zingiberis Officinalis, uncooked Rhizoma), 5 slices
Da Zao (Zizyphi Jujubae, Fructus), 5 pieces

MODIFICATIONS: Employing qi-dispersing medicinals makes a tremendous difference in this pattern, for "if qi moves, water moves." If *Shi Pi Yin* is not strong enough, Dr. Zhao[1] suggests using the following formula in addition: *Qian Niu Zi* (Pharbitidis, Semen), *Xiao Hui Xiang* (Foeniculi Vulgaris, Fructus), and uncooked *Da Huang* (Rhei, Radix Et Rhizoma). Grind equal amounts of the preceding three medicinals into a powder and mix together. Take 3.6 grams per day in four servings. One may also add modified *Wu Ling San* (Five [Ingredients] Poria Powder) instead: *Fu Ling* (Poriae Cocos, Sclerotium), 12g, *Zhu Ling* (Polypori Umbellati, Sclerotium), 12g, *Gui Zhi* (Cinnamomi Cassiae, Ramulus), 6-9g, *Bai Zhu* (Atractylodis Macrocephalae, Rhizoma), 12g, *Ze Xie* (Alismatis Orientalis, Rhizoma), 9g, *Shu Fu Zi* (Aconiti Carmichaeli, Radix Lateralis Praeparatus), 6-9g, *Yi Mu Cao* (Leonuri Heterophylli, Herba), 12g, and *Ze Lan* (Lycopi Lucidi, Herba), 9g. Both these formulas quicken blood and disinhibit water.[2]

ACUMOXIBUSTION: Choose points to moxa from *Pi Shu* (Bl 20), *Shen Shu* (Bl 23), *Ming Men* (GV 4), *Guan Yuan* (CV 4), *Qi Hai* (CV 6), *Zhong Wan* (CV 12), *Tai Bai* (Sp 3), *San Yin Jiao* (Sp 6), *Yin Ling Quan* (Sp 9), *Tai Xi* (Ki 3), *Zhao Hai* (Ki 6), and *Fu Liu* (Ki 7).

Case history of Dr. Er Shun-jiang: Zou, a 46 year-old male[3]

Four months prior to visiting Dr. Er, Zou began to have edema on his face. This edema gradually progressed to cover his whole body. Zou also had nausea, vomiting, abdominal distention, and low backache. All these symptoms worsened in the two weeks immediately preceding his first visit. Zou went to several Western doctors who had tried chemotherapy, cortisone, diuretics, and Western antihypertensive drugs without success. On June 8, 1977, Zou's blood pressure was 145/100mmHg, his waist was 93cm in circumference, his testicles were the size of a baby's head, and his lower extremities were swollen. His urine protein level was high, his blood cholesterol was 737mg%, his blood protein was low, and his BUN was 51.9mg%. Dr. Er noted that previous Chinese doctors had tried *Wu Ling San* (Five [Ingredients] Poria Powder), *Zhen Wu Tang* (True Warrior Decoction), and *Liu Jun Zi Tang* (Six Gentlemen Decoction), alternating these formulas. This regimen had increased Zou's urination and had reduced his blood pressure but had not reduced the size of his waist. At times, it expanded up to 101cm. On July 14, Dr. Er decided to start Zou on *Kong Xian Dan* (Drool-controlling Elixir): *Gan Sui* (Euphorbiae Kansui, Radix), *Hong Da Ji* (Euphorbiae Seu Knoxiae, Radix), and *Bai Jie Zi* (Sinapis Albae, Semen), equal amounts ground into powder and made into small pills. Zou's urine ou-put increased remarkably to about 2600-2800ml/day. His waist reduced in size to 77cm in one week. After one course of this formula, Dr. Er added *Zhen Wu Tang* (True Warrior Decoction) and *Liu Jun Zi Tang* (Six Gentlemen Decoction): *Shu Fu Zi* (Aconiti Carmichaeli, Radix Lateralis Praeparatus), *Bai Zhu* (Atractylodis Macrocephalae, Rhizoma), *Fu Ling* (Poriae Cocos, Sclerotium), *Bai Shao* (Paeoniae Lactiflorae, Radix Albus), *Sheng Jiang* (Zingiberis Officinalis, uncooked Rhizoma), *Ren Shen* (Panacis Ginseng, Radix), mix-fried *Gan Cao* (Glycyrrhizae Uralensis, Radix), *Ban Xia* (Pinelliae Ternatae,

Rhizoma), and *Chen Pi* (Citri Reticulatae, Pericarpium) in undisclosed amounts.

Zou took this combination for 15 days and had no side effects. Dr. Er decided to suspend the use of *Kong Xian Dan* and have Zou take *Liu Jun Zi Tang*, *Jin Gui Shen Qi Wan* (*Golden Cabinet* Kidney Qi Pills), and *Ba Zhen Tang* (Eight Pearls Decoction). *Ba Zhen Tang* consists of: *Ren Shen* (Panacis Ginseng, Radix), 9g, *Bai Zhu* (Atractylodis Macrocephalae, Rhizoma), 9g, *Fu Ling* (Poriae Cocos, Sclerotium), 9g, mix-fried *Gan Cao* (Glycyrrhizae Uralensis, Radix), 3g, *Shu Di Huang* (Rehmanniae Glutinosae, cooked Radix), 9g, *Dang Gui* (Angelicae Sinensis, Radix), 9g, *Bai Shao* (Paeoniae Lactiflorae, Radix Albus), 9g, and *Chuan Xiong* (Ligustici Wallichii, Radix), 9g. By Aug. 11, 1978, Zou's edema had dissipated, he was urinating about one liter per day, his blood pressure was normal, and his waist reduced to 70cm. His urinalysis was normal and his blood cholesterol was 256 mg%. Zou's only remaining problem was low blood protein.

2. SPLEEN-KIDNEY QI & YIN VACUITY

SIGNS & SYMPTOMS: A pale facial complexion, fatigue, shortness of breath, low back and knee soreness and limpness, dry mouth, heat in the five hearts, dry stool, scanty, yellow urination. The tongue is pale with teeth-marks on its edges, and the pulse is fine, forceless, and deep.

TREATMENT PRINCIPLES: Fortify the spleen and boost the qi, supplement the kidney and enrich yin

REPRESENTATIVE FORMULA: *Liu Wei Di Huang Wan* (Six Flavors Rehmannia Pills) plus *Ju Yuan Jian* (Origin-lifting Brew)

Shu Di Huang (Rehmanniae Glutinosae, cooked Radix), 12g
Shan Yao (Radix Dioscoreae Oppositae), 12g
Shan Zhu Yu (Corni Officinalis, Fructus), 12g
Ze Xie (Alismatis Orientalis, Rhizoma), 9g
Fu Ling (Poriae Cocos, Sclerotium), 12g
Mu Dan Pi (Moutan, Cortex Radicis), 9g
Huang Qi (Astragali Membranacei, Radix), 12g

Ren Shen (Panacis Ginseng, Radix), 6-9g
Bai Zhu (Atractylodis Macrocephalae, Rhizoma), 12g
mix-fried *Gan Cao* (Glycyrrhizae Uralensis, Radix), 3g
Sheng Ma (Cimicifugae, Rhizoma), 6g

MODIFICATIONS: If there is chronic lung yin vacuity with symptoms such as sore throat, add *Xuan Shen* (Scrophulariae Ningpoensis, Radix), *Mai Men Dong* (Ophiopogonis Japonici, Tuber), *Jie Geng* (Platycodi Grandiflori, Radix), and *Sha Shen* (Glehniae Littoralis, Radix). If there is heart qi and yin vacuity, add *Mai Men Dong* (Ophiopogonis Japonici, Tuber), *Wu Wei Zi* (Schisandrae Chinensis, Fructus), *Yuan Zhi* (Polygalae Tenuifoliae, Radix), and *Huang Jing* (Polygonati, Rhizoma). If there is dry stool, add *Rou Cong Rong* (Cistanchis Deserticolae, Herba). This yang-supplementing medicinal balances the yin-supplementing medicinals and counteracts their tendency to create dampness. It is the best medicinal for spleen and kidney qi vacuity constipation. One may also use *Hu Ma Ren* (Sesami Indici, Semen) and *Hei Zhi Ma* (Sesami Indici, black Semen). If there is low back soreness and coldness with frequent night-time urination, this indicates the patient has some concurrent yang vacuity and one should add *Fu Zi* (Aconiti Carmichaeli, Radix Lateralis Praeparatus), *Rou Gui* (Cinnamonmi Casiae, Cortex), and *Ba Ji Tian* (Morindae Officinalis, Radix).

ACUMOXIBUSTION: Choose from *Pi Shu* (Bl 20), *Shen Shu* (Bl 23), *Tai Xi* (Ki 3), *Zhao Hai* (Ki 6), *Fu Liu* (Ki 7), *Tai Bai* (Sp 3), *Gong Sun* (Sp 4), *Zu San Li* (St 36), *Guan Yuan* (CV 4), *Qi Hai* (CV 6), and *Zhang Men* (Liv 13).

Case history of Dr. Can Bing-fu: Bai, a 30 year-old male[4]

Bai had been suffering with chronic nephritis for years. He first experienced low back pain and tried Chinese medicine for half a year. The Chinese medical therapy relieved his low back pain for a while, but then it would worsen again. His other symptoms would also fluctuate, getting better and worse without resolution. One-half month before coming to see Dr. Can, Bai's face and eyes became edematous. Two days later, his entire body became edematous. He tried Western diuretics but these did not help. His blood pressure was high, his BUN was 120mg%, and his urine protein was 2+. He had dizziness, fatigue, insomnia, low back distention, a bitter taste in his mouth, vexation, nausea, and lack of appetite. Based on these signs and symptoms, Dr. Can reasoned as follows: Chronic nephritis is usually due to internal damage. Internal damage may be vacuity of former heaven yin and yang or the latter heaven constructive and defensive. No matter what the cause, the kidney becomes vacuous with kidney and bladder qi transformation failure. Water accumulates and becomes edema. If there is spleen damage, the constructive and defensive cannot nourish the five viscera. Whether there is initial yang or yin vacuity, long-term vacuity of either of these causes vacuity of the other.

Dr. Can's pattern identification was spleen and kidney yin and yang vacuity, yin vacuity being the most egregious. His treatment strategy was to nourish kidney yin, fortify the spleen, and harmonize the stomach. His prescription was augmented *Liu Wei Di Huang Wan* (Six Flavors Rehmannia Pills): *Shu Di Huang* (Rehmanniae Glutinosae, cooked Radix), *Shan Yao* (Radix Dioscoreae Oppositae), *Shan Zhu Yu* (Corni Officinalis, Fructus), *Ze Xie* (Alismatis Orientalis, Rhizoma), *Fu Ling* (Poriae Cocos, Sclerotium), *Mu Dan Pi* (Moutan, Cortex Radicis), *Tu Si Zi* (Cuscutae Chinensis, Semen), *Gou Qi Zi* (Lycii Chinensis, Fructus), *Nu Zhen Zi* (Ligustri Lucidi, Fructus), *Han Lian Cao* (Ecliptae Prostratae, Herba), *Sang Piao Xiao* (Mantidis, Ootheca), *Ban Xia* (Pinelliae Ternatae, Rhizoma), *Chen Pi* (Citri Reticulatae, Pericarpium), and *Zhu Ru* (Bambusae In Taeniis, Caulis), amounts not given. Bai took this formula for 10 days and his edema and other symptoms abated. He continued on it for three months and completely recovered.

Case history of Dr. Can Bing-fu: Chou, a 35 year-old female[5]

Chou had been experiencing recurrent edema and low back pain for five years. During this time, her urine protein fluctuated from 3+-5+. She was diagnosed with chronic nephritis. She often felt dizzy and had tinnitus, insomnia, fatigue, low appetite,

and loose stools. Chinese doctors had tried treating her for spleen-kidney yang vacuity, but this made her dizziness and insomnia worse. When Chou came to Dr. Can, her blood pressure was 160/110mmHg, her urine protein was 3+, and her BUN was 55mg%. Dr. Can's treatment strategy was to harmonize and supplement the spleen and kidney, nourish yin and enrich kidney essence. His formula consisted of variations of augmented *Liu Wei Di Huang Wan* (Six Flavors Rehmannia Pills): *Shu Di Huang* (Rehmanniae Glutinosae, cooked Radix), *Shan Yao* (Radix Dioscoreae Oppositae), *Shan Zhu Yu* (Corni Officinalis, Fructus), *Ze Xie* (Alismatis Orientalis, Rhizoma), *Fu Ling* (Poriae Cocos, Sclerotium), *Mu Dan Pi* (Moutan, Cortex Radicis), *Ren Shen* (Panacis Ginseng, Radix), *Wu Wei Zi* (Schisandrae Chinensis, Fructus), *Du Zhong* (Eucommiae Ulmoidis, Cortex), *Gou Qi Zi* (Lycii Chinensis, Fructus), *Nu Zhen Zi* (Ligustri Lucidi, Fructus), *Han Lian Cao* (Ecliptae Prostratae, Herba), and *Zhu Ru* (Bambusae In Taeniis, Caulis), amounts not given. Dr. Can's strategy and formula successfully resolved Chou's condition. After 10 months, her blood pressure was normal and her BUN was 45mg%.

3. BLOOD STASIS WITH DAMP HEAT

SIGNS & SYMPTOMS: Nausea, vomiting, vexation, headache, fever, dizziness, fatigue, itching skin, dry mouth, purple lips. There is also anemia and high blood pressure. The tongue is purple, and the pulse is bowstring and slippery.

TREATMENT PRINCIPLES: Clear heat and eliminate dampness, resolve toxins and quicken the blood

REPRESENTATIVE FORMULA: Modified *Qing Wen Bai Du Yin* (Scourge-clearing, Toxin-vanquishing Beverage)

Shi Gao (Gypsum Fibrosum), 9-30g
Zhi Mu (Anemarrhenae Asphodeloidis, Rhizoma), 6-12g
Gan Cao (Glycyrrhizae Uralensis, Radix), 3-6g
Shui Niu Jiao (Bubali, Cornu), 12-24g
Xin Yi (Magnoliae, Flos), 9-12g
Sheng Di Huang (Rehmanniae Glutinosae, uncooked Radix), 9-15g

Mu Dan Pi (Moutan, Cortex Radicis), 6-12g
Chi Shao (Paeoniae Lactiflorae, Radix Rubrus), 6-12g
Xuan Shen (Scrophulariae Ningpoensis, Radix), 6-12g
Huang Lian (Coptidis Chinensis, Rhizoma), 6-12g
Huang Qin (Scutellariae Baicalensis, Radix), 3-9g
Zhi Zi (Gardeniae Jasminoidis, Fructus), 6-12g
Lian Qiao (Forsythiae Suspensae, Fructus), 6-12g
Jie Geng (Platycodi Grandiflori, Radix), 3-6g

MODIFICATIONS: When treating blood stasis in patterns with heat or damp heat, the medicinal's qi is the most important consideration. One should choose cool blood-quickening, stasis-dispelling medicinals. The strength of the medicinal is second in importance. Mild medicinals that quicken the blood include *Dang Gui* (Angelicae Sinensis, Radix) and *Chuan Xiong* (Ligustici Wallichii, Radix). Strong medicinals that quicken blood and dispel stasis include *E Zhu* (Curcumae Zedoariae, Rhizoma) and *San Leng* (Sparganii Stoloniferi, Rhizoma). The strongest medicinals break blood and disperse nodulation. These include the "insect" or "worm" products *Shui Zhi* (Hirudo Seu Whitmania), *Tu Bie Chong* (Eupolyphga Seu Opisthoplatia), and *Meng Chong* (Tabanus). If there is long-term or very severe blood stasis, one should transform stasis, not just quicken blood, using medicinals such as *San Qi* (Notoginseng, Radix), *Tao Ren* (Pruni Persicae, Semen), and *Shui Zhi* (Hirudo Seu Whitmania).

ACUMOXIBUSTION: Choose from *Qu Chi* (LI 11), *He Gu* (LI 4), *Tai Chong* (Liv 3), *Xue Hai* (Sp 10), *Yin Ling Quan* (Sp 9), *Yang Ling Quan* (GB 34), *Ge Shu* (Bl 17), *Da Zhui* (GV 14), *Zhi Gou* (TB 6), *Wei Yang* (Bl 53), and *Nei Guan* (Per 6).

Case history of Dr. Qi Chiang: Ma, a 25 year-old female[6]

Five years prior to Ma's first visit on Nov. 9, 1976, she was diagnosed with acute nephritis. One month before her first visit, she suddenly became extremely nauseous. She went to a hospital where she had blood tests. The Western doctor's diagnosis was chronic nephritis and stage two chronic renal failure. When she saw Dr. Qi, Ma was pale and irritable. She was nauseous and often vomited, had no appetite,

and could not eat. Her urine was scanty but she had no edema. Her tongue had purple sides with thin, dry fur, and her pulse was bowstring and slippery. Dr. Qi's pattern identification was heat in the blood aspect with blood stasis. His prescription[7] consisted of: *Lian Qiao* (Forsythiae Suspensae, Fructus), 25g, *Tao Ren* (Pruni Persicae, Semen), 15g, *Hong Hua* (Carthami Tinctorii, Flos), 15g, *Dang Gui* (Angelicae Sinensis, Radix), 15g, *Ge Gen* (Puerariae, Radix), 25g, *Chi Shao* (Paeoniae Lactiflorae, Radix Rubrus), 15g, *Sheng Di Huang* (Rehmanniae Glutinosae, uncooked Radix), 20g, *Bai Hua She She Cao* (Oldenlandiae Diffusae, Herba), 50g, *Pu Gong Ying* (Taraxaci Mongolici, Herba Cum Radice), 50g, *Mu Dan Pi* (Moutan, Cortex Radicis), 15g, *Xuan Shen* (Scrophulariae Ningpoensis, Radix), 20g, *Gan Cao* (Glycyrrhizae Uralensis, Radix), 10g, and *Da Huang* (Rhei, Radix Et Rhizoma), 5g.

Ma took this formula for five days. She had dark stools at first that then became pale yellow. Her urine increased to 2000ml with a pale yellow color. Her nausea stopped and her vexation disappeared. Her blood work improved, her BUN changing from 82mg% to 61mg%. Dr. Qi's second prescription consisted of: *Lian Qiao* (Forsythiae Suspensae, Fructus), 20g, *Tao Ren* (Pruni Persicae, Semen), 15g, *Hong Hua* (Carthami Tinctorii, Flos), 15g, *Dang Gui* (Angelicae Sinensis, Radix), 15g, *Ge Gen* (Puerariae, Radix), 25g, *Chi Shao* (Paeoniae Lactiflorae, Radix Rubrus), 20g, *Sheng Di Huang* (Rehmanniae Glutinosae, uncooked Radix), 20g, *Chai Hu* (Bupleuri, Radix), 15g, *Bai Hua She She Cao* (Oldenlandiae Diffusae, Herba), 50g, *Da Huang* (Rhei, Radix Et Rhizoma), 5g, *Mu Dan Pi* (Moutan, Cortex Radicis), 15g, and *Gan Cao* (Glycyrrhizae Uralensis, Radix), 10g.

Ma's third visit was on November 28. She had used the formula for six days and all her symptoms had diminished. Although she felt much better, her blood work was about the same. So Dr. Qi decided to give her the following prescription: *Tu Si Zi* (Cuscutae Chinensis, Semen), 50g, *He Shou Wu* (Polygoni Multiflori, Radix), 50g, *Dang Gui* (Angelicae Sinensis, Radix), 50g, *Shu Di Huang*

(Rehmanniae Glutinosae, cooked Radix), 50g, *Sheng Di Huang* (Rehmanniae Glutinosae, uncooked Radix), 30g, *Jin Yin Hua* (Lonicerae Japonicae, Flos), 40g, *Bai Shao* (Paeoniae Lactiflorae, Radix Albus), 40g, *Hong Shen* (Panacis Ginseng, Radix Rubrus), 50g, *Dan Shen* (Salviae Miltiorrhizae, Radix), 25g, *Tian Men Dong* (Asparagi Cochinensis, Tuber), 25g, *Shan Zhu Yu* (Corni Officinalis, Fructus), 25g, *Fu Ling* (Poriae Cocos, Sclerotium), 25g, *Mu Dan Pi* (Moutan, Cortex Radicis), 25g, *Ze Xie* (Alismatis Orientalis, Rhizoma), 25g, *Shan Yao* (Radix Dioscoreae Oppositae), 50g, *Gou Qi Zi* (Lycii Chinensis, Fructus), 25g, and *Bai Zhu* (Atractylodis Macrocephalae, Rhizoma), 25g. These medicinals were to be ground up and made into pills with honey, with every pill about 15g. Ma was to take one pill two times per day.

By April 18, Ma's BUN was down to 35mg%, and her symptoms had disappeared. Dr. Qi then gave her: *Huang Qi* (Astragali Membranacei, Radix), 40g, *Dang Shen* (Codonopsitis Pilosulae, Radix), 30g, *Bai Hua She She Cao* (Oldenlandiae Diffusae, Herba), 50g, *Pu Gong Ying* (Taraxaci Mongolici, Herba Cum Radice), 50g, *Sheng Di Huang* (Rehmanniae Glutinosae, uncooked Radix), 30g, *Mai Men Dong* (Ophiopogonis Japonici, Tuber), 20g, *Bai Mao Gen* (Imperatae Cylindricae, Rhizoma), 50g, and *Gan Cao* (Glycyrrhizae Uralensis, Radix), 15g. Ma took this prescription as a decoction for seven days and all tests returned to normal. On June 8, Ma came in for a follow-up visit and all her blood work was normal with urine protein at 1+ and blood pressure at 140/90mmHg.

UREMIA[8]

In uremia, fluid and electrolyte balance are disturbed, azotemia increases, and systemic manifestations occur. GFR is below 10% of normal. Symptoms include nausea, vomiting, bleeding, anemia, and hypertension. In the patterns of uremia, vacuity and replete toxicity vary in importance. Toxicity is the tip, but if it is very severe, one must focus on it. If toxicity is not so severe, one may focus on supplementing vacuity, the root. There are six common patterns: turbid yin rebelling, heat entering the constructive/blood, evils sinking into the pericardium, interior heat stirring wind, interior wind caused by vacuity, and yang debilitation or desertion.[9]

1. TURBID YIN UPWARD COUNTERFLOW

SIGNS & SYMPTOMS: Chronic, long-term edema, a heavy feeling in the body, a heavy head, or dizziness, or headache, nausea, vomiting, thirst without desire to drink, no appetite, abdominal distention, constipation or loose stools. The tongue has white, slimy fur, and the pulse is slippery.

TREATMENT PRINCIPLES: Upbear the clear and downbear the turbid, warm the stomach and stop nausea

REPRESENTATIVE FORMULA: *Sheng Qing Jiang Zhuo Tang* (Upbear the Clear & Downbear the Turbid Decoction)

Wu Zhu Yu (Evodiae Rutaecarpae, Fructus), 3g
Ban Xia (Pinelliae Ternatae, Rhizoma), 9g
stir-fried *Bai Zhu* (Atractylodis Macrocephalae, Rhizoma), 6g
Hou Po (Magnoliae Officinalis, Cortex), 6g
Gan Jiang (Zingiberis Officinalis, dry Rhizoma), 9g
Chen Xiang (Aquilariae Agallochae, Lignum), 2.5g
Fu Ling (Poriae Cocos, Sclerotium), 25g
Ze Xie (Alismatis Orientalis, Rhizoma), 12g
Sheng Jiang (Zingiberis Officinalis, uncooked Rhizoma), 3g
He Ye (Nelumbinis Nuciferae, Folium), 6g

MODIFICATIONS: If there is loose stools, a puffy tongue with white fur, and a soggy pulse, add *Ren Shen* (Panacis Ginseng, Radix). If there are abdominal cramps, constipation, nausea, and the pulse is deep and bowstring, add *Fu Zi* (Aconiti Carmichaeli, Radix Lateralis Praeparatus) and *Shu Di Huang* (Rehmanniae Glutinosae, cooked Radix). If the tongue has yellow, slimy fur and the pulse is fast, add *Huang Lian* (Coptidis Chinensis, Rhizoma). If there is headache and the pulse is bowstring, add *Tian Ma* (Gastrodiae Elatae, Rhizoma) and *Gou Teng* (Uncariae Cum Uncis, Ramulus).

ACUMOXIBUSTION: Choose points to moxa from *Zu San Li* (St 36), *San Yin Jiao* (Sp 6), *Pi Shu* (Bl 20), *Zhong Wan* (CV 12), *Qi Hai* (CV 6), needle *He Gu* (LI 4), *Jian Shi* (Per 5), *Nei Guan* (Per 6), *Feng Long* (St 40), *Yin Ling Quan* (Sp 9), and *Tai Xi* (Ki 3).

Case history of Dr. Jing Ze-zao: Yang, a 69 year-old male[10]

Yang first came to see Dr. Jing on Aug. 16, 1980. In 1972, he experienced edema in his lower extremities. The Western medical diagnosis was chronic nephritis. The patient lived in the hospital for three months, and his condition improved somewhat. He then began taking a course of Chinese medicinals, but his condition would exacerbate and remit without resolution. By June 2, 1980, Yang was in the hospital for the second time. His BUN was 36mg%, his blood creatinine was 3.8mg%, and he had low blood protein. Ultrasound showed that his right kidney surface had nodules, both his kidneys were prolapsed, and that his liver and spleen were slightly enlarged. The diagnosis was chronic nephritis with uremia. Yang then came in to see Dr. Jing. On his first visit, Yang's face was pale, his whole body was edematous with pitting, and both his legs were heavy, weak, and cold. He had chest oppression with shortness of breath and profuse, white, sticky phlegm, nausea, no appetite, one or two bowel movements per day that were sometimes loose and sometimes dry, and profuse, clear urine. He sweated easily, had heart palpitations, insomnia, and tinnitus, was thirsty in afternoon and evening, and had a sweet, sticky taste in his mouth. His tongue was pale and dark with a crack on the tip and with watery, glossy, white fur. His pulse was deep and slow. His Hb (hemoglobin) was 7.8-8g% and his blood pressure was 120/70mmHg.

Based on the above signs and symptoms, Dr. Jing's pattern identification was spleen, kidney, and lung qi and yang vacuity with damp stagnation. His treatment strategy was to supplement the spleen, kidney, and lung and transform dampness. His initial prescription consisted of: *Dang Shen* (Codonopsitis Pilosulae, Radix), 15g, *Bai Zhu* (Atractylodis Macrocephalae, Rhizoma), 12g, *Fu Ling* (Poriae Cocos, Sclerotium), 15g, *Gan Cao* (Glycyrrhizae

Uralensis, Radix), 6g, *Chen Pi* (Citri Reticulatae, Pericarpium), 9g, *Ban Xia* (Pinelliae Ternatae, Rhizoma), 9g, *Chen Xiang* (Aquilariae Agallochae, Lignum), 2g, *Yin Yang Huo* (Epimedii, Herba), 15g, *Gou Qi Zi* (Lycii Chinensis, Fructus), 15g, *Xing Ren* (Pruni Armeniacae, Semen), 9g, *Tu Si Zi* (Cuscutae Chinensis, Semen), 10g, and *Ze Xie* (Alismatis Orientalis, Rhizoma), 12g. Yang took this prescription for seven days and his edema reduced, his urination was easier, and his phlegm became easy to expectorate. After 20 days, his edema continued to dissipate and both his legs felt stronger. His shortness of breath was much better with much less copious, thinner phlegm. His stools became formed and his sleep improved. His tongue was now pale and puffy with thin, white fur and his pulse was slow and bowstring.

Therefore, Dr. Jing continued to prescribe the same basic formula, modifying it according to Yang's symptoms. When Yang's hands and feet were cold, Dr. Jing removed *Gan Cao* and added *Rou Gui* (Cinnamonmi Casiae, Cortex), 2g. When Yang's tongue had dark spots, he added *Chi Shao* (Paeoniae Lactiflorae, Radix Rubrus), 9g. If there were heart palpitations, he added *Yuan Zhi* (Polygalae Tenuifoliae, Radix), 6g. When there was coughing and wheezing, he added *Bai Bu* (Stemonae, Radix), 9g, and *Zi Su Zi* (Perillae Frutescentis, Fructus), 6g. If Yang's phlegm became yellow, he added *Yu Xing Cao* (Houttuyniae Cordatae, Herba Cum Radice), 20g. If Yang's flatulence began to smell bad, he added *Lai Fu Zi* (Raphani Sativi, Semen), 9g, and *Mai Ya* (Hordei Vulgaris, Fructus Germinatus), 15g. If Yang had vivid dreams, he added *Huang Bai* (Phellodendri, Cortex), 9g, *Sha Ren* (Amomi, Fructus), 4.5g, and *Ye Jiao Teng* (Polygoni Multiflori, Caulis), 20g. If Yang's tongue became red with no fur, he removed *Yin Yang Huo* and *Tu Si Zi* and added *Bei Sha Shen* (Glenhniae Littoralis, Radix), 12g, *Nu Zhen Zi* (Ligustri Lucidi, Fructus), 15g, and *Han Lian Cao* (Ecliptae Prostratae, Herba), 15g. If Yang's edema increased, he added *Che Qian Zi* (Plantaginis, Semen), 12g, and *Yi Mu Cao* (Leonuri Heterophylli, Herba), 15g. If he had loose teeth and bleeding gums, Dr. Jing added *Sheng Di Huang* (Rehmanniae Glutinosae, uncooked Radix), 9g. By Jan. 19, 1981, Yang's BUN was 40 mg% and his creatinine was 4.7mg%. By Feb. 16, 1981, Yang's urine protein was 3+, his ARF was 0-2, and his granular cast was 0-2. By

March 16, 1981, Yang's BUN was 21.5mg%, all his symptoms abated, and he was stable.

2. HEAT ENTERING THE CONSTRUCTIVE & BLOOD ASPECTS

SIGNS & SYMPTOMS: Fever, headache, irritability, confusion or delirium, bleeding, black stools, bloody urine, purple skin rashes or spots. The tongue is red and purple with dry, black fur, and the pulse is deep, fine, and fast.

TREATMENT PRINCIPLES: Clear the constructive and cool the blood, move the blood and resolve toxins

REPRESENTATIVE FORMULA: Modified *Liang Xue Jie Du Yin* (Blood-cooling, Toxin-resolving Beverage)

Shui Niu Jiao (Bubali, Cornu), 12-24g
Huang Lian (Coptidis Chinensis, Rhizoma), 4.5-9g
fresh *Sheng Di Huang* (Rehmanniae Glutinosae, uncooked Radix), 30-60g
Huang Bai (Phellodendri, Cortex), 4-12g
Mu Dan Pi (Moutan, Cortex Radicis), 6-12g
Chi Shao (Paeoniae Lactiflorae, Radix Rubrus), 9-18g
Jin Yin Hua (Lonicerae Japonicae, Flos), 15-30g
Xiao Ji (Cephalanoplos Segeti, Herba), 9-18g
Bai Mao Gen (Imperatae Cylindricae, Rhizoma), 15-30g

MODIFICATIONS: If there is scanty urine, add *Tu Fu Ling* (Smilacis Glabrae, Rhizoma). If the skin has purple or red spots, add *Da Qing Ye* (Daqingye, Folium), *Sheng Ma* (Cimicifugae, Rhizoma), and *Xuan Shen* (Scrophulariae Ningpoensis, Radix).

If there is copious bleeding, use *Zi Xue Dan* (Purple Snow Elixir), 3-9g, divided into three doses. *Zi Xue Dan* (Purple Snow Elixir) consists of the following medicinals: *Shi Gao* (Gypsum Fibrosum), 1500g, *Han Shui Shi* (Calcitum), 1500g, *Hua Shi* (Talcum), 1500g, *Xi Jiao* (Rhinocerotis, Cornu), 150g, *Xin Yi* (Magnoliae, Flos), 150g, *Ling Yang Jiao* (Antelopis Saiga-tatarici, Cornu), 150g, *She Xiang* (Moschi Moschideri, Secretio), 37.5g, *Xuan Shen* (Scrophulariae Ningpoensis, Radix), 500g, *Ci Shi* (Magnititum), 1500g, *Sheng Ma* (Cimicifugae, Rhizoma), 500g, mix-fried *Gan Cao* (Glycyrrhizae

Uralensis, Radix), 240g, *Qing Mu Xiang* (Aristolochiae, Radix), 150g, *Chen Xiang* (Aquilariae Agallochae, Lignum), 150g, *Ding Xiang* (Caryophylli, Flos), 30g, *Zhu Sha* (Cinnabar), 90g, *Mang Xiao* (Miribilitum), 5000g, *Xiao Shi* (Niter), 96g, and *Huang Jin* (Gold), 3000g.

If the patient is in a coma, use *Ju Fang Zhi Bao Dan* (Greatest Treasure Elixir) or *Shen Xi Dan* (Magical Rhinoceros Elixir). The ingredients in *Ju Fang Zhi Bao Dan* are: *Xi Jiao* (Rhinocerotis, Cornu), 30g, *Xin Yi* (Magnoliae, Flos), 30g, *Niu Huang* (Bovis, Calculus), 15g, *Dai Mao* (Eretmochelydis Imbricatae, Carapax), 30g, *Bing Pian* (Borneol), 0.3g, *She Xiang* (Moschi Moschiferi, Secretio), 0.3g, *An Xi Xiang* (Benzoinum), 45g, *Zhu Sha* (Cinnabar), 30g, *Hu Po* (Succinum), 30g, and *Xiong Huang* (Realgar), 30g.

The ingredients in *Shen Xi Dan* are: *Xi Jiao* (Rhinocerotis, Cornu), 180g, *Xin Yi* (Magnoliae, Flos), 180g, *Sheng Di Huang* (Rehmanniae Glutinosae, uncooked Radix), 450g, *Jin Yin Hua* (Lonicerae Japonicae, Flos), 450g, *Lian Qiao* (Forsythiae Suspensae, Fructus), 300g, *Ban Lan Gen* (Isatidis Seu Baphicacanthi, Radix), 270g, *Huang Qin* (Scutellariae Baicalensis, Radix), 180g, *Chang Pu* (Acori Graminei, Rhizoma), 180g, *Dan Dou Chi* (Sojae, Semen Praeparatum), 240g, *Tian Hua Fen* (Trichosanthis Kirilowii, Radix), 120g, *Xuan Shen* (Scrophulariae Ningpoensis, Radix), 210g, and *Zi Cao* (Arnebiae Seu Lithospermi, Radix), 120g. If there is fright reversal, add *Di Long* (Lumbricus), *Gou Teng* (Uncariae Cum Uncis, Ramulus), and *Ling Yang Jiao* (Antelopis Saiga-tatarici, Cornu).

ACUMOXIBUSTION: Bleed the well points and choose points to needle from *He Gu* (LI 4), *Qu Chi* (LI 11), *Da Zhui* (GV 14), *Ye Men* (TB 2), *Hou Xi* (SI 3), *Nei Guan* (Per 6), *Shen Men* (Ht 7) *Yin Xi* (Ht 6), *Jian Shi* (Per 5), *Da Ling* (Per 7), *Wei Zhong* (Bl 40), *Zhi Bian* (Bl 49), *San Yin Jiao* (Sp 6), *Xue Hai* (Sp 10), *Ge Shu* (Bl 17), *Tai Chong* (Liv 3), *Qu Quan* (Liv 8), and *Tai Xi* (Ki 3).

Case history of Dr. Yu Xian-zou: Dong, a 43 year-old male[11]

Dong's first visit to Dr. Yu was on July 16, 1970. He

had experienced fatigue and low back soreness for a few years. Then, at the beginning of July 1970, Dong started having fever and watery diarrhea. He had bowel movements over 20 times a day with stools that looked like soy sauce mixed with mucus. He was given antibiotics, his fever disappeared, and he had less frequent diarrhea, but then he started to vomit. His vomiting consisted of coffee-colored fluids. He had no appetite and his stools were black. The doctors thought he had upper respiratory bleeding. When he came to Dr. Yu, Dong's face and four extremities had slight edema. He also had a stomachache and scanty urination. His urine protein was 3+, his BUN was 183mg%, and his creatinine was 13mg/100mm. His blood potassium, sodium, and chlorine were all low. His tongue was pale purple. He was diagnosed with uremia and gastritis.

Dr. Yu's treatment strategy was to supplement the qi, clear summer heat, aromatically transform dampness, harmonize the stomach, and descend the stomach qi and eliminate dampness. His formula consisted of: fresh *He Ye* (Nelumbinis Nuciferae, Folium), 9g, *Huo Xiang* (Agastachers Seu Pogostemi, Herba), 9g, *Zi Su Ye* (Perillae Frutescentis, Folium), 9g, *Dang Shen* (Codonopsitis Pilosulae, Radix), 10g, *Shi Hu* (Dendrobii, Herba), 12g, *Huang Lian* (Coptidis Chinensis, Rhizoma), 3g, *Zhu Ru* (Bambusae In Taeniis, Caulis), 9g, *Fu Ling* (Poriae Cocos, Sclerotium), 15g, *Fo Shou* (Citri Sarcodactylis, Fructus), 9g, *Liu Yi San* (Six-to-One Powder),[12] 12g, *Hong Hua* (Carthami Tinctorii, Flos), 9g, and fresh *Lu Gen* (Phragmitis Communis, Rhizoma), 30g.

By July 18, Dong's second visit, he had less vomiting and had regained some appetite. His BUN was down to 114mg/100ml. Therefore, Dr. Yu changed the prescription: *Huang Qi* (Astragali Membranacei, Radix), 12g, *Dang Shen* (Codonopsitis Pilosulae, Radix), 15g, *He Ye* (Nelumbinis Nuciferae, Folium), 5g, *Huo Xiang* (Agastachers Seu Pogostemi, Herba), 6g, *Fu Ling* (Poriae Cocos, Sclerotium), 15g, *Shi Hu* (Dendrobii, Herba), 9g, *Bai Shao* (Paeoniae Lactiflorae, Radix Albus), 9g, *Huang Lian* (Coptidis Chinensis, Rhizoma), 2.4g, *Bian Dou Yi* (Dolichoris Lablab, Cortex Semenis), 12g, *Hong Hua* (Carthami Tinctorii, Flos), 9g, and fresh *Lu Gen* (Phragmitis Communis, Rhizoma), 60g.

By July 20, Dong's third visit, his appetite was better, he was not thirsty, his BUN was 90, and his electrolytes were almost back to normal. But he still had some stomach discomfort after eating and occasional nausea. His pulse was fine and fast and his blood pressure was 140/90mmHg. Dr. Yu changed the prescription again: *Zi Su Ye* (Perillae Frutescentis, Folium), 1.5g, *Huang Lian* (Coptidis Chinensis, Rhizoma), 2.4g, *Zhu Ru* (Bambusae In Taeniis, Caulis), 12g, *He Ye* (Nelumbinis Nuciferae, Folium), 5g, *Dang Shen* (Codonopsitis Pilosulae, Radix), 9g, *Fu Ling* (Poriae Cocos, Sclerotium), 12g, *Gou Qi Zi* (Lycii Chinensis, Fructus), 9g, *Zhi Mu* (Anemarrhenae Asphodeloidis, Rhizoma), 9g, *Huang Bai* (Phellodendri, Cortex), 3g, *Zhi Shi* (Citri Aurantii, Fructus Immaturus), 3g, and *Bai Zhu* (Atractylodis Macrocephalae, Rhizoma), 9g.

By July 22, Dong's fourth visit, his nausea was gone, his appetite was better, he had no stomacache, his stools were yellow, his urine was normal, his edema had dissipated, and his electrolytes were back to normal, but he still had insomnia. His tongue fur was thin and white. Therefore, Dr. Yu gave him the following formula: *Zi Su Ye* (Perillae Frutescentis, Folium), 0.9g, *Huang Lian* (Coptidis Chinensis, Rhizoma), 1.8g, *Dang Shen* (Codonopsitis Pilosulae, Radix), 12g, *Fu Ling* (Poriae Cocos, Sclerotium), 12g, fresh *He Ye* (Nelumbinis Nuciferae, Folium), 3g, *Huo Xiang* (Agastachers Seu Pogostemi, Herba), 5g, *Yi Yi Ren* (Coicis Lachryma-jobi, Semen), 12g, *Gou Qi Zi* (Lycii Chinensis, Fructus), 12g, *Bai Zhu* (Atractylodis Macrocephalae, Rhizoma), 5g, and *Chen Pi* (Citri Reticulatae, Pericarpium), 3g.

By July 28, Dong's firth visit, he was much better. In fact, he felt positively good. His BUN was 78mg/ml and his blood pressure was 140/96mmHg. Dr. Yu's pattern identification changed to spleen-kidney qi vacuity and liver blood vacuity. Thus he also changed the prescription: *Dang Shen* (Codonopsitis Pilosulae, Radix), 12g, *Fu Ling* (Poriae Cocos, Sclerotium), 12g, *Gou Qi Zi* (Lycii Chinensis, Fructus), 9g, *Ci Shi* (Magnititum), 9g, *Gu Sui Bu* (Gusuibu, Rhizoma), 9g, *Dang Gui* (Angelicae Sinensis, Radix), 9g, *Bai Shao* (Paeoniae Lactiflorae, Radix Albus), 9g, *E Jiao* (Asini, Gelatinum Corii), 3g, *Suan Zao Ren* (Zizyphi Spinosae, Semen), 9g, *Bai Zhu* (Atractylodis

Macrocephalae, Rhizoma), 5g, and *Chen Pi* (Citri Reticulatae, Pericarpium), 3g.

Dong took this formula until the middle of September and his urine and kidney function returned to normal. On November 11, Dong's sixth visit, Dr. Yu gave him the following formula: *Dang Shen* (Codonopsitis Pilosulae, Radix), 15g, *Fu Zi* (Aconiti Carmichaeli, Radix Lateralis Praeparatus), 3g, *Gou Qi Zi* (Lycii Chinensis, Fructus), 12g, *Dang Gui* (Angelicae Sinensis, Radix), 9g, *Dang Shen* (Codonopsitis Pilosulae, Radix), 9g, *Tao Ren* (Pruni Persicae, Semen), 9g, *Hong Hua* (Carthami Tinctorii, Flos), 9g, *Bai Zi Ren* (Biotae Orientalis, Semen), 12g, *Fu Ling* (Poriae Cocos, Sclerotium), 9g, *Yuan Zhi* (Polygalae Tenuifoliae, Radix), 6g, and *Gan Cao* (Glycyrrhizae Uralensis, Radix), 3g.

Dong took this until the end of November and then went back to physical work. However, in February 1973, Dong began to feel feverish and he started having low back pain, chest pain, and heart palpitations. Urinalysis showed pus at 2+, RBCs at 3+, and BUN at 57. His blood pressure was normal. Dr. Yu decided to give Dong a formula to supplement the qi and free the flow of the yang, fortify the spleen and transform dampness, move the blood and dispel stasis, nourish yin and quiet the heart: *Dang Shen* (Codonopsitis Pilosulae, Radix), 24g, *Xie Bai* (Allii, Bulbus), 5g, *Gua Lou Ren* (Trichosanthis Kirlowii, Semen), 9g, *Cang Zhu* (Atractylodis, Rhizoma), 5g, *Tao Ren* (Pruni Persicae, Semen), 9g, *Hong Hua* (Carthami Tinctorii, Flos), 9g, *Dan Shen* (Salviae Miltiorrhizae, Radix), 9g, *Fu Ling* (Poriae Cocos, Sclerotium), 9g, *Shi Hu* (Dendrobii, Herba), 15g, *Han Lian Cao* (Ecliptae Prostratae, Herba), 6g, *Nu Zhen Zi* (Ligustri Lucidi, Fructus), 6g, *Bai Shao* (Paeoniae Lactiflorae, Radix Albus), 9g, and fresh *Lu Gen* (Phragmitis Communis, Rhizoma), 60g.

After Dong finished this formula, all his symptoms disappeared and his blood work returned to normal. He continued on this formula until April and then went back to work. He was still easily fatigued and this fatigue lasted until 1976. Finally, six years after he first came to Dr. Yu, he felt completely healthy and could do heavy physical work. In May 1978, Dong felt strong, his color was good, and he had a good appetite. His blood work, blood pressure, and urinalysis were all normal.

3. EVILS SINKING INTO THE PERICARDIUM

SIGNS & SYMPTOMS: Fever, irritability, clouding of the spirit with delirious speech or coma. The tongue has dry, yellow fur, and the pulse is replete and fast.

TREATMENT PRINCIPLES: Clear heat, resolve toxins, open the orifices

REPRESENTATIVE FORMULA: Modified *Qing Shen Jie Du Yin* (Spirit-clearing, Toxin-resolving Beverage) plus *Niu Huang Qing Xin Wan* (Calculus Bovis Heart-clearing Pill)

Qing Shen Jie Du Yin

Shui Niu Jiao (Bubali, Cornu), 12-24g
Xin Yi (Magnoliae, Flos), 3-9g
Huang Lian (Coptidis Chinensis, Rhizoma), 3g
Lian Xin (Nelumbinis Nuciferae, Plumula), 2g
Shi Chang Pu (Acori Graminei, Rhizoma), 4.5g
Dan Zhu Ye (Lophatheri Gracilis, Herba), 6g
Lian Qiao (Forsythiae Suspensae, Fructus), 6g
Zhi Zi (Gardeniae Jasminoidis, Fructus), 9g
Xuan Shen (Scrophulariae Ningpoensis, Radix), 9g
Huang Bai (Phellodendri, Cortex), 9g

Niu Huang Qing Xin Wan, one three-gram pill consisting of:

Niu Huang (Bovis, Calculus), 0.75g
Zhu Sha (Cinnabar), 4.5g
uncooked *Huang Lian* (Coptidis Chinensis, Rhizoma), 15g
Huang Qin (Scutellariae Baicalensis, Radix), 9g
Zhi Zi (Gardeniae Jasminoidis, Fructus), 9g
Yu Jin (Curcumae, Tuber), 6g

Grind the above medicinals into powder and form into pills with honey.

MODIFICATIONS: If the patient is constipated, add *Zhi Shi* (Citri Aurantii, Fructus Immaturus) and *Da Huang* (Rhei, Radix Et Rhizoma). If the patient has fright reversal, add *Quan Xie* (Buthus Martensi),

Gou Teng (Uncariae Cum Uncis, Ramulus), and *Di Long* (Lumbricus).

ACUMOXIBUSTION: Choose from *Nei Guan* (Per 6), *Da Ling* (Per 7), *Lao Gong* (Per 8), *Shen Men* (Ht 7), *Ren Zhong* (GV 26), and *Bai Hui* (GV 20).

Case history of Dr. Qi Chang: Wang, a 14 year-old female student[13]

Wang's first visit was on Apr. 7, 1972. She had been sick for 14 months with symptoms of scanty urination and severe edema. She had tried Western diuretics for eight months and her edema had improved. Her symptoms had worsened, however, in the two weeks preceding her first visit. Wang began to have stomach discomfort, nausea, no desire to eat, and vomiting as soon as she tried to eat. She was vexed, with a pale facial complexion, fatigue, and dry, yellow hair that fell out. She also had heat in the five hearts. Her tongue was purple and dry with no fur, and her pulse was vacuous and fast. Her urine protein was 3+, her RBCs were 3-5, she had granular casts 2-3, and her BUN was 117mg%. She had low blood protein, and her blood pressure was 160/110mmHg. The Western diagnosis was uremia. Dr. Qi's pattern identification was qi and yin vacuity with damp heat in the blood aspect and evils sinking into the pericardium. His treatment strategy was to clear heat and resolve toxins, move and cool the blood. His prescription consisted of: *Lian Qiao* (Forsythiae Suspensae, Fructus), 30g, *Tao Ren* (Pruni Persicae, Semen), 15g, *Hong Hua* (Carthami Tinctorii, Flos), 15g, *Dang Gui Wei* (Angelicae Sinensis, Extremitas Radicis), 10g, *Ge Gen* (Puerariae, Radix), 15g, *Chi Shao* (Paeoniae Lactiflorae, Radix Rubrus), 20g, *Gan Cao* (Glycyrrhizae Uralensis, Radix), 7.5g, *Sheng Di Huang* (Rehmanniae Glutinosae, uncooked Radix), 20g, and *Mu Dan Pi* (Moutan, Cortex Radicis), 15g.

By April 11, Wang had taken the formula for three days. Her nausea and vomiting had stopped and she could eat a bit of food, but her appetite was not good and her urine was still scanty. Therefore, Dr. Qi modified the formula as follows: *Lian Qiao* (Forsythiae Suspensae, Fructus), 30g, *Tao Ren* (Pruni Persicae, Semen), 15g, *Hong Hua* (Carthami

Tinctorii, Flos), 15g, *Dang Gui Wei* (Angelicae Sinensis, Extremitas Radicis), 10g, *Ge Gen* (Puerariae, Radix), 15g, *Chi Shao* (Paeoniae Lactiflorae, Radix Rubrus), 15g, *Mai Men Dong* (Ophiopogonis Japonici, Tuber), 15g, *Sheng Di Huang* (Rehmanniae Glutinosae, uncooked Radix), 20g, *Mu Dan Pi* (Moutan, Cortex Radicis), 15g, and *Gan Cao* (Glycyrrhizae Uralensis, Radix), 10g.

By April 15, Wang's third visit, she had taken the new formula for three days and her nausea and vomiting were completely gone, her appetite was better, her vexation was reduced, and her urination increased. She still had edema. Her tongue was purple, and her pulse was now bowstring and slippery. Her BUN was 27mg%. Dr. Qi decided to continued to use a formula to clear heat, quicken blood, and eliminate dampness: *Lian Qiao* (Forsythiae Suspensae, Fructus), 30g, *Tao Ren* (Pruni Persicae, Semen), 15g, *Hong Hua* (Carthami Tinctorii, Flos), 15g, *Dang Gui Wei* (Angelicae Sinensis, Extremitas Radicis), 15g, *Ge Gen* (Puerariae, Radix), 15g, *Chi Shao* (Paeoniae Lactiflorae, Radix Rubrus), 20g, *Sheng Di Huang* (Rehmanniae Glutinosae, uncooked Radix), 20g, *Fu Ling* (Poriae Cocos, Sclerotium), 20g, *Ze Xie* (Alismatis Orientalis, Rhizoma), 15g, *Bai Zhu* (Atractylodis Macrocephalae, Rhizoma), 15g, *Hua Shi* (Talcum), 20g, *Gan Cao* (Glycyrrhizae Uralensis, Radix), 10g, and *Zhu Ling* (Polypori Umbellati, Sclerotium), 15g.

By April 19, Wang's fourth visit, her urine had increased to about one liter per day and her edema had dissipated, but she felt weak and had a dry mouth, heat in the five hearts, shortness of breath, and fatigue. Her pulse was bowstring and forceless. Her urine protein was 3+, her RBCs were 2-3, with a granular cast of 2. This indicated that the replete heat and damp were gone. Dr. Qi decided it was now time to boost the qi and nourish yin. His new prescription consisted of: *Huang Qi* (Astragali Membranacei, Radix), 30g, *Dang Shen* (Codonopsitis Pilosulae, Radix), 25g, *Shi Lian Zi* (Caesalpiniae, Semen), 15g, *Di Gu Pi* (Lycii Chinensis, Cortex Radicis), 15g, *Chai Hu* (Bupleuri, Radix), 15g, *Fu Ling* (Poriae Cocos, Sclerotium), 15g, *Mai Men Dong* (Ophiopogonis Japonici, Tuber), 15g, *Che Qian Zi* (Plantaginis, Semen), 15g, *Bai Mao*

Gen (Imperatae Cylindricae, Rhizoma), 50g, and *Gan Cao* (Glycyrrhizae Uralensis, Radix), 10g.

By May 15, Wang's fifth visit, she had taken the new formula for 12 days, and she felt her whole body was strong. Her edema did not return. Her dry mouth, reddish tongue, and urination were better. Her urine protein was 3+, RBCs were 1-2, granular casts were negative, blood protein was normal, and BUN was 38mg% (or normal). On June 27, 1976, Wang had symptoms of low back pain and came in to see Dr. Qi. Her urine protein was 1+, but everything else was normal. Her hair was moist with a natural color and her weight was stable. Follow-up visits over the next three years found the patient working and needing no medicinals or other treatment.

4. INTERIOR HEAT STIRRING WIND

SIGNS & SYMPTOMS: Edema, high blood pressure, headache, vomiting, coma, fright reversal, fever, a smell of urine in the breath, no urination or very scanty urination, and itchy skin. The tongue is purple with turbid or black fur, and the pulse is deep and fast or bowstring and fast.

TREATMENT PRINCIPLES: Level the liver and extinguish wind, clear heat and resolve toxins, supplement the liver and kidney

REPRESENTATIVE FORMULA: *Xi Feng Jie Du Yin* (Wind-extinguishing, Toxin-resolving Beverage)

Di Long (Lumbricus), 12g
Shi Jui Ming (Haliotidis, Concha), 30g
Gou Teng (Uncariae Cum Uncis, Ramulus), 12g
Tian Ma (Gastrodiae Elatae, Rhizoma), 9g
Quan Xie (Buthus Martensi), 6g
Bai Shao (Paeoniae Lactiflorae, Radix Albus), 9g
Gan Cao (Glycyrrhizae Uralensis, Radix), 3g
Shi Chang Pu (Acori Graminei, Rhizoma), 12g
Yu Jin (Curcumae, Tuber), 9g
Luo Shi Teng (Trachelospermi Jasminoidis, Caulis), 30g
Zhu Ru (Bambusae In Taeniis, Caulis), 15g
Jing Zhi (Excrementi Hominis, Liquidum Extractum), 30g

MODIFICATIONS: If there is constipation, add *Zhi Shi*

(Citri Aurantii, Fructus Immaturus) and *Da Huang* (Rhei, Radix Et Rhizoma). If there is no urination, add *Lou Gu* (Gryllotalpa Africana, Os).

If there is coma, add *Su He Xiang Wan* (Liquid Styrax Pill), one pill. This pill is made of: *Su He Xiang* (Liquidis, Styrax), 30g, *She Xiang* (Moschi Moschiferi, Secretio), 60g, *Bing Pian* (Borneol), 30g, *An Xi Xiang* (Benzoinum), 60g, *Mu Xiang* (Aucklandiae Lappae, Radix), 60g, *Tan Xiang* (Santali Albi, Lignum), 60g, *Chen Xiang* (Aquilariae Agallochae, Lignum), 60g, *Ru Xiang* (Olibani, Resina), 30g, *Ding Xiang* (Caryophylli, Flos), 60g, *Xiang Fu* (Cyperi Rotundi, Rhizoma), 60g, *Bi Ba* (Piperis Longi, Fructus), 60g, *Xi Jiao* (Rhinocerotis, Cornu), 10g, *Xin Yi* (Magnoliae, Flos), 60g, *Zhu Sha* (Cinnabar), 60g, *Bai Zhu* (Atractylodis Macrocephalae, Rhizoma), 60g, and *He Zi* (Terminaliae Chebulae, Fructus), 60g. These medicinals are ground into powder and formed into three-gram pills with honey. If there are problems with the vision, add *Qing Xiang Zi* (Celosiae Argenteae, Semen).

COMMENTARY: The root of this pattern is kidney vacuity due to damage by chronic illness, and, in this case, one must treat the root. The formulas given above focus on the tip and on controlling the symptoms. This is like chasing after the disease. One must stay ahead of the disease by improving kidney function. With improved kidney function, all the symptoms will abate. The last part of the treatment strategy, "supplement the liver and kidney," focuses on the root since "the liver and kidney share a common source." Supplementing the liver and kidney must include nourishing the liver and kidney yin and boosting kidney yang. Formulas such as *Liu Wei Di Huang Wan* (Six Flavors Rehmannia Pills) improve kidney function but only nourish yin. Formulas such as *Jin Gui Shen Qi Wan* (*Golden Cabinet* Kidney Qi Pills), which supplement yin and yang, are not strong enough for this condition. The most important single medicinal to supplement kidney yin and yang in CRF is *Dong Chong Xia Cao* (Cordyceps Sinensis). Chinese research and clinical experience have proven this medicinal's remarkable ability to improve kidney function and repair kidney damage. No other medicinal has proven as effective. However, *Dong Chong Xia Cao*'s main ingredient is an amino acid. Since limiting protein intake is vitally important when treating CRF patients, one must concentrate on the following: 1) Reduce the total amount of protein, using only high quality protein (such as in this medicinal).[14] 2) Carefully balance nutrient levels. Kidney function quickly deteriorates if nutrient levels are too high or low. 3) Limit the use of toxic drugs. 4) Focus on improving kidney function.

ACUMOXIBUSTION: Bleed the well points and choose points to needle from *He Gu* (LI 4), *Qu Chi* (LI 11), *Da Zhui* (GV 14), *Gan Shu* (Bl 18), *Yun Men* (Liv 2), *Feng Chi* (GB 20), *Tai Xi* (Ki 3), *Shen Shu* (Bl 23), *Yong Quan* (Ki 1), and *Bai Hui* (GV 20).

Case history of Dr. Song Lian-xu: Song, a 55 year-old female[15]

Song had a long history of chronic urinary tract infections. One year before her first visit in August 1977, she was diagnosed with renal failure. She could not eat because of extreme nausea and vomiting. She also had abdominal bloating and discomfort, vexation, and hypersomnia. She had no desire to talk and was in a lethargic state. Her face was pale (due to severe anemia). Her blood creatinine was 11.2mg%, her BUN was 125mg%, and her blood pressure was 134/90mmHg. She had slimy tongue fur and a fine pulse. Dr. Song's pattern identification was spleen-kidney vacuity with evil damp stagnation and phlegm misting the heart orifices. His treatment strategy was to warm the kidney and resolve toxins, drain dampness and open the orifices. His prescription consisted of: *Zi Su Ye* (Perillae Frutescentis, Folium), 30g, *Dang Shen* (Codonopsitis Pilosulae, Radix), 15g, *Huang Lian* (Coptidis Chinensis, Rhizoma), 4.5g, *Lu Dou* (Phaseoli Radiati, Semen), 30g, uncooked *Gan Cao* (Glycyrrhizae Uralensis, Radix), 6g, *Fu Ling* (Poriae Cocos, Sclerotium), 30g, *Ban Zhi Lian* (Scutellariae Barbatae, Herba), 30g, *Shu Fu Zi* (Aconiti Carmichaeli, Radix Lateralis Praeparatus), 9g, *Da Huang* (Rhei, Radix Et Rhizoma), 15g, *Ban Xia* (Pinelliae Ternatae, Rhizoma), 12g, *Ze Xie* (Alismatis Orientalis, Rhizoma), 15g, and *Fu Long Gan* (Terra Flava Usta), 30g. At the same time, Song also received Western electrolyte correction. The patient improved on this regimen, her mind became clearer, and her nausea and vomiting reduced. Continuing on this formula, her nausea and vomiting completely disappeared, but her appetite did not improve very much and she still had spasms in her lower extremities. Her Hb (hemoglobin) was now 7.2g%, her creatinine was 6.4mg%, and her BUN was 76mg%. A follow-up one and a half years later found her stable.

5. INTERIOR WIND CAUSED BY VACUITY

SIGNS & SYMPTOMS: Muscular spasms in the extremities, thinness or dehydration, no urination or scanty urination. The tongue is trembling or shrunken, and the pulse is fine, bowstring, and fast.

TREATMENT PRINCIPLES: Supplement yin and yang, extinguish wind and resolve toxins

REPRESENTATIVE FORMULA: *Da Ding Feng Zhu* (Major Stabilize Wind Pearls) plus *Niu Huang Qing Xin Wan* (Calculus Bovis Heart-clearing Pills)

Ji Zi Huang (Galli, Vitellus), 2 yolks
E Jiao (Asini, Gelatinum Corii), 9g
Bai Shao (Paeoniae Lactiflorae, Radix Albus), 18g
mix-fried *Gan Cao* (Glycyrrhizae Uralensis, Radix), 12g
Wu Wei Zi (Schisandrae Chinensis, Fructus), 6g
Sheng Di Huang (Rehmanniae Glutinosae, uncooked Radix), 18g
Mai Men Dong (Ophiopogonis Japonici, Tuber), 18g
Huo Ma Ren (Cannabis Sativae, Semen), 6g
Gui Ban (Testudinis, Plastrum), 12g
Bie Jia (Amydae Sinensis, Carapax), 12g
Mu Li (Ostreae, Concha), 12g
Niu Huang (Bovis, Calculus), 0.75g
Zhu Sha (Cinnabar), 4.5g
uncooked *Huang Lian* (Coptidis Chinensis, Rhizoma), 15g
Huang Qin (Scutellariae Baicalensis, Radix), 9g
Zhi Zi (Gardeniae Jasminoidis, Fructus), 9g
Yu Jin (Curcumae, Tuber), 6g

ACUMOXIBUSTION: Choose from *Yun Men* (Liv 2), *Tai Chong* (Liv 3), *Ge Shu* (Bl 17), *Gan Shu* (Bl 18), *Shen Shu* (Bl 23), *Tai Xi* (Ki 3), *San Yin Jiao* (Sp 6), *Xue Hai* (Sp 10), *Nei Guan* (Per 6), and *Qu Chi* (LI 11).

Case history of Dr. Can Bing-fu: Li, a 34 year-old male[16]

One and a half years prior to visiting Dr. Can, Li experienced fever and chills, low back pain, and less than normal urination. The Western medical diagnosis was nephritis. Li used hormonal treatment for a half a year and his symptoms were reduced, but then they recurred. The treatment lasted eight months but was unsuccessful. Li tried a different regimen for another five months but only got worse. When Li came to see Dr. Can, he had a dark facial complexion, his eyes were swollen, and his abdomen was distended and made a sloshing sound. His tongue was pale and puffy with white, slimy fur, and his pulse was deep, slow, and weak. X-rays showed edema in his chest. Li's urine protein was 4+, granular casts were 2+, blood cholesterol was 520mg%, BUN was 75mg%, blood protein was low, and urine protein was high at 9.52g/24 hours. Dr. Can's pattern identification was kidney yang vacuity with dampness. His treatment strategy was to warm and supplement the spleen and kidney and eliminate dampness. He used modified *Ling Gui Zhu Gan Tang* (Poria, Cinnamon Twigs, Atractylodes, and Licorice Decoction) with *Shen Qi Wan* (Kidney Qi Pills) as a follow-up. *Ling Gui Zhu Gan Tang* consists of: *Fu Ling* (Poriae Cocos, Sclerotium), *Gui Zhi* (Cinnamomi Cassiae, Ramulus), *Bai Zhu* (Atractylodis Macrocephalae, Rhizoma), and mix-fried *Gan Cao* (Glycyrrhizae Uralensis, Radix). Dosages and modifications were not specified.

After Li took these formulas, his appetite improved and his edema disappeared, but two months later he suddenly caught cold with a fever. He came to Dr. Can who prescribed medicinals to resolve the exterior and harmonize the middle burner. After five days, the fever abated, but, two weeks later, it returned. Li's whole body became tight and heavy and he became edematous. His face was pale and he had dizziness, tinnitus, heart palpitations, and shortness of breath, wheezing, severe nose-bleeding, nausea, vomiting, and spasms in both his hands and arms. His tongue was pale and puffy with thick, slimy fur and his pulse was fast and forceless. His RBC count was 1,210,000/cubic mm and his BUN was 99mg%. The Western medical diagnosis was uremia. Dr. Can's pattern identification was

spleen-kidney yang vacuity, liver yin and blood vacuity, and liver wind. His treatment strategy was to warm the spleen and kidney, nourish the liver, and extinguish wind. His prescription was augmented *Zhen Wu Tang* (True Warrior Decoction): *Fu Zi* (Aconiti Carmichaeli, Radix Lateralis Praeparatus), *Bai Zhu* (Atractylodis Macrocephalae, Rhizoma), *Fu Ling* (Poriae Cocos, Sclerotium), *Sheng Jiang* (Zingiberis Officinalis, uncooked Rhizoma), *Bai Shao* (Paeoniae Lactiflorae, Radix Albus), *Hong Ren Shen* (Panacis Ginseng, Radix Rubrus), *Du Zhong* (Eucommiae Ulmoidis, Cortex), *Gou Ji* (Cibotii Barometsis, Rhizoma), *Hong Tang* (Saccharum Granorum Rubrum), *Gou Teng* (Uncariae Cum Uncis, Ramulus), *Tian Ma* (Gastrodiae Elatae, Rhizoma), and *Dai Zhe Shi* (Haematitum).

After taking this formula for a week, Li's spasms stopped and all his other symptoms abated. Dr. Can continued to treat Li for another year. At the conclusion of treatment, Li's RBC count was 3,650,000/cubic mm, blood protein was normal, blood cholesterol was normal, BUN was 52mg%, and urine protein was 0.9/24 hours.

6. YANG DEBILITATION OR DESERTION

SIGNS & SYMPTOMS: Scanty urination, severe edema, fatigue, low blood pressure, hypersomnia, shortness of breath, sweating, feeling cold and/or cold extremities, weak legs, abdominal pain and distention. The tongue is big and puffy with black or white fur, and the pulse is deep and fine.

TREATMENT PRINCIPLES: Rescue yang and supplement the qi, warm the channels and eliminate dampness

REPRESENTATIVE FORMULA: *Zhen Wu Tang* (True Warrior Decoction)

Fu Zi (Aconiti Carmichael, Radix Lateralis Praeparatus), 9g
Bai Zhu (Atractylodis Macrocephalae, Rhizoma), 6g
Fu Ling (Poriae Cocos, Sclerotium), 9g
Bai Shao (Paeoniae Lactiflorae, Radix Albus), 9g
Sheng Jiang (Zingiberis Officinalis, uncooked Rhizoma), 9g

MODIFICATIONS: If there is coughing from water in the lung, add *Gan Jiang* (Zingiberis Officinalis, dry Rhizoma) and *Wu Wei Zi* (Schisandrae Chinensis, Fructus). If there are seizures, add *Tian Ma* (Gastrodiae Elatae, Rhizoma), *Quan Xie* (Buthus Martensis), or *Wu Gong* (Scolopendra Subspinipes). If there is constant sweating with a thin, weak, deep pulse, this indicates exhausted heart yang. In that case, add mix-fried *Gan Cao* (Glycyrrhizae Uralensis, Radix), calcined *Long Gu* (Draconis, Os), and calcined *Mu Li* (Ostreae, Concha).

If inappropriate sweating and/or precipitating have consumed the yin, this will not only damage yin, but yang as well. Symptoms of yin and yang vacuity will include edema, difficulty breathing, sweating, and shortness of breath and/or wheezing (the kidney cannot grasp the qi and the lung qi counterflows upwards). The pulse will be floating and vacuous or deep, fine, and fast. In this case, one must supplement yang, qi, and yin. A useful formula is *Zhe Shi Yi Qi Tang* (Hematite Boost the Qi Decoction): *Ren Shen* (Panacis Ginseng, Radix), 3-6g, *Dai Zhe Shi* (Haematitum), 15g, *Shu Di Huang* (Rehmanniae Glutinosae, cooked Radix), 12g, *Mu Dan Pi* (Moutan, Cortex Radicis), 9g, *Fu Ling* (Poriae Cocos, Sclerotium), 12g, *Shan Yao* (Radix Dioscoreae Oppositae), 12g, *Ze Xie* (Alismatis Orientalis, Rhizoma), 9g, *Shan Zhu Yu* (Corni Officinalis, Fructus), 12g, *Wu Wei Zi* (Schisandrae Chinensis, Fructus), 12g, *Gan Jiang* (Zingiberis Officinalis, dry Rhizoma), 3-6g, and *Fu Zi* (Aconiti Carmichaeli, Radix Lateralis Praeparatus), 3-6g.

ACUMOXIBUSTION: Choose points to moxibustion from *Shen Shu* (Bl 23), *Ming Men* (GV 4), *Zhong Ji* (CV 3), *Guan Yuan* (CV 4), *Qi Hai* (CV 6), *Zu San Li* (St 36), *San Yin Jiao* (Sp 6), and *Tai Xi* (Ki 3).

Case history of Dr. Jin Zie-zao: Song, a 50 year-old female[17]

Song's first visit was on Aug. 22, 1977. In 1974, this patient started to feel fatigued and began having frequent asthma attacks. She also developed edema in her lower extremities. In 1976, these symptoms started getting worse. She was pale, drank a lot of water, and urinated frequently. Urinalysis showed

her protein at 1-2+, Hb(hemoglobin) at 8.0% (which then lowered to 5.5%), BUN at 70mg%, and Ch at 223mg%. Western doctors diagnosed her with chronic nephritis and prescribed cortisone 30mg/day. By the time she came to Dr. Jin, Song's face was pale yellow and edematous. She had soreness in her back and extremities, shortness of breath, chilliness, nausea, scanty urination, loose stools, and pitting edema principally confined to her lower extremities. Her tongue was puffy and dark with thin, yellow fur. Her pulse was deep and fine.

Based on these signs and symptoms, Dr. Jin's pattern identification was spleen-kidney yang vacuity with damp stagnation and debilitation of triple burner qi transformation. His treatment strategy was to warm and supplement the spleen and kidney, eliminate dampness and downbear turbidity. For this purpose, he prescribed modified *Liu Jun Si Tang* (Six Gentlemen Decoction): *Dang Shen* (Codonopsitis Pilosulae, Radix), 12g, *Bai Zhu* (Atractylodis Macrocephalae, Rhizoma), 9g, *Fu Ling* (Poriae Cocos, Sclerotium), 12g, mix-fried *Gan Cao* (Glycyrrhizae Uralensis, Radix), 6g, *Ban Xia* (Pinelliae Ternatae, Rhizoma), 9g, *Bai Dou Kou* (Cardamomi, Fructus), 5g, *Gui Zhi* (Cinnamomi Cassiae, Ramulus), 6g, *Huang Qi* (Astragali Membranacei, Radix), 30g, *Xu Duan* (Dipsaci Asperi, Radix), 12g, *Lu Jiao Shuang* (Cervi, Cornu Degelatinum), 12g, *Niu Xi* (Achyranthis Bidentatae, Radix), 9g, *Mu Gua* (Chaenomelis Lagenariae, Fructus), 9g, and *Dan Shen* (Salviae Miltiorrhizae, Radix), 9g. Song took this formula for two years and gradually began to stabilize. Her nausea disappeared, her appetite improved, and her edema dissipated. Her Hb increased to 9.7%, and her BUN decreased to 23mg%.

CLINICAL TIPS

1. Western physicians generally recommend dialysis and consider a kidney transplant for CRF patients when the creatinine level is about 5mg/dL, but many CRF patients want to wait as long as possible before using these options. In China, patients have the choice of using Chinese medicine or Western medicine. Many use Chinese medicine first, and there are many studies showing the efficacy of Chinese medicinals in improving kidney function and in delaying dialysis. In early stages of CRF, Chinese medicine routinely improves kidney function. In some cases, Chinese medicine can re-establish and maintain normal kidney function for lengthy periods of time. Chinese medicine also treats the complications of kidney failure, including anemia, blood pressure problems, and abnormal urinalyses. However, some cases of CRF are intractable and do not respond to Chinese medicine adequately. These CRF patients need dialysis, and the Chinese practitioner should take care to refer them appropriately.

2. Chronic renal failure is often a terminal disease and also occurs in other terminal diseases. In this condition, all major organs are vacuous, but this vacuity is complicated by toxin accumulation. Because of the inhibition or failure of kidney qi transformation, toxins cannot be excreted through urination. Urine may be excreted, it may be profuse or scanty, but toxins are not excreted and are left behind to accumulate. Western medicine relies on dialysis to eliminate these toxins, and, indeed, when toxicity is reduced in this way, the organs have a better chance of recovery. In Chinese medicine, while there is still a strategy to resolve toxins, the main focus is on supplementing the organs to improve their functioning. When the organs function better, they are better able to eliminate toxins.

3. While the principle treatment strategy in CRF is supplementing the lung, spleen, and kidney, other strategies are also used with these viscera. For instance, it is extremely important to open the lung. The lung is in the upper burner, the kidney is in the lower burner, and channels connect them. The kidney is the source of water and sends water upward to the lung. The lung diffuses and depuratively downbears water. Each viscus's functions balance and support one another's. If the lung's diffusion and depurative downbearing is compromised, water accumulates. To open the lung, one may use *Zi Su Ye* (Perillae Frutescentis, Folium), *Fang Feng* (Ledebouriellae Divaricatae, Radix), or any of the warm, exterior-resolving medicinals to "open the hole in the teapot's lid." (This metaphor refers to promoting urination by improving the lung's functions of diffusion and depurative downbearing.)

Opening the lung is especially important in acute cases. In chronic cases, it is more important to supplement the lung. For this, one may use medicinals that supplement lung qi such as *Huang Qi* (Astragali Membranacei, Radix), *Dang Shen* (Codonopsitis Pilosulae, Radix), *Bai Zhu* (Atractylodis Macrocephalae, Rhizoma), and *Ren Shen* (Panacis Ginseng, Radix) as well as medicinals that warm the lung, such as *Xi Xin* (Asari, Herba Cum Radice), *Gan Jiang* (Zingiberis Officinalis, dry Rhizoma), and *Gui Zhi* (Cinnamomi Cassiae, Ramulus). Combinations of these medicinals strengthen the lung and transform dampness.

Supplementing the spleen is one of the most important ways of strengthening the lung and kidney. The spleen is the root of engenderment and transformation of the latter heaven qi, the source of qi and blood for the entire body. Supplementing the spleen fortifies its transformation of food and its ability to upbear the clear and, thereby, to downbear the turbid. The upbearing of the clear qi supplements the lung qi and, eventually, descends to enrich the kidney qi. Two fundamental formulas to upbear the spleen qi are Li Dong-yuan's *Bu Zhong Yi Qi Tang* (Supplement the Center & Boost the Qi Decoction) and Zhong Jing-yue's *Ju Yuan Jian* (Origin-lifting Brew).

Bu Zhong Yi Qi Tang (Supplement the Center & Boost the Qi Decoction): *Huang Qi* (Astragali Membranacei, Radix), 12g, *Ren Shen* (Panacis Ginseng, Radix), 9g, *Bai Zhu* (Atractylodis Macrocephalae, Rhizoma), 12g, mix-fried *Gan Cao* (Glycyrrhizae Uralensis, Radix), 3g, *Dang Gui* (Angelicae Sinensis, Radix), 9g, *Chen Pi* (Citri Reticulatae, Pericarpium), 6g, *Sheng Ma* (Cimicifugae, Rhizoma), 9g, and *Chai Hu* (Bupleuri, Radix) 6g.

Ju Yuan Jian (Origin-lifting Brew): *Huang Qi* (Astragali Membranacei, Radix), 12g, *Ren Shen* (Panacis Ginseng, Radix), 9g, *Bai Zhu* (Atractylodis Macrocephalae, Rhizoma), 12g, mix-fried *Gan Cao* (Glycyrrhizae Uralensis, Radix), 3g, and *Sheng Ma* (Cimicifugae, Rhizoma), 9g.

These formulas are usually modified by adding extra

qi-rectifying, aromatic, dampness-transforming medicinals, such as *Hou Po* (Magnoliae Officinalis, Cortex), *Chen Pi* (Citri Reticulatae, Pericarpium), *Sha Ren* (Amomi, Fructus), *Da Fu Pi* (Arecae Catechu, Pericarpium), and *Bai Mao Gen* (Imperatae Cylindricae, Rhizoma).

The kidney is in charge of storage. It stores essence in the essence chamber or life gate. When kidney disease causes edema, one must boost the kidney qi and invigorate kidney yang. (One must also be careful to enrich kidney yin to maintain the balance of the kidney's fire and water.) Kidney yang-supplementing medicinals include *Lu Rong* (Cornu Cervi Parvum), *Rou Cong Rong* (Cistanchis Deserticolae, Herba), *Ba Ji Tian* (Morindae Officinalis, Radix), *Yin Yang Huo* (Epimedii, Herba), *Xian Mao* (Curculinginis Orchioidis, Rhizoma), and *Xu Duan* (Dipsaci Asperi, Radix). To supplement kidney qi, one may use *Shen Qi Wan* (Kidney Qi Pills): *Fu Zi* (Aconiti Carmichaeli, Radix Lateralis Praeparatus), 3g, *Rou Gui* (Cinnamonmi Casiae, Cortex), 3g, *Shu Di Huang* (Rehmanniae Glutinosae, cooked Radix), 24g, *Shan Yao* (Radix Dioscoreae Oppositae), 12g, *Shan Zhu Yu* (Corni Officinalis, Fructus), 12g, *Ze Xie* (Alismatis Orientalis, Rhizoma), 9g, *Fu Ling* (Poriae Cocos, Sclerotium), 9g, and *Mu Dan Pi* (Moutan, Cortex, Radicis), 9g. In this formula, *Rou Gui* and *Fu Zi* invigorate kidney yang. The yin-nourishing medicinals, *i.e.*, the other ingredients which are the ingredients of *Liu Wei Di Huang Wan* (Six Flavors Rehmannia Pills), enrich kidney yin and nourish kidney essence. An invigorated kidney yang "steams" essence to generate kidney qi.

The viscera and bowels are mutually serving and mutually conductive in physiology and pathology. Therefore, in formulating treatment strategies, one should recognize these functions so that one can efficiently treat several organs at the same time. For instance, coughing and asthma often involve the spleen as well as the lung and one must treat both concurrently. When there is severe edema, one should treat both the kidney and spleen by warming and harmonizing the spleen and kidney and transforming dampness and water. When the kidney and lung have a dual pathology, the treatment strategy often involves supplementing yin and clearing heat

at the same time. (As mentioned above, the kidney is the viscus of water and fire. Therefore, when supplementing kidney yin, one must simultaneously supplement kidney yang.) In clinic, one often treats all three of these viscera concurrently.

The liver and heart may also become involved in kidney pathology. Liver involvement may be due to kidney essence vacuity. Kidney essence vacuity often causes blood vacuity which, in turn, engenders wind. The *Huang Di Nei Jing* (*Yellow Emperor's Inner Classic*) states, "All wind is related to the liver." Liver involvement may start with kidney qi and yang vacuity that damages kidney yin. Kidney yin vacuity, in turn, cannot nourish the liver, causing liver yin vacuity and ascendant liver yang hyperactivity. The heart becomes involved if kidney water does not balance heart fire and it flares upward. This process is exacerbated if the spleen does not supply latter heaven qi to these viscera.

To sum up, although the main viscera affected in kidney pathology are the kidney, spleen, and lung, all five viscera may eventually become involved.

4. Along with organ dysfunction, damp accumulation and blood stasis always occur in chronic renal failure. (In Western medical terms, this may mean that the capillary loops are narrowed, widened, or attacked by antibodies.) In some stages of CRF, one may focus on the blood stasis and dampness. In advanced stages, however, one must focus only on improving kidney function. The kidneys can lose up to 75% of tissue and still perform necessary functions under mild to normal physical activity. However, when there is extra stress from exertion, infection, or other causes, diseased kidneys cannot maintain normal functioning. Chinese medicine may be able to improve kidney function, but this does not mean the kidney itself is back to normal physical health.

Blood stasis is an important concern in diminished renal reserve and renal insufficiency CRF.[18] There are three major patterns: spleen-kidney qi and yang vacuity, spleen-kidney qi and yin vacuity, and blood stasis with damp heat. The first two may also be complicated with dampness and/or blood stasis. Blood stasis and water accumulation are mutually engendering. When spleen and kidney yang vacuity cause dampness and water accumulation, this accumulation blocks the qi, thus leading to qi stagnation and eventually to blood stasis. Qi stagnation and blood stasis limit the true qi's ability to disperse dampness and water accumulation, leading to more qi stagnation and blood stasis and, hence, to a vicious cycle.

Typical symptoms of blood stasis in CRF include fatigue, paleness, abdominal distention, edema, a pale tongue with dark, purple spots, and a deep, fine, choppy pulse. When treating CRF patterns with accompanying blood stasis, one will not achieve satisfactory results using yang-warming and dampness-transforming medicinals alone. One must add blood-quickening, stasis-dispelling medicinals. A typical prescription for blood stasis in CRF is Wang Qing-ren's *Xue Fu Zhu Yu Tang* (Blood Mansion Stasis-dispelling Decoction): *Tao Ren* (Pruni Persicae, Semen), 9g, *Hong Hua* (Carthami Tinctorii, Flos), 7g, *Chuan Xiong* (Ligustici Wallichii, Radix), 15g, *Dang Gui* (Angelicae Sinensis, Radix), 9g, *Chi Shao* (Paeoniae Lactiflorae, Radix Rubrus), 9g, *Niu Xi* (Achyranthis Bidentatae, Radix), 9g, *Chai Hu* (Bupleuri, Radix), 3g, *Sheng Di Huang* (Rehmanniae Glutinosae, uncooked Radix), 9g, *Jie Geng* (Platycodi Grandiflori, Radix), 9g, *Zhi Ke* (Citri Aurantii, Fructus), 6g, and *Gan Cao* (Glycyrrhizae Uralensis, Radix), 3g.

This formula may be augmented with additional warm, cool, or stronger blood-quickening, stasis-dispelling medicinals depending on the patient's pattern. Important cool blood-quickening medicinals include *Dan Shen* (Salviae Miltiorrhizae, Radix), *Yi Mu Cao* (Leonuri Heterophylli, Herba), and *Mu Dan Pi* (Moutan, Cortex Radicis). Important warm blood-quickening medicinals include *Ji Xue Teng* (Jixueteng, Radix Et Caulis) and *Ze Lan* (Lycopi Lucidi, Herba). *Ze Lan* and *Yi Mu Cao* also move water and disperse swelling. The strongest blood-quickening, stasis-dispelling medicinals are the insect or worm products. These include *Shui Zhi* (Hirudo Seu Whitmania), *Tu Bie Chong* (Eupolyphga Seu Opisthoplatia), and *Meng Chong* (Tabanus).

However, although quickening the blood and dis-pelling stasis may be necessary in CRF, strong supplementation must remain the crux of the treatment strategy.

5. SINGLE MEDICINALS FOR CHRONIC RENAL FAILURE

A. *Dong Chong Xia Cao* (Cordyceps Sinensis) has been used in China for millennia. In the past 15-20 years, there has been a great deal of research in China into its use to improve renal function in CRF. This medicinal contains cordyceptic acid, cordyceptin, histidine, phenylalanine, glutamin acid, arginine alanine, proline, valine, and oxyvaline. It also contains an ingredient known in China as *Dong Chong Xia Cao Su* or "Cordyceps Sinensis special element." According to the *Zhong Yi Ling Chuang Shen Zang Bing Xue* (*Clinical Nephrology in Chinese Medicine*),[19] *Dong Chong Xia Cao* has many important pharmaceutical functions. It improves the growth and repair of kidney cells, remarkably reduces gentamicin damage to the kidney, prevents and treats kidney damage caused by kanamycin. It improves kidney filter function and the kidney's ability to recycle trace elements. Contemporary Chinese clinicians prescribe *Dong Chong Xia Cao* to delay the need for dialysis or to defer it altogether. Theory has not kept up with practice, however, and its therapeutic mechanism is not entirely understood. Of many unproven theories, one posits that the particular amino acids and trace elements in *Dong Chong Xia Cao* help improve kidney metabolism. The Shanghai Medical University, the Anhui Medical University, and other research facilities have employed *Dong Chong Xia Cao* to treat thousands of CRF patients. Some patients were followed for over five years and had significant clinical improvement in their renal function.

In Chinese medicine, *Dong Chong Xia Cao* is said to supplement the lung and kidney, nourish essence, and boost the qi. While *Dong Chong Xia Cao* is yin, it supplements yin and yang. The literal English name of this medicinal is "winter worm, summer grass." The worm is the "root," while the "summer grass" (the sprouted fungus) is the "sprout." In the *Ben Cao Wen Da* (*Questions & Answers on the Materia Medica*), Rong Chuan-tang states that, to supplement the lower burner yang, one must use the root, while, to nourish the upper burner yin, one must use the root and sprout. In any case, *Dong Chong Xia Cao* is used for chronic illnesses caused by lung and kidney qi and essence vacuity. Symptoms include spontaneous perspiration, night sweats, impotence, asthma, and low back and knee soreness and limpness. The dosage is usually 3-5 grams per day. One should soak *Dong Chong Xia Cao* in hot water for 24 hours and then chew it and/or drink the infusion. One may also cook it with meat, boil it in tea, make it with soup, or grind it to a powder.

B. *Lu Rong* (Cervi, Cornu Parvum): The kidneys produce erythropoietin, a hormone that stimulates the bone marrow to produce red blood cells. Chronic renal failure damages the kidney and its production of erythropoietin and anemia is often a sequelae of CRF. Most blood-nourishing medicinals are not strong enough to effect the anemia in CRF. *Lu Rong*, on the other hand, stimulates the kidney to secrete erythropoietin and promote RBC production.[20] *Lu Rong* strongly supplements many tissues, especially the sinews and bones. It boosts kidney yang, nourishes kidney essence (and thus the bone marrow), and nourishes the blood. For patterns of CRF with blood vacuity, one can use approximately one gram per day of *Lu Rong* powder.

C. *Fu Zi* (Aconiti Carmichaeli, Radix Lateralis Praeparatus) is hot, acrid, and moderately poisonous. It enters the kidney, spleen, and heart channels. It is listed in the interior-warming category, not the yang-supplementing category. There is a significant difference between these two categories. It arouses the life gate fire, but it does not supplement kidney yang. In clinic, one should only use it to warm the interior and eliminate cold. Even though some modern research shows prepared *Fu Zi* can increase the adrenal function, one should not substitute it for medicinals that invigorate kidney yang, and most CRF patients have patterns of yang vacuity with egregious water accumulation. Water is a yin evil that readily damages yang qi. For instance, water accumulates when the yang qi is not strong enough to disperse it. To treat this pattern, yang qi needs to be stimulated or aroused to move and drain water. *SFu Zi* is remarkable at doing this.[21] *Fu Zi* also sends more yang qi to the extremities to warm the patient.

There are two major ways toxic substances are discharged from the body: via the stool and via the urine. The liver must metabolize toxins for them to be discharged through the stool (via the bile). The kidney must metabolize toxins for them to be discharged through the urine. At present, there is no research indicating exactly where *Fu Zi* is metabolized, *i.e.*, what percentage of it is metabolized by the liver or by the kidney. If the kidney is involved in metabolizing *Fu Zi* to a large degree, CRF patients will take a longer time to metabolize it than normal individuals. Several books recommend high dosages of *Fu Zi* in formulas for CRF. However, in view of the above, one should be cautious with the dosage of *Fu Zi*. One should first determine how well the kidney is functioning, and then lower the dosage accordingly. To be safe, one should begin prescribing *Fu Zi* at no more than one-third to one-half the normal dose. Even when prescribing low dosages, one must carefully monitor the patient for signs of toxicity. These include burning mouth or tongue numbness, excess salivation, nausea, vomiting, diarrhea, dizziness, numbness of the extremities or the whole body, cold clammy skin, blurred vision, dyspnea, or heart arrhythmia. An overdose can lead to coma and death.[22]

D. *Da Huang* (Rhei, Radix Et Rhizoma) is bitter, cold, dispels blood stasis, and frees the flow of the stool. It is used for acute renal failure, chronic renal failure, and uremia in which the evils are the primary concern and the righteous vacuity is only secondary and where there is dry stool. According to Western pharmacodynamics, *Da Huang* has many beneficial physiological actions in terms of the treatment of CRF. It causes the intestines to absorb less amino acids resulting in less urea. It depresses the ability of the body to break down proteins reducing BUN and creatinine levels. It raises blood essential amino acids levels allowing the body to use BUN to make protein. It also decreases the liver and kidney's production of urea, improves urea recycling, increases creatinine discharge, reduces blood phosphorus, and increases blood calcium.

Da Huang may be uncooked or processed. The uncooked is stronger and its dosage is 3-6 grams per day in decoction. The dosage for processed *Da*

Huang is 5-10 grams per day in decoction. One should choose the type of *Da Huang* according to the strength of the patient and number of the patient's bowel movements. In most circumstances, 1-2 movements per day is optimum.

Western physicians may have concerns about the loss of fluids and consequences to potassium balance when Chinese practitioners prescribe *Da Huang*. Western physicians consider the monitoring of electrolyte balance to be a primary concern and will have their patients on a regular schedule for evaluation. Renal failure and nephritic patients usually have an established regimen of tests before they present to Chinese medical practitioners. It is incumbent on the Chinese medical practitioners to understand these tests. This is especially critical when prescribing diuretics or purgatives. If Chinese medical practitioners choose to use *Da Huang* as a form of dialysis, they should consult with the patient's attending Western physician to assure them both that electrolyte balance will be checked and corrected on a daily basis.

6. USING YIN-SUPPLEMENTING & BLOOD-QUICKENING, STASIS-DISPELLING MEDICINALS IN CRF

One must be careful when prescribing yin supplements for CRF patients with patterns of yang qi vacuity. Yin supplements are often cold and slimy and may cause or exacerbate dampness. Dampness is a yin evil that readily taxes yang qi. Therefore, one should not prescribe yin supplements until one has drained water swelling. One must be careful even with *Shen Qi Wan* (Kidney Qi Pills). *Shen Qi Wan* supplements kidney yang qi, an important strategy to dispel water and is often used for the treatment of edema. But, when there is egregious water dampness, one should not initially prescribe it because it contains a large amount of yin supplements. Nevertheless, *Shen Qi Wan* remains an important formula to supplement kidney yin, yang, and qi after water has been drained.

In general, one should not prescribe blood-quickening, stasis-dispelling medicinals for longer than two weeks. Overuse can cause anemia. (This anemia usually disappears after the patient discontinues the medicinals.) Chronic renal failure patients already have anemia, and these medicinals can exacerbate the anemia by too strongly dispersing blood and causing blood vacuity. One must be especially careful with female patients as these medicinals can cause heavy bleeding during menstruation. Processing and/or preparation will alter the function of blood-quickening, stasis-dispelling medicinals. For example, uncooked medicinals are usually stronger in quickening the blood and dispelling stasis, while charred medicinals often stanch bleeding.

To use blood-quickening, stasis-dispelling medicinals successfully, one must carefully consider their dosage, strength, qi, and blood-stanching ability. One must consider not only the dosage of individual blood-quickening, stasis-dispelling medicinals, but also their aggregate number and weight in relation to the supplements in formulas for CRF. One must assiduously analyze the patient's constitution and the degree of blood stasis to choose medicinals with the appropriate strength. Strength is usually described metaphorically. The mildest blood-quickening, stasis-dispelling medicinals harmonize the blood. The next strongest quicken the blood, while the strongest, crack the blood. One must use medicinals or combinations of medicinals with the appropriate qi: cool, cold, or warm. Finally, one must employ those that have the function of stanching bleeding when they are appropriate.

7. ENEMAS

A Chinese medicinal enema is a traditional way to treat patterns associated with CRF. A typical prescription consists of: uncooked *Da Huang* (Rhei, Radix Et Rhizoma), 15-30g (added later), *Fu Zi* (Aconiti Carmichaeli, Radix Lateralis Praeparatus), 9g, calcined *Mu Li* (Ostreae, Concha), 50g, *Pu Gong Ying* (Taraxaci Mongolici, Herba Cum Radice), 50g, and uncooked *Gan Cao* (Glycyrrhizae Uralensis, Radix), 6g. Within this formula, uncooked *Da Huang*, the ruling medicinal, precipitates stagnation, disperses blood stasis, and clears qi and blood aspect heat. *Fu Zi* is hot. When combined with *Da Huang*, it changes a cold precipitating formula to a warm one. *Mu Li* is a securing and astringing medicinal. It constrains yin. It also neutralizes toxicity in the intestines. *Mu Li* protects the righteous qi when one uses *Da Huang* to precipitate evils. *Pu Gong Ying* clears heat and resolves toxins. It works synergistically with *Da Huang* to help dispel toxins. Uncooked *Gan Cao* harmonizes the formula. It reduces abdominal cramping caused by *Da Huang*.

This formula is used for CRF and uremic patients with dry stool and no more than 1-2 bowel movements per day. One should use 200ml of the decoction at 37-38°C and administer the enema after a bowel movement. One should inject it slowly, at about 60 drops per minute. The patient should retain the enema for 45 minutes once a day. If the patient is strong and the condition is serious, one can use this enema twice a day. Five to seven days constitute one course. One must be cautious and modify this regimen according to the patient's constitution. If the patient is weak, one can administer this enema every other day or only two times a week. This enema is contraindicated if the patient is very weak or has over three bowel movements a day, hemorrhoids, a fistula, or bleeding.

The Anhui College of Chinese Medicine uses the following enema: uncooked *Da Huang* (Rhei, Radix Et Rhizoma), 15-30g, calcined *Long Gu* (Draconis, Os), 15-30g, calcined *Mu Li* (Ostreae, Concha), 15-30g, *Rou Gui* (Cinnamonmi Casiae, Cortex), 6-12g, *Huai Hua Mi* (Sophorae Japonicae, Flos Immaturus), 30-60g, and *Qing Dai* (Indigonis, Pulvis), 6-9g. These medicinals are decocted and administered in 150-200ml doses once a day. This enema should be retained in the colon for 1-2 hours. Two weeks constitute one treatment course, after which the patient should rest for one week. In 1986, 25 CRF patients were treated with this enema. There were remarkable results in 15 patients and effective results in five, with the total effective rate being 80%. Chang Chuan Chinese Medical College used this enema with 1000 CRF patients with an effective rate of 87.7%.

8. EXTERNAL FORMULAS FOR RENAL FAILURE

One can also put medicinals on acupuncture points to treat uremia according to the principle of treating internal disease by external application. One formula, reported in *Clinical Nephrology in Chinese Medicine*[23] consists of equal parts of: *Fu Zi* (Aconiti Carmichaeli, Radix Lateralis Praeparatus), *Yin Yang Huo* (Epimedii, Herba), *Tao Ren* (Pruni Persicae, Semen), *Hong Hua* (Carthami Tinctorii, Flos), *Chuan Xiong* (Ligustici Wallichii, Radix), and *Chen Xiang* (Aquilariae Agallochae, Lignum). These medicinals are ground into a powder, soaked in 95% alcohol, and then diluted. The infusion is placed on a gauze dressing and applied to *Shen Shu* (Bl 23) and *Guan Yuan* (CV 4). The gauze should be moistened with the infusion every day and should be changed once every three days. A treatment course consists of four applications of the dressing. A patient usually needs 2-4 courses. In one study, eight patients were treated with this formula. Four patients had remarkable results, three had effective results, and one had no change. There were no toxic reactions.

9. MEDICATED BATH FORMULAS FOR RENAL FAILURE

Clinical Nephrology in Chinese Medicine[24] reports using the following bath formula to treat nephritis: *Fu Ping* (Lemnae Seu Spirodelae, Herba), *Gui Zhi* (Cinnamomi Cassiae, Ramulus), *Sang Ye* (Mori Albi, Folium), *Sang Bai Pi* (Mori Albi, Cortex Radicis), *Fu Zi* (Aconiti Carmichaeli, Radix Lateralis Praeparatus), *Chuan Xiong* (Ligustici Wallichii, Radix), *Tao Ren* (Pruni Persicae, Semen), *Hong Hua* (Carthami Tinctorii, Flos), *Chi Shao* (Paeoniae Lactiflorae, Radix Rubrus), *Yi Mu Cao* (Leonuri Heterophylli, Herba), *Liu Yue Xue Ye* (Eupatorium Chinensis, Folium), *Tu Fu Ling* (Smilacis Glabrae, Rhizoma), *Ku Shen* (Sophorae Flavescentis, Radix), and *Bai Xian Pi* (Dictamni Dasycarpi, Cortex Radicis). Make a concentrated decoction using equal parts of these medicinals and fill a bathtub until the decoction covers the patient's body. The patient should soak for 15-30 minutes until sweat appears but must not feel enervated after the treatment. The patient should be treated once a day, two weeks constituting one course. Usually, 2-3 courses are needed. One must be cautious when applying this treatment and not allow the patient to catch cold. If the bath gets cold, add more hot water. Do not allow the patient to sweat too much and become fatigued. Thirty-four patients were treated with this medicated bath along with internal formulas appropriate for their patterns. The effective rate was 88.4%. This formula is especially effective for hypertension and remarkably reduces BUN.

10. MODERN CHINESE RESEARCH ON MEDICINALS FOR CRF[25]

Dr. Ping Dong-zheng used *Wen Pi Tang* (Warm the Spleen Decoction) to treat CRF in rats. *Wen Pi Tang* consists of: *Da Huang* (Rhei, Radix Et Rhizoma), *Ren Shen* (Panacis Ginseng, Radix), *Gan Cao* (Glycyrrhizae Uralensis, Radix), *Gan Jiang* (Zingiberis Officinalis, dry Rhizoma), and *Fu Zi* (Aconiti Carmichaeli, Radix Lateralis Praeparatus). Dr. Ping began his experiment by using toxic chemicals to cause renal failure in rats. He then gave the rats *Wen Pi Tang*. He found that this reduced the kidney weight and certain chemical toxins. There was also remarkable control of BUN and of phosphorus and calcium levels. The rats' morbidity rate was also reduced. Dr. Ping also tried *Da Huang Gan Cao Tang* (Rhubarb & Licorice Decoction) and *San Huang Xie Xin Tang* (Three Yellows Drain the Heart Decoction) but found *Wen Pi Tang* to be most effective.

The Shanghai College of Chinese Medicine conducted a study using *Da Huang Ling Pi Chong Ji* (Rhubarb & Epimedium Soluble Granules). This formula consisted of: *Tai Zi Shen* (Pseudostellariae Heterophyllae, Radix), *Fu Zi* (Aconiti Carmichaeli, Radix Lateralis Praeparatus), *Yin Yang Huo* (Epimedii, Herba), *Xian Mao* (Curculiginis Orchioidis, Rhizoma), *Ba Ji Tian* (Morindae Officinalis, Radix), processed *Da Huang* (Rhei, Radix Et Rhizoma), *Huang Bai* (Phellodendri, Cortex), *Zhi Mu* (Anemarrhenae Asphodeloidis, Rhizoma), *Dan Shen* (Salviae Miltiorrhizae, Radix), and *Mu Li* (Ostreae, Concha). No dosages were given and there were other medicinals in the formula that were not described. Altogether, 36 human subjects were treated with this protocol. Eighteen of these had remarkable results. This formula slowed the development of renal failure, and balanced calcium and phosphorus levels.

Dr. Qing Fa-zhou used a Chinese medicinal formula as a dialysis fluid by ingestion. That is, he attempted to remove toxic substances from the blood through the intestines. The formula was proprietary. Four of the ingredients were: *Huang Qi* (Astragali Membranacei, Radix), *Da Huang* (Rhei, Radix Et Rhizoma), *Chuan Xiong* (Ligustici Wallichii, Radix), and *Dang Shen* (Codonopsitis Pilosulae, Radix). Two hundred milliliters of the formula was ingested two times a day or a 200ml enema was given one or two times per day. One month constituted one course of treatment, and patients usually needed 2-3 courses. There were remarkable results in 11 patients and some positive effects in 16, for a total effective rate of 84%. This formula was also used in an experiment with rats with CRF. There was a remarkable improvement in the rats' kidney function.

11. DIET

Although CRF patients need to limit the amount of protein[26] in their diets, they do need a certain amount of high quality protein. (High quality protein contains all the essential amino acids and is usually found in animal products, not in plant products.) If patients' diets are too high in protein, regular metabolism will produce a great deal of waste nitrogen. If they eliminate all protein from their diets, they will begin to metabolize their own body's protein, also producing waste nitrogen. In either case, kidney function will be compromised. Stabilizing protein intake in relation to kidney function must be a primary concern. Chronic renal failure patients also need to limit the amount of salt[27] in their diet. As is the case with protein, too much or too little salt will damage kidney function.

12. BLOOD PRESSURE

Chronic renal failure patients usually have hypertension[28] due to nephron damage. The nephrons are the functional units of the kidneys responsible for filtering, secreting, and reabsorbing waste products of the body. Nephron damage results in decreased blood flow through the filters. The kidneys release hormones that encourage the heart to pump more forcefully in order to increase the blood flow to the kidneys and through the filters. These hormones also cause the body to retain body fluids longer. Both the increased heart function and fluid retention increase the pressure against arterial walls resulting in hypertension. In addition, when the blood pressure is too high, the kidney releases hormones that constrict the blood vessels and ultimately reduce the blood supply to the kidney. A blood pressure that is too low also reduces the blood supply to the kidney. A decreased blood supply results in decreased kidney function. The blood pressure control range should be 120-160/70-90mmHg.

13. TOXIC DRUGS

Chronic renal failure patients often have to take Western drugs that cause many adverse complications and side effects. While it is difficult to protect the kidney against the toxicity of these drugs, one can apply acupuncture and prescribe *Dong Chong Xia Cao* (Cordyceps Sinensis). *Dong Chong Xia Cao* has been shown to improve the growth and repair of kidney cells, remarkably reducing gentamicin damage to the kidney, and preventing and treating kidney damage caused by kanamycin.[29]

ENDNOTES

[1] Yu Guang-shi, *op. cit.*, p. 289
[2] Modern research has found that both these medicinals reduce protein in the urine.
[3] Yu Guang-shi, *op. cit.*, p. 222
[4] *Ibid.*, p. 285
[5] *Ibid.*, p. 286
[6] *Ibid.*, p. 267
[7] Warning: The dosages in Dr. Qi's formula are too large. One should use normal or even low dosages of medicinals to guard against any negative reactions (allergic or other) in kidney-compromised patients.
[8] Western medicine delineates diminished renal reserve, renal insufficiency, and uremia as three functional effects of chronic renal failure. In the modern TCM clinic one uses these functional effects as rubrics for determining treatment by patterns

identified (*bian zheng lun zhi*). Combining the first two functional effects and placing them into one category or rubric facilitates analysis. Therefore, the rubrics are titled "diminished renal reserve and renal insufficiency" and "uremia."
[9] These patterns were modified from Ping Dong's list in *Dong Dai Ming Lao Zhong Yi Ling Zheng Hui Cui* (*Modern Famous Doctors Clinical Experience*), Qing He-chen, Guandong Science Technique Publishing Company, Guandong, 1991, p. 391
[10] Yu Guan-shi, *op. cit.*, p. 281
[11] *Ibid.*, p. 243
[12] *Liu Yi San* (Six-to-One Powder) consists of six parts *Hua Shi* (Talcum) and one part *Gan Cao* (Glycyrrhizae Uralensis, Radix).
[13] Yu Guang-shi, *op. cit.*, p. 264
[14] The patient must limit protein to 0.38 gm/Kg of body weight or about 20g/day.
[15] Yu Guang-shi, *op. cit.*, p. 289
[16] *Ibid.*, p. 283
[17] *Ibid.*, p. 279
[18] Western medicine delineates diminished renal reserve, renal insufficiency, and uremia as three functional effects of chronic renal failure. In the modern Chinese medical clinic one uses these functional effects as rubrics for determining treatment by patterns identified. Combining the first two functional effects and placing them into one category and rubric facilitates analysis. Therefore, the rubrics are titled "diminished renal reserve and renal insufficiency" and "uremia."
[19] Qing Fa-shen, *Zhong Yi Lin Chuang Shen Zang Bing Xue* (*Clinical Nephrology in Chinese Medicine*), Shanghai Science and Technology Publishing Company, Shanghai, 1998, p. 321
[20] In research in China, *Lu Rong* (Cervi, Cornu Parvum) powder was given to healthy mature rabbits after which all blood cells and especially RBC and hemoglobin were increased.
[21] In Western medical terms, *Fu Zi* (Aconiti Carmichaeli, Radix Lateralis Praeparatus) dilates the blood vessels, even cardiac blood vessels. As a result, more fluid reaches the kidney and is excreted, thus ridding the body of excess fluids.
[22] Antidotes include 1-2% tannic acid, emetics, activated charcoal, IV Glucose-Saline. Use stimulants and keep the patient warm.
[23] Qing Fa-shen, *op. cit.*, p. 305
[24] *Ibid.*, p. 305
[25] *Ibid.*, p. 325
[26] The patient must limit protein to 0.38 gm/Kg of body weight or about 20g/day.
[27] This is dependent on blood Na level.
[28] Please see the section on hypertension in Part 2, Chapter 13.
[29] Qing Fa-shen, *op. cit.*, p. 321

CHAPTER 8

TUBULOINTERSTITIAL NEPHRITIS

Tubulointerstitial nephritis is a condition of inflammation of the kidney tubules and the spaces between the tubules. It is also known by the name interstitial allergic nephritis.

NOSOLOGY

The two main types of tubulointerstitial nephritis are acute tubulointerstitial nephritis (ATN) and chronic tubulointerstitial nephritis (CTN).

EPIDEMIOLOGY

Tubulointerstitial nephritis accounts for 20-30% of end-stage renal disease and 15-25% of acute renal failure.

ETIOLOGY & PATHOPHYSIOLOGY

Acute tubulointerstitial nephritis is typically due to hypersensitivity or an adverse reaction to a medication. Analgesics such as acetaminophen and aspirin and certain antibiotics are the major offending drugs. Acute tubulointerstitial nephritis may also result from snakebite poisoning, certain fish's bile, and chemical toxins or may be caused by urinary tract infections.

Several different diseases may cause chronic tubulointerstitial nephritis. These include ATN, diabetes mellitus, chronic pyelonephritis, systemic lupus erythematous and other autoimmune disorders, late stage hepatitis, and hypertension. End-stage kidney disease is often characterized by hardening and damage to the tubular interstitium. Chronic damage to the glomerular structures, from a variety of different diseases, is thought to unduly exhaust the tubules from unfiltered proteins. This contributes to their eventual demise.

SYMPTOMATOLOGY

If ATN is caused by an adverse drug reaction, symptoms include fever, rash, pruritis, joint pain and hematuria. If toxins are the cause, symptoms include nausea, vomiting, headache, oliguira or anuria, and local or systemic edema. Onset is variable when due to a drug reaction. ATN may occur within days of taking a medication or as long as several weeks after the initial exposure.

DIAGNOSIS

The Western medical diagnosis of tubulointerstitial

nephritis follows the routine lab tests used for other types of kidney disease. Urine tests may reveal protein, though not as severe as in nephrotic syndrome. Red blood cell casts may be found both with urine analysis and blood testing. Blood urea nitrogen and creatinine are assessed to gauge overall kidney function. Kidney biopsy is the standard to confirm ATN and the extent of the damage to the kidneys.

WESTERN MEDICAL TREATMENT

Western medical treatment for this condition often focuses on the identification and removal of the offending medications. Signs and symptoms may rapidly disappear by implementing such a change. Treatments specific to the kidneys include electrolyte, fluid, and protein management, and dialysis if needed. In most cases, ATN is a short-term condition, which can be remedied with a general treatment strategy for the kidney system.

PROGNOSIS & COMPLICATIONS

If ATN causes renal failure, complete recovery is unlikely. If ATN occurs due to a drug reaction and the kidney function is not damaged, patients should fully recover within 4-8 weeks.

CHINESE MEDICAL DISEASE CATEGORIZATION

In Chinese medicine, the clinical manifestations of tubulointerstitial nephritis correspond to the following traditional disease categories: kidney wind, block and repulsion, dribbling urinary block, bloody urine, and strangury.

TREATMENT BASED ON PATTERN IDENTIFICATION

ACUTE TUBULOINTERSTITIAL NEPHRITIS

1. DAMP HEAT IN THE LOWER BURNER

SIGNS & SYMPTOMS: Fever and chills, lower back pain, nausea and vomiting, frequent or urgent and painful, dark, yellow or red urine, and constipation. The tongue is red with thick, yellow fur, and the pulse is bowstring and slippery.

TREATMENT PRINCIPLES: Clear heat and eliminate dampness from the lower burner

REPRESENTATIVE FORMULAS: If dampness is more prominent, use modified Ba Zheng San (Eight [Ingredients] Rectification Powder)[1]

Qu Mai (Dianthi, Herba), 3g
Bian Xu (Polygoni Avicularis, Herba), 3g
Hua Shi (Talcum), 3g
Deng Xin Cao (Junci Effusi, Medulla), 3g
Che Qian Zi (Plantaginis, Semen), 3g
Zhi Zi (Gardeniae Jasminoidis, Fructus), 3g
processed Da Huang (Rhei, Radix Et Rhizoma), 3g
Gan Cao (Glycyrrhizae Uralensis, Radix), 3g

If heat is more prominent, use Huang Lian Jie Du Tang (Coptis Resolve Toxins Decoction)

Huang Lian (Coptidis Chinensis, Rhizoma), 9g
Huang Qin (Scutellariae Baicalensis, Radix), 9g
Huang Bai (Phellodendri, Cortex), 9g
Zhi Zi (Gardeniae Jasminoidis, Fructus), 9g

MODIFICATIONS: If heat and dampness are both severe, one can combine these two formulas. If the patient has blood in the urine, add Sheng Di Huang (Rehmanniae Glutinosae, uncooked Radix) and Mu Dan Pi (Moutan, Cortex Radicis) plus some cool, blood-staunching medicinals in small doses. If the patient feels feverish, add Zhi Mu (Anemarrhenae Aspheloidis, Rhizoma), Shi Gao (Gypsum Fibrosum), Zhi Zi (Gardeniae Jasminoidis, Fructus), and Dan Zhu Ye (Lophatheri Gracilis, Herba). For nausea and vomiting, add Zhu Ru (Bambusae In Taeniis, Caulis) and Huo Xiang (Agastachis Seu Pogostemi). For constipation, add Da Huang (Rhei, Radix Et Rhizoma). Finally, the patient should drink lots of watermelon juice. Watermelon juice drains heat, cools the kidney, and frees the flow of the water passageways. This diet therapy is extremely important. Because watermelon juice can drain too much and cause constipation, one may add Feng Mi (Mel, honey) to the formula or the juice to moisten dryness.

NOTE: In this pattern, one should use small dosages of medicinals because the kidney function is compromised and it may not be able to metabolize and excrete any potentially harmful medicinal constituents.

ACUMOXIBUSTION: Choose from *Wei Zhong* (Bl 40), *Zhong Ji* (CV 3), *Fu Liu* (Ki 7), *Pang Guang Shu* (Bl 28), *Yin Ling Quan* (Sp 9), *San Yin Jiao* (Sp 6), *Guan Yuan* (CV 4), *Shui Dao* (St 28), *Ci Liao* (Bl 32), *Nei Ting* (St 44).

Case history from Dr. Wei Li's private practice: Chao, a 23 year-old female

Chao first visited Dr. Li in 1992. Chao married a few months before this visit. Shortly after being married, she developed symptoms of frequent, urgent, painful, incomplete urination, fever and chills, low back pain, and night sweats. Chao went to a Western doctor who requested a urinalysis. It was positive for RBCs, pus and WBCs, and granular casts at 1-2+. The doctor's diagnosis was pyelonephritis with ATN, and he prescribed antibiotics for two weeks. Chao's symptoms improved, but she still had low back pain, slightly difficult urination, and night sweats. Therefore, Dr. Li was consulted and found a pattern of damp heat in the lower burner. She prescribed modified *Zhi Bai Di Huang Wan* (Anemarrhena & Phellodendron Rehmannia Pills) plus *Ba Zheng San* (Eight [Ingredients] Rectification Powder): *Zhi Mu* (Anemarrhenae Asphodeloidis, Rhizoma), 9g, *Huang Bai* (Phellodendri, Cortex), 9g, *Shu Di Huang* (Rehmanniae Glutinosae, cooked Radix), 12g, *Shan Yao* (Radix Dioscoreae Oppositae), 12g, *Shan Zhu Yu* (Corni Officinalis, Fructus), 12g, *Ze Xie* (Alismatis Orientalis, Rhizoma), 9g, *Fu Ling* (Poriae Cocos, Sclerotium), 9g, *Mu Dan Pi* (Moutan, Cortex Radicis), 9g, *Qu Mai* (Dianthi, Herba), 9g, *Che Qian Zi* (Plantaginis, Semen), 9g, and *Bei Xie* (Dioscoreae Hypolagucae, Rhizoma), 9g. Chao took this formula for two weeks. She then continued on *Zhi Bai Di Huang Wan* alone for one more month. She completely recovered.

2. TOXINS ATTACKING THE KIDNEY

SIGNS & SYMPTOMS: Fever, rash, pruritus, achy joints, low back pain, bloody urine, vexation and agitation, a dry mouth, and thirst. The tongue is red with thin, yellow fur, and the pulse is fast, bowstring, and slippery.

TREATMENT PRINCIPLES: Expel wind and resolve toxins

REPRESENTATIVE FORMULA: Modified *Xiao Feng San* (Eliminate Wind Powder), *Ba Zheng San* (Eight [Ingredients] Rectification Powder), and *Xiao Ji Yin Zi* (Cephalanoplos Beverage)

Jing Jie Sui (Schizonepetae Tenuifoliae, Herba Seu Flos), 3g
Fang Feng (Ledebouriellae Divaricatae, Radix), 3g
Ku Shen (Sophorae Flavescentis, Radix), 3g
Mu Tong (Akebiae Mutong, Caulis), 1.5g
Xiao Ji (Cephalanoplos Segeti, Herba), 3g
Pu Huang (Typhae, Pollen), 3g
Ou Jie (Nelumbinis Nuciferae, Nodus Rhizomatis), 3g
Hua Shi (Talcum), 3g
Deng Xin Cao (Junci Effusi, Medulla), 3g
Che Qian Zi (Plantaginis, Semen), 3g
Zhi Zi (Gardeniae Jasminoidis, Fructus), 3g

NOTE: The most important strategy in this pattern is to eliminate toxins, *i.e.*, to get them out of the body. Second in importance is helping the kidney recover from the attack. Symptomatic relief follows these in importance. We have chosen some medicinals from three formulas to eliminate toxins. However, the practitioner should review these formulas, using them as models for treating various aspects of this pattern, and choose the appropriate medicinals from each formula for their particular patient.

The complete representative formulas are as follows:

Xiao Feng San

Jing Jie Sui (Schizonepetae Tenuifoliae, Herba Seu Flos), 9g
Fang Feng (Ledebouriellae Divaricatae, Radix), 9g
Niu Bang Zi (Arctii Lappae, Fructus), 6g
Chan Tui (Cicadae, Periostracum), 9g
Cang Zhu (Atractylodis, Rhizoma), 9g
Ku Shen (Sophorae Flavescentis, Radix), 9g

Mu Tong (Akebiae Mutong, Caulis), 6g

Shi Gao (Gypsum Fibrosum), 6g

Zhi Mu (Anemarrhenae Aspheloidis, Rhizoma), 9g

Sheng Di Huang (Rehmanniae Glutinosae, uncooked Radix), 9g

Dang Gui (Angelicae Sinensis, Radix), 9g

Hei Zhi Ma (Sesami Indici, Semen), 9g

Gan Cao (Glycyrrhizae Uralensis, Radix), 3g

Xiao Ji Yin Zi

Xiao Ji (Cephalanoplos Segeti, Herba), 9g

Pu Huang (Typhae, Pollen), 9g

Ou Jie (Nelumbinis Nuciferae, Nodus Rhizomatis), 9g

Hua Shi (Talcum), 3g

Mu Tong (Akebiae Mutong, Caulis), 9g

Sheng Di Huang (Rehmanniae Glutinosae, uncooked Radix), 9g

Dang Gui (Angelicae Sinensis, Radix), 6g

Zhi Zi (Gardeniae Jasminoidis, Fructus), 9g

Dan Zhu Ye (Lophatheri Gracilis, Herba), 9g

Gan Cao (Glycyrrhizae Uralensis, Radix), 3g

Ba Zheng San

Mu Tong (Akebiae Mutong, Caulis), 9g

Qu Mai (Dianthi, Herba), 9g

Bian Xu (Polygoni Avicularis, Herba), 9g

Hua Shi (Talcum), 6g

Deng Xin Cao (Junci Effusi, Medulla), 9g

Che Qian Zi (Plantaginis, Semen), 9g

Zhi Zi (Gardeniae Jasminoidis, Fructus), 9g

processed *Da Huang* (Rhei, Radix Et Rhizoma), 9g

Gan Cao (Glycyrrhizae Uralensis, Radix), 9g

One should choose as few medicinals as possible and start with very low dosages. In ATN, the kidney is swollen and its function is compromised. When the kidney function is compromised, medicinals that are normally metabolized easily in the kidney may cause a toxic reaction. One must be extremely careful with the medicinals necessary for clearing and dispersing, using as few as possible and assiduously monitoring their dosage. In addition, one should avoid yang supplements following basic yin-yang theory. In this case, there is egregious heat and toxins, and, therefore, warming medicinals must be kept to a minimum. One must rid the body

of the toxins before attempting to supplement. One should also employ diet therapy in this pattern. The patient should be advised to drink plenty of water to flush out the toxins and to drink watermelon juice every day. Watermelon juice is a safe and especially effective alternative to Western diuretics. Watermelon juice is nontoxic. It clears heat, drains dampness, and provides essential vitamins.

MODIFICATIONS: It is extremely important to add medicinals to treat four aspect heat. One should choose medicinals from *Yin Qiao San* (Lonicera & Forsythia Powder) for the defensive aspect, from *Huang Lian Jie Du Tang* (Coptis Toxin-resolving Decoction) for the qi aspect, from *Qing Ying Tang* (Clear the Constructive Decoction) for the constructive aspect, and from *Xiao Ji Di Huang Tang* (Rhinoceros Horn & Rehmannia Decoction) for the blood aspect.

Yin Qiao San

Jin Yin Hua (Lonicerae Japonicae, Flos), 9-15g

Lian Qiao (Forsythiae Suspensae, Fructus), 9-15g

Jie Geng (Platycodi Grandiflori, Radix), 3-6g

Niu Bang Zi (Arctii Lappae, Fructus), 9-12g

Bo He (Menthae Haplocalycis, Herba), 3-6g

Dan Dou Chi (Sojae, Semen Praeparatum), 3-6g

Jing Jie Sui (Schizonepetae Tenuifoliae, Herba Seu Flos), 6-9g

Dan Zhu Ye (Lophatheri Gracilis, Herba), 3-6g

fresh *Lu Gen* (Phragmitis Communis, Rhizoma), 15-30g

Gan Cao (Glycyrrhizae Uralensis, Radix), 3-6g

Qing Ying Tang

Xi Jiao (Rhinocerotis, Cornu), 9g

Xuan Shen (Scrophulariae Ningpoensis, Radix), 9g

Sheng Di Huang (Rehmanniae Glutinosae, uncooked Radix), 15g

Mai Men Dong (Ophiopogonis Japonici, Tuber), 9g

Jin Yin Hua (Lonicerae Japonicae, Flos), 9g

Lian Qiao (Forsythiae Suspensae, Fructus), 6g

Huang Lian (Coptidis Chinensis, Rhizoma), 4.5g

Dan Zhu Ye (Lophatheri Gracilis, Herba), 3g

Dan Shen (Salviae Miltiorrhizae, Radix), 6g

Modified *Xi Jiao Di Huang Tang*

Shui Niu Jiao (Rhinocerotis, Cornu), 12-24g
Sheng Di Huang (Rehmanniae Glutinosae, uncooked Radix), 24g
Chi Shao (Paeoniae Lactiflorae, Radix Rubrus), 9g
Mu Dan Pi (Moutan, Cortex Radicis), 6g

ACUMOXIBUSTION: Choose from *Da Zhui* (GV 14), *Qu Chi* (LI 11), (LI 4), *Zhong Ji* (CV 3), *Shen Shu* (Bl 23), *Pang Guang Shu* (Bl 28), *Wei Zhong* (Bl 40), *Zhao Hai* (Ki 6), *Fu Liu* (Ki 7), and *Tai Xi* (Ki 3).

CLINICAL TIPS

1. The most important principle in the treatment of ATN is to resolve toxins, *i.e.*, to get them out of the body. Second in importance is helping the kidney recover from the attack. Symptomatic relief follows these in importance. In ATN, the kidney is swollen and its function is compromised. When the kidney function is compromised, medicinals that are normally metabolized easily in the kidney may cause a toxic reaction. One must be extremely careful with the medicinals necessary for clearing and dispersing, using as few as possible and assiduously monitoring their dosage.

2. DIETARY THERAPY FOR ANY PATTERN OF ATN

The *Nei Jing (Inner Classic)*, Chapter 70, "*Wu Chang Zheng Da Lun* (Great Treatise on the Five Invariable Administrators)" states:

> . . . when administering medicine, once the health is 60% recovered, discontinue the extremely toxic medicinals. Once the health is 70% recovered, discontinue the moderately toxic medicinals. Once the health is 80% recovered, discontinue the mildly toxic medicinals. Once the health is 90% recovered, discontinue the nontoxic medicinals. Follow up with diet therapy to consolidate and regenerate. If the physician follows this principle, success is assured.

Diet therapy is highly recommended for acute tubulointerstitial nephritis, especially when it is caused by a drug reaction. It is very safe, having little or no toxicity, and often provides faster results than Western diuretics. The following are especially efficacious:

A. *Liang Pi Jian* (Double Skin Beverage). This consists of watermelon skin, 60g, and winter melon skin, 60g. Cook this beverage as a tea and take one time a day.[2]

B. *Yi Yi Ren Lu Dou Tang* (Coix & Mung Bean Soup). This consists of 30 grams of these two medicinals. Cook as a decoction and take once a day.[3]

C. *Che Qian Zhu* (Plantain Boil). Cook fresh *Che Qian Cao* (Plantaginis, Herba), 100g, with white rice, 100g, to make porridge and take once a day.[4]

D. *Xi Gua Zhi* (Citrulli, Succus Fructi, watermelon juice). Juice one half of a watermelon and drink over one day. Watermelon juice is a safe and especially effective alternative to Western diuretics. Watermelon juice is non-toxic. It clears heat, percolates dampness, and provides essential vitamins.

E. *Feng Mi* (Mel, honey). Give 50-150 grams of honey three times a day.

CHRONIC TUBULOINTERSTITIAL NEPHRITIS

1. SPLEEN-KIDNEY QI VACUITY WITH DAMPNESS

SIGNS & SYMPTOMS: Fatigue, low back and knee soreness and limpness, insomnia, low appetite, loose stools, dribbling urination, cold hands and feet, a pale facial complexion. The tongue is pale and puffy with thin fur, and the pulse is deep, fine, and slow.

TREATMENT PRINCIPLES: Supplement the kidney and fortify the spleen, percolate dampness

REPRESENTATIVE FORMULA: *Bu Zhong Yi Qi Tang* (Supplement the Center & Boost the Qi Decoction) plus *Jin Gui Shen Qi Wan* (*Golden Cabinet* Kidney Qi Pills)

Huang Qi (Astragali Membranacei, Radix), 6g
Ren Shen (Panacis Ginseng, Radix), 3g
Bai Zhu (Atractylodis Macrocephalae, Rhizoma), 3g
mix-fried *Gan Cao* (Glycyrrhizae Uralensis, Radix), 1g

Dang Gui (Angelicae Sinensis, Radix), 3g

Chen Pi (Citri Reticulatae, Pericarpium), 3g

Sheng Ma (Cimicifugae, Rhizoma), 3g

Chai Hu (Bupleuri, Radix), 3g

Shu Fu Zi (Aconiti Carmichaeli, Radix Lateralis Praeparatus), 1g

Rou Gui (Cinnamonmi Casiae, Cortex), 1g

Shu Di Huang (Rehmanniae Glutinosae, cooked Radix), 6g

Shan Yao (Radix Dioscoreae Oppositae), 6g

Shan Zhu Yu (Corni Officinalis, Fructus), 3g

Ze Xie (Alismatis Orientalis, Rhizoma), 3g

Fu Ling (Poriae Cocos, Sclerotium), 3g

Mu Dan Pi (Moutan, Cortex Radicis), 3g

NOTE: Patients with this pattern are close to renal failure. Therefore, one must eliminate unnecessary medicinals, use low dosages of the remaining medicinals, and carefully monitor the patient's kidney function.

MODIFICATIONS: The best medicinal to boost kidney function is *Dong Chong Xia Cao* (Cordyceps Sinensis). For bloody urine, add *San Qi* (Notoginseng, Radix) and *Xu Duan* (Dipsaci Asperi, Radix). If the patient has proteinuria, please review the section on proteinuria in Part 4 for suggestions on how to treat it.

ACUMOXIBUSTION: Choose from *Pi Shu* (Bl 20), *Shen Shu* (Bl 23), *Pang Guang Shu* (Bl 28), *Tai Bai* (Sp 3), *San Yin Jiao* (Sp 6), *Yin Ling Quan* (Sp 9), *Tai Xi* (Ki 3), *Zhao Hao* (Ki 6), *Fu Liao* (Ki 7), *Zhong Ji* (CV 3), *Guan Yuan* (CV 4), *Qi Hai* (CV 6), and *Zu San Li* (St 36).

Case history from Dr. Wei Li's private practice: Yu, a 52 year-old female

Yu suffered for years with recurring urinary tract infections, and she often had uncomfortable urination and urgency. She was given six courses of antibiotics, but the infection always returned. Because of egregious low back pain, doctors recommended the patient have an x-ray. This revealed an enlarged renal pelvis due to fluid accumulation and a great deal of scar tissue due to recurrent infections. Urine had accumulated in the scar tissue and formed cysts. When Dr. Li saw this woman, she learned that Yu always felt tired and often

needed to lie down. She could not work. Her tongue was pale, puffy, and swollen with a red tip and her pulse was fine and forceless. Dr. Li decided that Yu's pattern was more vacuous than replete. Therefore, she prescribed modified *Shi Quan Da Bu Tang* (Ten [Ingredients] Completely & Greatly Supplementing Decoction): *Huang Qi* (Astragali Membranacei, Radix), 15g, *Ren Shen* (Panacis Ginseng, Radix), 5g, *Shu Di Huang* (Rehmanniae Glutinosae, cooked Radix), 12g, *Dang Gui* (Angelicae Sinensis, Radix), 5g, *Bai Shao* (Paeoniae Lactiflorae, Radix Albus), 5g, *Chi Shao* (Paeoniae Lactiflorae, Radix Rubrus), 4g, *Gui Zhi* (Cinnamomi Cassiae, Ramulus), 3g, and *Gan Jiang* (Zingiberis Officinalis, dry Rhizoma), 3g. The ruling medicinals in this formula are *Huang Qi* and *Shu Di Huang* which are used to supplement the qi, blood, and yin. *Gui Zhi* and *Gan Jiang* strengthen kidney yang so it can steam kidney yin to produce kidney qi. Yu took this formula for one week and was 50% better. In two weeks she was 80% better. She took variations of this formula for half a year and completely recovered.

2. LIVER-KIDNEY YIN VACUITY WITH ASCENDANT LIVER YANG HYPERACTIVITY

SIGNS & SYMPTOMS: Dizziness, headaches, tinnitus, dry mouth, low back and knee soreness and limpness, and irascibility. The tongue is red with no fur, and the pulse is fine and fast.

TREATMENT PRINCIPLES: Nourish liver and kidney yin, clear the liver and subdue yang

REPRESENTATIVE FORMULA: Modified *Qi Ju Di Huang Wan* (Lycium & Chrysanthemum Rehmannia Pills)

Shu Di Huang (Rehmanniae Glutinosae, cooked Radix), 12g

Shan Zhu Yu (Corni Officinalis, Fructus), 12g

Shan Yao (Radix Dioscoreae Oppositae), 12g

Fu Ling (Poriae Cocos, Sclerotium), 12g

Ze Xie (Alismatis Orientalis, Rhizoma), 9g

Mu Dan Pi (Moutan, Cortex Radicis), 12g

Zhu Ling (Polypori Umbellati, Sclerotium), 9g

Gou Qi Zi (Lycii Chinensis, Fructus), 12g

Ju Hua (Chrysanthemi Morifolii, Flos), 15g

MODIFICATIONS: If the patient has high blood pressure, add *Niu Xi* (Achyranthis Bidentatae, Radix), *Shi Jue Ming* (Haliotidis, Concha), *Huang Qin* (Scutellariae Baicalensis, Radix), *Tian Ma* (Gastrodiae Elatae, Rhizoma), and *Gou Teng* (Uncariae Cum Uncis, Ramulus). For bloody urine, add *Han Lian Cao* (Ecliptae Prostratae, Herba), *Pu Huang* (Typhae, Pollen), *Bai Mao Gen* (Imperatae Cylindricae, Rhizoma), *Xiao Ji* (Cepahalanoplos Segeti, Herba), and substitute half the *Shu Di Huang* with *Sheng Di Huang* (Rehmanniae Glutinose, uncooked Radix). For night sweats, add *Huang Bai* (Phellodendri, Cortex), *Zhi Mu* (Anemarrhenae Aspheloidis, Rhizoma), and *Di Gu Pi* (Lycii Chinensis, Cortex Radicis). For headache, add *Chuan Xiong* (Ligustici Wallichii, Radix), *Chai Hu* (Bupleuri, Radix), and *Man Jing Zi* (Viticis, Fructus).

ACUMOXIBUSTION: Choose from *Tai Xi* (Ki 3), *San Yin Jiao* (Sp 6), *Zhong Zhu* (TB 3), *Tai Chong* (Liv 3), *Qu Quan* (Liv 8), *Qi Men* (Liv 14), *Gan Shu* (Bl 18), *Feng Chi* (GB 20), *Bai Hui* (GV 20), and *He Gu* (LI 4).

3. KIDNEY YIN & YANG VACUITY

SIGNS & SYMPTOMS: Fatigue, cold in the morning but hot in the evening with night sweats, no appetite, loose stools, low back and knee soreness and limpness. The pulse is bowstring and slippery, and the tongue is pale red with thin, white fur.

TREATMENT PRINCIPLES: Supplement kidney yin and yang

REPRESENTATIVE FORMULAS: In the morning, take modified *Bu Zhong Yi Qi Tang* (Supplement the Center & Boost the Qi Decoction)

Huang Qi (Astragali Membranacei, Radix), 6g
Ren Shen (Panacis Ginseng, Radix), 3g
Bai Zhu (Atractylodis Macrocephalae, Rhizoma), 3g
mix-fried *Gan Cao* (Glycyrrhizae Uralensis, Radix), 1g
Dang Gui (Angelicae Sinensis, Radix), 3g
Chen Pi (Citri Reticulatae, Pericarpium), 3g
Sheng Ma (Cimicifugae, Rhizoma), 3g
Chai Hu (Bupleuri, Radix), 3g
Dong Chong Xia Cao (Cordyceps Sinensis), 3g
Gan Jiang (Zingiberis Officinalis, dry Rhizoma), 3g

In the evening, take *Zhi Bai Di Huang Wan* (Anemarrhena & Phellodendron Rehmannia Pills)

Zhi Mu (Anemarrhenae Aspheloidis, Rhizoma), 3g
Huang Bai (Phellodendri, Cortex), 3g
Sheng Di Huang (Rehmanniae Glutinosae, uncooked Radix), 6g
Shan Zhu Yu (Corni Officinalis, Fructus), 3g
Shan Yao (Radix Dioscoreae Oppositae), 3g
Fu Ling (Poriae Cocos, Sclerotium), 3g
Ze Xie (Alismatis Orientalis, Rhizoma), 3g
Mu Dan Pi (Moutan, Cortex Radicis), 3g

NOTE: Patients presenting this pattern are close to renal failure. Therefore, one must eliminate unnecessary medicinals, use low dosages of the remaining medicinals, and carefully monitor the patient's kidney function. One can use both the above formulas, but one should focus on the more prominent vacuity. Patient's presenting this pattern frequently and quickly change from more yang vacuity to yin vacuity and vice versa. Thus one must always monitor the level of each vacuity and change the focus of treatment accordingly. The best indication of the relative vacuity of yin and yang is the condition of the tongue and pulse.

MODIFICATIONS: If the patient is edematous, add *Gui Zhi Fu Ling Wan* (Cinnamon Twig & Poria Pills) plus *Ze Lan* (Lycopi Lucidi, Herba) and *Yi Mu Cao* (Leonuri Heterophylli, Herba). For insomnia, add *He Huan Pi* (Albizziae Julibrissinis, Cortex), *Ye Jiao Teng* (Polygoni Multiflori, Caulis), and *Suan Zao Ren* (Zizyphi Spinosae, Semen). For proteinuria, add *Wu Bei Zi* (Rhois Chinensis, Galla) administered as a granular extract due to its bad taste in decoction. Some sources report success with *Shi Wei* (Pyrrosiae, Folium). One may also use *Dong Chong Xia Cao* (Cordyceps Sinensis), but the patient must avoid consuming too much protein. Please review the section on proteinuria in Part 4.

ACUMOXIBUSTION: Choose from *Tai Xi* (Ki 3), *Zhao Hai* (Ki 6), *Fu Liu* (Ki 7), *Shen Shu* (Bl 23), *Ming Men* (GV 4), and *Guan Yuan* (CV 4).

4. DAMP OBSTRUCTION

SIGNS & SYMPTOMS: A pale facial complexion,

fatigue, scanty or profuse urination, edema, abdominal distention, coma (in severe cases). The tongue has thick, slimy white or yellow fur, and the pulse is fine, slippery, or fast.

TREATMENT PRINCIPLES: Eliminate dampness, harmonize the spleen and kidney

REPRESENTATIVE FORMULA: Modified *Er Chen Tang* (Two Aged [Ingredients] Decoction)

Ban Xia (Pinelliae Ternatae, Rhizoma), 9g
Chen Pi (Citri Reticulatae, Pericarpium), 6g
Fu Ling (Poriae Cocos, Sclerotium), 9g
mix-fried *Gan Cao* (Glycyrrhizae Uralensis, Radix), 3g
Sheng Jiang (Zingiberis Officinalis, uncooked Rhizoma), 6g
Wu Mei (Pruni Mume, Fructus), 5 pieces

MODIFICATIONS: If dampness is mixed with cold, use *Shi Pi Yin* (Bolster the Spleen Beverage) instead: *Shu Fu Zi* (Aconiti Carmichaeli, Radix Lateralis Praeparatus), 30g, *Gan Jiang* (Zingiberis Officinalis, dry Rhizoma), 30g, *Fu Ling* (Poriae Cocos, Sclerotium), 30g, *Bai Zhu* (Atractylodis Macrocephalae, Rhizoma), 30g, *Mu Gua* (Chaenomelis Lagenariae, Fructus), 30g, *Hou Po* (Magnoliae Officinalis, Cortex), 30g, *Mu Xiang* (Aucklandiae Lappae, Radix), 30g, *Da Fu Pi* (Arecae Catechu, Pericarpium), 30g, *Cao Guo* (Amomi Tsao-ko, Fructus), 30g, and mix-fried *Gan Cao* (Glycyrrhizae Uralensis, Radix), 15g. Grind into a powder and take 12 gram doses as a draft with five slices of *Sheng Jiang* (Zingiberis Officinalis, uncooked Rhizoma) and one piece of *Da Zao* (Zizyphi Jujubae, Fructus).

ACUMOXIBUSTION: Choose from *Jian Shi* (Per 5), *Nei Guan* (Per 6), *Zu San Li* (St 36), *Feng Long* (St 40), *Yin Ling Quan* (Sp 9), *San Yin Jiao* (Sp 6), *Tai Bai* (Sp 3), *Zhang Men* (Liv 13), *Tai Xi* (Ki 3), *Qi Hai* (CV 6), and *Zhong Wan* (CV 12).

CLINICAL TIPS

1. Dietary therapy for any pattern of CTN:[5]

A. *Shen Yuan Tang* (Ginseng & Longan Soup).

Cook six grams of *Ren Shen* (Panacis Ginseng, Radix) and 10 pieces of *Long Yan Rou* (Euphoriae Longanae, Arillus)[6] together and take over one day. This is for anemia, heart palpitations, and insomnia.

B. *Bian Dou Shan Yao Zhu* (Dolichos & Discorea Porridge). Cook 15 grams of *Bai Bian Dou* (Dolichoris Lablab, Semen) and 30 grams of *Shan Yao* (Dioscoreae Oppositae, Radix) with 30 grams of rice to make porridge. This is for spleen qi vacuity with dampness.

C. *Lu Gen Lu Dou Zhu* (Phragmites & Mung Bean Porridge). Cook 100 grams of fresh *Lu Gen* (Phragmitis Communis, Rhizoma), 100 grams of *Lu Dou* (Phaseoli Radiati, Semen), 10 grams of *Sheng Jiang* (Zingiberis Officinalis, uncooked Rhizoma), and 15 grams of *Zi Su Ye* (Perillae Frutescentis, Folium) together to make porridge and eat over one day. This is for damp heat causing nausea. *Lu Gen* stops nausea.

D. *Tu Fu Ling Zhu Gu Tang* (Smilax & Pig Bone Soup). Cook 500 grams of the pork spine in eight cups of water down to four cups. Remove the spine and skim any oil off the top. Add 15 grams of *Tu Fu Ling* (Smilacis Glabrae, Rhizoma) and cook down to two cups. Take one cup two times per day. This is for spleen-kidney qi vacuity with dampness.

E. *Dong Chong Xia Cao* (Cordyceps Sinensis). Take three grams daily. This is for renal failure.

ENDNOTES

[1] *Mu Tong* (Akebiae Mutong, Caulis), 9g has been removed from this and other formulas because one of its ingredients, aristolochic acid, has been implicated in some cases of kidney failure.
[2] Qing Guo-hong, *Shen Zhang Bing Zhen Duan Zhi Liao* (*The Diagnosis and Treatment of Kidney Disease*), Guangdong Science & Technology Publishing Company, Guangzhou, 2001, p. 196
[3] *Ibid.*, p. 196
[4] *Ibid.*, p. 196
[5] *Ibid.*, p. 207
[6] *Long Yan Rou* (Euphoriae Longanae, Arillus) is also known as *Gui Yuan*.

Polycystic kidney disease (PKD) is a genetic disorder marked by progressive cystic growth in the kidneys. These cysts are filled with fluid and can slowly replace much of the mass of the kidneys, reducing kidney function and leading to kidney failure. Polycystic kidney disease can also cause cysts in the liver and problems in other organs, such as the heart and blood vessels in the brain. These complications help doctors distinguish PKD from the usually harmless "simple" cysts that often form in the kidneys in later years of life.

NOSOLOGY

There are two types of inherited PKD, and one type of noninherited PKD. The two types of inherited PKD are autosomal dominant polycystic kidney disease (ADPKD) and autosomal recessive polycystic kidney disease (ARPKD). Of these two types, autosomal dominant is the more common. Acquired cystic kidney disease (ACKD) develops in association with long-term kidney problems, especially in patients who have kidney failure and who have been on dialysis for a long time. Even though it is not a genetic condition and we defined PKD above as a genetic disorder, it is still generally considered a form of PKD.

EPIDEMIOLOGY

In the United States, about 600,000 people have PKD, while 12.5 million people suffer from this condition worldwide. Its incidence is unrelated to sex, race, or ethnic origin. Autosomal dominant polycystic kidney disease affects one in 400 to one in 1,000 adults. Autosomal recessive polycystic kidney disease affects one in 10,000 and at a far younger age, including newborns, infants, and children. Thus it is sometimes referred to as infantile PKD. The onset of ADPKD is slow and symptoms are generally not noticed until middle-age, i.e., the fourth and fifth decades. Therefore, this form of PKD is sometimes referred to as adult polycystic kidney disease (APKD). In all forms of PKD, as the cysts grow within the renal structures, they have the potential to compromise kidney function. Approximately 50% of those with PKD will develop renal failure and need dialysis. Polycystic kidney disease is the most common genetic disease in the United States and is the fourth leading cause of kidney failure.

ETIOLOGY & PATHOPHYSIOLOGY

In 1994, the European Polycystic Kidney Disease Consortium isolated a gene from chromosome 16 that was disrupted in a family with adult polycystic kidney disease. The protein encoded by the PKD1 gene is an integral membrane protein involved in cell-cell interactions and cell-matrix interactions. Since then, it has been established that mutations in at least three genes play a role in PKD. The role of PKD1 in the normal cell may be linked to micro-tubule-mediated functions, such as the placement of Na(+), K(+)-ATPase ion pumps in the membrane. Programmed cell death, or apoptosis, may also be invoked in APKD. Further clarification of the patho-genesis of the disease await further research. The so-called "cpk mouse" is a well-known model for the human disease, and studying the molecular basis of this disease in this mouse is expected to provide a better understanding of the human disease which is hoped to lead to more effective therapies.

SYMPTOMATOLOGY

Patients with PKD are most affected by back and side pain and have frequent headaches. Polycystic kidney disease cysts may migrate to a number of different organs, including the brain, liver, heart, and intestines. In addi-tion, patients may present with urinary tract infections, hematuria, or kidney stones. Hypertension is common especially as the cysts weaken the kidney function.

DIAGNOSIS

The diagnosis of PKD is dependent on establishing bilateral renal cysts and enlargement. Therefore, imaging of the kidneys is the main way that practi-tioners of Western medicine diagnose this disease. If there is a parental history of PKD, gene linkage stud-ies may be performed to determine if the disease is present in the children. This is an expensive diag-nostic option and is not readily done. More fre-quently, a patient will present with symptoms with-out knowledge of family history, and a screening diagnosis will be made by ultrasound. Often, CT scan or MRI is used to look for possible cerebral aneurysms. Initially diagnosis will be made to distin-guish multiple bilateral cysts and tuberous sclerosis from multiple simple cyst disease. With childhood onset of PKD, examination is made of the liver to identify possible congenital hepatic fibrosis.

DIFFERENTIAL DIAGNOSIS

Multiple simple cyst disease
Hydronephrosis, for instance, due to retroperitoneal fibrosis
Tuberous sclerosis
Von Hippel-Lindau syndrome

WESTERN MEDICAL TREATMENT

Conventional Western medical treatment for PKD focuses on nutrition, pain management, and control of urinary tract infections and hypertension. Dietary changes are meant to reduce the strain on the kidneys to reduce waste, with low protein recommendations being the norm. Recent developments in pain man-agement include the use of laparoscopic surgery to col-lapse the cysts. Analgesic medications are prescribed with great caution due to the decreased ability of the kidneys to metabolize these drugs. Patients with PKD may be considered candidates for transplant surgery.

PROGNOSIS & COMPLICATIONS

As stated above, PKD also affects other organs. The liver may develop cysts secondary to the kidneys and have impaired function. The incidence of mitral valve pro-lapse increases in patients with PKD, as do both inguinal and umbilical hernias. Cerebral aneurysms are also common and may have a familial tendency. Ultimately, the most serious complication of PKD is renal failure.

CHINESE MEDICAL DISEASE CATEGORIZATION

In Chinese medicine, the clinical manifestations of PKD correspond to the following traditional disease categories: bloody urine, lumbar pain, rib-side pain, accumulations and gatherings, vacuity taxation, and dizziness.

TREATMENT BASED ON PATTERN IDENTIFICATION

1. COLD DAMP STAGNATION

SIGNS & SYMPTOMS: Chest oppression, abdominal distention, low back soreness, a pale facial complexion, lack of appetite, bloating after meals, loose stools or diarrhea, edema in the lower extremities. The tongue is pale, puffy, or has teeth-marks on its edges and white, slimy fur. The pulse is soggy and slow or deep, fine, and slippery.

The chest oppression, abdominal distention, bloating after meals, loose stools or diarrhea, and edema in the lower extremities are a result of dampness. The pale face, low back soreness, and lack of appetite are a result of spleen-kidney vacuity. The tongue and pulse reflect the cold and dampness.

TREATMENT PRINCIPLES: Warm yang, transform dampness, and disperse stagnation

REPRESENTATIVE FORMULA: Modified *Er Chen Tang* (Two Aged [Ingredients] Decoction)

Ban Xia (Pinelliae Ternatae, Rhizoma), 9g
Chen Pi (Citri Reticulatae, Pericarpium), 6g
mix-fried *Gan Cao* (Glycyrrhizae Uralensis, Radix), 3g
Sheng Jiang (Zingiberis Officinalis, uncooked Rhizoma), 6g
Wu Mei (Pruni Mume, Fructus), 5 pieces
Xiang Fu (Cyperi Rotundi, Rhizoma), 9g
Dong Chong Xia Cao (Cordyceps Sinensis), 3g
Shu Di Huang (Rehmanniae Glutinosae, uncooked Radix), 9g

MODIFICATIONS: To rectify the qi more, add *Qing Pi* (Citri Reticulatae Viride, Pericarpium), *Mu Xiang* (Aucklandiae Lappae, Radix), and/or *Jie Geng* (Platycodi Grandiflori, Radix). Add *San Qi* (Notoginseng, Radix) to dispel stasis, and *Xiang Fu* (Cyperi Rotundi, Rhizoma) to warm and open the channels. If there are loose stools due to spleen vacuity, add *Dang Shen* (Codonopsitis Pilosulae, Radix), *Bai Zhu* (Atractylodis Macrocephalae, Rhizoma), *Bai Bian Dou* (Dolichoris Lablab, Semen), *Shen Qu* (Massa Medica Fermentata), and *Lian Zi* (Nelumbinis Nuciferae, Semen). If there is low back soreness due to kidney vacuity, add *Gan Jiang* (Zingiberis Officinalis, dry Rhizoma), *Yin Yang Huo* (Epimedii, Herba), and *Gou Ji* (Cibotii Barometsis, Rhizoma).

ACUMOXIBUSTION: Choose points to needle from *Yin Ling Guan* (Sp 9), *Zu San Li* (St 36), *Zhong Ji* (CV 3), *San Yin Jiao* (Sp 6), *Xue Hai* (Sp 10), *Ge Shu* (Bl 17), *Pang Guang Shu* (Bl 28), and *Shui Fen* (CV 9). Also moxibustion *Shen Shu* (Bl 23), *Ming Men* (GV 4), *Pi Shu* (Bl 20), and *Guan Yuan* (CV 4).

2. QI STAGNATION & BLOOD STASIS

SIGNS & SYMPTOMS: Very low body weight, facial edema, abdominal and low back distention and pain. Patients feel an uneven lump in their abdomen. The lump may even push the lung, causing difficult breathing and difficulty lying down. The tongue is pale and dark purple and the pulse is choppy.

TREATMENT PRINCIPLES: Quicken the blood and transform stasis, soften the hard and scatter nodulation

REPRESENTATIVE FORMULA: Modified *Bie Jia Jian Wan* (Carapax Amydae Decocted Pills)

Dong Chong Xia Cao (Cordyceps Sinensis), 3g
Ren Shen (Panacis Ginseng, Radix), 7-9g
Bie Jia (Amydae Sinensis, Carapax), 9g
Sheng Di Huang (Rehmanniae Glutinosae, uncooked Radix), 3g
Shu Di Huang (Rehmanniae Glutinosae, cooked Radix), 9g
Mu Dan Pi (Moutan, Cortex Radicis), 5g
Bai Shao (Paeoniae Lactiflorae, Radix Albus), 5g
Bai Zhu (Atractylodis Macrocephalae, Rhizoma), 9g
Tao Ren (Pruni Persicae, Semen), 6g
San Qi (Notoginseng, Radix), 3g
Chi Shao (Paeoniae Lactiflorae, Radix Rubrus), 4g
Chai Hu (Bupleuri, Radix), 2g
Xiang Fu (Cyperi Rotundi, Rhizoma), 4g

MODIFICATIONS: If there is egregious qi and blood vacuity, add *Huang Qi* (Astragali Membranacei, Radix). If there is dark blood in the urine with clots, add *Han Lian Cao* (Ecliptae Prostratae, Herba), *Pu Huang* (Pollen, Typhae), and *Xian He Cao* (Agrimoniae Pilosae, Herba).

COMMENTARY: In this pattern, true qi vacuity underlies the qi stagnation, blood stasis with kidney channel obstruction, and damp stagnation. Supplementation is still the key, dispersing too strongly will cause more vacuity and more damp stagnation.

ACUMOXIBUSTION: Choose from *He Gu* (LI 4), *Tai Chong* (Liv 3), *San Yin Jiao* (Sp 6), *Xue Hai* (Sp 10), *Ge Shu* (Bl 17), and *Shen Shu* (Bl 23).

3. TRUE (QI) VACUITY WITH EVIL REPLETION

SIGNS & SYMPTOMS: Feeling extremely cold, low appetite, emaciation, a dark face, edema, nausea, and vomiting. The abdomen has a big, hard mass that is tender upon pressure. Urination is difficult and profuse. The tongue is puffy and pale and the pulse is deep and fine.

TREATMENT PRINCIPLES: Supplement qi, blood, yin, and yang, expel evils and transform stasis

REPRESENTATIVE FORMULAS: If there is yang vacuity, use augmented *You Gui Wan* (Restore the Right [Kidney] Pills).

Shu Fu Zi (Aconiti Carmichaeli, Radix Lateralis Praeparatus), 3g
Rou Gui (Cinnamonmi Casiae, Cortex), 3g
Lu Jiao Jiao (Cervi, Gelatinum Cornu), 9g
Shu Di Huang (Rehmanniae Glutinosae, cooked Radix), 12g
Shan Zhu Yu (Corni Officinalis, Fructus), 6-9g
Gou Qi Zi (Lycii Chinensis, Fructus), 9g
Tu Si Zi (Cuscutae Chinensis, Semen), 9g
Du Zhong (Eucommiae Ulmoidis, Cortex), 9g
Dang Gui (Angelicae Sinensis, Radix), 6-9g
Dong Chong Xia Cao (Cordyceps Sinensis), 6-9g
Ban Xia (Pinelliae Ternatae, Rhizoma), 6g
Xiang Fu (Cyperi Rotundi, Rhizoma), 6g

If there is yin vacuity, use *Zuo Gui Wan* (Restore the Left [Kidney] Pill)

Shu Di Huang (Rehmanniae Glutinosae, cooked Radix), 12g
Shan Yao (Radix Dioscoreae Oppositae), 9g
Gou Qi Zi (Lycii Chinensis, Fructus), 9g
Shan Zhu Yu (Corni Officinalis, Fructus), 120g
Chuan Niu Xi (Cyathulae, Radix), 6g
Tu Si Zi (Cuscutae Chinensis, Semen), 9g
Lu Jiao Jiao (Cervi, Gelatinum Cornu), 9g
Gui Ban Jiao (Testudinis, Gelatinum Plastri), 9g
Dong Chong Xia Cao (Cordyceps Sinensis), 6-9g

Ban Xia (Pinelliae Ternatae, Rhizoma), 6g
Xiang Fu (Cyperi Rotundi, Rhizoma), 6g

MODIFICATIONS: Usually, one can add *San Qi* (Notoginseng, Radix) and *Dang Gui* (Angelicae Sinensis, Radix) to either of the above formulas. These medicinals disperse stagnation but will not cause more vacuity or make the patient fatigued. If there is serious cold add *Gan Jiang* (Zingiberis Officinalis, dry Rhizoma) and *Fu Zi* (Aconiti Carmichaeli, Radix Lateralis Praeparatus). For yin vacuity with ascendant yang, add *Ju Hua* (Chrysanthemi Morifolii, Flos), *Bie Jia* (Amydae Sinensis, Carapax), *Gui Ban* (Testudinis, Plastrum), *Bai Shao* (Paeoniae Lactiflorae, Radix Albus), *Huai Niu Xi* (Achyranthis Bidentatae, Radix), and/or *He Shou Wu* (Polygoni Multiflori, Radix). These medicinals subdue yang and nourish yin. If yin vacuity heat burns the network vessels causing scanty urine with streaks of blood, add *Huang Bai* (Phellodendri, Cortex), *Zhi Mu* (Anemarrhenae Asphodeloidis, Rhizoma), *Han Lian Cao* (Ecliptae Prostratae, Herba), *Bai Mao Gen* (Imperatae Cylindricae, Rhizoma), and *Xiao Ji* (Cephalanoplos Segeti, Herba) to cool blood and stop bleeding. If there are concurrent liver cysts, add *Chai Hu* (Bupleuri, Radix), *Yu Jin* (Curcumae, Tuber), *Yuan Hu Suo* (Corydalis Yanhusuo, Rhizoma), *Zhi Ke* (Citri Aurantii, Fructus), and *Xiang Fu* (Cyperi Rotundi, Rhizoma) to disperse the qi and stop pain.

ACUMOXIBUSTION: Choose from *Shen Shu* (Bl 23), *Tai Xi* (Ki 3), *Zu San Li* (St 36), *Qi Hai* (CV 6), *Guan Yuan* (CV 4), *San Yin Jiao* (Sp 6), *Ge Shu* (Bl 17), *Xue Hai* (Sp 10), *He Gu* (LI 4), and *Tai Chong* (Liv 3).

Case history from Dr. Wei Li's private practice: Ynez, a 44 year-old female

Ynez's first visit was in February 2002. Her diagnosis was polycystic kidney disease. Ultrasound showed that both kidneys were enlarged with cysts. It also showed that the liver had three cysts, one 7 by 11 centimeters and two other small ones. The large liver cyst caused severe pain and Ynez was unable to work. Her blood work and kidney function were normal. Ynez's tongue was puffy and pale purple with moderately thick, white fur. Her pulse was bowstring, forceless, and vacuous. Based on these signs and symptoms, Dr. Li's pattern identification was true vacuity with evil repletion and qi, blood, and damp stagnation in the kidney and liver. Her prescription was modified *You Gui Wan* (Restore the Right [Kidney] Pills): *Dong Chong Xia Cao* (Cordyceps Sinensis), 3g, *Sheng Di Huang* (Rehmanniae Glutinosae, uncooked Radix), 6g, *Shu Di Huang* (Rehmanniae Glutinosae, cooked Radix), 14g, *Chi Shao* (Paeoniae Lactiflorae, Radix Rubrus), 5g, *Bai Shao* (Paeoniae Lactiflorae, Radix Albus), 4g, *Xiang Fu* (Cyperi Rotundi, Rhizoma), 5g, *Xuan Shen* (Scrophulariae Ningpoensis, Radix), 6g, *Mu Li* (Ostreae, Concha), 9g, *Dang Gui* (Angelicae Sinensis, Radix), 5g, *Gui Ban* (Testudinis, Plastrum), 7g, *Gui Zhi* (Cinnamomi Cassiae, Ramulus), 3g, *Fu Ling* (Poriae Cocos, Sclerotium), 9g, *Shan Zhu Yu* (Corni Officinalis, Fructus), 7g, *Shan Yao* (Radix Dioscoreae Oppositae), 9g, *Yin Yang Huo* (Epimedii, Herba), 7g, and *Tu Si Zi* (Cuscutae Chinensis, Semen), 5g. Ynez took this formula for one week and felt her pain remarkably reduced. After two weeks, her pain was gone. Ynez took variations of this formula for two months. Ultrasound showed the biggest liver cyst had reduced in size by one-third. Although there was little change in her kidneys, Ynez felt good, her energy was good, and she had no pain. At the time of this writing, she has returned to work and is continuing to take variations of this formula.

CLINICAL TIPS

1. In Chinese medicine, polycystic kidney disease is often discussed under accumulations and gatherings. Accumulations and gatherings can be caused by external evils or internal damage and are usually identified as qi stagnation, dampness, phlegm, and/or blood stasis. However, these patterns are the tip. The root is true qi vacuity and visceral disharmony. *Ling Shu*, Chapter 81, "*Yong Ju* (Welling & Flat Abscesses)" states, "If cold invades a channel, the channel will become obstructed and the blood becomes stagnant . . ." Again, in Chapter 62 of the *Su Wen*, "*Tiao Jing Lun*" (Treatise on Regulating the Channels)," it states, ". . . replete evils in the grandchild network vessels may overflow and cause the retention of blood in the network vessels." Chapter 11 of the *Jin Gui Yao Lue* states:

Accumulations are a disease of the viscera. They do not change their location. Gatherings are a disease of the bowels with sporadic attacks and changes of location.

The *Jing Yue Quan Shu* (*Jing Yue's Complete Book*) states that accumulation and gathering diseases can be caused by diet, qi stagnation, blood stasis, wind, and cold.

Nevertheless, in diseases with accumulations and gatherings, there is a combination of true qi vacuity and evil repletion. Therefore, one must combine strategies, supporting the righteous while dispelling evils. (In this instance, dispelling evils equates to dispersing the accumulations and gatherings.) True qi vacuity is the major cause of accumulations and gatherings and supporting the righteous is the most important treatment principle. However, one must use a combined treatment strategy in all stages of PKD even while emphasizing supporting the righteous.

2. Dr. Li has treated adult PKD, successfully stabilizing the size of the cysts and even significantly reducing their size in some cases. In her experience, one must employ three key strategies. First, one must emphasize supplementation. Polycystic kidney disease patients generally have former heaven kidney essence vacuity that leads to damp accumulation and, ultimately, to kidney cysts. Medicinals that boost the qi, nourish the blood, and supplement kidney yin and yang must constitute 60-70% of one's formula.

Second, one must transform stasis instead of simply quickening the blood and rectifying the qi. The latter uses mild stasis-dispelling, blood-quickening and qi-rectifying medicinals and may actually weaken PKD patients, thus resulting in greater stasis and stagnation. In PKD, there is a substantial accumulation, not just stagnant qi. One must break up and dissolve this accumulation, not just move the humors around the area of the accumulation. Transforming stasis accomplishes this by using stronger stasis-dispelling, blood-quickening medicinals, such as *Yi Mu Cao* (Leonuri Heterophylli, Herba), *Dan Shen* (Salviae Miltiorrhizae, Radix), *San Qi* (Notoginseng, Radix),

Tao Ren (Pruni Persicae, Semen), *San Leng* (Sparganii Stoloniferi, Rhizoma), *E Zhu* (Curcumae Zedoariae, Rhizoma), and *Xue Jie* (Draconis, Sanguis). The best single medicinal is *San Qi*. This medicinal transforms stasis without causing bleeding or greater stasis. One may strengthen the effect of *San Qi* by combining it with other medicinals that transform stasis and rectify the qi or with medicinals that supplement the qi and blood. Both of these strategies are important in treatment. One must support the righteous and transform stasis. However, one must be extremely careful with any medicinals that have the potential of weakening the patient. The rate at which cysts are stabilized or reduced is directly dependent on the patient's health and strength. The best guide to the relative strength of the patient, their righteous qi, or the presence of evils at any point in the course of treatment is the patient's tongue and pulse.

Third, do not use water-disinhibiting, dampness-percolating medicinals. These cause water to move, but, since the water has no easy exit, their use may just increase the size of the cysts.

3. When dispersing accumulations and gatherings, the treatment principles are to rectify the qi, transform stasis, and transform phlegm. Dr. Li has designed a basic formula that accomplishes this treatment strategy by modifying *Er Chen Tang* (Two Aged [Ingredients] Decoction): *Ban Xia* (Pinelliae Ternatae, Rhizoma), 9g, *Chen Pi* (Citri Reticulatae, Pericarpium), 6g, mix-fried *Gan Cao* (Glycyrrhizae Uralensis, Radix), 3g, *Sheng Jiang* (Zingiberis Officinalis, uncooked Rhizoma), 6g, *Wu Mei* (Pruni Mume, Fructus), 5 pieces, *Xiang Fu* (Cyperi Rotundi, Rhizoma), 9g, *Dong Chong Xia Cao* (Cordyceps Sinensis), 3g, *Shu Di Huang* (Rehmanniae Glutinosae, cooked Radix), 9g, *Du Zhong* (Eucommiae Ulmoidis, Cortex), 9g, *San Qi* (Notoginseng, Radix), 3g, *Dang Gui* (Angelicae Sinensis, Radix), 6g, *Shan Yao* (Radix Dioscoreae Oppositae), 9g, and *Bai Zhu* (Atractylodis Macrocephalae, Rhizoma), 9g. One should further modify this formula by adding additional medicinals that supplement kidney yin and yang and medicinals that transform stasis.

4. Caution: The causes of this disease are the affects, overexertion, taxation fatigue, and improper diet. Any of these can also exacerbate the symptoms. A good diet is especially important. Food should be fresh and nutritious. Too much salt and protein can burden the kidney. The patient needs to limit protein and salt intake and may have to eliminate salt entirely. The patient must also be careful to avoid trauma to the cyst, which might cause it to burst.

PART 4

INTEGRATING WESTERN & CHINESE MEDICINE

EDEMA

Edema is an abnormal accumulation of body fluids in the intercellular spaces. It can be caused by a variety of factors, including hypoproteinemia, poor lymphatic drainage, increased capillary permeability (*i.e.*, as in inflammatory responses), and congestive heart failure. The Western concept of edema is roughly equivalent to water swelling in Chinese medicine. Signs and symptoms are similar in both medicines, although theories about etiology and pathophysiology are poles apart. Please see Part 2, Chapter 5 for a discussion of water swelling.

Su Wen, Chapter 14, "*Tang Ye Lao Li Lun* (On Rice Soup, Aged & Sweet Wine)" indicates the therapeutic principles for water swelling:

> In treating this condition, one should eliminate water by dispelling static blood and make the patient exercise his extremities gently to cause the yang qi to spread gradually . . . Then strongly promote sweating and free the flow of urination.

Therefore, according to the authors of the *Nei Jing (Inner Classic)*, the most important treatment principles for water swelling are: 1) to eliminate water by dispelling stagnant blood, 2) to strongly promote sweating, and 3) to free the flow of urination.

1. ELIMINATE WATER BY DISPELLING STATIC BLOOD

Edema often presents patterns of dampness and/or blood stasis at the tip. Damp heat causes obstruction of the water passageways with water accumulation and stagnation. If the disease progresses, damp heat impediment eventually causes qi stagnation and blood stasis. (In the chronic stage, even if the damp heat has been cleared, the qi stagnation and blood stasis remain.) Yang qi propels water. As expressed in the saying, "If qi moves, water moves." Therefore, if qi and blood are stagnant, water accumulates and stagnates. Water accumulation blocks the qi, thus causing even greater qi stagnation and blood stasis. Moreover, blood stasis hinders the formation of new blood, causing more blood vacuity. The result is egregious qi stagnation and blood stasis with qi and blood vacuity. Qi and blood vacuity cause righteous qi vacuity and damp heat may easily invade again. This becomes a vicious cycle. (See Figure 4.1.) To break this cycle, one must use qi-rectifying and blood-quickening, stasis-dispelling medicinals.

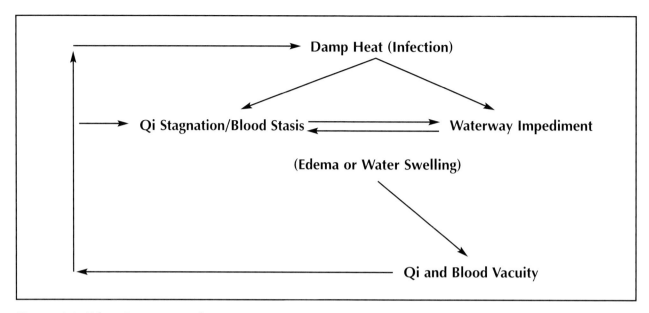

Figure 4.1. Edema's vicious cycle

When a patient with edema has blood and casts in the urine, this indicates that blood stasis has caused the blood to be diverted from its normal course to the urinary tract. On the other hand, if there is only protein in the urine, this may indicate that there is only vacuity. In most cases, however, there is still some qi stagnation and blood stasis. In all edema with blood stasis, quickening the blood and dispelling stasis is necessary to fully eliminate the edema, and the most important medicinals for eliminating water by dispelling stasis are *Yi Mu Cao* (Leonuri Heterophylli, Herba) and *Ze Lan* (Lycopi Lucidi, Herba). Their usual dosage is nine grams per day. Both of these have the functions of dispersing blood, percolating dampness, and dispersing (water) swelling. In addition, *Yi Mu Cao* regulates the menstruation. Other important medicinals that quicken the blood and dispel stasis are *Tao Ren* (Pruni Persicae, Semen), *Chuan Xiong* (Ligustici Wallichii, Radix), *Dang Gui* (Angelicae Sinensis, Radicis), and *Dan Shen* (Salviae Miltiorrhizae, Radix). In severe cases, one can use the "insect" or 'worm" products *Shui Zhi* (Hirudo Seu Whitmania) and *Di Long* (Lumbricus).

ACUMOXIBUSTION: Choose from *He Gu* (LI 4), *Tai Chong* (Liv 3), *Ge Shu* (Bl 17), *Xue Hai* (Sp 10), *Yin Ling Quan* (Sp 9), *Yang Ling Quan* (GB 34), *Pang Guan Shu* (Bl 28), *Zhong Ji* (CV 3).

Case history of Dr. He Ho-ling: Xu, a four year-old boy[1]

Xu had suffered chronic nephritis for over one year. Three months previous to his first visit, he caught a cold. This elicited a recurrence of the nephritis. He had edema over his entire body, a pale facial complexion, fatigue, abdominal bloating, loose stools, and scanty urination. His tongue was pale with thin white fur and purple stasis speckles on the sides. His pulse was fine and deep. Dr. He's pattern identification was spleen-kidney yang vacuity with water stagnation. His formula consisted of: *Dang Shen* (Codonopsitis Pilosulae, Radix), 9g, *Bai Zhu* (Atractylodis Macrocephalae, Rhizoma), 9g, *Yi Yi Ren* (Coicis Lachryma-jobi, Semen), 9g, *Chi Xiao Dou* (Phaseoli Calcarati, Semen), 9g, *Huang Qi* (Astragali Membranacei, Radix), 9g, *Dan Shen* (Salviae Miltiorrhizae, Radix), 9g, *Rou Gui* (Cinnamonmi Casiae, Cortex), 3g, *Bai Hua She She Cao* (Oldenlandiae Diffusae, Herba), 15g, *Ban Bian Lian* (Lobeliae Chinensis, Herba Cum Radice), 15g, *Pu Gong Ying* (Taraxaci Mongolici, Herba Cum Radice), 5g, and *Gan Cao* (Glycyrrhizae Uralensis, Radix), 2g.

Xu took this formula for 15 days, but there was no change in the edema. Urinalysis showed his urine protein at 3+ and WBCs at 0-6. Dr. He realized he had underestimated the importance of blood stasis in Xu's disease. To address the blood stasis, he removed *Pu Gong Ying* and *Yi Yi Ren* from his prescription and added *Fu Zi* (Aconiti Carmichaeli, Radix Lateralis Praeparatus), 5g, *Yi Mu Cao* (Leonuri Heterophylli, Herba), 9g, and *Tao Ren* (Pruni Persicae, Semen), 7g. Xu took this new formula for seven days and his edema completely dissipated. His urine protein went down to 1+, and his urine WBCs returned to normal. To consolidate the treatment, Dr. He advised Xu to take *Jin Gui Shen Qi Wan* (*Golden Cabinet* Kidney Qi Pills). Xu took this formula for six months and completely recovered. His urinalysis was taken three times and was always negative. A follow-up one and a half years later showed no recurrence.

2. STRONGLY PROMOTE SWEATING

This treatment principle uses the sweating method to open the lung. The lung governs the water passageways and is the upper source of water. The lung must function properly for urine to flow unobstructed. (It may be noted that animals that eliminate urine through a bladder and urethra generally have lungs.) A simile, mentioned above, involves a teapot. Ancient potters found that a teapot's lid must be made with a hole in it to allow the tea to flow out of the spout unobstructed.[2] The lung is like the hole in the teapot's lid. All formulas that open the pores and promote sweating also open the lungs. This, in turn, promotes the free flow of urine. Representative formulas that strongly promote sweating for acute edema include *Yue Bi Tang* (Maidservant from Yue Decoction) and *Ma Huang Lian Qiao Chi Xiao Dou Tang* (Ephedra, Forsythia & Red Bean Decoction).

Yue Bi Tang (Maidservant from Yue Decoction)

Ma Huang (Ephedrae, Herba), 9g
Shi Gao (Gypsum Fibrosum), 48g
Sheng Jiang (Zingiberis Officinalis, Rhizoma), 9g
Gan Cao (Glycyrrhizae Uralensis, Radix), 6g
Da Zao (Zizyphi Jujubae, Fructus), 10 pieces

Ma Huang Lian Qiao Chi Xiao Dou Tang (Ephedra Forsythia & Red Bean Decoction)

Ma Huang (Ephedrae, Herba), 6g

Lian Qiao (Forsythiae Suspensae, Fructus), 6g
Chi Xiao Dou (Phaseoli Calcarati, Semen), 18g
Sang Bai Pi (Mori Albi, Cortex Radicis), 9g
Xing Ren (Pruni Armeniacae, Semen), 6g
Da Zao (Zizyphi Jujubae, Fructus), 3 pieces
Sheng Jiang (Zingiberis Officinalis, uncooked Rhizoma), 6g
Gan Cao (Glycyrrhizae Uralensis, Radix), 6g

Because *Ma Huang* may cause negative side effects, one may substitute *Fu Ping* (Lemnae Seu Spirodelae, Herba) at 10-15g per day.

ACUMOXIBUSTION: *He Gu* (LI 4), *Wai Guan* (TB 5), and *Fu Liu* (Ki 7).

Case history 1: Huang, a 12 year-old boy [3]

Huang's first visit was in April 1980. Previously, he had caught cold and had chills, fever, and a sore throat for a week. Subsequently, his whole body became edematous. Urinalysis showed protein 2+ and RBCs 2+. Granular casts were 0-1. The Western medical diagnosis was acute nephritis. Huang was referred to a Chinese medical clinic for treatment to which Huang presented with symptoms of fever without sweating, sore throat, generalized edema, yellow, scanty urination, and constipation. His tongue had thin, yellow, slimy fur and his pulse was floating and fast. The Chinese medical diagnosis was wind heat kidney wind. The treatment strategy was to clear and diffuse the lung, transform water, and percolate dampness. The prescription was *Ma Huang Lian Qiao Chi Xiao Dou Tang* (Ephedra, Forsythia & Red Bean Decoction) plus *Huang Lian Jie Du Tang* (Coptis Toxin-resolving Decoction) with modifications: *Ma Huang* (Ephedrae, Herba), 10g, *Lian Qiao* (Forsythiae Suspensae, Fructus), 20g, *Sang Bai Pi* (Mori Albi, Cortex Radicis), 20g, *Xing Ren* (Pruni Armeniacae, Semen), 8g, *Huang Qin* (Scutellariae Baicalensis, Radix), 10g, *Zhi Zi* (Gardeniae Jasminoidis, Fructus), 10g, *Da Huang* (Rhei, Radix Et Rhizoma), 5g, *Jie Geng* (Platycodi Grandiflori, Radix), 15g, *Bo He* (Menthae Haplocalycis, Herba), 10g, uncooked *Gan Cao* (Glycyrrhizae Uralensis, Radix), 8g, and *Chi Xiao Dou* (Phaseoli Calcarati, Semen), 20g. After two days, Huang experienced a slight sweat over his entire body and his fever came down. He was able to pass more urine, the edema greatly decreased, and his constipation abated. His doctor then removed *Da Huang* from Huang's prescription. After taking this altered prescription for two days, the edema completely dissipated. His doctor then gave him a new prescription to harmonize the middle burner and clear heat. He took this last prescription for three weeks and had a complete recovery.

3. FREE THE FLOW OF URINATION

The most important route of elimination for the excess fluids in edema is through urination. Therefore, it is vitally important that urination be free-flowing or disinhibited. Representative formulas for freeing the flow of urination include *Wu Ling San* (Five [Ingredients] Poria Powder), *Fang Ji Huang Qi Tang* (Stephania & Astragalus Decoction), *Huang Qi Chi Xiao Dou Tang* (Astragalus & Red Bean Decoction), *Shi Pi Yin* (Bolster the Spleen Beverage), and *Zhen Wu Tang* (True Warrior Decoction).

Wu Ling San (Five [Ingredients] Poria Powder)

Ze Xie (Alismatis Orientalis, Rhizoma), 9g
Fu Ling (Poriae Cocos, Sclerotium), 9-12g
Zhu Ling (Polypori Umbellati, Sclerotium), 9g
Bai Zhu (Atractylodis Macrocephalae, Rhizoma), 9-12g
Gui Zhi (Cinnamomi Cassiae, Ramulus), 6-9g

Fang Ji Huang Qi Tang (Stephania & Astragalus Decoction)

Huang Qi (Astragali Membranacei, Radix), 9-12g
Han Fang Ji (Stephaniae Tetrandrae, Radix), 9g
Bai Zhu (Atractylodis Macrocephalae, Rhizoma), 9-12g
mix-fried *Gan Cao* (Glycyrrhizae Uralensis, Radix), 3g
Sheng Jiang (Zingiberis Officinalis, uncooked Rhizoma), 4 pieces
Da Zao (Zizyphi Jujubae, Fructus), 3 pieces

Huang Qi Chi Xiao Dou Tang (Astragalus & Red Bean Decoction)

Huang Qi (Astragali Membranacei, Radix), 100g

Chi Xiao Dou (Phaseoli Calcarati, Semen), 30g, cooked at a low temperature until completely soft

Shi Pi Yin (Bolster the Spleen Beverage)

Shu Fu Zi (Aconiti Carmichaeli, Radix Lateralis Praeparatus), 3g
Gan Jiang (Zingiberis Officinalis, dry Rhizoma), 3g
Fu Ling (Poriae Cocos, Sclerotium), 9g
Bai Zhu (Atractylodis Macrocephalae, Rhizoma), 9g
Mu Gua (Chaenomelis Lagenariae, Fructus), 9g
Hou Po (Magnoliae Officinalis, Cortex), 9g
Mu Xiang (Aucklandiae Lappae, Radix), 3g
Da Fu Pi (Arecae Catechu, Pericarpium), 9g
Cao Guo (Amomi Tsao-ko, Fructus), 3g
mix-fried *Gan Cao* (Glycyrrhizae Uralensis, Radix), 3g
Sheng Jiang (Zingiberis Officinalis, uncooked Rhizoma), 5 slices
Da Zao (Zisyphi Jujubae, Fructus), 5 pieces

Zhen Wu Tang (True Warrior Decoction)

Shu Fu Zi (Aconiti Carmichaeli, Radix Lateralis Praeparatus), 9g
Bai Zhu (Atractylodis Macrocephalae, Rhizoma), 6g
Fu Ling (Poriae Cocos, Sclerotium), 9g
Bai Shao (Paeoniae Lactiflorae, Radix Albus), 9g
Sheng Jiang (Zingiberis Officinalis, uncooked Rhizoma), 9g

An important single medicinal is *Yu Mi Xu* (Zeae Maydis, Stylus). The dosage of this medicinal must be decided on a case to case basis.

Typically, 3-6 months constitutes one course of treatment. Goat milk is important in Chinese dietary therapy. Drinking goat milk, 500ml twice a day for 3-5 weeks, can reduce edema and lower blood pressure. However, because goat milk has a high-protein content, it is contraindicated if the patient has a high BUN or renal failure.

ACUMOXIBUSTION: Choose from *San Yin Jiao* (Sp 6), *Yin Ling Quan* (Sp 9), *Zhong Ji* (CV 3), *Guan Yuan* (CV 4), *Qi Hai* (CV 6), *Fu Liu* (Ki 7), *Shen Shu* (Bl 23), and *Pang Guan Shu* (Bl 28).

Case history of Dr. Ke Wan-chen: Yong, a 45 year-old male[4]

Yong had suffered chronic nephritis for 10 years. He was treated for half a year without any change in the abnormal level of his urine protein. He had edema in both legs and his kidney function was compromised. Dr. Ke prescribed *Huang Qi Chi Xiao Dou Tang* (Astragalus & Red Bean Decoction): *Huang Qi* (Astragali Membranacei, Radix), 100g, *Chi Xiao Dou* (Phaseoli Calcarati, Semen), 30g, cooked at a low temperature until completely soft. This formula was divided into two servings and taken twice a day. Yong took this formula every day for approximately one and a half months. His edema completely dissipated and his proteinuria disappeared. Then he continued on it for another month and a half to consolidate the results. Yong recovered completely. In fact he passed his entrance exam for graduate school and became a college teacher. Follow-up examinations once a year revealed no recurrence.

PROTEINURIA

Proteinuria is an abnormal amount of protein in the urine.

> The major mechanisms producing proteinuria are elevated plasma concentrations of normal or abnormal proteins . . . increased tubular cell secretion . . . decreased tubular resorption of normal filtered proteins; and an increase of filtered proteins caused by altered glomerular capillary permeability.

> In adults, proteinuria is usually found incidentally during a routine physical examination. Proteinuria may be intermittent, orthostatic (occurring only when upright), or constant (persistent). Most patients with intermittent or orthostatic proteinuria do not show any deterioration of renal function, and in about 50% the proteinuria ceases after several years. Constant proteinuria is more serious. Although the course is indolent without other indicators or renal disease (*e.g.*, microscopic hematuria), most patients demonstrate proteinuria over many years; many develop an abnormal urine sediment and hypertension; and a few progress to renal failure.[5]

Proteinuria is the most difficult and important issue in nephritis. Nephritis patients with proteinuria are divided into two groups: 1) patients with protein, casts, and blood cells in the urine, and 2) protein only in the urine. Patients with protein, casts, and blood cells in their urine usually have either spleen-kidney qi and yang vacuity or yin vacuity. Both these patterns may be complicated with patterns of dampness or damp heat. Yin vacuity may also be complicated with patterns of blood stasis. Patients with protein only in their urine usually have one of the following patterns: spleen-kidney qi vacuity, spleen-kidney yang vacuity, or kidney yin and yang vacuity. Any of these may be complicated with patterns of dampness or damp heat.

In modern Chinese medicine, proteinuria indicates the body is losing essence. Patients will experience fatigue and weakness. Qi, blood, yin, and yang are all vacuous. When there is great vacuity, qi cannot contain the essence and cannot descend and drain the turbid. The separation of the clear and turbid involves the absorption of the clear (the essence of grain and water) and the elimination of the turbid (solid and liquid wastes) from the body. The absorption of the clear takes place in the small intestine under the governance of the spleen. The elimination of the turbid is the transference of waste products to and removal from the large intestine and bladder. The separation of the clear and turbid relies on the proper functioning of the lung, spleen, and kidney. These viscera must provide the necessary qi transformation. The lung must downbear the qi, the spleen must upbear the qi, and the kidney must control opening and closing (of the lower orifices). If any of these viscera are or become vacuous, this process may be compromised.

The lung may become vacuous due to contraction of wind heat or damp heat evils that exhaust the lung qi. If the lung qi is vacuous, it cannot contain evils in the upper burner. In that case, these evils may then move down to the lower burner and damage the kidney. Lung qi vacuity may also be due to spleen qi vacuity, since the spleen is the mother of the lung in the five phase engenderment cycle.

Spleen qi vacuity is most often caused by irregular diet, *i.e.*, irregular amounts of food or eating at irregular times. Certain foods, such as greasy, deep fried foods, overly sugary foods, or chilled, uncooked foods, damage the spleen. Excessive concentration, such as studying too much, or constant worrying and obsessing, also taxes the spleen.

Kidney qi vacuity may be due to any of the three causes: contraction of external evils, internal damage by the seven affects, or neither external nor internal causes. Among the neither external nor internal causes, taxation and sexual indiscretion can especially damage the kidney. In addition, the spleen and kidney are the sources of qi. The kidney is the former heaven root and provides essential qi, while the spleen is the latter heaven root and provides grain qi. Because these two viscera are mutually interdependent, damage to one viscus usually affects the other.

Case history from Dr. Wei Li's private practice: David, an 18 year-old male

Urinalysis revealed that David had proteinuria. His tongue was pale and his pulse was vacuous. Dr. Li treated David for three months using *Liu Wei Di Huang Wan* (Six Flavors Rehmannia Pills) plus *Huang Qi* (Astragali Membranacei, Radix). His condition improved but did not completely resolve. Therefore, Dr. Li decided to prescribe the following medicinal porridge in addition to the original formula: *Huang Qi* (Astragali Membranacei, Radix), 10g, *Dang Shen* (Codonopsitis Pilosulae, Radix), 10g, *Da Zao* (Zizyphi Jujubae, Fructus), 10g, and white rice, 20g. These medicinals were cooked with the white rice as porridge, discarding the medicinals, and eating the porridge with honey. After two days of this new regimen, David's condition resolved. He looked completely healthy and had more energy.

COMMENTARY: In proteinuria, spleen and lung vacuity have to be addressed as well as kidney vacuity. If the central qi is strong, the upper and lower burners can recover. The spleen upbears the clear and the stomach downbears the turbid. This function facilitates the lung's downbearing and the kidney's opening and closing.

However, even though lung, spleen, and kidney vacuity are at the root of proteinuria, one must also address the tip, such as damp heat, qi stagnation and blood stasis, yin vacuity, etc. Many famous doctors have empirical formulas for a variety of Chinese

medical patterns as well as Western medical conditions. Following are some of these formulas that may have value for specific problems:

1. *Huang Qi Chi Xiao Dou Tang* (Astragalus & Red Bean Decoction)[6]

Huang Qi (Astragali Membranacei, Radix), 100g
Chi Xiao Dou (Phaseoli Calcarati, Semen), 30g-50g, cooked at a low temperature until completely soft

This formula is for qi vacuity. It must be taken for three months or for one month after the proteinuria has disappeared.

2. *Shi Wei* (Pyrrosiae, Folium), 15 grams per day.[7] This medicinal is for cases of replete damp heat only and should be taken for three months. According to the *Chinese Medicinal Handout*,[8] this medicinal is able to stanch bleeding as well as percolate dampness. This implies *Shi Wei* separates the clear and turbid, since it secures and astringes and drains at the same time.

3. Dr. Han Xiang-wu[9] suggests the following soup: 10 grams of *Shang Lu* (Phytolaccae, Radix) and 100 grams of lean pork put into 500ml of water and simmered down to 300ml of soup. The soup is strained and divided into three parts and eaten in one day. This regimen should be followed for four months.

WARNING: *Shang Lu* is very draining and should only be used for patients with severe replete edema caused by qi stagnation and blood stasis or damp heat.

4. One may use *Bei Xie Wan* (Dioscorea Hypolaguca Pills)[10] for proteinuria in chronic nephritis:

Bei Xie (Dioscoreae Hypoglaucae, Rhizoma), 9g
saltwater stir-fried *Huang Bai* (Phellodendri, Cortex), 9g
Zhi Mu (Anemarrhenae Asphodeloidis, Rhizoma), 9g
Ze Xie (Alismatis Orientalis, Rhizoma), 9g
Fu Ling (Poriae Cocos, Sclerotium), 9g
Mu Dan Pi (Moutan, Cortex Radicis), 6g
saltwater stir-fried *Yi Zhi Ren* (Alpiniae Oxyphyllae, Fructus), 3g

This formula is for cases of replete damp heat. In one study, 70% of patients taking this pill were better within seven days.

5. Dr. Wei Zu-liu[11] suggests using *Gui Shen Tang* (Stabilize the Kidney Decoction), *Shen Yi Feng* (Kidney Formula Number One), *Shen Er Feng* (Kidney Formula Number Two), and *Shen San Feng* (Kidney Formula Number Three):

Gui Shen Fang (Stabilize the Kidney Decoction)

Chan Tui (Cicadae, Periostracum), 15-25g
Yi Mu Cao (Leonuri Heterophylli, Herba), 50g
Da Ji (Euphorbiae Seu Knoxiae, Radix), 50g
Xiao Ji (Cephalanoplos Segeti, Herba), 50g
He Shou Wu (Polygoni Multiflori, Radix) or *Huang Jing* (Polygonati, Rhizoma), 25g
Du Zhong (Eucommiae Ulmoidis, Cortex), 25g
Hu Tao Rou (Juglandis Regiae, Semen), 25g
Bu Gu Zhi (Psoraleae Corylifoliae, Fructus), 25g
Xi Xin (Asari, Herba Cum Radice), 5g
Fu Pen Zi (Rubi Chingii, Fructus), 50g

This formula is only for patients with damaged kidney function, little or no edema, and protein in their urine. The patients should have no blood or casts in their urine.

Warning: The medicinal dosages in the above formula are much too high. For example, *Yi Mu Cao* has a low toxicity, but, in high dosages, it may cause generalized weakness, soreness, aching, or numbness, paralysis of the lower extremities, chest oppression, sweating, low back pain, proteinuria, blood in the urine, blood in the stool, a drop in blood pressure, shortness of breath, damage to kidney function, and even death.[12] A dosage of 10-30 grams is best. *Xi Xin* is toxic due to its containing aristolochic acid, a nephrotoxin. Therefore, caution must be used with this medicinal when the kidney function is compromised. Alternative warming medicinals may be substituted for *Xi Xin*, such as *Gan Jiang* (Zingiberis Officinalis, dry Rhizoma) and *Rou Gui* (Cinnamomi Cassiae, Cortex).

Shen Yi Fang (Kidney Formula Number One)

Di Yu (Sanguisorbae Officinalis, Radix), 50g
Lu Han Cao (Pyrolae Rotundifoliae, Herba), 50g
Ma Bian Cao (Verbenae Officinalis, Herba), 50g
Yi Mu Cao (Leonuri Heterophylli, Herba), 50g
Hai Jin Sha (Lygodii Japonici, Spora), 50g
Guan Zhong (Guanzhong, Rhizoma), 25g
Tu Si Zi (Cuscutae Chinensis, Semen), 25g
Tian Kui Zi (Semiaquilegiae, Fructus), 25g
Chan Tui (Cicadae, Periostracum), 15g
Da Zao (Zizyphi Jujubae, Fructus), 8 pieces

Dr. Wei indicates this formula for patients with stubborn proteinuria and bloody urine. The patients should have no edema or only slight edema. This is a very strong draining and dispersing formula and is not appropriate for patients with vacuity. It is only for patients with strong constitutions who have bloodstasis.

Warning: *Yi Mu Cao* may be toxic at high dosages; see above.

Shen Er Fang (Kidney Formula Number Two)

Huang Qi (Astragali Membranacei, Radix), 5g
Fang Ji (Stephaniae Tetrandrae, Radix), 50g
Ting Li Zi (Tinglizi, Semen), 50g
Ma Huang (Ephedrae, Herba), 15g
Fang Feng (Ledebouriellae Divaricatae, Radix), 25g
Cang Zhu (Atractylodis, Rhizoma), 25g
Da Fu Pi (Arecae Catechu, Pericarpium), 25g
Hou Po (Magnoliae Officinalis, Cortex), 10g
Chi Xiao Dou (Phaseoli Calcarati, Semen), 50g
fresh *Bai Mao Gen* (Imperatae Cylindricae, Rhizoma), 50g
Cha Shu Gen (Camelliae Sinensis, Radix), 50g
Shu Fu Zi (Aconiti Carmichaeli, Radix Lateralis Praeparatus), 15g

This formula is for proteinuria patients with severe edema, high cholesterol, low blood protein, and high levels of urine protein. Blood pressure must be normal.

Warning: There are two medicinals called *Fang Ji*: *Guang Fang Ji* (Aristolochiae Seu Cocculi, Radix) and *Han Fang Ji* (Stephaniae Tetrandrae, Radix). *Guang Fang Ji* has been implicated in kidney damage and is not approved by the FDA. *Ting Li Zi* at 50 grams is too high a dosage to be used safely.

Shen San Fang (Kidney Formula Number Three):

Chan Tui (Cicadae, Periostracum), 15g
Bai Hua She She Cao (Oldenlandiae Diffusae, Herba), 50g
Qi Ye Yi Zhi Hua (Paridis Polyohyllae, Rhizoma), 50g
Da Ji (Cirsii Japonici, Herba Seu Radix), 50g
Pu Gong Ying (Taraxaci Mongolici, Herba Cum Radice), 50g
Yi Mu Cao (Leonuri Heterophylli, Herba), 50g
Shi Wei (Pyrrosiae, Folium), 25g
Xuan Shen (Scrophulariae Ningpoensis, Radix), 25g
Fang Ji (Stephaniae Tetrandrae, Radix), 25g
Zhi Mu (Anemarrhenae Asphodeloidis, Rhizoma), 20g
Huang Bai (Phellodendri, Cortex), 20g
Fu Pen Zi (Rubi Chingii, Fructus), 50g

This formula is for patients with nephritis and proteinuria with a concurrent upper respiratory infection.

WARNING: In Dr. Li's opinion, the dosages of all these medicinals are too high.

6. Dr. De Qiang-yan[13] recommends *Yi Shen Tang* (Boost the Kidney Decoction), *Long Feng Fang* (Solanum Nigrum & Wasp Nest Formula), *Jiang Can Fen* (Batryticated Silkworm Powder), *Su Feng Tang* (Search Wind Decoction), and *Da Ji Su Fang* (Hormone [Substitute] Formula).

Yi Shen Tang (Boost the Kidney Decoction)

Sheng Di Huang (Rehmanniae Glutinosae, uncooked Radix), 15g
Tai Zi Shen (Pseudostellariae Heterophyllae, Radix), 15g
Dang Shen (Codonopsitis Pilosulae, Radix), 10g
Huang Qi (Astragali Membranacei, Radix), 10g
Fu Ling (Poriae Cocos, Sclerotium), 9g
Ba Ji Tian (Morindae Officinalis, Radix), 9g
Bu Gu Zhi (Psoraleae Corylifoliae, Fructus), 9g
Hu Lu Ba (Trigonellae Foeni-graeci, Semen), 9g

This formula raises blood protein levels and eliminates proteinuria in patients with vacuity.

Long Feng Fang (Solanum Nigrum & Wasp Nest Formula)

Long Kui (Solani Nigri, Herba), 30g
Shu Yang Quan (Solani Lyrati, Herba), 30g
She Mei (Duchesneae Indicae, Herba), 30g
Lu Feng Fang (Vespae, Nidus), 9g

This formula clears heat and toxins, dispels wind, and drains water. It treats recurrent proteinuria and depresses the autoimmune response.

Jiang Can Fen (Batryticated Silkworm Powder)

Powder *Jiang Can* (Bombyx Batryticatus) and take 1.5 grams each time, three times per day. This medicinal lowers the autoimmune response and raises blood protein levels for any pattern of proteinuria. *Jiang Can* is often used for nephrotic syndrome.

Shu Feng Tang (Course Wind Decoction)

Zi Su Ye (Perillae Frutescentis, Folium), 9g
Jing Jie (Schizonepetae Tenuifoliae, Herba Seu Flos), 9g
Fang Feng (Ledebouriellae Divaricatae, Radix), 9g
Yuan Tou (Coriandri Sativi, Herba), 9g
Xi He Liu (Tamaricis, Ramulus Et Folium), 9g
Fu Ping (Lemnae Seu Spirodelae, Herba), 9g
Chan Tui (Cicadae, Periostracum), 6g
Bo He (Menthae Haplocalycis, Herba), 4.5g
Yi Yi Ren Gen (Coicis Lachryma-jobi, Radix), 30g

This formula is for long-term proteinuria.

If a patient has had proteinuria for a long time with frequent recurrences, Dr. De recommends *Long Feng Fang* (Solanum Nigrum & Wasp Nest Formula) or *Su Feng Tang* (Search Wind Decoction). If the patient's blood protein level is low, *Yi Shen Tang* (Boost the Kidney Decoction) is the one he suggests using. If the patient has been sick for a long time and the disease has penetrated deep into the channels and network vessels, he adds stasis-dispelling, blood-quickening medicinals, such as *Yi Mu Cao* (Leonuri Heterophylli, Herba), *Ze Lan* (Lycopi Lucidi, Herba), and *Shui Zhi* (Hirudo Seu Whitmania).

Da Ji Su Fang (Hormone [Substitute] Formula)

He Shou Wu (Polygoni Multiflori, Radix)
Shan Yao (Radix Dioscoreae Oppositae)
Huang Qi (Astragali Membranacei, Radix)
Tai Zi Shen (Pseudostellariae Heterophyllae, Radix)
Gan Cao (Glycyrrhizae Uralensis, Radix)
Zi He Che (Hominis, Placenta)

Grind equal amounts of each medicinal into a powder. Take 1.5 grams each time, three times per day.

ACUMOXIBUSTION: Choose from *Shui Dao* (St 28), *Wai Guan* (TB 5), *Guan Yuan* (CV 4), *Qi Hai* (CV 6), *Zu San Li* (St 36), *Tai Xi* (Ki 3), *Yin Ling Quan* (Sp 9), *Feng Chi* (GB 20), *Shen Shu* (Bl 23), and *Ming Men* (GV 4).

Case history of Dr. Chuan Hua-jiang: Chou, a 45 year-old male[14]

Ten years before his first visit, Chou had greatly overexerted himself and he gradually became edematous. A subsequent urinalysis revealed blood and protein in his urine with protein at 4+, granular casts at 2+, and the 24 hour urine protein at 8.65g. The Western medical diagnosis was acute nephritis. Chou was given Western medical treatment, such as hormone therapy, immunodepressant therapy, and diuretic drug therapy, but his condition did not improve. When Chou came to see Dr. Chuan, he had edema over his entire body. He also had a pale facial complexion, he felt cold, had no appetite, and he had thin and loose stools. His tongue was puffy and swollen with white, glossy fur, and his pulse was deep and fine. Based on these signs and symptoms, Dr. Chuan's pattern identification was spleen-kidney yang vacuity with damp accumulation. His treatment principles were to fortify the spleen and warm the kidney, free the flow of yang and eliminate dampness. His formula consisted of: *Hong Ren Shen* (Panacis Ginseng, Radix Rubrus), 6g, *Huang Qi* (Astragali Membranacei, Radix), 30g,

Shu Fu Zi (Aconiti Carmichaeli, Radix Lateralis Praeparatus), 12g, *Gui Zhi* (Cinnamomi Cassiae, Ramulus), 6g, *Bai Zhu* (Atractylodis Macrocephalae, Rhizoma), 9g, *Fu Ling* (Poriae Cocos, Sclerotium), 15g, *Xian Mao* (Curculiginis Orchioidis, Rhizoma), 9g, *Yin Yang Huo* (Epimedii, Herba), 9g, *Ba Ji Tian* (Morindae Officinalis, Radix), 12g, *Bai Shao* (Paeoniae Lactiflorae, Radix Albus), 9g, *Hu Lu Ba* (Trigonellae Foeni-graeci, Semen), 6g, *Che Qian Zi* (Plantaginis, Semen), 15g, and *Sheng Jiang* (Zingiberis Officinalis, uncooked Rhizoma), 3g.

Chou took this formula for 14 days and, on his second visit, his edema was much reduced, his urine output had increased, his appetite was better, he was warmer, and his stools were not so loose. His urine protein reduced to 1+, the granular casts were gone, and the 24 hour urine protein was reduced to 0.63g. Dr. Chuan decided to remove *Che Qian Zi* and add *Shan Yao* (Dioscoreae Oppositae, Radix), 9g, and *Chen Pi* (Citri Reticulatae, Pericarpium), 6g. Chou took this new formula for 21 days and, on his third visit, the edema had completely dissipated. His urine protein was negative and his 24 hour urine protein was 0.15g. Although his tongue was pale and his pulse was soggy, he had no more symptoms and Dr. Chuan discontinued treatment. Follow-ups over the next year found no recurrence.

Case history of Dr. Chuan Hua-jiang: Chen, a 35 year-old female[15]

Chen had suffered chronic nephritis for six years and often had edema. Urinalysis showed her urine protein at 1-2+, but she had neither hypertension nor uremia. When she first visited Dr. Chuan, she had a pale face, low back and knee soreness and limpness, fatigue, shortness of breath, dizziness, constipation, and a sore throat once a week. Her tongue was pale red, and her pulse was soggy. Dr. Chuan's pattern identification was spleen qi vacuity and kidney qi and essence vacuity. His treatment strategy was to fortify the spleen and supplement the qi, supplement the kidney and secure the essence, clear heat and disinhibit the throat. His formula consisted of: *Huang Qi* (Astragali Membranacei, Radix), 30g,

Cang Zhu (Atractylodis, Rhizoma), 15g, *Fu Ling* (Poriae Cocos, Sclerotium), 15g, *Hei Dou* (Phaseoli Vulgaris, Semen), 15g, *Du Zhong* (Eucommiae Ulmoidis, Cortex), 15g, *Jue Chuan*,[16] 15g, *Shan Yao* (Radix Dioscoreae Oppositae), 15g, *Shan Zhu Yu* (Corni Officinalis, Fructus), 10g, *Mu Dan Pi* (Moutan, Cortex Radicis), 10g, *Zhi Mu* (Anemarrhenae Asphodeloidis, Rhizoma), 10g, and *Huang Bai* (Phellodendri, Cortex), 15g.

Chen took this formula for 14 days. At Chen's second visit, her appetite was better, she had less fatigue, and her sore throat was gone, but she still had low back and knee soreness and weakness. Dr. Chuan modified her formula, adding *Dang Shen* (Codonopsitis Pilosulae, Radix), 15g, and *Gou Ji* (Cibotii Barometsis, Rhizoma), 15g. Chen took this new formula for another 14 days. At her third visit, all Chen's symptoms were better and her urine protein came down to 1+. Dr. Chuan modified the formula again, adding *Bu Gu Zhi* (Psoraleae Corylifoliae, Fructus), 9g, and *Tu Si Zi* (Cuscutae Chinensis, Semen), 9g. Chen continued this type of treatment with Dr. Chuan for half a year. She would take a formula for 14 days, Dr. Chuan would modify it, she would take the new formula for another 14 days, he would modify it again, and so on. Over the course of treatment, Chen's urine protein returned to normal, but she still had slight edema and low back soreness. Dr. Chuan's final modification was adding *Ze Xie* (Alismatis Orientalis, Rhizoma), 10g, and *Fang Ji* (Stephaniae Tetrandrae, Radix), 15g. After taking this new formula, Chen completely recovered.

7. According to Dr. Su Shen-chen,[17] there are three essential considerations when dealing with proteinuria. The first has to do with the treatment strategy, the most important of which he sums up in four words, "contain essence, drain turbid." In other words, both true qi vacuity and replete evils are present in proteinuria. It is extremely rare to see pure vacuity or repletion or pure hot or cold in most kidney diseases. These patterns are almost always mixed. Western hormone therapy or antibiotics complicate the pattern even more. Hormones create vacuity heat, while antibiotics damage the spleen. Therefore, one must use a treatment strategy that addresses both vacuity and repletion.

Second, the practitioner must understand that an extended course of treatment is necessary to achieve solid results. The practitioner must counsel the patient and assiduously follow the course of the patient's treatment.

Third, the treatment must not be too aggressive. The practitioner should aim for gradual, steady improvement using moderate methods, not immediate resolution using heroic methods.

Dr. Su's base formula is *Qiang Shen Xie Zhuo Jian* (Strengthen Kidney & Drain the Turbid Beverage)

Sang Ji Sheng (Sangjisheng, Ramulus), 12g
Xu Duan (Dipsaci Asperi, Radix), 12g
Gou Ji (Cibotii Barometsis, Rhizoma), 12g
Lu Han Cao (Pyrolae Rotundifolia, Herba), 12g
Tu Fu Ling (Smilacis Glabrae, Rhizoma), 30-60g
Ren Dong Teng (Lonicerae Japonicae, Caulis), 24-40g
Lian Qiao (Forsythiae Suspensae, Fructus), 9-12g
Bai Wei (Cynanchi Baiwei, Radix), 9-12g

Dr. Su provides the following analysis of the medicinals in his formula. The first four are yang supplements, but they also drain dampness. (He thinks that one should not start with yang medicinals that only supplement and do not drain, such as *Du Zhong* [Eucommiae Ulmoidis, Cortex] unless the urination is clear and copious.) *Tu Fu Ling* and *Ren Dong Teng* are especially useful for detoxification of heavy metals or chemicals. They can also be used for the long-term problems caused by antibiotics and hormones. *Lian Qiao* and *Bai Wei* clear heat and resolve toxins but do not harm the spleen qi.

Case history of Dr. Su Shen-chen: Zhuan, a 35 year-old male[18]

Zhuan had been suffering with chronic nephritis for more than two years. He also had chronic laryngitis. Urinalysis showed his urine protein at 3-4+. When he came to see Dr. Su, his symptoms included hypertension, fatigue, low back pain, recurrent sore throats, heart palpitations, insomnia, chest heat, and night sweats. Dr. Su's pattern identification was yin vacuity with ascendant yang, kidney failing to absorb the qi, and vacuity heat rising. He prescribed *Qiang Shen Xie Zhuo Jian* (Strengthen Kidney & Drain the Turbid Beverage). Zhuan took this formula with modifications to level the liver and subdue yang for two months. His urine protein fell to 1-2+. The chest heat and night sweats were better, but he still had a sore throat. Dr. Su continued to prescribe this formula with additions such as *Du Zhong* (Eucommiae Ulmoidis, Cortex), *Niu Xi* (Achyranthis Bidentatae, Radix), *Cang Zhu* (Atractylodis, Rhizoma), *Xuan Shen* (Scrophulariae Ningpoensis, Radix), *Ye Jiao Teng* (Polygoni Multiflori, Caulis), *He Huan Pi* (Albizziae Julibrissinis, Cortex), *Zhi Mu* (Anemarrhenae Asphodeloidis, Rhizoma), and *Gan Cao* (Glycyrrhizae Uralensis, Radix). He also added liver-nourishing, kidney-supplementing, spleen-fortifying medicinals, such as *Sha Yuan Zi* (Astragali Complanati, Semen), *Can Jian* (Bombycis Mori, Concha), *Huang Qi* (Astragali Membranacei, Radix), *Shan Yao* (Radix Dioscoreae Oppositae), and *Ze Xie* (Alismatis Orientalis, Rhizoma).

Zhuan continued on variations of Dr. Su's formula for six months. His energy and appetite continued to improve and his blood pressure returned to normal. After urinalyses and blood tests came back negative, he felt he had completely recovered and returned to work. Follow-ups over eight years found no recurrence.

8. Dr. Mei Zhong-yue[19] recommends a single medicinal, *Yu Mi Xu* (Zeae Maydis, Stylus) for proteinuria.

HYPERTENSION

Hypertension refers to the excessive pressure of blood against the arterial walls. Hypertension and kidney disease are closely related in Western medicine. High blood pressure can stress the kidney nephrons, and, over time, damage these filters and other microstructures. Conversely, kidney disease from factors other than hypertension may cause a cascade of events that ultimately raise the blood pressure. In many kidney diseases, the kidney nephrons are damaged which results in decreased blood flow through these filters. In that case, the kidneys release hormones that encourage the heart to pump more forcefully in order to increase the blood flow to the kidneys and through these filters. However, these same hormones also cause the body to retain body fluids longer, and both the increased heart function and fluid retention increase the pressure against arterial walls resulting in hypertension. Hypertensive patients usually present any of three patterns: 1) replete ascendant liver yang hyperactivity, 2) liver-kidney yin vacuity with ascendant liver yang hyperactivity, and 3) yin and yang vacuity with ascendant liver yang hyperactivity. In replete ascendant liver yang hyperactivity, liver-kidney yin is at a normal level, but liver yang is replete. In yin vacuity with ascendant yang, liver-kidney yin is vacuous, while liver yang is at a normal level but is relatively hyperactive compared to yin. In yin and yang vacuity with ascendant yang, liver-kidney yin and yang are both vacuous, but yin has the greater vacuity.

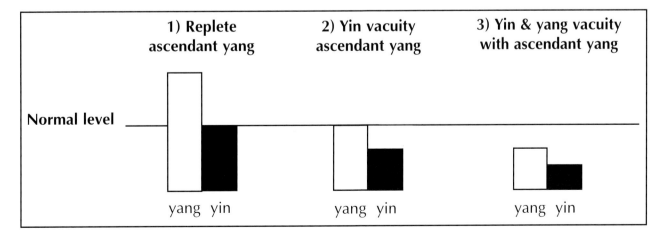

Figure 4.2. Comparison of replete ascendant yang, yin vacuity with ascendant yang, and yin & yang vacuity with ascendant yang

Therefore, yin fails to control what yang there is and yang floats upward. (Please see Figure 4.2.)

For replete ascendant yang, one should use heavy, settling, spirit-quieting medicinals and liver-levelling, wind-extinguishing medicinals, such as *Long Gu* (Draconis, Os), *Mu Li* (Ostreae, Concha), *Shi Jui Ming* (Haliotidis, Concha), *Ling Yang Jiao* (Antelopis Saiga-tatarici, Cornu), and *Gou Teng* (Uncariae Cum Uncis, Ramulus). For liver-kidney yin vacuity with ascendant yang, one should use relatively more yin-supplementing medicinals, such as *Gou Qi Zi* (Lycii Chinensis, Fructus), *Ju Hua* (Chrysanthemi Morifolii, Flos), *Bai Shao* (Paeoniae Lactiflorae, Radix Albus), *Gui Ban* (Testudinis, Plastrum), *Bie Jia* (Amydae Sinensis, Carapax), and *He Shou Wu* (Polygoni Multiflori, Radix), while clearing the liver and subduing yang. For yin and yang vacuity with ascendant yang, one should use the above medicinals plus yang-supplements, such as *Du Zhong* (Eucommiae Ulmoidis, Cortex) and *Niu Xi* (Achyranthis Bidentatae, Radix).

Hypertension in kidney diseases is often difficult to treat with Western medicine whether the hypertension has caused the kidney disease or vice versa. When using Chinese medicine, pattern identification is essential. For example, acute nephritis usually presents patterns of external evils and internal dampness. Thus the treatment strategy must include dispelling external evils and draining dampness. Chronic nephritis usually presents patterns of kidney vacuity with liver repletion and stagnation, and, therefore, the treatment strategy must include supplementing the kidney, soothing and draining the liver, and dispersing stagnation. When nephritis causes hypertension, there is usually a pattern of liver-kidney yin vacuity with ascendant liver yang hyperactivity. In some patients, yin vacuity has damaged the yang and there is a complex pattern of liver-kidney yin vacuity, kidney yang vacuity, and ascendant liver yang hyperactivity.

The representative formula for liver-kidney yin vacuity with ascendant liver yang is *Qi Ju Di Huang Wan* (Lycium & Chrysanthemum Rehmannia Pills), or *Er Zhi Wan* (Two Ultimates Pills) with the addition of blood-moving medicinals, such as *Yi Mu Cao* (Leonuri Heterophylli, Herba) and *Ze Lan* (Lycopi Lucidi, Herba). If there is concurrent kidney yang vacuity, the representative formula is *You Gui Wan* (Restore the Right [Kidney] Pills). If the hypertension is especially severe, one must add some draining medicinals, such as *Ling Yang Jiao* (Antelopis Saiga-tatarici, Cornu), *Gou Teng* (Uncariae Cum Uncis, Ramulus), *Mu Li* (Ostreae, Concha), and *Shi Jui Ming* (Haliotidis, Concha) even if there is vacuity.

Qi Ju Di Huang Wan consists of:

Gou Qi Zi (Lycium Chinensis, Fructus), 9g
Ju Hua (Chrysanthemi Morifolii, Flos), 7g
Shu Di Huang (Rehmanniae Glutinosae, cooked Radix), 15g
Shan Zhu Yu (Corni Officinalis, Fructus), 9g
Shan Yao (Radix Dioscoreae Oppositae), 9g
Fu Ling (Poriae Cocos, Sclerotium), 6g
Ze Xie (Alismatis Orientalis, Rhizoma), 6g,
Mu Dan Pi (Moutan, Cortex Radicis), 6g

Er Zhi Wan consists of:

Nu Zhen Zi (Ligustri Lucidi, Fructus), 9g
Han Lian Cao (Ecliptae Prostratae, Herba), 9g

You Gui Wan consists of:

Fu Zi (Aconiti Carmichaeli, Radix Lateralis Praeparatus), 3g
Rou Gui (Cinnamonmi Casiae, Cortex), 3g
Lu Jiao Jiao (Cervi, Gelatinum Cornu), 6g
Shu Di Huang (Rehmanniae Glutinosae, cooked Radix), 9-12g
Shan Zhu Yu (Corni Officinalis, Fructus), 9g
Gou Qi Zi (Lycii Chinensis, Fructus), 9g
Tu Si Zi (Cuscutae Chinensis, Semen), 9g
Du Zhong (Eucommiae Ulmoidis, Cortex), 9g
Dang Gui (Angelicae Sinensis, Radix), 6g

ACUMOXIBUSTION: Choose from *Feng Chi* (GB 20), *Feng Fu* (GV 16), *Qu Chi* (LI 11), *Zu San Li* (St 36), *Tai Chong* (Liv 3), *Yun Men* (Liv 2), *Yin Tang* (M-HN-3), *Yi Feng* (TB 17), *Shen Men* (Ht 7), *San Yin Jiao* (Sp 6), *Tai Xi* (Ki 3), *Yang Ling Quan* (GB 34), *Yin Ling Quan* (Sp 9), *Feng Long* (St 40), *Nei Guan* (Per 6), *Guan Yuan* (CV 4), and *Qi Hai* (CV 6).

In treating hypertension with kidney disease, treating the root is of paramount importance, and one should discover the disease causes and disease mechanisms in order to treat the underlying causes. An example of the etiology of hypertension in acute nephritis is as follows: Heat and toxins invade (often due to kidney, lung, and spleen vacuity) and damage the kidney. The resultant kidney dysfunction leads to water accumulation. The water accumulation then damages the spleen. The spleen, now replete with dampness, rebels against the liver causing ascendant liver yang hyperactivity (hypertension).

In chronic nephritis, any of the following: blood stasis, yang vacuity leading to water accumulation, blood vacuity and kidney yin vacuity, may lead to ascendant liver yang hyperactivity and hypertension. Each of these factors may also exacerbate the others. Blood stasis can prevent the formation of new blood, thus leading to more yin-blood vacuity or lead to more yang-qi vacuity. Yin-blood vacuity can cause more blood stasis. Yang-qi vacuity or water accumulation can also cause more blood stasis. (Please see Figure 4.3.)

Although treatment should aim at reducing hypertension, one should not try to drastically reduce it.

Reducing blood pressure below a certain level will damage kidney function. The kidney needs a certain amount of blood and blood pressure to function properly. In chronic nephritis, for example, low blood pressure can cause greater uremia. Some modern Chinese sources state that the blood pressure should not be below 140/90mmHg.

Labile blood pressure, *i.e.*, blood pressure that fluctuates frequently, is often due to spleen-kidney qi vacuity. Supplementing the qi often achieves positive results in this pattern, but one must be careful when using qi-supplementing medicinals. Some of these can cause hypertension. For example, *Huang Qi* (Astragali Membranacei, Radix) and *Ren Shen* (Panacis Ginseng, Radix) can only be used if the tongue and pulse confirm the vacuity. Even here one must be cautious, and one should use these medicinals only if appropriate Western drugs[20] or Chinese medicinals have already controlled the patient's hypertension. In addition, the practitioner must assiduously monitor the patient's blood pressure throughout the course of treatment.

AZOTEMIA

Azotemia refers to an increase in nitrogenous waste

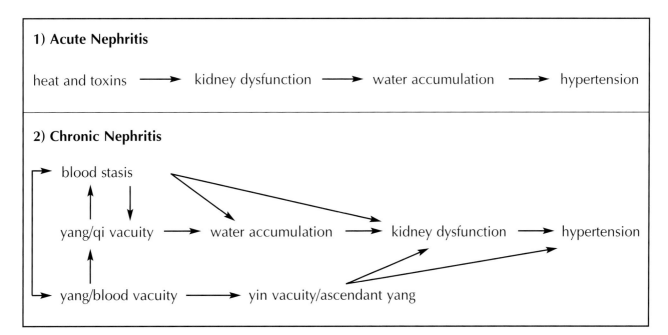

Figure 4.3. Examples of simplified disease mechanisms of kidney-caused hypertension

in the blood stream. It is caused by conditions that impair blood flow to the kidneys. As the glomerular filtration rate is reduced, the kidneys have less opportunity to clean the blood. Urine formation decreases, while waste products continue to increase. The waste is then reabsorbed into the blood. In such cases, urea is the primary nitrogenous body found in the blood. Hence, uremia is another term used for azotemia. Azotemia is diagnosed through laboratory tests showing elevated urea, creatinine, and BUN levels.

Chinese medicine considers the build up of nitrogenous waste to be a form of toxins. In terms of root and tip, the root of azotemia is kidney vacuity and the tip is toxins, *i.e.*, nitrogenous waste. The kidney vacuity can be of yin, yang, qi, and/or blood. However, both the root and the tip need to be treated simultaneously. Depending on the stage and severity of the azotemia, treatment should focus more on supplementing the kidney or resolving toxins.

ROOT TREATMENT: SUPPLEMENTATION

An important single medicinal is *Dong Chong Xia Cao* (Cordyceps Sinensis). Research and clinical trials in China have shown remarkable results using this medicinal for azotemia. In some cases, *Dong Chong Xia Cao* is used instead of dialysis.

When she was practicing at the Nephrology Department of the Anhui Medical University Hospital, Dr. Li treated a 47 year-old man with azotemia with remarkable results. This patient had a creatinine level of up to 5+. Dr. Li prescribed *Dong Chong Xia Cao* at six grams per day. This regimen reduced his blood creatinine to 2.5-3+, lowered his BUN, and maintained the lower levels for five years. The man improved so much, he was able to work a regular job.

One can also use *Ren Shen* (Panacis Ginseng, Radix) to supplement qi and blood. However, *Ren Shen* can raise blood pressure. Therefore, one should use it with caution and carefully monitor the patient's blood pressure.

The *Zhong Yao Da Ci Dian* (*The Great Dictionary of Chinese Medicinals*)[21] includes an experiment using modified *Liu Wei Di Huang Wan* (Six Flavors Rehmannia Pills) to treat azotemia. The ratio of the medicinals were as follows: *Shu Di Huang* (Rehmanniae Glutinosae, cooked Radix), 8 parts, *Shan Zhu Yu* (Corni Officinalis, Fructus), 4 parts, *Shan Yao* (Radix Dioscoreae Oppositae), 4 parts, *Fu Ling* (Poriae Cocos, Sclerotium), 3 parts, *Ze Xie* (Alismatis Orientalis, Rhizoma), 3 parts, *Mu Dan Pi* (Moutan, Cortex Radicis), 3 parts, and *Zhu Ling* (Polypori Umbellati, Sclerotium), 3 parts. The medicinals were ground and mixed to form the pills. The experimenters gave 1.5 grams per day per kilogram of weight to mice with azotemia and kidney disease-induced hypertension. After six days, the mice showed a remarkable reduction in their blood pressure and a remarkable improvement of their kidney function. With their improved kidney function, the mice's azotemia was reduced. The mice's death rate was also reduced.

COMMENTARY & CAVEAT: When treating vacuity in azotemia, one must use *Shu Di Huang* (Rehmanniae Glutinosae, cooked Radix), not *Sheng Di Huang* (Rehmanniae Glutinosae, uncooked Radix). There is a great deal of difference between these two medicinals even though they come from the same part of the same plant species. The former supplements yin and blood in vacuity patterns. After it is steamed, it also supplements the kidney qi. The latter is more for blood heat and is not as strong a supplement. In Western medical terms, *Sheng Di Huang* has more anti-inflammatory properties. For instance, one must use *Shu Di Huang* for hot flashes associated with menopause in turn associated with kidney yin vacuity. *Sheng Di Huang* does not work. Li Dong-yuan has stated that *Sheng Di Huang* nourishes kidney water and clears heat in the five hearts and blood heat with a surging, replete pulse. If the pulse is vacuous, on the other hand, one must use *Shu Di Huang*. Yuan Sui-jiang has said that *Shu Di Huang* supplements the kidney and is used for blood exhaustion. When there is lower abdominal pain, this implies blockage in the kidney channel, and one must use *Shu Di Huang*.

TIP TREATMENT: RESOLVING TOXINS

The major Chinese medicinal for resolving toxins in azotemia is *Da Huang* (Rhei, Radix Et Rhizoma). Although *Da Huang* is an extremely important medicinal in Chinese medicine, most Westerners are not used to it and its effects. Western patients who are unaccustomed to purgatives may have difficulty taking it. Western physicians may also have concerns about the loss of fluids and consequences to potassium balance when Chinese practitioners prescribe it. However, in extreme situations when the kidneys have shut down, toxins accumulate in the body. The kidneys cannot be used to drain these toxins because of their decreased function and because the toxins will further damage them. In Western medicine, hemodialysis and peritoneal dialysis are used to remove toxins from the blood. Hemodialysis refers to the direct removal of toxins from the blood. Peritoneal dialysis refers to the indirect removal of toxins via the peritoneal fluid. More generally, dialysis refers to the therapeutic elimination of toxins from the blood across a semipermeable membrane. When one uses *Da Huang* to evacuate fluids via the stools in order to remove blood toxins, this is also a form of therapeutic dialysis.

For patients who cannot receive hemodialysis or peritoneal dialysis, precipitation is the only way to eliminate toxins. In that case, *Da Huang* is the Chinese medicinal of choice. In Western medicine, drugs such as magnesium sulfate are used, but Chinese doctors generally believe that *Da Huang* achieves a better result. Most patients with serious kidney disease have tried Western purgatives and laxatives and are accustomed to therapeutic diarrhea. In cases where patients have not had good results, they may consider trying Chinese medicinals.

As stated above, Western physicians may have concerns about the loss of fluids and consequences to potassium balance when Chinese practitioners prescribe *Da Huang*. Western physicians consider the monitoring of electrolyte balance to be a primary concern and will have their patients on a regular schedule for evaluation. Renal failure and nephritic patients usually have an established regimen of tests before they present to Chinese medical practitioners. It is incumbent on the Chinese practitioners to understand these tests. This is especially critical when prescribing diuretics or purgatives. If Chinese practitioners choose to use *Da Huang* as a form of dialysis, they should consult with the patient's attending Western physician to assure them both that electrolyte balance will be checked and corrected on a daily basis.

In the treatment of azotemia, *Da Huang* can be used together with *Wang Bu Liu Xing* (Vaccariae Segetalis, Semen), *Gui Zhi* (Cinnamomi Cassiae, Ramulus), *Fu Ling* (Poriae Cocos, Sclerotium), *Yi Mu Cao* (Leonuri Heterophylli, Herba), *Che Qian Zi* (Plantaginis, Semen), *Bian Xu* (Polygoni Avicularis, Herba), and *Bi Xie* (Dioscoreae Hypoglaucae, Rhizoma). However, *Da Huang* may also be used alone and remains the most effective single medicinal for resolving toxins in azotemia. The author of *Zhong Xi Yi Jie He Shen Zhang Bing Zhen Duan Zhi Liao Xue* (*The Diagnosis & Treatment of Kidney Disease with Integrated Chinese-Western Medicine*)[22] states that *Da Huang* reduces the ability of the large intestine to absorb amino acids, and thus reduces the source of azotemia. One of the active ingredients in *Da Huang* stimulates the body's ability to manufacture proteins. This process uses nitrogen and thus also reduces azotemia. *Da Huang* also stimulates bone marrow to produce blood platelets. The blood platelets reduce bleeding. This improves capillary function that in turn improves kidney function. *Da Huang* also promotes diuresis to some extent, improves bile secretion (which increases lipid absorption), adjusts the body's immune function, improves the body's use of trace elements, and reduces catabolism. In 1960, researchers at the Jiangsu Provincial Chinese Medicine Hospital reported that *Da Huang* was effective in treating azotemia. This started its use in the rest of China as a single medicinal or as the principal medicinal in formulas for azotemia. It may be given orally, as an enema, or intravenously. Other examples of modern research follow.

In one study, *Da Huang* was given as a powder at three grams per day, with 20 days constituting one course. Seventy percent of the patients who followed this regimen improved.[23] Doctors at the Harbin Medical University Hospital (a Western medical hospital) used *Da Huang* intravenously in the treatment of 37 patients with azotemia. There were remarkable results in nine patients, 11 were much better, six had some improvement, and 11 were worse or had no results, for a total effective rate of 66%. At the Chong Qing City Chinese Medical Research Institute, researchers used 100-200ml of 50% fluid of *Da Huang* plus 250-500ml of 10% glucose fluid intravenously once a day. Seven to 14 days constituted one course. This regimen was tried with three patients for 2-3 courses with remarkable results. Dr. Zhen Qi-bi used *Da Huang* with calcined *Mu Li* (Ostreae, Concha) and *Pu Gong Ying* (Taraxaci Mongolici, Herba Cum Radice) cooked as a decoction and used as an enema. He treated 20 cases with very satisfactory results.

An important formula for azotemia is Dr. Jing Mingxiang's *Xiao Huang Fu Zi Tang* (Miribilitum, Rhubarb & Aconite Decoction):[24] *Mang Xiao* (Miribilitum), 15g, uncooked *Da Huang* (Rhei, Radix Et Rhizoma), 15g, *Fu Zi* (Aconiti Carmichaeli, Radix Lateralis Praeparatus), 30g, *Fu Ling* (Poriae Cocos, Sclerotium), 30g, *Ze Xie* (Alismatis Orientalis, Rhizoma), 30g, *Dang Shen* (Codonopsitis Pilosulae, Radix), 50g, *Huang Qi* (Astragali Membranacei, Radix), 50g, *Chen Pi* (Citri Reticulatae, Pericarpium), 20g, and *Gan Cao* (Glycyrrhizae Uralensis, Radix), 20g. Dr. Jing treated 100 cases of azotemia with this formula and achieved good results.

Dr. Li and her colleagues at the Anhui Medical University kidney department used *Da Cheng Qi Tang* (Major Order the Qi Decoction) as an enema to drain blood toxicity in azotemia with good results, while Dr. Yi Ping-chen[25] treated 45 cases of uremia with: *Da Huang* (Rhei, Radix Et Rhizoma), 15g, *Fu Zi* (Aconiti Carmichaeli, Radix Lateralis Praeparatus), 15g, *Fu Ling* (Poriae Cocos, Sclerotium), 15g, *Zi Su Ye* (Perillae Frutescentis, Folium), 10g, *Ban Xia* (Pinelliae Ternatae, Rhizoma), 10g, *Sheng Jiang* (Zingiberis Officinalis, uncooked Rhizoma), 10g, *Huang Lian* (Coptidis Chinensis, Rhizoma), 6g, and *Sha Ren* (Amomi, Fructus), 5g. All the patients in

this study experienced an improvement of their symptoms and all had their azotemia reduced to lower than 80mg%. Compared with Western drugs, 14 patients achieved remarkable improvement, 13 were better, 12 had no results, and six died.

Dr. Li Tian-chen[26] uses *Shen Yan Yi Huo* (Nephritis Formula #1): *Ban Xia* (Pinelliae Ternatae, Rhizoma), *Chen Pi* (Citri Reticulatae, Pericarpium), *Fu Ling* (Poriae Cocos, Sclerotium), *Gan Cao* (Glycyrrhizae Uralensis, Radix), *Da Huang* (Rhei, Radix Et Rhizoma), and *Hei Da Dou* (Glycines, Semen Atrum). He treated 30 cases of azotemia. Six patients had remarkable improvement, 15 were better, and nine had no results.

Dr. Yun He-liu[27] of the Air Force General Hospital used a combination therapy of 1) maintaining a low protein diet, 2) drinking *Shen An Tong Jiang* (Kidney Quiet Pain Syrup),[28] 14.5g per day, 3) ingesting a powder made of *Da Huang*, 1-2g, and *Mang Xiao* (Miribilitum), 1-2g per day, and 4) performing ultrasound over the kidney area for 30 minutes every day. He treated 53 cases of chronic renal failure and reported an effective rate of 86.7%.

Caveat: Although treatments are divided into root treatments and tip treatments, one should treat both root and tip at the same time. One may combine some of the protocols listed above.

Acumoxibustion: 1. To supplement the kidney, needle or moxa *Tai Xi* (Ki 3), *Zhao Hai* (Ki 6), *Shen Shu* (Bl 23), *Ci Liao* (Bl 32), *Jing Men* (GB 25), *Ming Men* (GV 4), *Guan Yuan* (CV 4). 2. To resolve toxins, needle *He Gu* (LI 4), *Qu Chi* (LI 11), *Da Zhui* (GV 14), *Lie Que* (Lu 7), *Ran Gu* (Ki 2), *Nei Guan* (Per 6), and *Yang Ling Quan* (GB 34).

Heart failure

Heart failure may affect the left and/or right sides of the heart. The left side of the heart receives blood from the lungs. Pulmonary edema occurs when either the atrium or the ventricle loses its contractility and blood back-flows into the lungs. Congestive heart failure occurs when a chamber of the heart loses contractility and enlarges in size. In that case, the pumping action of the heart decreases, the flow of blood decreases, and fluid accumulates throughout the body. The right atrium of the heart receives blood from the body and sends it to the lungs through the right ventricle. If the left side of the heart has become enlarged and blood is forced back into the lungs, the blood will eventually back up into the right ventricle. This will cause right-sided engorgement and decreased contractility, as on the left. Ultimately, the right side may lose effective pumping action and blood will flow back into the veins of the body. The result is swelling of the legs and ankles. Heart failure corresponds to water qi intimidating the heart in Chinese medicine.

For left-sided heart failure, Dr. Han Xiang-wu[29] uses modified *Zhen Wu Tang* (True Warrior Decoction) plus *Ting Li Da Zao Xie Fei Tang* (Descurainia & Dates Drain the Lung Decoction): *Shu Fu Zi* (Aconiti Carmichaeli, Radix Lateralis Praeparatus), 9-18g, *Fu Ling* (Poriae Cocos, Sclerotium), 15-30g, *Bai Zhu* (Atractylodis Macrocephalae, Rhizoma), 9g, *Bai Shao* (Paeoniae Lactiflorae, Radix Albus), 9g, *Sheng Jiang* (Zingiberis Officinalis, uncooked Rhizoma), 9g, *Da Zao* (Zizyphi Jujubae, Fructus), 5g, and *Ting Li Zi* (Descurainiae Seu Lepidii, Semen), 30-60g.

COMMENTARY & CAVEAT: Dr. Han's formula strengthens the heart, but it does not lower blood pressure. One must also lower the patient's blood pressure. Just strengthening the heart is like whipping a dead horse. Of course, Dr. Han's formula does have some medicinals that drain water, but these are not strong enough to effect hypertension. One must improve the kidney function to reduce water accumulation in order to treat the root of this disease. (For an explanation of how kidney diseases cause hypertension, please consult the section on hypertension in this chapter and the physiology section at the beginning of the book.)

For right-sided heart failure Dr. Han uses modified *Zhen Wu Tang* (True Warrior Decoction): *Shu Fu Zi* (Aconiti Carmichaeli, Radix Lateralis Praeparatus), 9-18g, *Fu Ling* (Poriae Cocos, Sclerotium), 15-30g, *Bai Zhu* (Atractylodis Macrocephalae, Rhizoma), 9g, *Bai Shao* (Paeoniae Lactiflorae, Radix Albus), 9g, *Sheng Jiang* (Zingiberis Officinalis, uncooked Rhizoma), 9g, *Da Zao* (Zizyphi Jujubae, Fructus), 5g, *Ren Shen* (Panacis Ginseng, Radix), 9-15g, and *Wan Nian Qing Gen* (Rhodeae Japonicae, Radix), 30g.

For right-sided heart failure in kidney diseases, one must do more than just make the heart stronger. In these cases, reduced kidney function has led to the water accumulation that has overburdened the heart. The kidney is the root. Therefore, one must treat both the heart and the kidney, with a focus on improving kidney function. Just using water-disin-hibiting, dampness-percolating medicinals is not enough. Most of these just increase urination without strengthening the kidney itself. Strengthening the kidney is the root treatment.

For difficult heart failure cases, the authors of the *Zhong Yao Da Ci Dian (The Great Dictionary of Chinese Medicinals)*[30] advise the use of *Yu Zhu* (Polygonati Odorati, Rhizoma) at 15 grams per day. In two cases, *Yu Zhu* was successful in improving heart function even when Western drugs failed. Compared to *Shu Fu Zi* (Aconiti Carmichaeli, Radix Lateralis Praeparatus), *Yu Zhu* is safe. If patients are on Western drug therapy, one must be cautious with or avoid *Shu Fu Zi*. *Shu Fu Zi* may increase the toxicity of the Western drugs when both are used. There is only a small dosage difference between the effective and toxic range of some Western heart drugs. Although *Shu Fu Zi* strengthens the heart, it may cause reduced toler-ance for these Western drugs. Again, the combination of *Shu Fu Zi* and Western drugs may also overburden the heart by too greatly increasing the strength of the heartbeat. On the other hand, one may prescribe *Yu Zhu* without these problems.

ACUMOXIBUSTION: Choose from *Xin Shu* (Bl 15), *Nei Guan* (Per 6), *Xi Men* (Per 4), *Shen Men* (Ht 7), *Shan Zhong* (CV 17), *Shui Fen* (CV 9), *Qi Hai* (CV 6), and *Shen Shu* (Bl 23).

ANEMIA

Anemia is defined as a decrease in the number of cir-culating red blood cells (RBCs) and hemoglobin.

Hemoglobin is found in the RBCs and is primarily responsible for carrying oxygen from the lungs to the tissues of the body. A decrease in the body's oxygen-carrying capacity commonly results in fatigue. One aspect of healthy kidney function is the production of a cytokine called erythropoietin. Cytokines are white blood cell proteins the body uses for the cell growth and renewal. Erythropoietin is used in the bone marrow for the proliferation of new red blood cells. Decreased kidney function inevitably leads to a decrease in both erythropoietin production and release. As a result, new red blood cells are not produced, and the patient becomes anemic.

When kidney disease causes anemia, it is because of lowered kidney function (and output of erythropoietin). The pattern identification usually involves vacuity of the spleen-kidney qi and blood. Supplementing medicinals such as *Ren Shen* (Panacis Ginseng, Radix), *Bai Zhu* (Atractylodis Macrocephalae, Rhizoma), *Fu Ling* (Poriae Cocos, Sclerotium), mix-fried *Gan Cao* (Glycyrrhizae Uralensis, Radix), *Chen Pi* (Citri Reticulatae, Pericarpium), *Rou Gui* (Cinnamonmi Casiae, Cortex), *Shu Di Huang* (Rehmanniae Glutinosae, cooked Radix), *Shan Zhu Yu* (Corni Officinalis, Fructus), *Bu Gu Zhi* (Psoraleae Corylifoliae, Fructus), *Tu Si Zi* (Cuscutae Chinensis, Semen), *E Jiao* (Asini, Gelatinum Corii), and *Lu Jiao Jiao* (Cervi, Gelatinum Cornu) supplement the qi to nourish blood or nourish the blood directly. But these medicinals, according to Dr. Han Xiang-wu,[31] cause an increase in azotemia. He feels that one must supplement and drain at the same time by combining formulas such as *Si Jun Zi Tang* (Four Gentlemen Decoction) or *Dang Gui Bu Xue Tang* (Dang Gui Supplement the Blood Decoction) with *Gou Qi Zi* (Lycii Chinensis, Fructus), *Rou Cong Rong* (Cistanchis Deserticolae, Herba), *Xian He Cao* (Agrimoniae Pilosae, Herba), *Zhu Ru* (Bambusae In Taeniis, Caulis), *Chuan Xiong* (Ligustici Wallichii, Radix), *Xuan Fu Hua* (Inulae Racemosae, Flos), *Tian Ma* (Gastrodiae, Elatae, Rhizoma), *Ji Nei Jin* (Gigeriae Galli, Endothelium Corneum), etc. These sorts of combinations can nourish the blood without raising the azotemia levels.

Si Jun Zi Tang consists of:

Ren Shen (Panacis Ginseng, Radix), 9g

Bai Zhu (Atractylodis Macrocephalae, Rhizoma), 9g
Fu Ling (Poriae Cocos, Sclerotium), 9g
mix-fried *Gan Cao* (Glycyrrhizae Uralensis, Radix), 3g

Dang Gui Bu Xue Tang consists of:

Huang Qi (Astragali Membranacei, Radix), 30g
Dang Gui (Angelicae Sinensis, Radix), 6g

COMMENTARY: Dr. Li has definitely seen cases where the use of supplements has caused higher azotemia. Many factors, such as over-activity, infection, diet, and even unstable blood pressure, can also increase azotemia, and it is not always clear which causes the higher nitrogen levels. Glue products and animal medicinals are almost 100% protein and will directly increase protein and thus azotemia. In view of this, one cannot use *Shu Fu Zi* (Aconiti Carmichaeli, Radix Lateralis Praeparatus), *Rou Gui* (Cinnamonmi Casiae, Cortex), *Ren Shen* (Panacis Ginseng, Radix), etc., in combinations with *Jiao* (medicinal gelatins). These combinations will almost always cause high azotemia. Again, many of the supplementing medicinals that increase the metabolism and higher catabolism of proteins may cause higher azotemia. This process is quite variable in patients, and correct pattern identification is essential. (The best guide is the patient's tongue and pulse.) If the pattern identification indicates that supplementation is appropriate, the practitioner may supplement. However, Dr. Li agrees that a combined strategy, supplementing and draining at the same time, is the best strategy. A combined strategy builds up the blood slowly with less risk of increasing azotemia.

ACUMOXIBUSTION: Choose from *Zu San Li* (St 36), *San Yin Jiao* (Sp 6), *Qi Hai* (CV 6), *Ge Shu* (Bl 17), *Gan Shu* (Bl 18), *Pi Shu* (Bl 20), *Shen Shu* (Bl 23), and *Xue Hai* (Sp 10).

ENDNOTES

[1] *Shui Zhong Guan Ge Jun* (*Water Swelling and Block & Repulsion*, Volume 2), Chinese Medicine Publishing Company, Beijing, 1998, p. 107

[2] The treatment strategy of diffusing the lung to free the flow of the urine is also called "raising the pot and removing the lid" (*ti hu jie gai fa*).

[3] Yu Wong-shi, *Dong Dai Ming Yi Ling Zhen Jing Hua* (*Modern Famous Doctors Clinic Collection*), Chinese Ancient Book

Publishing Co., Beijing, 1991, p. 8

[4] *Shui Zhong Guan Ge Jun* (*Water Swelling and Block & Repulsion, Volume 2*), *op. cit.*, p. 176

[5]Beers and Berkow, *The Merck Manual*, 17th edition, Merck RL, Whitehouse Station, NJ, 1999, p. 1807

[6] *Shui Zhong Guan Ge Jun* (*Water Swelling and Block & Repulsion*), Vol. 2, *op. cit.*, p. 176

[7] *Ibid.*, p. 16

[8] *Zhong Yao Xue Jian Yi* (*Chinese Medicinal Handout*), People's Health Publishing Co., Beijing, 1950, p. 149. This is a textbook used at the Beijing, Nanjing, Shanghai, Guanzhou, and Chendu Chinese Medicine Colleges.

[9] *Ibid.*, p. 16

[10] *Ibid.*, p. 16

[11] *Ibid.*, p. 95

[12]Qian Guo-hong, *Zhong Xi Yi Jie He Shen Zhang Bing Zhen Duan Zhi Liao Xue* (*Combined Chinese and Western Diagnosis and Treatment of Kidney Diseases*), Guandong Science and Technology Publishing Company, Guandong, 2001. p. 363

[13]*Shui Zhong Guan Ge Jun* (*Water Swelling and Block & Repulsion*), Vol. 2, *op. cit.*, p. 204

[14] *Ibid.*, p. 37

[15] *Ibid.*, p. 41

[16] The authors were unable to find this common folk medicinal in any Chinese source.

[17]*Shui Zhong Guan Ge Jun* (*Water Swelling and Block & Repulsion*), Vol. 2, *op. cit.*, p. 83

[18] *Ibid.*, p. 86

[19] *Ibid.*, p. 123

[20] If there is a choice of Western drugs, one should choose one that does not reduce blood flow to the kidney.

[21] *Zhong Yao Da Zi Dian* (*The Great Dictionary of Chinese Medicinals*), Shanghai Science & Technology Publishing Co., 1991, p. 2626 and p. 74

[22] Qian Guo-hong, *Zhong Xi Yi Jie He Shen Zhang Bing Zhen Duan Zhi Liao Xue* (*Combined Chinese and Western Diagnosis and Treatment of Kidney Diseases*), Guangdong Science & Technology Publishing Company, Guandong, 2001, p. 495

[23] Qing Fa-shen, *Zhong Yi Lin Chuang Shen Zang Bing Xue* (*Clinical Nephrology in Chinese Medicine*), Shanghai Science & Technology Publishing Co., 1998, p. 312

[24] *Ibid.*, p. 312

[25] *Ibid.*, p. 312

[26] *Ibid.*, p. 312

[27] *Ibid.*, p. 314

[28] The composition of this syrup was not given.

[29]*Shui Zhong Guan Ge Jun* (*Water Swelling and Block & Repulsion*), Vol. 2, *op. cit.*, p. 19

[30]*Zhong Yao Da Zi Dian* (*The Great Dictionary of Chinese Medicinals*), *op. cit.*, p. 309

[31]*Shui Zhong Guan Ge Jun* (*Water Swelling and Block & Repulsion*), Vol. 2, *op. cit.*, p. 19

BIBLIOGRAPHY

ENGLISH LANGUAGE BIBLIOGRAPHY

Acupuncture, A Comprehensive Text, Shanghai College of Chinese Medicine, trans. & edit. by John O'Connor & Dan Bensky, Eastland Press, Chicago, 1981

"Are Aristolochia Plants Dangerous?" Subhuti Dharmananda, Institute for Traditional Medicine, Portland, OR, 2002

Basic Pathology, 3rd ed., Stanley Robbins *et al.*, W.B. Saunders Co., Philadelphia, 1981

Chinese Herbal Medicine: Formulas & Strategies, Dan Bensky & Randall Barolet, Eastland Press, Seattle, 1990

Chinese Herbal Medicine: Materia Medica, Dan Bensky & Andrew Gamble, Eastland Press, Seattle, 1986

The Classic of Difficulties, trans, by Bob Flaws, Blue Poppy Press, Boulder, CO, 1999

Dui Yao, An Introduction to the Use of Processed Chinese Medicinals, Philippe Sionneau, Blue Poppy Press, Boulder, CO, 1997

English-Chinese Chinese-English Dictionary of Chinese Medicine, Nigel Wiseman, Hunan Science & Technology Publishing Co., Changsha, 1995

Essentials of Chinese Acupuncture, Beijing College of Chinese Medicine, Foreign Languages Press, Beijing, 1980

Fluid Physiology and Pathology in Traditional Chinese Medicine, Steven Clavey, Churchill Livingstone, Edinburgh, 1995

Fundamentals of Chinese Medicine, revised edit., trans. by Nigel Wiseman & Andrew Ellis, Paradigm Publications, Brookline, MA, 1995

Handbook of Chinese Herbs and Formulas, Vol. 1, Him-che Yeung, Institute of Chinese Medicine, Los Angeles, 1983

The Merck Manual, 17th edit., Mark H. Beers & Robert Berkow, Merck Research Laboratories, Whitehouse Station, NJ, 1999

Pharmacology, Examination & Board Review, 3rd edit., B.G. Katzung & Anthony J. Trevor, Appleton & Lange, Norwalk, CT, 1993

A Practical Dictionary Of Chinese Medicine, Nigel Wiseman & Feng Ye, Paradigm Publications, Brookline, MA, 1998

Shang Han Lun, On Cold Damage, Translation and Commentaries, Zhang Zhong-jing, trans. by Craig Mitchell, Feng Ye & Nigel Wiseman, Paradigm Publications, Brookline, MA, 1999

Synopsis of Prescriptions of the Golden Chamber, Zhang Zhong-jing, trans. by Luo Xi-wen, New World Press, Beijing, 1987

Thousand Formulas and Thousand Herbs of Traditional Chinese Medicine, Vol. 1 & 2, Huang Bing-shan *et al.*, Heilongjiang Educational Press, Harbin, 1993

Treatise On Febrile Diseases Caused By Cold, Zhang Zhong-jing, trans. by Luo Xi-wen, New World Press, Beijing, 1986

Warm Diseases, A Clinical Guide, Liu Guo-hui, Eastland Press, Seattle, 2001

The Yellow Emperor's Classic Of Medicine, trans. by Maoshing Ni, Shambala, Berkeley, CA, 1995

Yellow Empero's [sic] *Canon Internal Medicine*, trans. by Nelson Liansheng Wu & Andrew Qi Wu, China Science & Technology Press, Beijing, 1997

CHINESE LANGUAGE BIBLIOGRAPHY

Ben Cao Wen Da (Materia Medica Questions & Answers), Tong Zhong-hai, a.k.a. Tang Rong-chuan, Qing dynasty

Chang Qi Lin Chuang Jin Yen Ji Yao (The Gathered Essentials of the Clinical Experiences of Chang Qi), Chang Qi, China Medical Science Publishing Company, Beijing, 1999

"Cytological Study of the Prevention & Treatment of Primary Osteoporosis with Chinese Medicinals to Supplement the Kidney," Shi Yin-yu, *Zhong Yi Za Zhi (Journal of Chinese Medicine)*, #1, 1997, p. 621

Dan Xi Xin Fa (Dan-xi's Heart Methods), Zhu Zhen-heng, 1481

Dong Dai Ming Yi Lin Zhen Jing Hua (A Collection of the Clinical Experiences of Famous Modern Doctors), Yu Wong-shi, Chinese Ancient Book Publishing Company, Beijing, 1991

Dong Dai Ming Lao Zhong Yi Lin Zheng Hui Cui (A Collection of Modern Famous Old Chinese Doctors' Clinical Experiences), Qing He-chen, Guandong Science & Technology Publishing Company, Guanzhou, 1991

Dong Dai Ming Lao Zhong Yi Lin Zheng Hui Cui (A Collection of Modern Famous Chinese Doctors' Clinical Experiences), Guandong Science & Technology Publishing Company, Guanzhou, 1987

Dong Dai Ming Yi Lin Zheng Jing Hua (The Efflorescence of Clinical Case Histories of Modern Famous Doctors), Yu Guan-shi & Shui Jian-shen, Ancient Chinese Medicine Book Publishing Company, Beijing, 1998

Dao De Qing (The Way & Its Power), attributed to Lao Zi, Zhou dynasty

Du Yi Sui Bi (Random Notes While Reading Medicine), Zhou Xue-hai, 1895

Fu Qing Zhu Nu Ke (Fu Qing-zhu's Gynecology), Fu Qing-zhu, Qing dynasty

Hua Shi Zhong Zang Jing (Master Hua's Central Treasury Classic), attributed to Hua Tuo, probably Six Dynasties

Jin Gui Yao Lue (Essentials from the Golden Cabinet), Zhang Zhong-jing, Eastern Han dynasty

Jin Gui Yi (Supplements to [Essentials From] the Golden Cabinet), You Yi, Qing dynasty

Jing Yue Quan Shu (Jing-yue's Complete Book [i.e., Writings]), Zhang Jie-bing, a.k.a. Zhang Jing-yue, 1624

Lei Jing (Systematic Classic), Zhang Jing-yue, Ming dynasty

Li Jin Yong Lin Chuang Jing Yen Ji Yao (Collected Essentials of the Clinical Experience of Li Jin-yong), Beijing Chinese Medical Science Publisher, Beijing, 1998

Nan Jing (The Classic of Difficulties), attributed to Qin Yue-ren, late Han dynasty

"On the Kidney in Chinese Medicine, Ancient & Modern", Shen Zi-yin, *Zhong Yi Za Zhi (Journal of Chinese Medicine)*, #1, 1997, p. 49

Qian Jin Yao Fang (Essential Formulas [Worth] a Thousand [Pieces of] Gold), Sun Si-miao, 652 A.D.

Qian Guo-hong, *Zhong Xi Yi Jie He Shen Zhang Bing Zhen Duan Zhi Liao Xue (Combined Chinese and Western Diagnosis and Treatment of Kidney Diseases)*, Guangdong Science & Technology Publishing Company, Guandong, 2001, p. 196

San Yin Ji Yi Bing Zheng Fang Lun (Treatise on Diseases, Patterns & Formulas Related to the Unification of the Three Causes), Wu Ze-chen, a.k.a. Chen Yan, 1174

Shang Han Lun (Treatise on Damage [Due to] Cold), Zhang Zhong-jing, Eastern Han dynasty

Shen Nong Ben Cao Jing (Divine Farmer's Materia Medica Classic), anonymous, late Han dynasty

Shen Shi Qun Sheng Shu (Master Shen's Book for Recovering Life), Shen Jin-ao, 1773

Shen Yan Liao Du Zhen Zhuan Ji (Treatise on Nephritis & Chronic Renal Failure), Yu Guan-shi, Ancient Chinese Medical Book Publishing Co., Beijing, 1991

Shui Zhong Guan Ge Lun (Treatise on Water Swelling and Block & Repulsion), Vol. 1 & 2, Chinese Medicine Publishing Company, Beijing, 1998

Song Yuan Ming Qing (Song, Yuan, Ming, Qing [Famous Doctors' Case Histories), Vol. 111, Wu Qing, Qing dynasty

"The Experience of Jian Hua-hu Using *Yin Yang Huo* (Epimedii, Herba) & *Rou Cong Rong* (Cistanchis Deserticolae, Herba)", Yu Ping-gong, *Zhong Yi Za Zhi (Journal of Chinese Medicine)*, #6, 1998, p. 334

Wen Re Lun (Treatise on Warm Heat [Diseases]), Ye Gui, a.k.a. Ye Tian-shi or Ye Xiang-yan, 1746

Xue Zheng Lun (Treatise on Bleeding Conditions), Tang Zong-hai, a.k.a. Tang Rong-chuan, Qing dynasty

Yi Guan ([Key] Link of Medicine), Zhao Xian-ke, Ming dynasty

Yi Jian Fang Lun (Treatise on Simple Formulas), Nu Xin-chen, Ming dynasty

Yi Lin Gai Cuo (Errors in the Forest of Medicine Corrected), Wang Qing-ren, a.k.a. Wang Xun-chen, Qing dynasty

Yi Xue Zhong Zhong Can Xi Lu (Records of Heart-felt Experiences in Medicine with Reference to the West), Zhang Xi-chun, Qing dynasty

Yi Zong Jin Jian (Golden Mirror of Ancestral Medicine), Wu Qian et al., 1742

Yin Xue Xin Wu (Medical Revelations), Cheng Guo-peng, 1731

Yu Guang-shi, Dong Dai Ming Yi Ling Zheng Jing Hua (Modern Famous Doctors Clinical Experience), Chinese Medical Classics Publishing Company, Beijing, 1991

Zhong Xi Yi Jie He Shen Zhang Bing Zhen Duan Zhi Liao Xue (The Integrated Chinese-Western Medicine Diagnosis & Treatment of Kidney Diseases), Qian Guo-hong, Guandong Science & Technology Publishing Co., Guanzhou, 2001

Zhong Yao Da Zi Dian (The Great Dictionary of Chinese Medicinals), Shanghai Science & Technology Publishing Co., 1991

Zhong Yao Xue Jian Yi (Chinese Medicinal Handout), People's Health Publishing Co., Beijing, 1950

Zhong Yi Lin Chuang Shen Zang Bing Xue (Clinical Nephrology in Chinese Medicine), Xi Ming-wang, Chinese Medicine Publishing Co., Beijing, 1997

Zhong Yi Lin Chuang Shen Zang Bing Xue (Clinical Nephrology in Chinese Medicine), Qing Fa-shen, Shanghai Science & Technology Publishing Co., 1998

Zhu Bing Yuan Hou Zong Lun (Treatise on the Origin & Symptoms of All Diseases), Chao Yuan-fang, 610 A.D.

GENERAL INDEX

A

A *Practical Dictionary Of Chinese Medicine*, 57
abdomen, cramping that shoots to the lower, 163
abdomen, hypertonicity in the lower, 109
abdominal aneurysm, 229
abdominal distention, 23, 42, 51-52, 60-61, 64, 68,
 75, 77-78, 82, 93, 103, 117, 120-122, 126,
 129-131, 142,163, 165-166, 174, 176-178,
 185-187, 199, 210, 228, 230, 242-243, 247,
 259, 272, 274-275
abdominal distention and fullness, rib-side and, 61,
 176
abdominal pain, acute lower, 144
abdominal x-ray, 111
ACE inhibitors, 184, 228, 240-241
acquired cystic kidney disease (ACKD), 273
acupuncture, 191, 262, 264
ADPKD, 273
agility, 9
AGN, 197-199, 208, 210, 228
Air Force General Hospital, 294
alcohol toxicity, 229
aldosterone, 4
allergic reactions, 191, 264
Alport syndrome, 240
aminoglycosides, 155
amoxicillin, 155
amyloidosis, 184
analgesic nephropathy, 153, 184, 240
anemia, 67, 153-154, 183, 199, 229, 239-241, 245,
 247, 254, 257, 260-261, 272, 295-296
anger, excessive, 20

angina pectoris, 145
angioedema, 199
angiotensin II, 4, 184
angiotensin-converting enzyme inhibitors, 184, 241
Anhui Medical University, 231, 259, 292, 294
anorexia, 184, 198
antibiotics, 71, 81, 111, 123, 153-155, 157, 168,
 171-172, 174-175, 179, 181, 197, 199, 208,
 229, 250, 265, 267, 270, 288
antidiuretic hormone, 4
antiglomerular basement membrane disease, 198
antineutrophil cytoplasmic antibody, 198
antistreptolysin O, 199
anuria, 227-229, 232, 265
anxiety, 133, 146, 174, 232, 234
appetite, lack of, 45, 64, 72, 77, 80, 83, 99, 187,
 242, 245, 274-275
appetite, large, 177
appetite, no, 42, 55, 161, 167, 185-186, 204, 210-
 211, 215-216, 246-248, 250, 271, 287
aristolochic acid, 35-36, 228, 237, 272, 285
ascendant liver yang hyperactivity, 52, 54, 94, 138,
 258, 270, 289-291
ascites, 80, 92, 184, 194, 211, 216, 228
ASO, 199
asthma, 22, 63, 188, 202, 256, 258, 260
asymptomatic bacteriuria, 152
atherosclerosis, 184, 228, 240-241
ATN, 265-269
atrial diuretic peptide, 4
attacking medicinals, 211
autoimmune disease, 228
autosomal dominant polycystic kidney disease, 273

azotemia, 227, 235, 240, 247, 291-294, 296

B

back, difficulty lying down on one's, 90
back, lower and upper aching and, 9, 90
back pain, 42, 44-45, 69-70, 72-73, 77, 89, 94, 105, 109-110, 117-119, 121, 123, 146, 157, 160, 164, 167-169, 171, 189, 201, 203, 207, 218-219, 228, 230-231, 244-245, 251, 253, 255, 266-267, 270, 285, 288
back pain, lower and upper, 9, 89-90
back, upper, 9, 89-90, 98, 105
bacterial colonization, 154
bad breath, 55, 126, 178
balanitis, 154
bath formulas, medicated, 262
Ben Cao Wen Da (Materia Medica Questions & Answers), 259
bend, inability to, 107
benign prostatic hypertrophy, 153-154
Berger disease, 198
bladder cancer, 153-154
bladder infections, 151
bladder, malposition of the, 153
bladder, prolapse of the, 153
bleeding, 23, 25, 28, 41, 57, 68-73, 80, 84, 90, 117-118, 137, 146, 158-160, 173, 187, 211, 219-220, 229, 231, 233, 240, 247-250, 261-262, 276, 278, 284, 293
bloating after meals, 274-275
block and repulsion, 19, 49-51, 53-57, 59, 184, 195, 199, 208, 226, 230, 241, 266, 296-297
blood aspect, 29, 73, 81, 84, 126, 145, 191, 202, 215-216, 232, 246, 252, 261, 268
blood cholesterol, 45, 226, 243-244, 255
blood disharmony, 94
blood pressure, high, 51, 94, 146, 211, 217, 219, 245, 253, 271, 289
blood protein, 45-46, 214-215, 224, 226, 243-244, 248, 252-253, 255, 285-286
blood stasis, 17, 22-23, 25, 27-30, 41, 52, 57, 65-66, 68, 73, 79, 84, 105, 108-109, 111-114, 121, 129-130, 135, 137, 141-148, 158, 163, 166, 172, 176, 178-179, 181, 194, 217, 219-221, 225-226, 230, 232, 235, 238, 245-246, 258-261, 275, 277, 279-281, 283-285, 291
blood urea nitrogen, 53, 228, 266

blood vacuity, 21, 23, 54, 71, 81, 88, 93, 122, 135, 137, 141-142, 144, 158, 177, 250, 255, 258, 260-261, 275, 279-280, 291
blood volume, 4
bloody strangury, 67, 110
bodily aching, pain, and heaviness, 101
bodily exhaustion, 135
bodily fatigue, 88
body aches, 203
body, emaciated, thin, 101
body, heavy, 77, 83, 136
body weight, very low, 275
bone steaming, 90
borborygmus, 131
breast distention, 142, 176
breath, shortness of, 62, 71, 77, 79, 89, 92, 97-98, 101-103, 108, 118-119, 122, 134-136, 142, 144, 161, 170, 190, 198, 210, 215, 218, 228, 242, 244, 248, 252, 255-256, 285, 287
breath, smell of urine in the, 253
breathing, short, hasty, 61
breathing, uneasy, 100
Brucella suis, 198
bruising, easy, 142, 209
BUN, 52, 55, 92, 187, 199, 205-206, 209, 225, 228, 241, 243, 245-256, 260, 263, 282, 292

C

calyces, 4
Can Bing-fu, 244-245, 255
Candida albicans, 152
cardiotonic drugs, 85
catheterization, 63-66, 152-153, 228, 241
causes, neither external nor internal, 18, 21, 23, 87, 141, 284
cephalexin, 155
CGN, 209-210
Chang Qi, 111-112, 114, 139, 148, 157, 168, 172, 252
Chang Qi Lin Chuan Jin Yen Ji Yao (The Collected Essentials of the Clinical Experience of Chang Qi), 114
cheeks and lips, red, 179
chemical toxins, 263, 265
Chen Yan, 18
cherry hemangiomas, 142
chest and stomach fullness and oppression, 120

chest and rib-side propping fullness, 98
chest distention and vexation, 126
chest ECG monitoring, 229
chest fullness and pain, 87, 90
chest oppression, 77, 83, 89, 100-102, 122, 126,
    136, 145, 176, 248, 274-275, 285
chest oppression and discomfort, 100
chest pain, burning, 100
chills, 23, 40-41, 43-44, 52, 82, 87, 90-92, 99, 103,
    116, 130, 137, 153, 175, 199-200, 202-204,
    230-231, 236, 255, 266-267, 281
chills, severe, 40, 91
chills, slight, 41
Chinese Herbal Medicine: Materia Medica, 36
chlamydia, 151, 154
cholesterol, high, 224, 226, 240, 285
Chong Qing City Chinese Medical Research
    Institute, 294
Chuan Hua-jiang, 287
cigarette smoking, 153
cirrhosis, 80, 85, 194, 229
The Classic of Difficulties, 6
clitoris, 4
CO2, 240
cold, aversion to, 39, 68, 75-76, 79, 99, 101, 105,
    118, 121, 136, 143-144, 179, 201
cold, fear of, 62, 78, 88, 102, 108
cold, feeling, 45-46, 50, 171, 186, 189, 211, 213,
    215-216, 242, 255
cold, upper back, 98
coma, 228, 232, 240, 249, 251, 253, 260, 272
common cold, susceptibility to, 177
computed tomography, 229
confusion, 153, 198, 249
congestion, nasal, 40-41, 61, 230-231
congestive heart failure, 210, 227, 229, 279, 294
consciousness, sudden loss of, 145
constipation, 10, 23, 41-42, 44, 50, 52, 60-61, 67,
    69, 77, 82, 92, 99, 102, 111, 116-117, 119,
    121, 126-127, 131, 134, 156, 163, 174-175,
    177-179, 190, 197, 200-201, 203-204, 206,
    215, 217, 219, 225, 234, 244, 247, 253,
    266, 281-282, 287
constructive aspect, 268
convulsions, 22, 145
corticosteroids, 184, 210
costovertebral tenderness, 198
cough, 42, 61, 76, 82, 87, 90, 92, 97, 99-101, 177,

199, 201-202, 231, 235
cough, dry, 90, 235
cough, oppressive, 100
cough, severe, 90
coughing and panting, 77, 101-102
coughing, 22, 41, 76-77, 97, 99-103, 147, 230, 248,
    256, 258
coughing, occasional, 100
cramping, lower leg, 102
creatinine, 52-53, 55, 199, 206, 209, 225, 227-228,
    239-241, 248, 250, 254, 256, 260, 266, 292
creatinine clearance, 239
CRF, 185, 239-241, 243, 245, 247, 249, 251, 253-
    263
cryoglobulinemia, 198
CT, 36, 229, 274
CTN, 265
cyclosporine, 228
cystitis, 151-155, 173-175, 177, 179-181
cystitis, chronic, 152, 155
cystitis, initial, 152
cystitis, recurrent, 152, 155
cystitis, reinfection, 152
cytokines, 296

D

damp cold, 18-20, 27, 40, 42, 44, 46, 50, 64, 98,
    106, 185, 189-190, 204, 274
damp heat, 11, 19-20, 22-23, 25-26, 28, 31, 39-40,
    42, 44, 47-48, 60-61, 65, 68, 71, 77, 81,
    83, 86, 107, 115-118, 120, 123, 125-126,
    128, 141,156-159, 162-163, 167-169, 171,
    174-175, 180, 185, 188-190, 200-201, 204,
    206, 215-216, 218, 221, 230, 233-234, 245-
    246, 252, 258, 266-267, 272, 279-280, 283-
    285
Dan Xi Xin Fa (Dan-xi's Heart Methods), 82, 125, 201
Dan Zhu-li, 207
De Qian-yan, 224
deafness, 136
defecation, uneasy, 60, 126
defensive aspect, 46, 84, 94, 191, 201, 215, 268
dehydration, 227-229, 254
delirium, 249
desires, unfulfilled, 142
Dharmananda, Subhuti, 36
diabetes, 153-154, 183-184, 240, 265

dialysis, 191, 199, 208, 210, 229, 231, 239, 241,
    256-257, 259, 261, 263, 266, 273, 292-293
dialysis complications, 229
diarrhea, 10, 52, 77, 88, 93, 100, 121, 128, 131, 136,
    153, 160, 180, 228-229, 250, 260, 275, 293
diarrhea, cockcrow, 88
dietary irregularities, 18, 22
disease, minimal change, 183-184
disease, multiple simple cyst, 274
diuretics, 81, 184, 199, 229, 240, 243-244, 252,
    261, 268-269, 293
diuretics, potassium-sparing, 229, 240
dizziness, 9, 52, 70, 73, 78, 89-90, 93-94, 97-98,
    102, 108, 120-121, 127-128, 133-139, 142,
    159-162, 165-171, 176, 179-180, 185, 190,
    199, 210, 217-220, 225, 228, 232-233, 242,
    245, 247, 255, 260, 270, 274, 287
dizziness and vertigo, 78, 98, 102, 134-136,
dizziness, severe, 136
dizziness when standing up, 142
DNA gyrase, 155
drugs, immune-suppressant, 45
dry heat, 19-20, 141
dry heaves, 52, 99, 101, 131
*Du Yi Sui Bi (Random Notes While Reading
    Medicine)*, 16
dysmenorrhea, 144
dyspnea on exertion, 198

E

E. coli, 152-155
eating and drinking, devitalized, 50, 62
edema, 35, 41, 43-46, 51, 63, 75-83, 85, 88-89, 97-
    98, 101-103, 110, 130, 134, 146-147, 169,
    171, 176, 180, 183-190, 194, 197-208, 210-
    213, 215, 217-219, 224-226, 228-231, 235-
    237, 240, 242-248, 250, 252-253, 255-256,
    258-259, 261, 265, 272, 275-276, 279-285,
    287-288, 294
edema, enduring, 78
edema, focal, 184
edema, generalized, 44-45, 77, 88, 199-200, 204, 281
edema in the lower extremities, 83, 171, 217, 248,
    275
edema, lower limb superficial, 88
edema of the four extremities, 77
edema, pitting, 44-45, 78-79, 201, 212-213, 256

edema, pulmonary, 228-229, 294
edema, severe, 41, 76-78, 89, 98, 110, 194, 224,
    252, 255, 258, 285
edema, sudden onset of, 76
efferent arterioles, 4
18 incompatibilities, 34-35
electroacupuncture, 162-166
electrolyte balance, 184, 238, 241, 247, 261, 293
electrolytes, 238, 241, 250
emaciation, 120, 276
emergencies, hypertensive, 199
emotional depression, 61, 133, 142,
emotional disturbance, 122
endocarditis, 198, 228-229
endometriosis, 154, 174
enemas, 261
enuresis, 176, 180
epigastric glomus and fullness, 77
epigastric fullness, 136, 142
EPO, 241
Er Shun-jiang, 243
erythropoietin, recombinant, 241
ESRD, 239-240
essence, 4-16, 19, 21-22, 30, 43, 48, 49, 63, 85-88,
    91-92, 105, 120, 125, 127, 133, 135,160-
    161, 190, 192, 213, 222, 225-226, 236, 245,
    258-260, 277, 283, 287-288
essence turbidity, 125, 127
estrogen deficiencies, 154
European Polycystic Kidney Disease Consortium,
    273
external causes, 18, 23
external contraction, 98
external formulas, 262
extremities, cold, 92, 167, 203, 233, 255
extremities, superficial edema in the, 101
extremities, upper, 213
extremities, weakness of the, 71
eyelids, puffiness of the, 198
eyelids, swollen, 73, 92
eyes, dark circles around the, 142
eyes, distention of the 134
eyes, dry, 165, 217
eyes, dry, rough, 89
eyes, rubbing of the, 134
eyes, upward staring of the, 145

F

facial complexion, bright white, 108, 110, 122, 180
facial complexion, dark, 55, 69, 255
facial complexion, pale, 45, 50, 68, 80, 118-119, 176, 185-186, 188, 190, 203, 210, 212, 215, 217, 224, 242, 244, 252, 269, 271, 274, 280, 287
facial complexion, red, 133, 137, 169, 231
facial complexion, sallow yellow, 135
facial complexion, somber white, 50, 62, 71, 77-78, 88-89
facial complexion, sooty, 142
facial edema, 77, 176, 188, 198, 204, 275
falling hair, 142
fatigue, 8, 17-18, 21-22, 40, 42, 44, 52, 62, 70, 73, 77-79, 81, 88, 92, 98, 110, 118-119, 122, 127, 134, 142, 146-147, 153, 157-158, 161, 166-167, 170-171, 174, 176-177, 185-186, 188-190, 198, 204, 206, 210-211, 213, 215-216, 218-219, 224-225, 228, 230, 234, 240, 242, 244-245, 250-252, 255, 259, 269, 271-272, 278, 280, 283, 287-288, 296
feet, superficial edema of the, 102
fever, 23, 41-45, 55, 68-70, 75-76, 81-82, 84, 87, 90, 99, 101, 103, 105-107, 116-119, 127, 130, 137, 146, 153, 156-157, 163, 171, 175, 179, 198-206, 215, 218-220, 231-232, 234, 241, 245, 249-251, 253, 255, 265-267, 281
fever and chills, alternating, 99, 116, 175
fever, high, 55, 76, 84, 107, 200, 202, 204-205, 231
fever, low-grade, 55, 68, 70, 206, 220
fever, rheumatic, 199
fever unresolved by sweating, 99
fever without sweating, 44, 200, 205, 281
fevers, night, 144
filariasis, 198
fingernails, somber white, 50
fingertips and lips, cyanotic, 143
fire, immaterial, 5-6
five hearts, heat in the, 45, 52, 71-73, 89, 107, 111, 127,157, 160, 165, 169, 179, 218, 244, 252, 292
fluid overload, 210, 229
food intake, reduced, 77, 135, 176
food stagnation, 129, 141, 177
formulas, drastic, 85, 193-194
formulas, mildly draining, 85, 194

four aspects, 46-47, 81, 83, 94-95, 201
four extremities, reversal chilling of the, 51
four limbs, heaviness and encumbrance of the, 51
four limbs, lack of warmth of the, 50, 78, 176
fright, easy, 89
fright reversal, 249, 251, 253
FSGS, 183
furosemide, 229

G

gallbladder, 16, 136
gastritis, 250
generalized heaviness, 202
genital herpes, 154
gentamicin, 16, 55, 259, 264
glomerular capillary thrombosis, 228
glomerular filtration rate, 3, 227, 239-240, 292
glomerular permeability, 183
glomerulonephritis, chronic, 209-210
glomerulonephritis, fibrillary, 183
glomerulonephritis, idiopathic rapidly progressive, 198
glomerulonephritis, membranous, 183, 210
glomerulonephritis, mesangial proliferatie, 183
glomerulonephritis, poststreptococcal, 197-198
glomerulonephritis, rapidly progressive, 183, 198, 228
glomerulosclerosis, focal segmental, 183, 210
glomerulus, 3, 240
glomus and hardness below the heart, 99
glomus lumps, 51
glomus and oppression below the heart, 98
GN, 183
gonorrhea, 151
Goodpasture syndrome, 198
granular casts, 43, 45-46, 55, 92, 187, 198, 207, 228, 252-253, 255, 267, 281, 287
Guillain-Barré syndrome, 199

H

half exterior, half interior, 13
Han Xiang-wu, 296
hands and feet, cold, 129, 211, 213, 215-216, 269
hands and feet, heat in the hearts of the, 63, 101
hands and feet, lack of warmth in the, 108
He Ho-ling, 212, 280
head distention, 133

head, empty sensation in the, 135
head, heavy, 136, 247
headache, 9, 44, 52, 61, 92, 110, 121-122, 133, 136, 138, 146, 198, 201, 203, 217, 231, 245, 247, 249, 253, 265, 271
headache, distending, 110, 231
hearing loss, 9, 165
heart, 4-5, 11, 13-14, 16, 21, 60-61, 63, 69, 71, 78, 81-82, 85, 88-89, 97-99, 101, 103, 108, 115-118, 120, 125, 131, 133-135, 137-138, 141, 144, 147, 156, 159, 167, 178-180, 185, 194, 199, 201, 210, 215, 217, 226-227, 229, 233-234, 240, 244, 248, 251, 254-256, 258, 260, 263, 272-274, 279, 288-289, 294-295
heart failure, 85, 194, 199, 210, 227, 229, 279, 294-295
heart palpitations, 71, 78, 89, 97-99, 108, 134-135, 137-138, 144, 147, 179-180, 185, 210, 215, 233-234, 248, 251, 255, 272, 288
heartbeat, 85, 194, 295
heat, 10-11, 16,18-20, 22-23, 25-26, 28-31, 35, 39-42, 44-48, 49-50, 52, 55, 60-61, 63, 65, 67-69, 71-73, 76-77, 81-87, 89-91, 94-95, 99-101, 107-109, 111-112, 115-123, 125-128, 130-131, 133-138, 141-146, 156-160, 162-163, 165-169, 171-172, 174-181, 185, 188-191, 195, 199-202, 204-207, 215-218, 220-221, 223, 230-231, 233-235, 237-238, 244-247, 249-253, 258, 261-262, 266-269, 272, 276, 279-289, 291-292
heat strangury, 115-116, 156, 174, 180
heatstroke, 19, 228
heavenly water, 7-8, 10, 16, 21
HELLP syndrome, 228
hematuria, 41, 43, 127, 145, 62, 69, 71, 77, 117, 119-120, 153, 174-175, 178-179, 197-198, 206, 209-210, 228, 265, 274, 283
hematuria, enduring, 71
hematuria, idiopathic recurrent, 210
hematuria, profuse, 117
hemolytic uremic syndrome, 229
Henoch-Schönlein purpura, 198
hepatitis, 23, 183, 198, 265
hernia, 153
hormone therapy, 187, 194-195, 221-224, 287-288
hormones, 3-4, 186-187, 222-224, 263-264, 288-289
Hua Tuo, 115, 231
Huang Di, 4, 15-16, 23, 30, 43, 47-48, 127-128, 134-138, 144-146, 51, 60, 62-63, 66, 68-71, 73, 77, 81, 84, 86, 89-95, 102, 107, 109, 111-112, 117-122, 157-161, 163, 165-166, 168-171, 175, 177, 179-180, 186, 188-192, 201-202, 204-205, 207, 212-214, 216-220, 222, 224-225, 231-234, 242, 244-249, 252-254, 256, 258-259, 266-271, 275-278, 284, 286, 290, 292, 296
Huang Di Nei Jing (Yellow Emperor's Inner Classic), 4, 86, 258
hungering, rapid, 177
hydronephrosis, 274
hypercoagulability, 183-184
hyperhomocysteinemia, 241
hyperkalemia, 227-229, 241
hyperlipidemia, 183-184, 241
hypermagnesemia, 229
hyperparathyroidism, 240-241
hypertension, 42, 65, 183, 190, 197-199, 209-210, 223, 228-230, 240-241, 247, 263-265, 274, 283, 287-292, 295
hypertension, malignant, 183, 210, 228
hypoalbuminemia, 183
hyponatremia, 229
hypotension, 184, 228, 241
hypothalamus, 4, 8, 222-223

I

IC, non-ulcerative, 173
IC, ulcerative, 173
IgA nephropathy, 183, 198, 210
immune complexes, 198
impetigo, 199
impotence, 128, 135-136, 118-119, 121, 168-170, 180, 260
incontinence, 6, 10, 144-145, 65, 153, 156, 176, 180, 228
indigestion, 51
infections, sexually transmitted, 154
infection, susceptibility to, 152-153, 210
infections, upper respiratory tract, 223
injury, history of, 108
injury, iatrogenic, 227
insomnia, 9, 11, 42, 127, 134-135, 146, 55, 69-71, 79, 81, 87, 90-91, 98, 108, 117-118, 120-121, 157, 159-161, 165, 171, 179, 185, 194, 210, 217-219, 232-234, 245, 248, 250, 269,

271-272, 288
interior wind caused by vacuity, 247, 254
interior heat stirring wind, 247, 253
internal causes, 17-18, 20-21, 67, 87, 284
internal damage, 67, 85,133, 245, 277, 284
intercourse, pain with, 153
interstitial cystitis, 154, 173-175, 177, 179-181
intestines, 10, 13-14, 22, 53-54, 97, 99, 177, 225, 260, 262-263, 274
intestines, water sounding within the, 99
intrarenal ARF, 227-228
intravenous pyelography, 240
intravesical DMSO, 174
irascibility, 61, 133, 137-138, 146, 217-219, 270
irritability, 45, 77, 92, 109, 136-138, 142, 144-145, 147, 176, 231, 233, 249, 251
ischemia, 228
itchiness, 207
IV drug use, 228

J

Jin Zie-zao, 256
Jing Ming-xiang, 294
Jing Yue Quan Shu (Jing-yue's Complete Book), 115
Jing Ze-zao, 248
joints, aching, 76, 230
joy, excessive, 21
jue yin, 89, 105, 133

K

Ke Wan-chen, 186, 211, 282
ketoacidosis, 229
kidney and heart, 11, 13-14, 89, 115, 260, 295
kidney and liver, 11-13, 30, 59, 64, 81, 86, 89, 93, 112, 253, 260, 270, 277
kidney and lung, 12-13, 20, 22, 59, 75, 82-84, 97, 201-202, 248, 257-260, 283-284, 291
kidney and spleen, 12, 20, 22, 27, 29, 31, 39-40, 49-50, 56, 59, 75, 80-82, 84, 86, 88, 94-95, 97, 102-103, 115-116, 129, 156, 190-191, 193, 202, 206-208, 211, 213, 221, 237, 242, 244-245, 248, 255-260, 272, 283-284, 291
kidney area, cramping in the, 162-163
kidney essence, 6, 9-13, 15, 21, 30, 48, 87, 92, 133, 135, 190, 225-226, 236, 245, 258, 260, 277
kidney qi, 6-11, 14, 16, 19-23, 27, 29-32, 39, 46,

52, 56, 62, 79-80, 83, 86-87, 91-92, 94-95, 102-103, 111-112, 116, 119-122, 126-127, 147, 156, 165, 168, 170-171, 177, 187, 189-191, 194, 201, 203, 206, 211-214, 216, 218, 221, 237, 242, 244, 253, 255, 257-258, 260-261, 269-270, 281, 284, 287, 292
kidney self-regulation, 3
kidney stone(s), 115, 154, 155, 164, 174, 229, 240, 274
kidney taxation, 19, 21, 23, 87-89, 91, 93-95, 184, 199, 210, 242
kidney tenderness and pain, 228
kidney vacuity, 9-10, 14, 40, 45, 50, 54, 56, 71, 86, 88, 94, 106-107, 109-110, 115, 119-120, 129, 131, 135, 138, 174-175, 189, 207-208, 230, 253, 258, 275, 284, 290-292
kidney yang, 5-6, 10-11, 14, 16, 19-22, 27, 29-30, 32, 40, 53, 62, 66, 75, 78, 85-86, 108, 111, 116, 118, 136, 156, 163, 168-169, 171, 179-180, 213, 221, 224, 237, 242, 253, 255, 258-261, 270, 288, 290
kidney yin, 5, 10-14, 16, 19-21, 29-30, 32, 127, 146, 60, 63, 66, 72-73, 81, 86, 91-92, 94, 107, 116, 118, 120-121, 156, 160, 163, 165, 168-169, 171, 179, 207, 212-215, 217-219, 221, 223, 226, 245, 253, 258, 261, 270-271, 277-278, 283, 291-292

L

Lao Zi, 5
laparoscopic surgery, 274
large intestine, 7, 13, 46, 55, 283, 293
Lasix, 229
legs, weak, 167, 207, 255
lethargy, 52, 228
leukemia, 183-184
Li Shi-zhen, 138
Li Jin-yong, 137, 139
life-gate, 5-6, 9-10, 12-14, 16, 27, 82, 85, 91-92, 115, 138,
life-gate fire, 5-6, 9-10, 12-14, 16, 85, 91-92, 115, 138
lifting, heavy, 153
limbs, chilled, 78-79, 88, 102, 136
Ling Shu (Spiritual Axis), 7
lips, pale, 50, 135, 176
liver, 5, 8, 11-13, 16, 20-22, 30, 35, 52-54, 59, 61-

62, 64-65, 68-70, 80-82, 85-90, 93-94, 103, 105, 109, 112, 115-116, 121, 133-138, 142, 156, 166, 174-180, 194, 218, 228, 234, 241, 248, 250, 253, 255, 258, 260, 270, 273-274, 276-277, 289-291

liver and spleen, 5, 88, 93, 248
liver and stomach, 176, 218
liver blood vacuity, 21, 54, 88, 137, 250
liver depression qi stagnation, 20-21, 54, 61, 80, 109, 121, 137, 166, 180
liver enzymes, elevated, 228
liver fire, 69-70, 134,
liver wind, 133, 137, 255
low appetite, 129, 185, 187, 189, 194, 202, 206, 213-214, 233, 245, 269, 276
low back and knee aching and chilliness, 79
low back and knee chill, pain, and lack of strength, 62
low back and knee pain and soreness, 127, 170
low back and knee pain and weakness, 135, 170
low back and knee soreness and limpness, 50, 70, 88-89, 118, 120, 170, 179, 190, 206, 210, 215, 217, 242, 244, 260, 269-271, 287
low back and knees, lack of strength in the, 180
low back, hot sensation in the, 107
low back pain, 42, 44-45, 69-70, 73, 77, 94, 105, 109-110, 117-119, 121, 123, 146, 157, 160, 164, 167-168, 171, 189, 201, 203, 207, 218-219, 230-231, 244-245, 251, 253, 255, 267, 270, 285, 288
low back pain, severe, 69
low platelets, 228
low blood pressure, 146, 233, 255, 291
low blood protein, 224, 244, 248, 252, 285
lower abdominal cramping and distention, 116, 118
lower abdominal distention and fullness, 60, 174, 176
lower abdominal distention and pain, 60-61, 68, 116-118, 121-122, 163, 165-166, 168, 176, 178
lower abdominal sagging and distention, 62, 122
lower abdomen, 5, 10, 64, 69, 72, 82, 91, 105, 109, 111, 118, 143, 162-164, 178
lower back and knee weakness, 159
lower back distention and pain, 168, 204
lower back pain, 72, 163, 168-169, 218, 266
lower burner, 5, 7, 10-11, 13-14, 19, 39, 53-54, 60, 63, 65, 67, 72, 81-82, 116, 123, 126, 143,

147-148, 156-157, 159, 167, 169, 220, 257, 259, 266-267, 283
lowered immunity, 191
lumbar pain, 19, 105-114, 120, 185, 199, 210, 242, 274
lung, 5, 7, 10-14, 19-22, 26-27, 31, 39-40, 43-45, 59, 61, 66, 68, 75-76, 82-84, 86, 88, 90, 94, 97-100, 102-103, 122, 187-189, 191, 195, 200-206, 216, 230-231, 235-236, 244, 248, 256-260, 275, 281, 283-284, 291, 295-296
lung and kidney, 12-13, 20, 22, 39, 59, 75, 82-84, 97, 201-202, 248, 257-260, 283-284, 291
lusterless facial complexion, 51, 62
lymph glands, swollen, 205

M

malar flushing, 70, 89, 101, 169
malaria, 23, 208
marrow, 5-9, 12, 19, 22, 48, 133, 160, 260, 293, 296
mask muscle wasting, 184
MCD, 183
memory, impaired, 9, 71, 135, 234
menses, 137, 143
menstrual irregularity, 109
menstrual pain, 142, 176
menstruation, irregular, 10, 144
menstruation, scanty, 121, 127, 179
mental clarity, decreased, 209
The Merck Manual, 297
mercury toxicity, 209
metabolic acidosis, 227-229
MGN, 183
micturition, 4, 153
middle burner, 12-13, 19, 22, 40, 43-44, 52-53, 55, 82, 133, 147-148, 175, 192, 201, 203, 255, 282
ministerial fire, stirring of, 138
mouth, bitter taste in the, 60, 69, 99, 110, 116-117, 122, 133, 136, 175-176, 178
mouth, deviation of the, 145
mouth, dry, with a bitter taste, 51, 215
mouth, sores in the, 69
mouth, sticky, dry, 169, 174
moxibustion, 50, 52, 62-63, 70, 78-79, 89, 99, 101-102, 106, 108, 110, 120-122, 128, 135, 144, 177, 180, 203, 214, 230, 232-233, 235, 256, 275

MPGN, 183
mucous membranes, dry, 228
mutual counteraction, 35
mutual accentuation, 35
mutual enhancement, 35
mutual incompatibility, 35
mutual suppression, 35
mutual antagonism, 35

N

Nan Jing (Classic of Difficulties), 6
natriuresis, 4
nausea, 22, 42, 50-53, 55-57, 59, 63-64, 77, 79, 99,
        110, 116-118, 130-131, 133, 136, 153, 160,
        162, 174-175, 185, 187-188, 197-198, 228,
        232-233, 240, 243, 245-248, 250, 252, 254-
        256, 260, 265-266, 272, 276
nausea and vomiting, 50-53, 55-56, 59, 77, 99,
        116-118, 130-131, 133, 136,153, 175, 232,
        240, 252, 254-255, 266, 276
navel, palpitations below the, 102
neck veins, collapsed, 228
necrotizing fasciitis, 199
Nei Jing (Inner Classic), 269, 279
nephritis, 23, 31-32, 43, 45, 52, 57, 71, 73, 80, 92,
        147, 186, 191, 197-201, 203, 205, 207-213,
        215-217, 219-225, 228, 244-246, 248, 255-
        256, 262, 265-267, 269, 271, 280-281, 283-
        284, 286-288, 290-291, 294
nephritis, acute, 43, 45, 71, 197-201, 203, 205, 207-
        208, 212, 222-223, 246, 281, 287, 290-291
nephritis, acute tubulointerstitial, 265-266, 269
nephritis, chronic, 32, 45, 52, 71, 73, 80, 92, 186,
        209-213, 215, 217, 219-223, 225, 244-246,
        248, 256, 280, 283-284, 287-288, 290-291
nephritis, chronic tubulointerstitial, 265, 269
nephrons, 3-4, 199, 209, 239, 241, 263, 289
nephrosis, 184
nephrotic syndrome, 183-185, 187, 189-195, 197,
        210, 229, 241, 266, 286
nephrotoxic medications, 229
neural regulation, 3
neurogenic bladder, 229
neurological dysfunction, 154
19 antagonisms, 34-35
nitrofurantoin, 155
nocturia, 79, 121, 153, 180

nosebleeds, 209
NSAIDs, 209, 228
numbness, 89, 94, 106, 144, 232, 260, 285

O

oliguria, 184, 197, 199, 209, 227-228
orthostatic hypotension, 184, 228
orthostatic proteinuria, 283
osteodystrophy, 240-241
ovaries, 5
over-diuresis, 229
overdose, 260
overexertion, 21-22, 278
oxygen-carrying capacity, 296

P

pain, burning, 60, 170-171, 179
pain, dull lumbar, 107-108
pain, dull, lingering lumbar, 108
pain, flank, 153
pain, heart, 89
pain, heavy lumbar, 110
pain, hollow, 108, 119, 122
pain, hypochondriac, 97, 147
pain, penis, 153
pain, piercing, in the chest and rib-side, 99
pain, severe, spasmodic, 119
pain, stabbing, 121
pain, urethral 164
palms and soles, hot, 217
panting and hasty breathing, 77, 79, 102
panting and wheezing, 79, 100
panting counterflow, 180
papillary necrosis, 154, 240
paralysis, 285
parasites, 18, 129, 198, 208
pelvic inflammatory disease, 154
penetrating vessel, 7, 10, 12
penetrating vessels, conception and, 7, 10
penicillin, 205
pericardium, 67, 138-139, 247, 251-252
pericardium, evils sinking into the, 247, 251-252
peripheral neuropathy, 240
peristalsis, 4
perspiration, spontaneous, 76, 106-107, 135-136,
        180, 260

pH, 153
pharyngitis, 199
phimosis, 154
phlegm, 18, 22, 28-29, 41-42, 55, 87, 90, 92, 94-
     95, 97-103, 123, 133, 136, 141, 142, 145,
     177, 184, 202, 205, 210, 242, 248, 254,
     277-278
phlegm, cough with scanty, 90, 99
phlegm dampness, 133, 136, 177, 205, 277
phlegm heat, 94-95, 133, 141-142, 205
phlegm, profuse, 102, 145
phlegm, profuse, white, frothy, 101
phlegm rheum, 28, 97-99, 101, 103, 184, 210, 242
phlegm, sound of, in the back of the throat, 145
phlegm, thick, sticky, 90, 101
phlegmy drool, 98
pituitary gland, 4
PKD, 273-274, 277
placenta, 46, 93, 135, 192, 224, 242, 287
plasma sodium, 240
Plasmodium falciparum, 198
Plasmodium malariae, 198
poison, 22, 232
poisoning, snakebite, 265
polyarteritis nodosa, 198
polycystic kidney disease, 28, 240, 273-277
prednisone, 18
pregnancy, 12, 21, 152, 154-155, 183-184
premature greying, 135
prostate, 4-5, 65, 151-152
prostatitis, 123, 151, 153, 174
protein loss, 211-212, 214, 225
proteinuria, 184, 186, 191, 197, 199, 209, 211-212,
     214, 221, 225, 228, 270-271, 283-286, 288-
     289
Proteus mirabilis, 152
pruritus, 240, 267
pubic symphysis, 4
purpura, 72, 198-199, 219-220, 229
pyelonephritis, 151-152, 154-155, 167-168, 171,
     184, 218, 228-229, 241, 265, 267
pyelonephritis, chronic, 151, 155, 167-168, 171,
     218, 241, 265

Q

qi aspect, 126, 84, 94-95, 191, 202, 215-216, 268
Qi Bo, 15, 39

Qi Chiang, 246
qi panting, 90
qi, scanty, 88
qi, shortage of, 176, 180
qi strangury, 116, 121-122, 156, 166, 174
Qing He-chen, 48, 66, 86, 96, 226, 264
Qing Guo-hong, 272

R

RA, 183
rash, 199, 205, 265, 267
RBC casts, 198
RBCs, 43-45, 52, 71-73, 93, 111, 171, 187-188,
     190, 200-201, 204-207, 217-218, 220, 228,
     251-253, 267, 281, 295-296
rectum, 4
renal biopsy, 184, 210, 229
renal blood vessels, 4
renal deposition, 198
renal disease, end-stage, 210, 239
renal failure, 9, 23, 35, 52, 55, 57, 81, 85, 155, 184-
     185, 192, 194, 198-199, 208, 210, 227-231,
     233, 235-237, 239-241, 243, 245-247, 249,
     251, 253-255, 257-266, 270-274, 282-283,
     293-294
renal failure, acute, 184, 199, 227-231, 233, 235-
     237, 240, 260, 265
renal failure, chronic, 52, 57, 81, 155, 185, 210,
     239-241, 243, 245-247, 249, 251, 253, 255,
     257-261, 263-264, 294
renal failure, progressive oliguric, 198
renal interstitium, 228
rennin, 4
restlessness, 69, 144
rib-side discomfort, 176
rib-side distention, 70, 121, 134, 142
rib-side pain, 97, 99, 122, 176, 178, 274

S

Salmonella typhosa, 198
scarlet fever, 199, 205
Schistosoma mansoni, 198
seizures, 228, 256
semen, 4, 16, 26-29, 34-35, 40-46, 50-51, 54, 56-
     57, 60-63, 68-73, 76-82, 84, 88-94, 98-100,
     102-103, 107-114, 116, 118-123, 127-128,

131, 134-138, 142-144, 146-147, 152, 156-171, 174-180, 185-190, 192-193, 200-204, 206-207, 211-220, 222, 225-226, 230, 232-237, 242-246, 248-254, 259, 262, 266-268, 271-272, 275-278, 280-290, 293-296

seminal emission, 70, 88-90, 108, 121, 127, 135-136, 160-161, 168-170, 179-180, 203

sensation like sitting in water, 186

sepsis, 228-229, 241

serum parathyroid hormone, 239

serum sickness, 199

seven interactions, 34-35

sex, 7, 21, 87, 92, 98, 115, 126, 155, 273

sexual desire, decreased, 79, 179-180

sexual intercourse, dribbling after, 168-169

Shang Han Lun (Treatise on Damage [Due to] Cold), 27

shao yang, 7, 13-14, 16, 105

shao yin, 5, 7, 14, 55, 91

Shen Yian Liao Du Zhen Zhuan Ji (Treatise on Nephritis & Chronic Renal Failure), 57

Shen Zhang Bing Zhen Duan Zhi Liao (Kidney Disease Diagnosis & Treatment), 272, 293, 297

shock, 21, 184, 228

Shui Jian-shen, 96, 172, 208

Shui Zhong Guan Ge Jun (Water Swelling and Block & Repulsion), 57, 195, 208, 226, 296-297

sickle-cell anemia, 153

sighing, frequent, 110, 122, 176

single effect, 35

Sjögren's syndrome, 183

skin, dry, 42, 142, 205, 245

skin, dry, scaly, 142

skin, itchy, 253

skin, local red swollen, 42

skin rashes, purple, 249

skin turgor, poor, 228

SLE, 183

sleep, dream-disturbed, 133-134

small intestine, 10, 69, 116, 156, 159, 283

Song Lian-xu, 254

sorrow, excessive, 21, 67

source qi, 5, 8-9, 11-12, 14, 16

spasms, muscular, 254

speak, disinclination to, 62, 71, 88

speech, deranged, 144

sperm, 6, 8, 12, 21, 125

spider nevi, 142

spinal cord, lower, 4

spirit, clouding of the, 251

spirit, lassitude of the, 50-51, 62, 71, 78, 88, 102, 110, 118, 120, 122, 134-136, 176

spitting, 101

spleen, 5-7, 12-14, 18-22, 27, 29, 31-32, 39-40, 42, 45-46, 48, 49-54, 56, 59, 64, 68-69, 71, 75-78, 80-86, 88, 93-95, 97-98, 100, 102-103, 115-117, 121-122, 129-131, 133, 135-136, 142-143, 148, 156, 161, 167, 176-180, 185-193, 202, 206-208, 211-214, 216-217, 221, 223-224, 226, 234, 236-237, 242-245, 248, 251, 255-260, 263, 269, 272, 275, 282-284, 287-288, 291

spleen qi vacuity, 20-21, 40, 77, 115, 121, 130-131, 176, 179, 187, 214, 221, 236, 272, 283-284, 287

spleen, straitened, 177

spleen yang vacuity, 75, 78, 80, 98, 187, 213

spots, purple, 72-73, 220, 259

sprain, 108

stenosis, 154, 228

stomach, 6-7, 10, 12-14, 19, 22, 40, 46, 52-55, 59, 77, 82, 84, 86, 98-100, 106, 110, 120, 129-131, 133, 148, 176-177, 188, 202, 205, 218, 223, 225, 245, 247, 250, 252, 284

stomach heat, 130-131, 86, 218

stomach, water sloshing in the, 98

stone strangury, 110, 116, 118-119, 156, 162, 174, 179

stone strangury, enduring, 119

stones, lower urethra, 162

stones, upper urethra, 162

stool, dry, 43, 54, 126, 130, 178-179, 188, 244, 260, 262

stools, 40, 43, 45, 61, 72, 78-79, 83, 88, 92-93, 98, 106-108, 110, 126, 135, 146-147, 52, 161, 174, 176-179, 185-187, 189, 207, 212-213, 215, 240, 242, 245-250, 256, 269, 271, 275, 280, 287, 293

stools, black, 249

stools, bloody, 72, 249

stools, dry, hard, 177

stools, dry, with a bad smell, 126

stools, loose, 40, 45, 52, 78-79, 83, 88, 92-93, 98, 106-108, 110, 126, 135, 147, 161, 174, 176, 185-187, 189, 207, 212-213, 215, 242, 245,

247, 256, 269, 271, 274-275, 280, 287
stools, sticky, 126
strain, 108, 153, 274
strangury, 10, 25, 50, 62, 67, 110, 115-123, 128, 131, 155-156, 158-159, 162, 166-169, 171-172, 174, 179-180, 266
strength, lack of, 50-51, 62, 69-71, 77-78, 107, 134-135, 142, 176, 180
stress and frustration, 142
Su Shen-chen, 288
summerheat, 18, 20, 23
Sun Lian-xu, 215-216
suprapubic discomfort, 153
sweating, 19-20, 25-26, 39, 44-45, 48, 76, 84, 89, 99, 101, 106, 110, 118, 200, 202, 205-206, 212, 230-231, 233, 236-238, 255-256, 279, 281, 285
sweating, inappropriate, 256
sweating, profuse, 19, 39, 84, 110, 118, 202
sweating, proper, 19, 236
sweats, night, 43, 89-91, 101, 107-108, 118, 120-121, 134, 160-161, 165, 171, 175, 179, 206, 213-214, 217-219, 226, 232, 260, 267, 271, 288-289
syncope, 133, 145
systemic bacteremia, 155
systemic lupus erythmatosus, 183, 265

T

tai yin, 105
tai yang, 5, 7, 14
talk, reluctance to, 166
taste, sweet, 51
taxation fever, 179
taxation strangury, 10, 116, 156, 167-168, 174
taxation wind, 87-91, 93-95, 184, 199, 210, 242
thinking, excessive, 21, 129
thirst, 4, 23, 42, 44, 52, 60-61, 69, 76-78, 84, 92, 98, 101, 103, 107, 117, 120-121, 126, 136, 144, 146, 156-159, 163, 165, 170-171, 174, 179, 187-188, 201-202, 204, 206, 215, 218-220, 228, 234-235, 240, 242, 247, 267
thirst but no desire to drink, 60, 98
thirst center, 4
thirst with desire to drink, 92, 159, 165, 174
three yin, 7
three yang, 7

throat, 5, 23, 41-44, 49, 55, 61, 63, 70, 76, 82, 89, 91, 99, 101, 107-108, 116-117, 121,145, 171, 175-176, 179, 189-191, 199-201, 204-207, 214-215, 217-218, 228, 231, 234-235, 244, 281, 287-289
throat, chronic sore, 42
throat, parched, 89, 99, 101
throat, red, sore, 76, 189
throat, sore, 23, 41-44, 55, 70, 76, 82, 91, 108, 190, 199-201, 204-207, 214-215, 228, 231, 244, 281, 287-289
thrombocytopenia, 228
thrombocytopenic purpura, 199
tidal heat, 90, 179
tinnitus, 9, 70, 78, 89-90, 108, 133-136, 160-161, 165, 168-169, 171, 179-180, 217-219, 245, 248, 255, 270
tip treatment principles, 25
TMP-SMX, 155
tongue, sores on the, 60, 69, 117
tonsillitis, 71, 216
tonsils, 71, 205
torpid intake, 52, 71, 77-78, 126,
toxic reactions, 23, 85, 194, 262
toxins, 3, 9, 17-18, 22-23, 25-26, 31, 44, 55-56, 60, 71, 83, 87, 90, 94, 171-172, 190-191, 197, 201, 204-207, 212, 217, 223, 228, 231-232, 237, 240, 245, 249, 251-252, 254, 257, 260, 262-263, 265-269, 286, 288, 291-294
transcutaneous electrical stimulation(TENS), 174
transplant rejection, 183
treatment strategies, combined, 30-32
Treponema pallidum, 198
trichinosis, 198
trimethoprin-sulfamethoxazole, 155
triple burner, 5-6, 10-14, 16, 20, 27, 39, 50, 56, 59, 75, 82-83, 201, 226, 235-236, 256
true fire, 5
true yin, 5
true water, 5-6
trypanosomes, 198
tuberous sclerosis, 274
tubular necrosis, acute, 228
tubulointerstitial disease, 210
turbid urination, 120, 174
turbidity condition, 125, 127-128
two yin, 9, 27
type IV collagen, 198

U

ultrasound, 55, 111, 162, 164, 199, 240, 248, 274, 276-277, 294

unctuous strangury, 116, 120, 128, 156, 169

uremia, 55, 92, 227, 239-240, 247-248, 250, 252, 255, 260, 262, 264, 287, 291-292, 294

urethra, membranous, 4

urethra, prostatic, 4

urethra, spongy, 4

urethral discharge, purulent, 151

urethritis, 151, 154

urinary block, dribbling, 10, 50, 59-61, 63, 65-66, 184, 199, 202, 210, 230-231, 241, 266

urinary frequency, 11, 68, 166, 168-169, 173, 179, 240

urinary obstruction, 229, 241

urinary stoppage, 49

urinary stoppage, fecal and, 49

urinary tract infections, 23, 65, 115, 151-155, 157, 159, 161, 163, 165, 167, 169, 171, 174, 191, 210, 223, 254, 265, 270, 274

urinary turbidity, 10, 125-126

urinate, inability to, 62-63

urination, burning, 60, 117, 119-120, 127, 157-159, 166-167, 169, 175-176, 178

urination, clear, scanty, 78-79

urination, dark, scanty, 41, 77, 92, 157, 199, 201, 204

urination, difficult, 40, 44, 50, 73, 167, 185, 202, 204, 207, 220, 235, 267

urination, difficult but profuse, 186

urination, dribbling, 116, 121-122, 178, 180, 269

urination, dribbling and dripping, 61

urination, enduring, slightly painful, 118-119

urination, frequent, clear, 122, 127, 176, 180

urination, frequent, long, clear, 176, 180

urination, frequent night-time, 91, 180, 244

urination, frequent, urgent, and burning, 158, 163, 167

urination, hot, 68

urination, incomplete, 121, 175, 267

urination, inhibited, 19, 26, 102, 117-121, 126, 189

urination, long, clear, 108, 110, 176, 180

urination, non-freely flowing, 61-62

urination, painful, 19-20, 59, 69, 107, 110-111, 117-120, 122-123, 146, 156-157, 160, 162, 164-165, 168, 174, 178, 215

urination, painful, burning, 160, 165-167, 169

urination, painful, urgent, frequent, short, hot, dark yellowish, 116

urination, pale red, 118, 159

urination, profuse, 20, 186, 192, 230, 233-234, 242, 272

urination, scanty, 41-42, 44, 60, 76-77, 79-80, 83, 101, 110, 146-147, 157, 159, 187, 199-201, 204, 207, 212-213, 227, 230-233, 238, 250, 252-256, 280-281

urination, severely painful, 111, 117

urine, 3-4, 6, 10-11, 23, 31, 42-46, 49, 52, 55-56, 59-62, 64-74, 77, 79-80, 82, 84-86, 92, 107-108, 110-111, 115, 117-121, 125-128, 144-147, 152-154, 157-165, 167-171, 178, 183-184, 186-187, 189-191, 194, 198-199, 201-202, 204-207, 209-211, 214-222, 224-228, 230-232, 234-235, 238, 240, 243, 245-253, 255, 257, 260, 264, 266-267, 270-271, 274-276, 280-283, 285, 287-289, 292, 296

urine, blood clots in the, 69, 117, 120

urine, bloody, 10, 42, 67-73, 77, 111, 146, 161, 199, 204, 210, 217, 230, 249, 266-267, 270-271, 274, 285

urine, bloody, with pink blood, 161

urine, dark, 42, 121, 153, 206, 234

urine, dark-colored, 110, 228

urine, foamy, 209

urine, fresh blood in the, 68-69, 158-159

urine, fresh red blood in the, 68-69, 159

urine, incontinence of, 144

urine like rice-washing water, 120, 126, 169-170

urine, pale yellow, 72, 165, 246

urine protein, 31, 45-46, 52, 147, 186-187, 190, 204-205, 214-215, 217-218, 224, 243, 245, 247-248, 250, 252-253, 255, 280-281, 283, 285, 287-289

urine, reddish, 69, 117

urine, sand in the, 164

urine sediment, abnormal, 283

urine, slightly hot, 121

urine, small stones in the, 162

urine stream, fine, 61

urine, sudden blockage of the, 162

urine, sudden stoppage of, 164

uterus, 4, 6, 10, 153

UTIs, lower, 151-152, 154-155

UTIs, upper, 151

V

vacuity vexation, 179
vagina, 4, 153
vaginal discharge, clear, thin, 78, 180
vaginal discharge, profuse, 121, 211, 128
vaginal pain, 153
vaginal infection, 154
varicosities, 142
vasculitis, 183, 198
vertigo, recurrent, 145
vesicoureteral reflux, 152-153, 155
vexation, 11, 60-61, 63, 69, 101, 117-118, 120, 126, 133-134, 137, 157, 159, 165, 169, 178-179, 201, 204, 245-246, 252, 254, 267
vexation and agitation, 101, 133, 137, 204, 267
vexatious heat of the five hearts, 118-121, 127, 179
vexatious thirst, 144, 61
vision, blurred, 70, 87, 90, 110, 134-135, 160, 165, 188, 260
vitamin D, 240-241
voice, weak, 62, 71, 88
vomiting, 22, 42, 49-57, 59, 66, 77-78, 98-103, 106, 111, 116-119, 130-131, 133, 136, 153, 175, 228-229, 232-233, 240, 243, 245, 247, 250, 252-255, 260, 265-266, 276
vomiting caused by drinking water, 98
vomiting of clear water, 98
Von Hippel-Lindau syndrome, 274

W

Wang Qing-ren, 28, 259
warm disease, 14, 18
warm drinks, preference for, 78
water swelling, 6, 19-20, 22-23, 32, 39-42, 44-45, 50, 57, 75-77, 79-86, 92, 97, 115, 129, 147, 168, 184, 186, 189, 195, 199, 201, 204, 207-208, 210-211, 216, 218, 226, 230, 242, 261, 279-280, 296-297
waves, dense-disperse, 162
WBCs, 73, 111, 154, 157, 168, 171, 198, 204-205, 207, 228, 241, 267, 280
weight loss, 209, 240
wheezing, 75-76, 79, 97, 100, 103, 187, 202-203, 236, 248, 255-256
wind, 18-20, 26, 39-46, 55-56, 67, 75-76, 83-91,
    93-95, 105-106, 109-110, 112-114, 133-134, 137, 141-142, 144-145, 175, 184, 189, 191, 199-207, 210, 223, 230-231, 235-237, 242, 247, 253-255, 258, 266-267, 277, 281, 283, 286
wind, aversion to, 19, 39, 45, 76, 87, 90, 106
wind and chill, aversion to, 76
wind cold, 19-20, 39-40, 43, 67, 76, 83-86, 105, 110, 112, 114, 142, 199-200, 202-203, 230-231, 236-237
wind cold damp, 40, 42
wind damp, 19, 106
wind heat, 19, 39-41, 44, 55, 76, 83-84, 86-87, 94-95, 141-142, 175, 189, 191, 199-202, 223, 230-231, 235, 237, 281, 283
wind phlegm, 184, 210, 242
Wiseman, 16, 57, 238
Wiseman and Ye, 57
Wu Qing, 96, 103
Wu Ze-chen, 18

X

x-ray, 111, 172, 229, 270
Xi Ming-wang, 16
Xi Shuan-chang, 217
Xin Jun-hang, 224

Y

yang qi, 6, 11-12, 18, 20-22, 27, 29, 46, 49, 63, 86, 98, 128, 157, 185-186, 190, 215-216, 221, 237, 242, 256, 260-261, 279, 291-292
yang ming, 7, 10, 234
Yi Guan ([Key] Link of Medicine), 6
Ye Tian-shi, 6, 85, 128
Yi Zong Jin Jian (Golden Mirror of Ancestral Medicine), 8
yin, former heaven, 5, 245
yin, latter heaven, 5
yin water, 82-83, 85-86, 98, 213
Yin Yu-shi, 16
Yu Ping-gong, 225-226
Yu Guan-shi, 57, 96, 172, 208, 264
Yu Wong-shi, 48, 148, 208, 226, 296
Yu Xian-zou, 249
Yu Xiong-zao, 205

Z

Zhang Jing-yue, 6
Zhang Zhong-jing, 17, 27
Zhao Xian-ke, 6, 138
Zhen Qi-bi, 294
Zhi Xian-gong, 218
Zhong Yao Da Ci Dian (The Great Dictionary of Chinese Medicinals), 292, 295

Zhong Yao Xue Jian Yi (Chinese Medicinal Handout), 297
Zhou Xue-hai, 16
Zhu Dan-xi, 48, 82, 125, 201
Zi Yi-shen, 16
zinc, 152-153

FORMULA INDEX

B

Ba Wei Shen Qi Wan (Eight Flavors Kidney Qi Pills), 111
Ba Wei Wan (Eight Flavors Pills), 92, 111
Ba Zhen Tang (Eight Pearls Decoction), 119, 122, 177, 233, 238, 244
Ba Zheng San (Eight [Ingredients] Rectification Powder), 60, 188
Ban Xia Xia Xin Tang (Pinellia Drain the Heart Decoction), 131
Bei Xie Fen Qing Yin (Dioscorea Hypolaguca Separate the Clear Beverage), 126, 169
Bei Xie Wan (Dioscorea Hypolaguca Pills), 284
Bu Tian Da Zao Wan (Supplement Heaven Great Creation Pills), 242
Bu Zhong Yi Qi Tang (Supplement the Center & Boost the Qi Decoction), 62, 71, 103, 122, 128, 135, 161, 166-167, 176, 185, 210, 234, 257, 269, 271

C

Can Jian (Bombycis Mori, Concha), 289
Chen Xiang San (Aquilaria Powder), 61, 121, 166
Cheng Qi Tang (Order the Qi Decoction), 144, 217, 230, 232, 238, 294
Chuan Ze Tang (Spring Pond Decoction), 188

D

Da Ban Xia Tang (Major Pinellia Decoction), 53
Da Chai Hu Tang (Major Bupleurum Decoction), 64
Da Cheng Qi Tang (Major Order the Qi Decoction), 230, 294
Da Huang Gan Cao Tang (Rhubarb & Licorice Decoction), 263
Da Huang Ling Pi Chong Ji (Rhubarb & Epimedium Soluble Granules), 263
Da Ji Su Fang (Hormone Substitute Formula), 286-287
Da Tu Si Zi Wan (Major Cuscuta Pills), 242
Dang Gui Bu Xue Tang (Dang Gui Supplement the Blood Decoction), 233, 238, 296
Dang Gui Si Ni Tang (Dang Gui Four Counterflows Decoction), 143
Dao Chi San (Abduct the Red Powder), 69, 159
Du Huo Ji Sheng Tang (Angelica Pubescens & Sangjisheng Decoction), 144

E

Er Chen Tang (Two Aged [Ingredients] Decoction), 29, 57, 110, 272, 275, 278
Er Zhi Wan (Two Ultimates Pills), 70, 94, 96, 121, 206, 208, 290

F

Fang Ji Huang Qi Tang (Stephania & Astragalus Decoction), 27, 32, 210, 282

G

Gua Lou Xie Bai Bai Jiu Tang (Trichosanthes,

Allium & Alcohol Decoction), 89
Gui Lu Di Huang Wan (Turtle, Deer & Rehmannia
    Pills), 92
Gui Pi Tang (Restore the Spleen Decoction), 103,
    122, 135
Gui Shen Tang (Stabilize the Kidney Decoction), 285
Gui Zhi Fu Ling Wan (Cinnamon Twig & Poria
    Pills), 29, 57, 271

H

Hai Zao Yu Hu Tang (Sargassium Jade Flask
    Decoction), 123
Hou Xiang Zheng Qi San (Agastaches Rectify the Qi
    Powder), 93
Huang Lian Jie Du Tang (Coptis Toxin-resolving
    Decoction), 25, 44, 83, 126, 159, 175, 189,
    200, 216, 268, 281
Huang Lian Tang (Coptis Decoction), 25, 44, 53-54,
    83, 126, 159, 175, 189, 200, 216, 266, 268,
    281
Huang Qi Chi Xiao Dou Tang (Astragalus & Red
    Bean Decoction), 186, 211, 282-284
Huang Qi Gui Zhi Wu Wu Tang (Astragalus &
    Cinnamon Twig Five Materials Decoction),
    142

J

Jiang Can Fen (Bombyx Batryticatus Powder), 286
Jin Qian Cao San (Lysimachia Powder), 163

K

Kong Xian Dan (Drool-controlling Elixir), 83, 85,
    193, 243

L

Li Zhong Wan (Rectify the Center Pills), 82, 98,
    129
Liang Pi Jian (Double Skin Beverage), 269
Liang Xue Jie Du Yin (Blood-cooling & Toxin-
    resolving Beverage), 249
Ling Gui Zhu Gan Tang (Poria, Cinnamon,
    Atractylodes & Licorice Decoction), 32,
    255
Liu Jun Zi Tang (Six Gentlemen Decoction), 243
Liu Wei Di Huang Wan (Six Flavors Rehmannia

Pills), 16, 30, 63, 86, 118, 159, 165, 169,
    190, 207, 213-214, 217, 222, 224, 244-245,
    253, 258, 284, 292
Liu Yi San (Six-to-One Powder), 206, 208, 219,
    250, 264
Long Feng Fang (Solanum Nigrum & Wasp Nest
    Formula), 286
Long Kui (Solani Nigri, Herba), 286
Lu Feng Fang (Vespae, Nidus), 286
Lu Han Cao (Pyrolae Rotundifoliae, Herba), 285

M

Ma Bian Cao (Verbenae Officinalis, Herba), 285
Ma Huang Fu Zi Xi Xin Tang (Ephedra, Aconite &
    Asarum Decoction), 44, 203-204
Ma Huang Jia Zhu Tang (Ephedra Plus Atractylodes
    Decoction), 40, 43, 202-203
Ma Huang Lian Qiao Chi Xiao Dou Tang (Ephedra,
    Forsythia & Red Bean Decoction), 41, 44,
    84, 200, 202, 281
Ma Huang Zhu Ling Tang (Ephedra & Polyporus
    Decoction), 230

N

Niu Huang Qing Xin Wan (Calculus Bovis Heart-
    clearing Pills), 251

Q

Qi Ju Di Huang Wan (Lycium & Chrysanthemum
    Rehmannia Pills), 89, 270, 290
Qing Hao Bie Jia Tang (Artemisia Annua &
    Carapax Amydae Sinensis Decoction), 45
Qing Shen Jie Du Yin (Spirit-clearing, Toxin-resolv-
    ing Beverage), 251
Qing Shen Xiao Du Yin (Kidney-clearing, Toxin-dis-
    persing Beverage), 42, 44, 201, 204
Qing Wen Bai Du Yin (Scourge-clearing, Toxin-van-
    quishing Beverage), 231, 245
Qing Ying Tang (Clear the Constructive Decoction),
    268

R

Replace Hormone Formula #1, 224
Replace Hormone Formula #2, 225

S

San Huang Xia Du Tang (Three Yellows Precipitate Toxins Decoction), 232

San Huang Xie Xin Tang (Three Yellows Drain the Heart Decoction), 263

Sang Ju Yin (Morus & Chrysanthemum Beverage), 215

Shao Fu Zhu Yu Tang (Lower Abdomen Dispel Stasis Decoction), 69, 178

She Mei (Duchesneae Indicae, Herba), 286

Shen Er Feng (Kidney Formula Number Two), 285

Shen Fu Tang (Ginseng & Aconite Decoction), 233

Shen Ling Bai Zhu San (Ginseng, Poria & Atractylodes Powder), 26, 31, 78, 187, 192

Shen Tong Zhu Yu Tang (Body Pain Dispel Stasis Decoction), 109

Shen Xi Dan (Magical Rhinoceros Elixir), 249

Shen Yan Yi Huo (Nephritis Formula #1), 294

Shen Yi Feng (Kidney Formula Number One), 285

Sheng Hua Tang (Generation & Transformation Decoction), 143

Sheng Mai San (Generate the Pulse Powder), 234

Sheng Qing Jiang Zhuo Tang (Upbear the Clear & Downbear the Turbid Decoction), 247

Shi Pi Yin (Bolster the Spleen Beverage), 29, 42, 51, 78, 83, 85, 98, 185-189, 193, 212-213, 216, 243, 272, 282

Shi Wei San (Pyrrosia Powder), 110, 118

Shu Yang Quan (Solani Lyrati, Herba), 286

Si Jun Zi Tang (Four Gentlemen Decoction), 192, 296

Si Ling San (Four [Ingredients] Poria Powder), 187

Si Mo Yin (Four Milled [Ingredients] Beverage), 53

Si Ni Tang (Four Counterflows Decoction), 143, 233

Si Wu Tang (Four Materials Decoction), 109, 179

Shu Feng Tang (Course Wind Decoction), 286

Su Feng Tang (Search Wind Decoction), 286

Suo Quan Wan (Shut the Sluice Pills), 64

T

Tao He Cheng Qi Tang (Persica Order the Qi Decoction), 144

Tian Kui Zi (Semiaquilegiae, Fructus), 285

Tu Si Zi Wan (Cuscuta Pills), 170, 242

W

Wan Nian Qing Gen (Rhodeae Japonicae, Radix), 295

Wei Ling Tang (Stomach Poria Decoction), 188

Wen Jing Tang (Warm the Menses Decoction), 143

Wen Pi Tang (Warm the Spleen Decoction), 50, 263

Wen Shen San (Warm the Kidney Powder), 242

Wu Ling San (Five [Ingredients] Poria Powder), 83, 164, 186, 193, 204, 243, 282

Wu Pi San (Five Peels Powder), 27

Wu Pi Yin (Five Peels Beverage), 27, 40, 77, 185, 202

Wu Zhi Yin (Five Juices Beverage), 53

Wu Zi Bu Shen Wan (Schisandra Supplement the Kidney Pills), 146

X

Xi Feng Jie Du Yin (Wind-extinguishing, Toxin-resolving Beverage), 253

Xi Jiao Di Huang Tang (Rhinoceros Horn & Rehmannia Decoction), 145

Xi Lei San (Tin-like Powder), 205

Xiao Ji Yin Zi (Cephalanoplos Drink), 73, 159

Xuan Fu Dai Zhe Tang (Inula & Hematite Decoction), 52-53

Xue Fu Zhu Yu Tang (Blood Mansion Dispel Stasis Decoction), 28, 146, 219

Y

Yi Shen Tang (Boost the Kidney Decoction), 286

Qi Ye Yi Zhi Hua (Paridis Polyohyllae, Rhizoma), 286

Yin Qiao San (Lonicera & Forsythia Powder), 41, 46, 83, 90, 94, 189, 191, 200, 215

You Gui Wan (Restore the Right [Kidney] Pills), 16, 180, 192, 203, 276-277, 290

You Gui Yin (Restore the Right [Kidney] Beverage), 192

Yu Ping Feng San (Jade Windscreen Powder), 224

Yue Bi Jia Zhu Tang (Maidservant from Yue Plus Atractylodes Decoction), 76

Yue Bi Tang (Maidservant from Yue Decoction), 26, 41, 76, 83, 85, 200, 281

Yun Nan Bai Yao (Yunnan White Medicine), 72, 109

Z

Zhe Shi Yi Qi Tang (Hematite Boost the Qi Decoction), 256
Zhen Wu Tang (True Warrior Decoction), 27, 32, 79, 83, 85, 88, 186, 193, 211, 216, 243, 255, 282, 295
Zhi Bai Di Huang Wan (Anemarrhena & Phellodendron Rehmannia Pills), 16, 43, 48, 70, 119-120, 127, 157, 159-160, 168, 175, 179, 192, 207, 214, 218-219, 267, 271
Zhi Shi Gua Lou Gui Zhi Tang (Aurantium Immaturus, Trichosanthes, & Cinnamon Twig Decoction), 145
Zhong Yi Qi Tang (Supplement the Center & Boost the Qi Decoction), 62, 71, 103, 122, 128, 135, 161, 166-167, 176, 185, 210, 234, 257, 269, 271
Zhou Che Wan (Vessel & Vehicle Pill), 85
Zhu Ling Tang (Polyporus Decoction), 63, 157, 165, 230
Zi Xue Dan (Purple Snow Elixir), 249
Zuo Gui Wan (Restore the Left [Kidney] Pills), 107, 135

CURING ARTHRITIS NATURALLY
WITH CHINESE MEDICINE
by Douglas Frank & Bob Flaws
ISBN 0-936185-87-2

CURING DEPRESSION NATURALLY
WITH CHINESE MEDICINE
by Rosa Schnyer & Bob Flaws
ISBN 0-936185-94-5

CURING FIBROMYALGIA NATURALLY
WITH CHINESE MEDICINE
by Bob Flaws
ISBN 1-891845-09-8

CURING HAY FEVER NATURALLY
WITH CHINESE MEDICINE
by Bob Flaws
ISBN 0-936185-91-0

CURING HEADACHES NATURALLY
WITH CHINESE MEDICINE
by Bob Flaws
ISBN 0-936185-95-3

CURING IBS NATURALLY WITH
CHINESE MEDICINE
by Jane Bean Oberski
ISBN 1-891845-11-X

CURING INSOMNIA NATURALLY
WITH CHINESE MEDICINE
by Bob Flaws
ISBN 0-936185-86-4

CURING PMS NATURALLY WITH
CHINESE MEDICINE
by Bob Flaws
ISBN 0-936185-85-6

THE DIVINE FARMER'S MATERIA MEDICA:
A Translation of the Shen Nong Ben Cao
translation by Yang Shou-zhong
ISBN 0-936185-96-1

THE DIVINELY RESPONDING CLASSIC:
A Translation of the Shen Ying Jing
from Zhen Jiu Da Cheng
trans. by Yang Shou-zhong & Liu Feng-ting
ISBN 0-936185-55-4

DUI YAO: THE ART OF COMBINING
CHINESE HERBAL MEDICINALS
by Philippe Sionneau
ISBN 0-936185-81-3

ENDOMETRIOSIS, INFERTILITY AND
TRADITIONAL CHINESE MEDICINE:
A Laywoman's Guide
by Bob Flaws
ISBN 0-936185-14-7

THE ESSENCE OF LIU FENG-WU'S
GYNECOLOGY
by Liu Feng-wu, translated by Yang Shou-zhong
ISBN 0-936185-88-0

EXTRA TREATISES BASED ON INVESTIGA-
TION & INQUIRY: A Translation of Zhu Dan-
xi's Ge Zhi Yu Lun
translation by Yang Shou-zhong
ISBN 0-936185-53-8

FIRE IN THE VALLEY: TCM Diagnosis &
Treatment of Vaginal Diseases
by Bob Flaws
ISBN 0-936185-25-2

FU QING-ZHU'S GYNECOLOGY
trans. by Yang Shou-zhong and Liu Da-wei
ISBN 0-936185-35-X

FULFILLING THE ESSENCE: A Handbook of
Traditional & Contemporary Treatments for
Female Infertility
by Bob Flaws
ISBN 0-936185-48-1

GOLDEN NEEDLE WANG LE-TING: A 20th
Century Master's Approach to Acupuncture
by Yu Hui-chan and Han Fu-ru,
trans. by Shuai Xue-zhong

A GUIDE TO GYNECOLOGY
by Ye Heng-yin,
trans. by Bob Flaws and Shuai Xue-zhong
ISBN 1-891845-19-5

A HANDBOOK OF MENSTRUAL DISEASES
IN CHINESE MEDICINE
by Bob Flaws
ISBN 0-936185-82-1

A HANDBOOK OF TCM PATTERNS &
TREATMENTS
by Bob Flaws & Daniel Finney
ISBN 0-936185-70-8

A HANDBOOK OF TCM PEDIATRICS
by Bob Flaws
ISBN 0-936185-72-4

A HANDBOOK OF TCM UROLOGY & MALE
SEXUAL DYSFUNCTION
by Anna Lin, OMD
ISBN 0-936185-36-8

A HANDBOOK OF TRADITIONAL CHINESE
DERMATOLOGY
by Liang Jian-hui, trans. by Zhang Ting-liang
& Bob Flaws
ISBN 0-936185-07-4

A HANDBOOK OF TRADITIONAL CHINESE
GYNECOLOGY
by Zhejiang College of TCM, trans. by Zhang Ting-liang
& Bob Flaws
ISBN 0-936185-06-6 (4th ed.)

A HANDBOOK OF CHINESE HEMATOLOGY
by Simon Becker
ISBN 1-891845-16-0

THE HEART & ESSENCE OF DAN-XI'S
METHODS OF TREATMENT
by Xu Dan-xi, trans. by Yang Shou-zhong
ISBN 0-926185-49-X

THE HEART TRANSMISSION OF MEDICINE
by Liu Yi-ren, trans. by Yang Shou-zhong
ISBN 0-936185-83-X

HIGHLIGHTS OF ANCIENT ACUPUNCTURE
PRESCRIPTIONS
trans. by Honora Lee Wolfe & Rose Crescenz
ISBN 0-936185-23-6

IMPERIAL SECRETS OF HEALTH
& LONGEVITY
by Bob Flaws
ISBN 0-936185-51-1

INSIGHTS OF A SENIOR
ACUPUNCTURIST
by Miriam Lee
ISBN 0-936185-33-3

INTRODUCTION TO THE USE OF
PROCESSED CHINESE MEDICINALS
by Philippe Sionneau
ISBN 0-936185-62-7

KEEPING YOUR CHILD HEALTHY
WITH CHINESE MEDICINE
by Bob Flaws
ISBN 0-936185-71-6

THE LAKESIDE MASTER'S STUDY
OF THE PULSE
by Li Shi-zhen, trans. by Bob Flaws
ISBN 1-891845-01-2

Li Dong-yuan's TREATISE ON THE SPLEEN &
STOMACH: A Translation of the Pi Wei Lun
trans. by Yang Shou-zhong
ISBN 0-936185-41-4

MANAGING MENOPAUSE NATURALLY
with Chinese Medicine
by Honora Lee Wolfe
ISBN 0-936185-98-8

MASTER HUA'S CLASSIC OF THE
CENTRAL VISCERA
by Hua Tuo, trans. by Yang Shou-zhong
ISBN 0-936185-43-0

MASTER TONG'S ACUPUNCTURE
by Miriam Lee
ISBN 0-926185-37-6

THE MEDICAL I CHING:
Oracle of the Healer Within
by Miki Shima
ISBN 0-936185-38-4

PATH OF PREGNANCY, VOL. I,
Gestational Disorders
by Bob Flaws
ISBN 0-936185-39-2

PATH OF PREGNANCY, Vol. II,
Postpartum Diseases
by Bob Flaws
ISBN 0-936185-42-2

THE PULSE CLASSIC:
A Translation of the Mai Jing
by Wang Shu-he, trans. by Yang Shou-zhong
ISBN 0-936185-75-9

RECENT TCM RESEARCH FROM CHINA
by Bob Flaws and Charles Chase
ISBN 0-936185-56-2

SEVENTY ESSENTIAL CHINESE HERBAL
FORMULAS
by Bob Flaws
ISBN 0-936185-59-7

SHAOLIN SECRET FORMULAS FOR
TREATMENT OF EXTERNAL INJURIES
by De Chan, trans. by Zhang Ting-liang & Bob Flaws
ISBN 0-936185-08-2

STATEMENTS OF FACT IN TRADITIONAL
CHINESE MEDICINE
by Bob Flaws
ISBN 0-936185-52-X

STICKING TO THE POINT 1: A Rational
Methodology for the Step by Step Formulation
& Administration of an Acupuncture Treatment
by Bob Flaws
ISBN 0-936185-17-1

STICKING TO THE POINT 2:
A Study of Acupuncture & Moxibustion
Formulas and Strategies
by Bob Flaws
ISBN 0-936185-97-X

A STUDY OF DAOIST ACUPUNCTURE
by Liu Zheng-cai
ISBN 1-891845-08-X

THE SYSTEMATIC CLASSIC OF ACUPUNC-
TURE & MOXIBUSTION: A translation of the
Jia Yi Jing
by Huang-fu Mi, trans. by Yang Shou-zhong & Charles Chace
ISBN 0-936185-29-5

THE TAO OF HEALTHY EATING
ACCORDING TO CHINESE MEDICINE
by Bob Flaws
ISBN 0-936185-92-9

TEACH YOURSELF TO READ MODERN
MEDICAL CHINESE
by Bob Flaws
ISBN 0-936185-99-6

THE TREATMENT OF DIABETES MELLITUS
WITH CHINESE MEDICINE
by Bob Flaws, Lynn Kuchinski & Robert Casañas, M.D.
ISBN 1-891845-21-7

THE TREATMENT OF DISEASE IN TCM, Vol. I:
Diseases of the Head & Face Including Mental
/Emotional Disorders
by Philippe Sionneau & Lü Gang
ISBN 0-936185-69-4

THE TREATMENT OF DISEASE IN TCM, Vol.
II: Diseases of the Eyes, Ears, Nose, & Throat
by Philippe Sionneau & Lü Gang
ISBN 0-936185-69-4

THE TREATMENT OF DISEASE, Vol. III:
Diseases of the Mouth, Lips, Tongue,
Teeth & Gums
by Philippe Sionneau & Lü Gang
ISBN 0-936185-79-1

THE TREATMENT OF DISEASE, Vol. IV:
Diseases of the Neck, Shoulders,
Back, & Limbs
by Philippe Sionneau & Lü Gang
ISBN 0-936185-89-9

THE TREATMENT OF DISEASE, Vol. V:
Diseases of the Chest & Abdomen
by Philippe Sionneau & Lü Gang
ISBN 1-891845-02-0

THE TREATMENT OF DISEASE, Vol. VI:
Diseases of the Urogential System & Proctology
by Philippe Sionneau & Lü Gang
ISBN 1-891845-05-5

THE TREATMENT OF DISEASE, Vol. VII:
General Symptoms
by Philippe Sionneau & Lü Gang
ISBN 1-891845-14-4

THE TREATMENT OF EXTERNAL DISEASES
WITH ACUPUNCTURE & MOXIBUSTION
by Yan Cui-lan and Zhu Yun-long,
trans. by Yang Shou-zhong
ISBN 0-936185-80-5

THE TREATMENT OF MODERN WESTERN
MEDICAL DISEASES WITH
CHINESE MEDICINE
by Bob Flaws & Philippe Sionneau
ISBN 1-891845-20-9

160 ESSENTIAL CHINESE HERBAL
PATENT MEDICINES
by Bob Flaws
ISBN 1-891945-12-8

230 ESSENTIAL CHINESE MEDICINALS
by Bob Flaws
ISBN 1-891845-03-9

630 QUESTIONS & ANSWERS ABOUT
CHINESE HERBAL MEDICINE:
A Workbook & Study Guide
by Bob Flaws
ISBN 1-891845-04-7

750 QUESTIONS & ANSWERS ABOUT
ACUPUNCTURE
Exam Preparation & Study Guide
by Fred Jennes
ISBN 1-891845-22-5